Managing Side Effects of Breast Cancer Treatment

Yeşim Bakar • Alper Tuğral
Editors

Managing Side Effects of Breast Cancer Treatment

Springer

Editors
Yeşim Bakar
Institute of Postgraduate Education
Izmir Bakircay University
Izmir, Türkiye

Alper Tuğral
Department of Physical Therapy
and Rehabilitation
Izmir Bakircay University
Izmir, Türkiye

ISBN 978-3-031-75479-1 ISBN 978-3-031-75480-7 (eBook)
https://doi.org/10.1007/978-3-031-75480-7

This Springer imprint is published by the registered company Springer Nature Switzerland AG
The registered company address is: Gewerbestrasse 11, 6330 Cham, Switzerland

Contents

About the Editors

Yeşim Bakar graduated from the School of Physiotherapy and Rehabilitation at Hacettepe University in 1997, completed her Master of Science degree in the Physiotherapy and Rehabilitation Department at Hacettepe University in 2000, and earned her Doctor of Philosophy degree in the Physiotherapy and Rehabilitation Department at Hacettepe University in 2005. Dr. Bakar worked as a physical therapist at Baskent Hospital from 1997 to 1998 and then served as a Research Assistant at the School of Physiotherapy and Rehabilitation at Hacettepe University from 1998 to 2005. Subsequently, she held academic positions at Abant Izzet Baysal University, first as an Assistant Professor in 2005, then as an Associate Professor in 2011, and finally as a Professor in 2016.

Yeşim Bakar has worked as a physical therapist and academic staff member for over 25 years. In 2001, she received training in Manual Lymph Drainage and Complex Decongestive Physiotherapy at Földischule in Germany, becoming a certified lymphedema therapist. After that, she won the German Academic Exchange Service Award and spent 6 months as a researcher at the Földiclinic Germany (European Centre for Lymphology) in 2001. She then returned to her country and opened the first lymphedema unit at Hacettepe University in Turkey. She can be regarded as one of the first pioneers of lymphology knowledge in Turkey.

She is also currently a Senior Instructor for Manual Lymph Drainage/Complex Decongestive Physiotherapy at Földischule, Germany, where she is responsible for teaching postgraduate courses that include manual lymph drainage techniques for managing lymphedema, chronic venous insufficiency, and compression techniques. Nearly 700 postgraduate physiotherapists in Turkey have been trained and certified as a result of her efforts. Dr. Yeşim Bakar has dedicated most of her time to teaching and, in particular, to conducting research projects focused on lymphedema and physiotherapy.

Specifically, her studies are associated with oncological rehabilitation, lymphedema, women's health, and chronic venous insufficiency. She has authored over 200 international publications and research papers in peer-reviewed journals, presented papers at international congresses, and contributed to more than 20 book chapters, focusing on lymphology, phlebology, and oncologic physiotherapy. Her publications have been cited more than 1500 times. In addition to her academic pursuits, Dr. Bakar has accumulated extensive administrative experience, having held various positions, including Dean of the Faculty of Health Sciences, Head of the Department of

Physiotherapy and Rehabilitation, Member of the University Senate and Board of Directors, and Member of the Ethics Committee. She is the Founding President of the Lymphedema Association in Turkey, established in 2008, and the Lymphology Association, established in 2014. She is a member of the European Society of Lymphology and the Turkish Physiotherapists Association. She has been working at a private clinic since January 2024.

Alper Tuğral is working as an academician in the Department of Physical Therapy and Rehabilitation at Izmir Bakırçay University, Türkiye. He earned his PhD in 2021, with his doctoral dissertation focusing on the evaluation of upper extremity functionality in breast cancer survivors. His scholarly and research activities are focused on several key areas within physiotherapy and rehabilitation. These include, but are not limited to, the management and therapeutic approaches for lymphedema and its rehabilitation processes; comprehensive rehabilitation strategies in oncological care; therapeutic interventions and rehabilitative measures for venous diseases; and the principles and practices of complex decongestive physiotherapy. Dr. Tuğral's research is crucial for advancing both theoretical knowledge and clinical practice in these specialized areas. His published works cover a range of topics, including breast cancer, the role of exercise in cancer treatment, and functional outcomes in cancer rehabilitation. In addition, he contributes to the academic community by teaching various lectures, including kinesiology, biostatistics, prosthetics and orthotics, and lymphedema management, as part of the Bachelor of Science degree program. He has been attending international scientific congresses, such as those of the European Society of Lymphology (ESL) and the International Society of Lymphology (ISL), since 2015. His works were awarded the "Young Lymphologist Prize" at ESL 2019, Czech Republic, and "Best Oral Presentation" at ESL 2016, France.

Part I

Medical Management of Breast Cancer

Breast Cancer: General Overview

1

Gözde Kavgacı and Sercan Aksoy

1.1 Introduction

Breast cancer is the second most common cancer worldwide, accounting for 11.6% of all new cancer diagnoses after lung cancer [1]. The incidence of breast cancer has steadily risen over the years and is projected to surpass 3.1 million new cases by 2045 [1]. However, this rise is not uniform across geographic regions; developed countries have a higher incidence of breast cancer [2, 3]. Advancements in screening and treatment have led to declining mortality rates in high-income countries. However, there are significant disparities that emphasize the need for targeted interventions and equitable access to care [4]. Breast cancer has a multifactorial etiology that encompasses hormonal, genetic, dietary, lifestyle, and environmental factors. At least 50% of cases lack identifiable risk factors beyond age and gender. Comprehensive screening and prevention strategies are imperative to reduce the burden of breast cancer. Mammography screening programs have shown efficacy in reducing mortality, although implementation and participation rates vary [5]. Personalized surveillance and prevention approaches can be enabled by identifying high-risk individuals through genetic testing and risk assessment models [6, 7]. The treatment of breast cancer requires a multidisciplinary approach that is tailored to the individualized characteristics of a patient and disease stage. Both locoregional management and systemic therapy are essential to minimize the risk of relapse in the early stages. In recurrent or metastatic settings, systemic treatments prioritize both survival and quality of life. This necessitates collaborative decision making and integration of supportive care. Addressing the multifaceted challenges posed by breast cancer requires concerted efforts emphasizing the prevention, early detection, and personalized treatment approaches across healthcare systems.

1.2 Anatomy of the Female Breast

The female breast is located on the anterior thoracic wall, extending from the second through the sixth ribs and from the edge of the sternum to the midaxillary line. The majority of the breast tissue is located above the pectoralis major muscle, while the remainder is in contact with the serratus anterior and oblique abdominal muscles. Spence's axillary tail is an extension of breast tissue into the axilla. The breast is composed of breast tissue, subcutaneous tissue, and skin. The breast tissue is located within the superficial fascia, which is attached to the skin by Cooper's suspensory fibrous ligaments that run perpendicular

G. Kavgacı (✉) · S. Aksoy
Department of Medical Oncology, Hacettepe University Cancer Institute, Ankara, Turkey
e-mail: saksoy@hacettepe.edu.tr

Y. Bakar, A. Tuğral (eds.), *Managing Side Effects of Breast Cancer Treatment*,
https://doi.org/10.1007/978-3-031-75480-7_1

to the dermis. When contracted, they may cause skin dimpling, which is often indicative of breast cancer. The breast tissue is composed of approximately 15% epithelium and the rest is stromal elements (Fig. 1.1). Each breast contains glandular tissue divided into lobes, which are further divided into lobules containing branching tubuloalveolar glands. Adipose tissue fills the interlobar space, contributing to variations in breast size. The breast is divided into four quadrants: superior medial, inferior medial, superior lateral, and inferior lateral. The superior lateral quadrant contains the majority of breast volume and is the most common site for tumors.

Three major arterial routes supply blood to the breast. The medial blood supply is derived from the internal mammary artery, which predominantly supplies the medial and central areas, accounting for 60% of the blood supply. The breast receives lateral blood supply from the lateral thoracic artery and the thoracoacromial artery. These arteries supply the superior lateral quadrant of the breast and provide 30% of the blood supply. The remaining blood supply comes from the posterior intercostal arteries. Venous drainage follows the course of the arteries, with drainage directed primarily toward the axilla.

Lymphatic drainage occurs predominantly through axillary lymph nodes, with over 95% of drainage transferred via this route (Fig. 1.2). Axillary lymph nodes are divided into three levels based on their relationship to the pectoralis minor muscle. Sentinel nodes are typically located in level 1. Nodes located lateral to the pectoral muscle are level I, superficial and deep to the muscle are level II, and medial to the muscle are level III. The internal mammary nodes are involved in the lymphatic drainage of the medial side of the breast and are located in the first six intercostal spaces near the sternum. Communication with the contralateral breast may occur via superficial lymphatics [8–11].

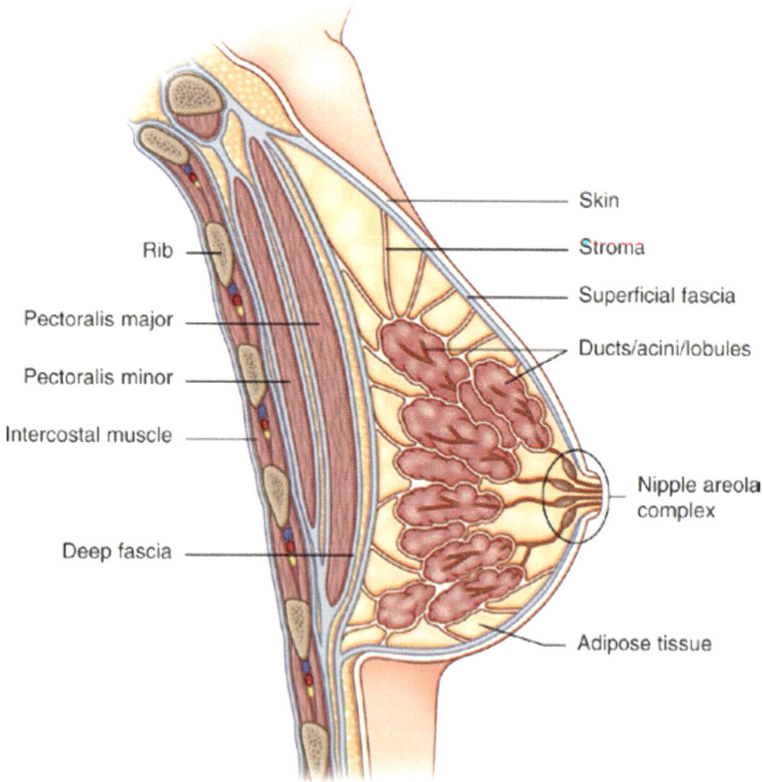

Fig. 1.1 Anatomical compositions of breast tissue

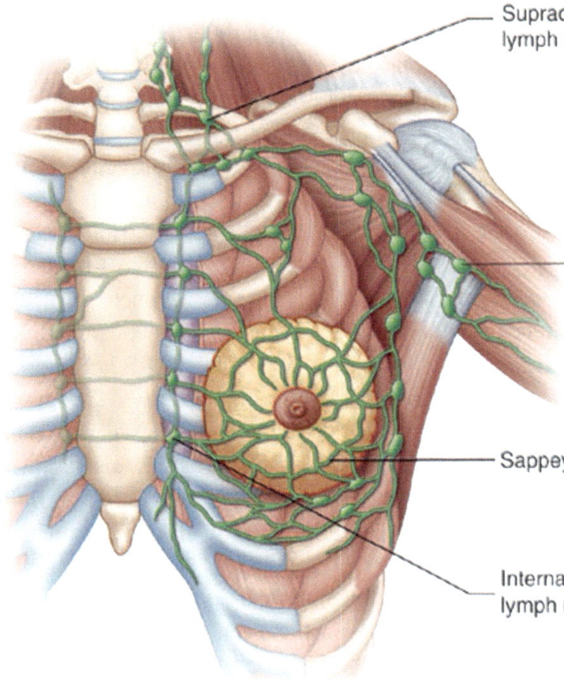

Fig. 1.2 Lymphatic drainage of the breast

1.3 Epidemiology

1.3.1 Incidence and Mortality of Breast Cancer

Breast cancer is the second most common cancer among both sexes, accounting for 11.6% of all new cancer diagnoses after lung cancer. In 2022, 2,310,051 new cases of breast cancer and 669,846 deaths were reported globally, ranking breast cancer as the fourth leading cause of cancer-related deaths worldwide, accounting for 6.9% of all cancer deaths. Breast cancer was the most common cancer in women, with 2,296,640 new cases in 2022, representing 23.8% of all female cancer diagnoses [1]. The incidence of breast cancer has consistently increased globally over the years, with 641,000 cases reported in 1980 and over 1.5 million in 2010 [12]. It is projected to exceed 3.1 million new cases by 2045 [1]. However, breast cancer incidence rates vary across geographical regions. Developed Western nations tend to have higher rates compared to low-incidence regions like Africa and Asia [2, 3]. The introduction of screening programs and the widespread use of hormone replacement therapy led to a sustained increase in breast cancer cases into the early twenty-first century but advances in screening techniques and adjuvant systemic treatments have consistently reduced breast cancer mortality rates in recent decades [4]. The United States has experienced a reduction in breast cancer mortality between 1950 and 2020 at the rate of 40%, which is consistent with trends observed in other countries [2, 13, 14]. However, significant disparities persist, with the rates of mortality and incidence varying up to fourfold and over tenfold between high-incidence and low-incidence areas, respectively. In low- and middle-income countries, breast cancer is frequently detected at advanced stages, leading to poorer survival rates, as evidenced by mortality statistics. Additionally, patients diagnosed with breast cancer in developing countries tend to be approximately a decade younger than those in developed nations. The percentage of patients under the age of 35 varies from approximately 10% to 25% in developed and certain developing

Asian countries, respectively [15, 16]. The burden of breast cancer can be mitigated globally through targeted interventions and equitable access to screening, diagnosis, and treatment services.

1.3.2 Risk Factors

Breast cancer is the result of a complex interaction of hormones, genes, diet, lifestyle, and environmental factors. However, at least 50% of women with breast cancer have no known risk factors.

1.3.3 Hormonal Factors

The length of time exposed to endogenous estrogen is important in developing breast cancer. Risk factors for breast cancer include early onset of menstruation, late onset of menopause, nulliparity, and delayed age at first pregnancy [17, 18]. Conversely, early oophorectomy reduces the risk [19]. Nulliparous women have a higher risk than women who have given birth [18]. Furthermore, women who give birth to their first child after the age of 30 face a higher risk of developing breast cancer compared to those who give birth before the age of 18. After pregnancy, there is a temporary increase in risk for about 10 years, which declines thereafter. Conversely, breastfeeding, especially for extended periods, lowers the risk. The influence of reproductive history may contribute significantly to the observed differences in breast cancer risk between countries with different income levels. In addition, hormone replacement therapy with estrogen and progesterone, especially in combination, has been associated with an increased risk [20, 21].

1.3.4 Genetic Factors

A family history of breast cancer significantly increases the risk, with approximately 10% of breast cancer cases attributed to inheritance. BRCA1 and BRCA2 mutations are associated with an increased risk of breast and ovarian cancer. Individuals with pathogenic mutations in BRCA genes have a lifetime risk estimate for breast cancer ranging from 26% to 85%. BRCA1 mutations correlate with an increased incidence of triple-negative breast cancers, whereas BRCA2-related cancers show no significant difference from sporadic tumors [22, 23]. Other genetic mutations, including TP53, PTEN, and PALB2, also contribute to breast cancer susceptibility. The risk of developing HER2-positive breast cancer is higher in women with TP53 mutations, also known as Li-Fraumeni syndrome [24]. Carriers of germline loss-of-function mutations in PALB2, a nuclear partner of BRCA2, have an increased risk of breast cancer, with an estimated cumulative risk of developing breast cancer by age 70 of 35%. The CHEK2 mutation is responsible for 1.9% of breast cancer cases [25, 26]. CDH1 mutations are associated with an autosomal dominant predisposition to diffuse gastric cancer and lobular breast cancer [27]. Genetic testing and counseling are important to assess the risk and guide preventive measures. Patients are increasingly utilizing multigene panels for genetic testing, which include genes associated with breast cancer such as BRCA1, BRCA2, PALB2, BARD1, CHEK2, CDH1, ATM, P53, and PTEN. This helps to clarify some cases of familial cancer while also increasing the detection of variants whose significance is uncertain.

1.3.5 Dietary and Lifestyle Factors

Diet and lifestyle choices have a significant impact on breast cancer risk. High alcohol consumption is associated with an increased risk that increases linearly with the amount of alcohol consumed [28]. Conversely, a lower risk of breast cancer is associated with a diet high in fruits and vegetables, whole grains, and fiber [29]. Regular physical activity has been shown to reduce the risk. Obesity, especially in postmenopausal women, is strongly associated with increased breast cancer risk and mortality. Weight gain during adulthood, especially after the age of 18, further increases this risk [30].

1.3.6 Benign Breast Lesions

Certain benign breast lesions, especially those with proliferative characteristics, are associated with an increased risk. Lesions such as atypical hyperplasia and lobular carcinoma in situ significantly increase the risk and often require close surveillance or preventive measures [31–34].

1.3.7 Breast Density

Mammographic breast density is a significant indicator of breast cancer risk. A higher density is associated with an increased risk. Breast density is measured by assessing the proportion of glandular and stromal tissue to adipose tissue in the breast. While it can complicate the detection of breast cancer, however, it is a strong predictor of breast cancer risk [35].

1.3.8 Environmental Factors

Exposure to ionizing radiation, especially during adolescence, increases the likelihood of developing breast cancer. This risk has been noted in atomic bomb survivors, individuals who have undergone diagnostic X-ray procedures, and those who have received therapeutic chest irradiation [36]. Although studies have investigated other environmental factors, such as electromagnetic fields and organochlorine pesticides, conclusive evidence linking these exposures to breast cancer is still lacking. Tailored preventive interventions, including lifestyle modifications, genetic screening, and awareness of potential environmental factors, hold immense promise in reducing the burden of breast cancer and improving outcomes for individuals at risk for breast cancer. It is important to comprehensively address multifaceted risk factors to achieve this goal.

1.4 Screening and Prevention

Breast cancer screening programs aim to detect early-stage diseases in women at average risk of developing breast cancer, utilizing noninvasive and accurate tests that are acceptable to the individuals being screened, with mammography screening serving as a secondary prevention strategy. Screening mammography has been shown to reduce the death rate from breast cancer by 20%. This efficacy is most pronounced in women aged 50–69 years; however, the results of the UK Age study underscore the importance of annual screening for women to reduce breast cancer mortality between the ages of 40 and 49 [5]. Although screening mammography is widely implemented in developed health systems, the organization of screening services and women's participation rates vary from country to country. The United States Preventive Services Task Force updated its preliminary recommendations for 2023, proposing routine screening to begin at the age of 40 [37]. The NCCN Panel continues to endorse its longstanding recommendation of annual screening starting at the age of 40, emphasizing its significant effect on reduction in mortality and improved survival [38]. The European Society for Medical Oncology (ESMO) and the European Commission Initiative on Breast Cancer (ECIBC) recommend screening mammography every 2 years between the ages of 50 and 69 [39, 40].

Identifying individuals at high risk for developing breast cancer is essential for implementing personalized screening and prevention strategies. Guidelines often consider a lifetime risk of breast cancer of ≥20%, primarily assessed through family history models, as a threshold for identifying potential candidates for risk reduction strategies and guiding screening approaches [38]. High-risk factors for breast cancer include carrying mutations in the BRCA1, BRCA2, PALB2, and CHEK2 genes, having a family history consistent with hereditary breast cancer, prior mantle irradiation (typically for lymphoma), or the presence of lobular carcinoma in situ or atypical hyperplasia. It is recommended to consult an expert in cancer genetics to assess of an individual's lifetime risk using models such as Gail, Tyrer-Cuzick, BRCAPRO, BOADICEA, Claus, and others. However, it is important to note that these models have limitations. For example, the Gail model accounts for factors such as early onset of menstruation, delayed age at first full-term pregnancy, family history, and biopsies, but may underestimate risk in women with a strong family history or atypical hyperplasia [41]. Conversely, the Claus model includes comprehensive family history but does not account for other risk factors [42]. Other models, such as BRCAPRO, BOADICEA, and Tyrer-Cuzick, incorporate additional factors, such as benign breast histology and mammographic breast density [6, 7, 43, 44]. Surveillance measures for high-risk women typically include annual screening mammography. However, the effectiveness of mammography in high-risk women is limited due to higher rates of interval cancer diagnoses. Magnetic resonance imaging (MRI) has shown promise in reducing node-positive disease at diagnosis, especially in women at very high risk. Some experts suggest alternating mammograms and MRIs every 6 months to identify potentially interval cancers earlier [45]. High-risk women have several risk reduction options, including chemoprevention with medications like tamoxifen, raloxifene, or aromatase inhibitors (AIs), depending on menopausal status and individual risk factors [46–48]. For those at highest risk, prophylactic bilateral mastectomy or bilateral salpingo-oophorectomy can significantly reduce the risk of developing breast cancer and ovarian cancer [49, 50]. To effectively manage breast cancer risk in high-risk women, tailored screening and prevention strategies are necessary. Healthcare providers should consider risk-reduction options based on individualized risk assessments and discussions with patients.

1.5 Diagnosis and Staging

1.5.1 Clinical Presentation

Breast cancer is usually asymptomatic and is often detected by preventive or regular screening for breast cancer. However, it can be present with different signs and symptoms. The most common symptomatic presentation is the presence of a palpable, painless, solid breast lump with indistinct margins. Rare signs and symptoms of breast cancer include nipple retraction, skin changes such as edema, nipple discharge or bleeding, and palpable, indurated lymph nodes in the axilla, occasionally associated with arm lymphedema. Inflammatory carcinoma presents with diffuse breast involvement and signs of inflammation.

1.5.2 Clinical Breast Examination

Clinical breast examination is a comprehensive physical assessment that includes inspecting and palpating the neck, breasts, chest wall, and axilla. The examiner visually inspects for asymmetry, skin changes, nipple abnormalities, and any discharge without manipulation. Palpation is performed with the patient seated and involves examining the entire circumference of the breasts to detect any abnormalities, including abnormal discharge. Regional lymph node examination involves evaluating the axillary lymph nodes while the patient is seated to allow for easier access to the deepest nodes. Additionally, it is important to examine the cervical, supraclavicular, infraclavicular, internal mammary nodes, and axillary nodal basins.

1.5.3 Imaging Methods in Breast Cancer Diagnosis

Mammography serves as the primary imaging modality for the diagnosis and screening of breast cancer. It typically detects breast neoplasms as radiolucent nodules with spiculated margins, sometimes accompanied by microcalcifications. Ultrasound complements mammography, particularly in individuals with dense breast tissue, by providing a characterization of an additional lesion and lymph node assessment. MRI is reserved for high-risk patients, multifocal lesions, or monitoring treatment response because of its increased sensitivity, albeit lower specificity, compared with mammography [51, 52].

1.5.4 Biopsy and Diagnosis

Definitive diagnosis of breast cancer requires tissue biopsy, which is commonly performed by fine needle aspiration (FNA), core needle biopsy, or excisional biopsy. While FNA is easy to perform, it requires a specialized pathologist for interpretation and may not differentiate invasive cancer from in situ carcinoma. Core needle biopsy provides histologic samples suitable for comprehensive analysis and biomarker testing. Surgical biopsy is reserved for cases where image-guided biopsy results are inconclusive or for specific lesions that warrant excision.

1.5.5 Breast Cancer Staging

The American Joint Committee on Cancer (AJCC) uses two primary groups for staging breast cancer: anatomic, based on tumor size (T), lymph node (N), and metastasis (M) (Tables 1.1 and 1.2); and prognostic, which includes anatomic criteria along with grade, hormone receptor (HR) and human epidermal growth factor receptor 2 (HER2) status. Ductal carcinoma in situ and early-stage breast cancers represent cancer confined to the breast or axillary lymph nodes. Because lobular carcinoma in situ is not a malignancy but a risk factor, it is excluded from the staging system. Accurate staging is critical for determining prognosis and guiding treatment decisions. Staging after neoadjuvant chemotherapy reflects treatment response, emphasizing the importance of effective therapy in determining prognosis. Pathologic complete response (pCR), meaning the absence of invasive cancer, is a favorable prognostic indicator. The assessment of residual disease after neoadjuvant chemotherapy helps to determine subsequent treatment strategies and assess patient prognosis. In addition, the updated AJCC staging system incorporates prognostic multigene signatures that provide additional insight into individual patient prognosis. These signatures allow for more precise stratification of patients based on their molecular profiles, enabling more personalized treatment approaches [53].

Table 1.1 Definitions for Primary Tumor (T), Regional Lymph Nodes (N), and Distant Metastasis (M)

Primary tumor (T)	
TX	Primary tumor cannot be assessed
T0	No evidence of primary tumor
Tis (DCIS)	Ductal carcinoma in situ
Tis (Paget)	Paget disease of the nipple
T1	Tumor ≤20 mm in greatest dimension
T1mi	Tumor ≤1 mm in greatest dimension
T1a	Tumor >1 mm but ≤5 mm in greatest dimension
T1b	Tumor >5 mm but ≤10 mm in greatest dimension
T1c	Tumor >10 mm but ≤20 mm in greatest dimension
T2	Tumor >20 mm but ≤50 mm in greatest dimension
T3	Tumor >50 mm in greatest dimension
T4	
T4a	Extension to the chest wall
T4b	Ulceration/ipsilateral macroscopic satellite nodules / edema (including peau d'orange) of the skin
T4c	Both T4a and T4b are present
T4d	Inflammatory carcinoma
Clinical nodes (cN)	
cNX	Regional lymph nodes cannot be assessed
cN0	No regional lymph node metastases (by imaging or clinical examination)
cN1	Metastases to movable ipsilateral level I, II axillary lymph node(s)
cN2	Metastases in ipsilateral level I, II axillary lymph nodes that are clinically fixed or matted; or in ipsilateral internal mammary nodes in the absence of axillary lymph node metastases
cN3	Metastases in ipsilateral infraclavicular (level III axillary) lymph node(s) with or without level I, II axillary lymph node involvement; or in ipsilateral internal mammary lymph node(s) with level I, II axillary lymph node metastases; or metastases in ipsilateral supraclavicular lymph node(s) with or without axillary or internal mammary lymph node involvement
Pathological nodes (pN)	
pNX	Regional lymph nodes cannot be assessed
pN0	No regional lymph node metastasis identified or ITCs only (malignant cells clusters no larger than 0.2 mm)

Table 1.1 (continued)

pN1	Micrometastases; or metastases in 1–3 axillary lymph nodes; and/or in clinically negative internal mammary nodes with micrometastases or macrometastases by sentinel lymph node biopsy
pN2	Metastases in 4–9 axillary lymph nodes; or positive ipsilateral internal mammary lymph nodes by imaging in the absence of axillary lymph node metastases
pN3	Metastases in 10 or more axillary lymph nodes; or in infraclavicular (level III axillary) lymph nodes; or positive ipsilateral internal mammary lymph nodes by imaging in the presence of one or more positive level I, II axillary lymph nodes; or in more than three axillary lymph nodes and micrometastases or macrometastases by sentinel lymph node biopsy in clinically negative ipsilateral internal mammary lymph nodes; or in ipsilateral supraclavicular lymph nodes
Distant metastasis (M)	
M0	No clinical or radiographic evidence of distant metastases
M1	Distant metastases

Modified from AJCC Cancer Staging Manual, Eighth Edition (2017) published by Springer International Publishing

Table 1.2 AJCC Anatomic Stage Groups

Stage 0	Tis N0 M0
Stage IA	T1 N0 M0
Stage IB	T0 N1mi M0 T1 N1mi M0
Stage IIA	T0 N1 M0 T1 N1 M0 T2 N0 M0
Stage IIB	T2 N1 M0 T3 N0 M0
Stage IIIA	T0 N2 M0 T1 N2 M0 T2 N2 M0 T3 N1 M0 T3 N2 M0
Stage IIIB	T4 N0 M0 T4 N1 M0 T4 N2 M0
Stage IIIC	Any T N3 M0
Stage IV	Any T Any N M1

Modified from AJCC Cancer Staging Manual, Eighth Edition (2017) published by Springer International Publishing

1.6 Pathology of the Breast Cancer

1.6.1 Ductal Carcinoma In Situ

The diagnosis of ductal carcinoma in situ (DCIS) has increased notably with the widespread use of screening. DCIS refers to the proliferation of epithelial cells confined to the basement membrane without stromal invasion and accounts for 80–85% of carcinoma in situ and is often considered a precursor to invasive breast cancer. DCIS may present as a mass, an incidental biopsy finding, or, most commonly, as mammographic calcifications. It is necessary to examine the entire lesion to reliably exclude invasive carcinoma. Two commercially available assays predict the risk of recurrence after conservative treatment for DCIS: the Oncotype DX DCIS Score and the DCIS Biologic Risk Profile [54, 55]. These assays use gene expression profiling and/or a combination of clinical and pathological characteristics to estimate the local recurrence risk.

1.6.2 Invasive Carcinoma

The classification of breast tumors is an evolving process as new research findings are rapidly incorporated into clinical protocols. Invasive breast cancer is initially assessed by examination of cells under a light microscope and is still classified based on their morphologic subtypes, architectural patterns, and cytologic features. The World Health Organization's classification system, updated in 2019, continues to use this approach, ensuring ongoing relevance in clinical practice [56].

Invasive breast carcinoma is a type of epithelial tumor that can be divided into several subtypes, including infiltrating ductal, lobular, lipid-rich, glycogen-rich, sebaceous, tubular, cribriform, invasive micropapillary, metaplastic carcinomas, and mucinous adeno and cystadenocarcinomas. Importantly, breast cancer typically arises from epithelial precursor cells in the terminal ductal lobular unit. The most common type of invasive breast carcinoma, accounting for 75–80%, is invasive ductal carcinoma. It is diagnosed by exclusion because it lacks the histologic features to be morphologically classified as a specific subtype called infiltrating ductal carcinoma, not otherwise specified (NOS) [56, 57]. Specific subtypes of breast cancer account for about 20% to 25% of all types of invasive breast cancer. The most common subtype is invasive lobular carcinoma, which comprises 10% of breast cancers. This type of carcinoma is characterized by a loss of cellular adhesion, resulting in a discohesive or single-file pattern. The invasiveness and loss of cellular cohesion are attributed to abnormalities in the adherens complex, which is composed of cadherins and catenins. Most lobular carcinomas show a loss of E-cadherin expression [58]. They often manifest as multifocal, multicentric, or bilateral lesions [59, 60]. Lobular carcinoma is more likely to spread to the leptomeninges, cerebrospinal fluid, gastrointestinal tract, uterus, ovary, and peritoneum than any other subtype [60]. Rare types have a different prognosis than ductal invasive carcinoma. The prognosis is generally more favorable for rare breast cancers with pure tubular, mucinous, papillary, or cribriform features. Micropapillary tumors have a higher incidence of lymphatic and vascular invasion and a higher incidence of axillary nodal metastases at initial diagnosis. Metaplastic carcinoma has a poor response to neoadjuvant chemotherapy [61–63]. Additional types of carcinomas, such as adenoid cystic carcinoma, secretory carcinoma, acinar cell carcinoma, and mucoepidermoid carcinoma, which are rare and salivary gland-like tumors, may also be present. To be categorized as a specific histologic type, a tumor must demonstrate more than 90% of the defining histological characteristics associated with that type.

1.6.3 Pathological Reporting

For cases of invasive carcinoma, the pathology report should include information on tumor histological type, grade, HR, HER2 status, Ki67 score, tumor size, and involvement of lymph nodes. Additionally, surgical specimens obtained during surgery should be assessed to determine peritumoral vascular invasion and surgical margin status [64].

The histological grade assessment follows the Elston and Ellis-modified Scarff–Bloom–Richardson system, which is endorsed by the AJCC staging. This grading system evaluates three tumor characteristics: tubule formation, nuclear pleomorphism, and the number of mitoses. Each feature is assigned a score, and the individual scores are summed to determine grades 1, 2, and 3. A high tumor grade indicates a poor prognosis [65].

In the diagnosis and treatment of breast cancer, hormone receptors, including the estrogen receptor (ER) and progesterone receptor (PR), play a critical role. Immunohistochemistry (IHC) is the standard method used to evaluate these markers obtained from preoperative core needle biopsies. Based on the guidelines established by the American Society of Clinical Oncology (ASCO) and the College of American Pathologists, any nuclear staining observed in over 1% of invasive tumor cells indicates HR positivity (ER and/or PR). This determination is important because approximately 80% of breast cancers are classified as hormone receptor-positive based on this criterion. However, it is noteworthy that tumors classified as ER low/PR low, defined by 1%–9% ER and/or PR expression, exhibit behavior and clinical outcomes similar to triple-negative breast cancer. The expression of ER and PR serve as valuable prognostic indicators in the management of breast cancer [66]. HER2 is overexpressed in 15–20% of breast cancers, which is often associated with amplification of the HER2 gene. Overexpression of HER2 typically correlates with higher tumor grade, lower expression or absence of HRs, increased tumor proliferation rates, and more extensive nodal tumor burden. HER2 status can be assessed using IHC or fluorescence in situ hybridization (FISH). HER2 status can be classified as positive, negative, or equivocal based on the results obtained from either one or both of these technical approaches [67]. In clinical practice, tumors eligible for treatment with anti-HER2 therapies are those classified as HER2 3+ by IHC or exhibiting HER2 gene amplification, with a copy number greater than 6 or a HER2/CEP17 ratio of ≥2 [67, 68]. HER2 low status is characterized by an IHC score of 1+ or 2+ and negativity on ISH testing in metastatic disease [69].

Proliferation markers, such as Ki-67 expression and mitotic index, are robust prognostic factors in the early stages. IHC is typically employed to evaluate tumor cell proliferation. For Ki-67, the most commonly utilized cutoff value is staining in 20% or more of invasive tumor cell nuclei, with staining below or above this threshold indicative of low proliferation or high proliferation, respectively. However, the lack of standardized thresholds for clinical prognosis and the variability among observers limit the reliability of these measures which are the sole determinants of treatment decisions [70, 71]. A decline in Ki-67 levels (≤10%) following a brief preoperative endocrine therapy within 4–6 weeks among postmenopausal individuals with HR-positive breast cancer carries prognostic significance and may indicate a favorable response to endocrine treatment [72]. Tumor-infiltrating lymphocytes (TILs) scoring offers valuable prognostic and predictive insights. However, specific TILs thresholds for guiding medical decisions have yet to be defined, and they are not solely relied upon for treatment determinations [73].

Vascular invasion around the tumor is strongly associated with lymph node metastasis and local recurrences. A positive tumor margin, where cancer cells extend beyond the excision edge (referred to as a 0-mm margin or "ink on tumor"), significantly increases the risk of recurrence after surgery. Most guidelines recommend achieving a clear margin without any ink on the tumor for invasive breast cancer, while for DCIS, a margin of 2 mm without abnormal cells around the specimen is suggested [74–76].

1.6.4 Molecular Classification

For prognostic and treatment decision purposes, tumors are classified into intrinsic subtypes based on histology and IHC data, including luminal A, luminal B, HER2-positive, and basal-like subtypes [77–80]. Breast cancer is biologically heterogeneous, with each subtype having specific clinical characteristics and treatment options.

Luminal A is the most common subtype, accounting for over 50% of all breast cancers. It is characterized by high expression of estrogen receptor-related genes and often has low Ki67 and histologic grade. Patients with luminal A breast cancer generally have a favorable prognosis, with a significantly lower recurrence rate compared to other subtypes. Recurrences often occur in bone, with less frequent visceral metastases.

Luminal B accounts for 10–20% of all breast cancers. It is characterized by higher histologic grade, increased proliferation rate, and poorer prognosis. Luminal B tumors are more likely to have HER2 overexpression than luminal A tumors. Although bone remains the most frequent site of recurrence, metastasis to visceral organs, such as the liver, is more likely. Luminal B tumors are more sensitive to chemotherapy.

HER2-enriched breast cancer is identified by high expression of HER2 and HER2-related genes at the RNA and protein levels. Biologically aggressive, HER2-enriched breast cancer inherently carries a poor prognosis; however, the introduction of HER2-targeted treatments has significantly improved survival.

Approximately 15% of all breast cancers are classified as basal-like subtypes. These tumors exhibit elevated expression of genes associated with proliferation and keratins typically found in the basal layer of the skin while displaying minimal expression of genes related to luminal characteristics. Basal-like tumors generally have a higher grade, higher mitotic index, and lack expression of hormone receptors, and HER2.

Patients diagnosed with basal-like breast cancer typically have a dismal prognosis and shorter survival.

1.7 Treatment

Breast cancer treatment should be carried out with a multidisciplinary team. The selection of a treatment approach, which is determined by the size, location, and biological characteristics of the tumor, as well as the patient's age and preexisting health conditions, should be reviewed with the patient. In addition, patient preferences should be considered in this discussion. Treatment approaches differ based on the stage of breast cancer, including DCIS, early-stage breast cancer, and metastatic breast cancer (MBC). This section provides a brief introduction to breast cancer treatment, which will be discussed in more detail in the following chapters.

1.7.1 Treatment of DCIS

For most DCIS patients, standard options include local management through excision, with the consideration of adjuvant radiation therapy (RT) or mastectomy. Mastectomy is curative in about 98% of patients, regardless of various factors such as age, DCIS presentation, size, or grade [81]. Mastectomy is primarily indicated for DCIS lesions that cannot be excised with clear margins while maintaining a cosmetic appearance [82]. For localized DCIS, excision of the lesion followed by RT is an alternative to mastectomy. Studies suggest that a 2-mm margin is associated with low rates of local recurrence and is generally considered to be adequate in DCIS treated with RT [83]. Studies investigating the role of adjuvant RT after DCIS excision have shown that RT significantly decreases the risk of local recurrence without affecting overall survival [84, 85]. Younger age, insufficient margins, and larger disease volume have been linked to an increased risk of local recurrence following breast-conserving surgery. In cases of low-risk DCIS, where the tumor size is less than 1 cm, nuclear grade is low, and surgical margins are adequate, the possibility of omitting RT may be considered a viable option [83]. Axillary staging and the routine use of sentinel lymph node biopsy (SLNB) are usually not recommended [86]. However, SLNB in high-risk cases or cases with suspected coexistent invasive carcinoma may be appropriate. Endocrine therapy, particularly with tamoxifen or aromatase inhibitors (AIs), has shown benefits in reducing local recurrence and preventing new primary breast cancer in ER-positive DCIS. Tamoxifen has been shown to reduce ipsilateral and contralateral events, especially in patients not receiving RT [87]. AI therapy is an option instead of tamoxifen for DCIS for postmenopausal women [88].

1.7.2 Treatment of Early Breast Cancer

The primary focus for early breast cancer treatment is locoregional management and systemic therapy to minimize recurrence and eradicate micrometastases. Surgery aims to radically excise macroscopic disease and perform local staging of the disease. RT is used to target any remaining tumor cells in the breast and lymph nodes, and systemic treatment is used to eliminate systemic micrometastases, both of which reduce recurrence. The use of ER, PR, HER2, and Ki-67 as predictive biomarkers and gene expression signatures is widely recognized to effectively guide treatment recommendations. There is no difference in overall survival between a Halsted radical mastectomy, involving the removal of the breast, chest wall muscles, and regional lymph nodes, and total mastectomy, which involves the removal of the breast alone. The rates of local recurrence were comparable between lumpectomy with RT and mastectomy [89]. Breast-conserving surgery (BCS) followed by adjuvant RT, known as breast-conserving therapy, is a suitable option for most breast cancer patients to achieve optimal clinical and cosmetic outcomes. Margin status is reported, aiming for clear margins (no tumor at the inked margin) for invasive cancer [83]. SLNB is the standard staging procedure for clinically negative axillary lymph nodes. It provides reliable prognostic information with less morbidity [90]. Micrometastases do not alter treatment decisions, except in cases where neoadjuvant chemotherapy was administered [91]. In cases where the SLN shows macrometastatic spread, results from the ACOSOG Z0011 trial suggest similar outcomes without ALND for patients diagnosed with invasive breast cancer with clinical tumors less than 5 cm and no evidence of clinical nodal involvement [92]. In cases where patients have up to two positive SLNs with metastases, treatment typically includes BCS, postoperative RT, and adjuvant systemic chemotherapy. However, for patients who do not meet these specific criteria or who have more than two positive SLNs, ALND is recommended. The role of ALND after positive SLNB following neoadjuvant chemotherapy is under investigation. In cases where axillary nodes are clinically and imaging negative, SLNB after neoadjuvant chemotherapy is usually preferred. However, if any SLN is found to be positive, complete ALND is recommended [93]. For individuals who initially present with positive axillary lymph nodes but transition to clinically negative status after neoadjuvant treatment, SLNB may be considered, although ALND may still be required [94]. Whole breast RT after BCS significantly reduces locoregional or distant recurrence and mortality [95]. Regional nodal irradiation following BCS or mastectomy results in reduced local and distant recurrence, especially in patients with axillary lymph node involvement [96].

Systemic treatment decisions for hormone receptor (HR)-positive, HER2-negative early breast cancer are influenced by factors such as tumor stage, biological characteristics, menopausal status, and available therapeutic options, including endocrine therapy, chemotherapy, and targeted therapy. Surgery remains the primary treatment option for most HR-positive, HER2-negative breast cancers detected through screening. However, in cases of larger tumors or clinical lymph node involvement, neoadjuvant chemotherapy has been shown to be effective in reducing tumor size prior to surgery, although achieving a complete pCR is rare [97]. As effective in reducing locoregional and distant metastatic recurrence and contralateral breast cancer, and increasing overall survival, endocrine therapy is recommended for all HR-positive breast cancer patients [98]. Adjuvant chemotherapy also reduces the risk of recurrence and improves survival, with genomic signatures helping to guide patient selection. Low-risk genomic scores may indicate that endocrine therapy alone is sufficient, while higher-risk scores may benefit from chemotherapy. Adjuvant chemotherapy does not significantly reduce recurrence for postmenopausal women diagnosed with node-negative disease or fewer than four positive nodes, and exhibiting low-risk genomic scores [99]. In premenopausal women with similar node status and low-risk genomic scores, adjuvant chemotherapy reduces recurrence rates. This reduction may be due to chemotherapy-induced amenorrhea [100]. In addition, premenopausal women with higher risk benefit from ovarian function suppression combined with an AI or tamoxifen, which reduces recurrence and improves overall survival compared with tamoxifen alone [101]. Treatment with cyclin-dependent kinases 4 and 6 (CDK4/6) inhibitors such as abemaciclib and ribociclib has shown efficacy in reducing recurrence, particularly in high-risk disease [102, 103]. Furthermore, adjuvant olaparib for 1 year improves disease-free survival and overall survival in patients with germline BRCA1/2 mutations and high-risk HER2-negative tumors [104].

In HER2-positive early breast cancer, adjuvant treatment encompasses HER2-directed therapy, chemotherapy, and endocrine therapy if HR-positive. Tumors that have undergone surgery initially benefit from adjuvant HER2-directed therapy and chemotherapy with anthracycline and taxane-based regimens [105]. The duration of trastuzumab therapy is 12 months. For patients diagnosed with pathological stage pT1 N0 disease, adjuvant treatment with weekly paclitaxel for up to 3 months in combination with 12 months of trastuzumab is recommended [106].

In cases of clinical stage II-III disease, neoadjuvant treatment followed by surgery is preferred. Neoadjuvant chemotherapy in combination with trastuzumab and pertuzumab is associated with higher rates of pCR than trastuzumab alone, particularly in patients with lymph node-positive disease [107]. Patients who achieve pCR after neoadjuvant treatment have a significantly lower risk of disease recurrence. Therefore, it is recommended to continue anti-HER2 therapy for a total duration of 1 year. However, in patients with residual disease, adjuvant treatment with trastuzumab emtansine (T-DM1) instead of trastuzumab significantly decreases the risk of recurrence [108]. Extended therapy with neratinib for 1 year after completing 1 year of adjuvant trastuzumab demonstrates an overall improvement in disease-free survival, particularly in the subgroup of HR-positive tumors [109].

Neoadjuvant treatment is the preferred option for triple-negative breast cancer (TNBC) cases with tumors larger than 10 mm or positive lymph nodes. Adjuvant treatment decisions are guided by pathologic response. Anthracycline-based regimens followed by taxanes are the main treatment. Additionally, adjuvant capecitabine has been shown to benefit patients with residual disease after neoadjuvant treatment [110]. For patients diagnosed with stage two and three TNBC, a chemotherapy regimen comprising taxane and carboplatin followed by doxorubicin-cyclophosphamide or epirubicin-cyclophosphamide, all conjunctive with pembrolizumab, has shown improved pCR rates and event-free survival [111]. The efficacy of pembrolizumab is not affected by PD-L1 status. In patients with high-risk TNBC and germline BRCA1/2 mutations, adjuvant olaparib for 1 year has been shown to improve survival [104].

1.7.3 Treatment of Recurrent/Metastatic Breast Cancer

Addressing the systemic treatment of MBC extends survival and improves quality of life albeit without offering a complete cure. Therefore, treatments with minimal toxicity profiles are prioritized. While systemic therapy stands as the cornerstone in managing MBC, adjunct locoregional treatments may be considered based on individual disease status, underscoring the importance of a multidisciplinary team for optimal care. When making treatment decisions, patient age should not be the sole determining factor; instead, comorbidities, patient characteristics, and preferences should be factored in a collaborative decision-making process [112]. For geriatric patients, a comprehensive evaluation can provide valuable insights [113]. In addition, it is important to include supportive care in the treatment plan, such as involving specialized palliative care early on, to effectively manage symptoms and improve the overall well-being of the patient. Biopsy should be performed to confirm histology and reassess HR, and HER2 status in patients with newly diagnosed or recurrent MBC [112]. In the presence of bone metastasis, it is recommended to consider treatment with zoledronic acid, or denosumab [112, 114].

Patients diagnosed with HR-positive and HER2-negative recurrent or MBC, who experience disease progression within a year after completing adjuvant endocrine treatment or present with de novo MBC, typically receive first-line therapy consisting of endocrine treatment combined with targeted agents. Combining CDK4/6 (palbociclib, ribociclib, or abemaciclib) inhibitors with endocrine treatment has become the standard-of-care for ER-positive, HER2-negative MBC, demonstrating improved progression-free survival with a favorable toxicity profile across several trials [115–118]. Notably, at 3.5 years, ribociclib demonstrated an improvement in overall survival [119]. In the first-line setting, endocrine treatment alone should only be considered in patients with comorbidities that prevent the use of CDK4/6 inhibitor combinations. Premenopausal women receiving endocrine treatment should also undergo ovarian function suppression. Patients benefit from sequential administration of endocrine therapies upon progression. Second-line endocrine therapy is recommended for cases where patients experience progression during or within 12 months of completing adjuvant endocrine therapy or while on first-line endocrine therapy for MBC. For postmenopausal patients, the recommended second-line treatment is to combine fulvestrant with a CDK4/6 inhibitor, particularly for those who have not previously received a CDK4/6 inhibitor. Both ribociclib and abemaciclib have demonstrated improved overall survival when used in combination with fulvestrant compared to fulvestrant alone, particularly in patients who have received prior endocrine therapy [120–123]. Second-line therapy options include fulvestrant, fulvestrant, and alpelisib (if the tumor is PIK3CA mutant), exemestane and everolimus, tamoxifen and everolimus, fulvestrant and everolimus, AI, tamoxifen, chemotherapy, or poly ADP-ribose polymerase (PARP) inhibitors for tumors harboring germline BRCA mutations [124–127]. In situations where endocrine-sensitive tumors progress beyond the second line, continued endocrine therapy with agents not previously used may be an alternative. For tumors that exhibit endocrine resistance, chemotherapy is a consideration. Typically, sequential single-agent chemotherapy is preferred over combination approaches. However, in cases of impending organ failure requiring a rapid response, combination chemotherapy may be preferred.

For patients diagnosed with HER2-positive MBC, the treatment strategy is HER2-targeted therapy in combination with chemotherapy. Standard first-line treatment typically consists of pertuzumab, trastuzumab, and a taxane [128]. For patients with HR-positive tumors, endocrine therapy may be added to trastuzumab-pertuzumab maintenance after upfront taxane chemotherapy. Until progression, maintenance pertuzumab-trastuzumab is given. In cases where chemotherapy is contraindicated due to patient comorbidities, personal preference, or performance status, endocrine therapy in combination with trastuzumab or trastuzumab-pertuzumab is considered. For patients with HR-negative breast cancer who are contraindicated for chemotherapy, HER2-targeted therapy without chemotherapy is used [129]. For patients with metastatic recurrence within 6–12 months following adjuvant trastuzumab and pertuzumab, second-line recommendations are considered. T-DM1 has traditionally been considered the standard in the second-line setting, supported by consistent survival data [130]. However, trastuzumab deruxtecan offers improved progression-free survival compared to T-DM1 [131]. Trastuzumab deruxtecan is, therefore, the preferred second-line treatment after progression on trastuzumab and a taxane. In patients with brain metastases, tucatinib, capecitabine, trastuzumab, or trastuzumab deruxtecan may be considered as second-line options [131, 132].

For patients with metastatic TNBC, combination chemotherapy may be considered as the initial treatment option in cases of rapidly progressing visceral metastases. If the patient has a combined positive score (CPS) of ≥10, pembrolizumab in combination with chemotherapy is recommended [133]. In cases of PD-L1-negative and germline BRCA-wild-type metastatic TNBC, chemotherapy is the preferred initial treatment. For monotherapy, taxanes or anthracyclines may be considered. In the case of patients with germline BRCA mutant metastatic TNBC, carboplatin may be preferred over docetaxel due to a slightly improved median progression-free survival, although without a significant overall survival benefit [134]. PARP inhibitors are recommended in this subgroup [135]. Sacituzumab govitecan is the recommended second-line treatment after taxanes [136]. After disease progression, standard chemotherapy options such as eribulin, capecitabine, and vinorelbine should be considered.

1.8 Conclusion

Breast cancer is a major global health challenge due to its increasing incidence and high mortality rate, particularly among women. Despite progress in screening, treatment, and awareness, it remains a leading cause of cancer-related deaths worldwide. Addressing disparities in incidence and outcomes across regions requires targeted interventions and equitable access to care. Developed countries have made progress in reducing breast cancer mortality rates through improved screening and treatment options. However, low- and middle-income countries still struggle with early detection and access to quality of care, resulting in lower survival rates. Breast cancer is a multifactorial disease, influenced by hormonal, genetic, dietary, lifestyle, and environmental factors, underscoring the importance of comprehensive prevention and screening strategies. Tailored strategies should be employed, incorporating genetic testing, risk assessment models, and lifestyle modifications to reduce the burden of the disease. Effective management requires a multidisciplinary approach based on tumor characteristics, disease stage, and patient preferences. Locoregional management and systemic therapy are essential for early-stage disease, with the aim of minimizing the risk of recurrence. In recurrent/metastatic settings, systemic treatments prioritize survival and quality of life, requiring collaborative decision making and integration of supportive care.

References

1. GLOBOCAN. Global cancer statistics. 2022. https://gco.iarc.who.int/media/globocan/factsheets/cancers/20-breast-fact-sheet.pdf.
2. Torre LA, Siegel RL, Ward EM, Jemal A. Global cancer incidence and mortality rates and trends—an update. Cancer Epidemiol Biomarkers Prev. 2016;25(1):16–27.
3. Ginsburg O, Bray F, Coleman MP, Vanderpuye V, Eniu A, Kotha SR, et al. The global burden of women's cancers: a grand challenge in global health. Lancet. 2017;389(10071):847–60.
4. Berry DA, Cronin KA, Plevritis SK, Fryback DG, Clarke L, Zelen M, et al. Effect of screening and adjuvant therapy on mortality from breast cancer. N Engl J Med. 2005;353(17):1784–92.
5. Duffy SW, Vulkan D, Cuckle H, Parmar D, Sheikh S, Smith RA, et al. Effect of mammographic screening from age 40 years on breast cancer mortality (UK age trial): final results of a randomized, controlled trial. Lancet Oncol. 2020;21(9):1165–72.
6. Antoniou AC, Pharoah P, Smith P, Easton DF. The BOADICEA model of genetic susceptibility to breast and ovarian cancer. Br J Cancer. 2004;91(8):1580–90.
7. Tyrer J, Duffy SW, Cuzick J. A breast cancer prediction model incorporating familial and personal risk factors. Stat Med. 2004;23(7):1111–30.
8. Moore KL, Dalley AF. Clinically oriented anatomy. Wolters Kluwer India; 2018.
9. Moore KL, Persaud TVN, Torchia MG. The developing human-e-book: clinically oriented embryology. Amsterdam: Elsevier Health Sciences; 2018.
10. Pandya S, Moore RG. Breast development and anatomy. Clin Obstet Gynecol. 2011;54(1):91–5.
11. Drew P, Cawthorn S, Michell M. Interventional ultrasound of the breast. Boca Raton, FL: CRC; 2007.
12. Bray F, Ferlay J, Laversanne M, Brewster D, Gombe Mbalawa C, Kohler B, et al. Cancer incidence in five continents: inclusion criteria, highlights from volume X and the global status of cancer registration. Int J Cancer. 2015;137(9):2060–71.
13. Siegel RL, Miller KD, Fuchs HE, Jemal A. Cancer statistics, 2022. CA Cancer J Clin. 2022;72(1):7–33.
14. Howlader N, Noone A, Krapcho M, Garshell J, Miller D, Altekruse S, et al. SEER cancer statistics review, 1975–2012. Bethesda, MD: National Cancer Institute; 2014.
15. Allemani C, Weir HK, Carreira H, Harewood R, Spika D, Wang X-S, et al. Global surveillance of cancer survival 1995–2009: analysis of individual data for 25 676 887 patients from 279 population-based registries in 67 countries (CONCORD-2). Lancet. 2015;385(9972):977–1010.
16. Agarwal G, Pradeep P, Aggarwal V, Yip CH, Cheung PS. Spectrum of breast cancer in Asian women. World J Surg. 2007;31(5):1031–40.
17. Bernstein L, Ross RK. Endogenous hormones and breast cancer risk. Epidemiol Rev. 1993;15(1):48–65.
18. Rosner B, Colditz GA, Willett WC. Reproductive risk factors in a prospective study of breast cancer: the Nurses' Health Study. Am J Epidemiol. 1994;139(8):819–35.
19. Trichopoulos D, MacMahon B, Cole P. Menopause and breast cancer risk. J Natl Cancer Inst. 1972;48(3):605–13.
20. Chlebowski RT, Hendrix SL, Langer RD, Stefanick ML, Gass M, Lane D, et al. Influence of estrogen plus progestin on breast cancer and mammography in healthy postmenopausal women: the Women's Health Initiative randomized trial. JAMA. 2003;289(24):3243–53.
21. Beral V, Banks E, Reeves G, Bull D. Breast cancer and hormone-replacement therapy: the million women study. Lancet. 2003;362(9392):1330–1.
22. Lakhani SR, Van De Vijver MJ, Jacquemier J, Anderson TJ, Osin PP, McGuffog L, et al. The pathology of familial breast cancer: predictive value of immunohistochemical markers estrogen receptor, progesterone receptor, HER-2, and p53 in patients with mutations in BRCA1 and BRCA2. J Clin Oncol. 2002;20(9):2310–8.
23. Incorvaia L, Fanale D, Bono M, Calò V, Fiorino A, Brando C, et al. BRCA1/2 pathogenic variants in triple-negative versus luminal-like breast cancers: genotype–phenotype correlation in a

cohort of 531 patients. Therapeut Adv Med Oncol. 2020;12:1758835920975326.
24. Masciari S, Dillon DA, Rath M, Robson M, Weitzel JN, Balmana J, et al. Breast cancer phenotype in women with TP53 germline mutations: a Li-Fraumeni syndrome consortium effort. Breast Cancer Res Treat. 2012;133:1125–30.
25. Consortium CBCC-C. CHEK2* 1100delC and susceptibility to breast cancer: a collaborative analysis involving 10,860 breast cancer cases and 9,065 controls from 10 studies. Am J Hum Genet. 2004;74(6):1175–82.
26. Antoniou AC, Casadei S, Heikkinen T, Barrowdale D, Pylkäs K, Roberts J, et al. Breast-cancer risk in families with mutations in PALB2. N Engl J Med. 2014;371(6):497–506.
27. Lynch HT, Kaurah P, Wirtzfeld D, Rubinstein WS, Weissman S, Lynch JF, et al. Hereditary diffuse gastric cancer: diagnosis, genetic counseling, and prophylactic total gastrectomy. Cancer. 2008;112(12):2655–63.
28. LoConte NK, Brewster AM, Kaur JS, Merrill JK, Alberg AJ. Alcohol and cancer: a statement of the American Society of Clinical Oncology. J Clin Oncol. 2018;36(1):83–93.
29. Prentice RL, Caan B, Chlebowski RT, Patterson R, Kuller LH, Ockene JK, et al. Low-fat dietary pattern and risk of invasive breast cancer: the Women's Health Initiative randomized controlled dietary modification trial. JAMA. 2006;295(6):629–42.
30. Willett WC, Tamimi R, Hankinson SE, Hazra A, Eliassen AH, Colditz GA. Nongenetic factors in the causation of breast cancer. Diseases of the breast. 5th ed. Wolters Kluwer Health Adis (ESP); 2014.
31. Fitzgibbons PL, Henson DE, Hutter RV. Benign breast changes and the risk for subsequent breast cancer: an update of the 1985 consensus statement. Arch Pathol Lab Med. 1998;122(12):1053.
32. Dupont WD, Page DL. Risk factors for breast cancer in women with proliferative breast disease. N Engl J Med. 1985;312(3):146–51.
33. Page DL, Kidd TE Jr, Dupont WD, Simpson JF, Rogers LW. Lobular neoplasia of the breast: higher risk for subsequent invasive cancer predicted by more extensive disease. Hum Pathol. 1991;22(12):1232–9.
34. Chuba PJ, Hamre MR, Yap J, Severson RK, Lucas D, Shamsa F, et al. Bilateral risk for subsequent breast cancer after lobular carcinoma-in-situ: analysis of surveillance, epidemiology, and end results data. J Clin Oncol. 2005;23(24):5534–41.
35. Boyd NF, Guo H, Martin LJ, Sun L, Stone J, Fishell E, et al. Mammographic density and the risk and detection of breast cancer. N Engl J Med. 2007;356(3):227–36.
36. Elkin EB, Klem ML, Gonzales AM, Ishill NM, Hodgson D, Ng AK, et al. Characteristics and outcomes of breast cancer in women with and without a history of radiation for Hodgkin's lymphoma: a multi-institutional, matched cohort study. J Clin Oncol. 2011;29(18):2466.
37. Tallent A. Start mammograms at 40, not 50, USPSTF suggests. Nature. 2023;617:312–24.
38. Bevers TB, Niell BL, Baker JL, Bennett DL, Bonaccio E, Camp MS, et al. NCCN guidelines® insights: breast cancer screening and diagnosis, version 1.2023: featured updates to the NCCN guidelines. J Natl Compr Canc Netw. 2023;21(9):900–9.
39. Canelo-Aybar C, Posso M, Montero N, Solà I, Saz-Parkinson Z, Duffy SW, et al. Benefits and harms of annual, biennial, or triennial breast cancer mammography screening for women at average risk of breast cancer: a systematic review for the European Commission Initiative on Breast Cancer (ECIBC). Br J Cancer. 2022;126(4):673–88.
40. Loibl S, André F, Bachelot T, Barrios C, Bergh J, Burstein H, et al. Early breast cancer: ESMO clinical practice guideline for diagnosis, treatment and follow-up☆. Ann Oncol. 2024;35(2):159–82.
41. Gail MH, Brinton LA, Byar DP, Corle DK, Green SB, Schairer C, et al. Projecting individualized probabilities of developing breast cancer for white females who are being examined annually. JNCI J Natl Cancer Inst. 1989;81(24):1879–86.
42. Claus EB, Risch N, Thompson WD. Autosomal dominant inheritance of early-onset breast cancer. Implications for risk prediction. Cancer. 1994;73(3):643–51.
43. Parmigiani G, Berry DA, Aguilar O. Determining carrier probabilities for breast cancer–susceptibility genes BRCA1 and BRCA2. Am J Hum Genet. 1998;62(1):145–58.
44. Frank TS, Deffenbaugh AM, Reid JE, Hulick M, Ward BE, Lingenfelter B, et al. Clinical characteristics of individuals with germline mutations in BRCA1 and BRCA2: analysis of 10,000 individuals. J Clin Oncol. 2002;20(6):1480–90.
45. Le-Petross HT, Whitman GJ, Atchley DP, Yuan Y, Gutierrez-Barrera A, Hortobagyi GN, et al. Effectiveness of alternating mammography and magnetic resonance imaging for screening women with deleterious BRCA mutations at high risk of breast cancer. Cancer. 2011;117(17):3900–7.
46. King M-C, Wieand S, Hale K, Lee M, Walsh T, Owens K, et al. Tamoxifen and breast cancer incidence among women with inherited mutations in BRCA1 and BRCA2: National Surgical Adjuvant Breast and Bowel Project (NSABP-P1) breast cancer prevention trial. JAMA. 2001;286(18):2251–6.
47. Vogel VG. The NSABP study of tamoxifen and raloxifene (STAR) trial. Expert Rev Anticancer Ther. 2009;9(1):51–60.
48. Goss PE, Richardson H, Chlebowski R, Johnston D, Sarto GE, Maunsell E, et al. National Cancer Institute of Canada clinical trials group MAP. 3 trial: evaluation of exemestane to prevent breast cancer in postmenopausal women. Clin Breast Cancer. 2007;7(11):895–900.
49. De Felice F, Marchetti C, Musella A, Palaia I, Perniola G, Musio D, et al. Bilateral risk-reduction mastec-

tomy in BRCA1 and BRCA2 mutation carriers: a meta-analysis. Ann Surg Oncol. 2015;22:2876–80.
50. Berek JS, Chalas E, Edelson M, Moore DH, Burke WM, Cliby WA, et al. Prophylactic and risk-reducing bilateral salpingo-oophorectomy: recommendations based on risk of ovarian cancer. Obstet Gynecol. 2010;116(3):733–43.
51. Senkus E, Kyriakides S, Ohno S, Penault-Llorca F, Poortmans P, Rutgers E, et al. Primary breast cancer: ESMO clinical practice guidelines for diagnosis, treatment and follow-up. Ann Oncol. 2015;26:v8–v30.
52. Katipamula R, Degnim AC, Hoskin T, Boughey JC, Loprinzi C, Grant CS, et al. Trends in mastectomy rates at the Mayo Clinic Rochester: effect of surgical year and preoperative magnetic resonance imaging. J Clin Oncol. 2009;27(25):4082.
53. Giuliano AE, Edge SB, Hortobagyi GN. Of the AJCC cancer staging manual: breast cancer. Ann Surg Oncol. 2018;25:1783–5.
54. Solin LJ, Gray R, Baehner FL, Butler SM, Hughes LL, Yoshizawa C, et al. A multigene expression assay to predict local recurrence risk for ductal carcinoma in situ of the breast. J Natl Cancer Inst. 2013;105(10):701–10.
55. Bremer T, Whitworth PW, Patel R, Savala J, Barry T, Lyle S, et al. A biological signature for breast ductal carcinoma in situ to predict radiotherapy benefit and assess recurrence risk. Clin Cancer Res. 2018;24(23):5895–901.
56. Tan PH, Ellis I, Allison K, Brogi E, Fox SB, Lakhani S, et al. The 2019 WHO classification of tumours of the breast. Histopathology. 2020;77:181.
57. Sinn H-P, Kreipe H. A brief overview of the WHO classification of breast tumors, focusing on issues and updates from the 3rd edition. Breast Care. 2013;8(2):149–54.
58. Rakha EA, Patel A, Powe DG, Benhasouna A, Green AR, Lambros MB, et al. Clinical and biological significance of E-cadherin protein expression in invasive lobular carcinoma of the breast. Am J Surg Pathol. 2010;34(10):1472–9.
59. van Bommel RM, Voogd AC, Nederend J, Setz-Pels W, Louwman MW, Strobbe LJ, et al. Incidence and tumour characteristics of bilateral and unilateral interval breast cancers at screening mammography. Breast. 2018;38:101–6.
60. Findlay-Shirras LJ, Lima I, Smith G, Clemons M, Arnaout A. Population trends in lobular carcinoma of the breast: the Ontario experience. Ann Surg Oncol. 2020;27:4711–9.
61. Al-Hilli Z, Choong G, Keeney MG, Visscher DW, Ingle JN, Goetz MP, et al. Metaplastic breast cancer has a poor response to neoadjuvant systemic therapy. Breast Cancer Res Treat. 2019;176:709–16.
62. Han M, Salamat A, Zhu L, Zhang H, Clark BZ, Dabbs DJ, et al. Metaplastic breast carcinoma: a clinical-pathologic study of 97 cases with subset analysis of response to neoadjuvant chemotherapy. Mod Pathol. 2019;32(6):807–16.
63. Hennessy B, Giordano S, Broglio K, Duan Z, Trent J, Buchholz TA, et al. Biphasic metaplastic sarcomatoid carcinoma of the breast. Ann Oncol. 2006;17(4):605–13.
64. Srigley JR, McGowan T, MacLean A, Raby M, Ross J, Kramer S, et al. Standardized synoptic cancer pathology reporting: a population-based approach. J Surg Oncol. 2009;99(8):517–24.
65. Elston E, Ellis I. Method for grading breast cancer. J Clin Pathol. 1993;46(2):189.
66. Allison KH, Hammond MEH, Dowsett M, McKernin SE, Carey LA, Fitzgibbons PL, et al. Estrogen and progesterone receptor testing in breast cancer: American Society of Clinical Oncology/College of American Pathologists guideline update. Arch Pathol Lab Med. 2020;144(5):545–63.
67. Wolff AC, Hammond MEH, Hicks DG, Dowsett M, McShane LM, Allison KH, et al. Recommendations for human epidermal growth factor receptor 2 testing in breast cancer: American Society of Clinical Oncology/College of American Pathologists clinical practice guideline update. Arch Pathol Lab Med. 2014;138(2):241–56.
68. Perez EA, Dueck AC, McCullough AE, Reinholz MM, Tenner KS, Davidson NE, et al. Predictability of adjuvant trastuzumab benefit in N9831 patients using the ASCO/CAP HER2-positivity criteria. J Natl Cancer Inst. 2012;104(2):159–62.
69. Denkert C, Seither F, Schneeweiss A, Link T, Blohmer J-U, Just M, et al. Clinical and molecular characteristics of HER2-low-positive breast cancer: pooled analysis of individual patient data from four prospective, neoadjuvant clinical trials. Lancet Oncol. 2021;22(8):1151–61.
70. Petrelli F, Viale G, Cabiddu M, Barni S. Prognostic value of different cut-off levels of Ki-67 in breast cancer: a systematic review and meta-analysis of 64,196 patients. Breast Cancer Res Treat. 2015;153:477–91.
71. Dowsett M, Nielsen TO, A'Hern R, Bartlett J, Coombes RC, Cuzick J, et al. Assessment of Ki67 in breast cancer: recommendations from the international Ki67 in breast cancer working group. J Natl Cancer Inst. 2011;103(22):1656–64.
72. Smith I, Robertson J, Kilburn L, Wilcox M, Evans A, Holcombe C, et al. Long-term outcome and prognostic value of Ki67 after perioperative endocrine therapy in postmenopausal women with hormone-sensitive early breast cancer (POETIC): an open-label, multicentre, parallel-group, randomised, phase 3 trial. Lancet Oncol. 2020;21(11):1443–54.
73. Salgado R, Denkert C, Demaria S, Sirtaine N, Klauschen F, Pruneri G, et al. The evaluation of tumor-infiltrating lymphocytes (TILs) in breast cancer: recommendations by an international TILs working group 2014. Ann Oncol. 2015;26(2):259–71.
74. Rakha EA, Martin S, Lee AH, Morgan D, Pharoah PD, Hodi Z, et al. The prognostic significance of lymphovascular invasion in invasive breast carcinoma. Cancer. 2012;118(15):3670–80.

75. Barrio AV, Morrow M. Appropriate margin for lumpectomy excision of invasive breast cancer. Chin Clin Oncol. 2016;5(3):35.
76. Chung A, Gangi A, Amersi F, Bose S, Zhang X, Giuliano A. Impact of consensus guidelines by the Society of Surgical Oncology and the American Society for Radiation Oncology on margins for breast-conserving surgery in stages 1 and 2 invasive breast cancer. Ann Surg Oncol. 2015;22:422–7.
77. Charles M, Network CGA. Comprehensive molecular portraits of human breast tumors. Nature. 2012;490(7418):61–70.
78. Sørlie T, Tibshirani R, Parker J, Hastie T, Marron JS, Nobel A, et al. Repeated observation of breast tumor subtypes in independent gene expression data sets. Proc Natl Acad Sci. 2003;100(14):8418–23.
79. Perou CM, Sørlie T, Eisen MB, Van De Rijn M, Jeffrey SS, Rees CA, et al. Molecular portraits of human breast tumours. Nature. 2000;406(6797):747–52.
80. Russo A, Peeters M, Incorvaia L, Rolfo C. Practical medical oncology textbook. Berlin: Springer; 2021.
81. Boyages J, Delaney G, Taylor R. Predictors of local recurrence after treatment of ductal carcinoma in situ: a meta-analysis. Cancer. 1999;85(3):616–28.
82. Burstein HJ, Polyak K, Wong JS, Lester SC, Kaelin CM. Ductal carcinoma in situ of the breast. N Engl J Med. 2004;350(14):1430–41.
83. Morrow M, Van Zee KJ, Solin LJ, Houssami N, Chavez-MacGregor M, Harris JR, et al. Society of Surgical Oncology–American Society for Radiation Oncology–American Society of Clinical Oncology consensus guideline on margins for breast-conserving surgery with whole-breast irradiation in ductal carcinoma in situ. Ann Surg Oncol. 2016;23:3801–10.
84. Bijker N, Meijnen P, Peterse JL, Bogaerts J, Van Hoorebeeck I, Julien J-p, et al. Breast-conserving treatment with or without radiotherapy in ductal carcinoma-in-situ: ten-year results of European Organisation for Research and Treatment of Cancer randomized phase III trial 10853—a study by the EORTC Breast Cancer Cooperative Group and EORTC Radiotherapy Group. J Clin Oncol. 2006;24(21):3381–7.
85. Wapnir IL, Dignam JJ, Fisher B, Mamounas EP, Anderson SJ, Julian TB, et al. Long-term outcomes of invasive ipsilateral breast tumor recurrences after lumpectomy in NSABP B-17 and B-24 randomized clinical trials for DCIS. J Natl Cancer Inst. 2011;103(6):478–88.
86. Julian TB, Land SR, Fourchotte V, Haile SR, Fisher ER, Mamounas EP, et al. Is sentinel node biopsy necessary in conservatively treated DCIS? Ann Surg Oncol. 2007;14:2202–8.
87. Cuzick J, Sestak I, Pinder SE, Ellis IO, Forsyth S, Bundred NJ, et al. Effect of tamoxifen and radiotherapy in women with locally excised ductal carcinoma in situ: long-term results from the UK/ANZ DCIS trial. Lancet Oncol. 2011;12(1):21–9.
88. Margolese RG, Cecchini RS, Julian TB, Ganz PA, Costantino JP, Vallow LA, et al. Anastrozole versus tamoxifen in postmenopausal women with ductal carcinoma in situ undergoing lumpectomy plus radiotherapy (NSABP B-35): a randomised, double-blind, phase 3 clinical trial. Lancet. 2016;387(10021):849–56.
89. Fisher B, Anderson S, Bryant J, Margolese RG, Deutsch M, Fisher ER, et al. Twenty-year follow-up of a randomized trial comparing total mastectomy, lumpectomy, and lumpectomy plus irradiation for the treatment of invasive breast cancer. N Engl J Med. 2002;347(16):1233–41.
90. Krag DN, Anderson SJ, Julian TB, Brown AM, Harlow SP, Costantino JP, et al. Sentinel-lymph-node resection compared with conventional axillary-lymph-node dissection in clinically node-negative patients with breast cancer: overall survival findings from the NSABP B-32 randomised phase 3 trial. Lancet Oncol. 2010;11(10):927–33.
91. Galimberti V, Cole BF, Zurrida S, Viale G, Luini A, Veronesi P, et al. Axillary dissection versus no axillary dissection in patients with sentinel-node micrometastases (IBCSG 23–01): a phase 3 randomised controlled trial. Lancet Oncol. 2013;14(4):297–305.
92. Giuliano AE, Ballman KV, McCall L, Beitsch PD, Brennan MB, Kelemen PR, et al. Effect of axillary dissection vs no axillary dissection on 10-year overall survival among women with invasive breast cancer and sentinel node metastasis: the ACOSOG Z0011 (Alliance) randomized clinical trial. JAMA. 2017;318(10):918–26.
93. Pilewskie M, Morrow M. Axillary nodal management following neoadjuvant chemotherapy: a review. JAMA Oncol. 2017;3(4):549–55.
94. Kuehn T, Bauerfeind I, Fehm T, Fleige B, Hausschild M, Helms G, et al. Sentinel-lymph-node biopsy in patients with breast cancer before and after neoadjuvant chemotherapy (SENTINA): a prospective, multicentre cohort study. Lancet Oncol. 2013;14(7):609–18.
95. Group EBCTC. Effect of radiotherapy after breast-conserving surgery on 10-year recurrence and 15-year breast cancer death: meta-analysis of individual patient data for 10 801 women in 17 randomised trials. Lancet. 2011;378(9804):1707–16.
96. Taylor C, Dodwell D, McGale P, Hills RK, Berry R, Bradley R, et al. Radiotherapy to regional nodes in early breast cancer: an individual patient data meta-analysis of 14 324 women in 16 trials. Lancet. 2023;402(10416):1991–2003.
97. Cortazar P, Zhang L, Untch M, Mehta K, Costantino JP, Wolmark N, et al. Pathological complete response and long-term clinical benefit in breast cancer: the CTNeoBC pooled analysis. Lancet. 2014;384(9938):164–72.
98. Group EBCTC. Aromatase inhibitors versus tamoxifen in early breast cancer: patient-level meta-analysis of the randomised trials. Lancet. 2015;386(10001):1341–52.

99. Kalinsky K, Barlow WE, Gralow JR, Meric-Bernstam F, Albain KS, Hayes DF, et al. 21-gene assay to inform chemotherapy benefit in node-positive breast cancer. N Engl J Med. 2021;385(25):2336–47.
100. Sparano JA, Gray RJ, Makower DF, Pritchard KI, Albain KS, Hayes DF, et al. Adjuvant chemotherapy guided by a 21-gene expression assay in breast cancer. N Engl J Med. 2018;379(2):111–21.
101. Bernhard J, Luo W, Ribi K, Colleoni M, Burstein HJ, Tondini C, et al. Patient-reported outcomes with adjuvant exemestane versus tamoxifen in premenopausal women with early breast cancer undergoing ovarian suppression (TEXT and SOFT): a combined analysis of two phase 3 randomised trials. Lancet Oncol. 2015;16(7):848–58.
102. Johnston SR, Toi M, O'Shaughnessy J, Rastogi P, Campone M, Neven P, et al. Abemaciclib plus endocrine therapy for hormone receptor-positive, HER2-negative, node-positive, high-risk early breast cancer (monarchE): results from a preplanned interim analysis of a randomised, open-label, phase 3 trial. Lancet Oncol. 2023;24(1):77–90.
103. Slamon DJ, Stroyakovskiy D, Yardley DA, Huang C-S, Fasching PA, Crown J, et al. Ribociclib and endocrine therapy as adjuvant treatment in patients with HR+/HER2-early breast cancer: primary results from the phase III NATALEE trial. J Clin Oncol. 2023;41(17_suppl):LBA500.
104. Geyer C Jr, Garber J, Gelber R, Yothers G, Taboada M, Ross L, et al. Overall survival in the OlympiA phase III trial of adjuvant olaparib in patients with germline pathogenic variants in BRCA1/2 and high-risk, early breast cancer. Ann Oncol. 2022;33(12):1250–68.
105. Romond EH, Jeong J-H, Rastogi P, Swain SM, Geyer CE Jr, Ewer MS, et al. Seven-year follow-up assessment of cardiac function in NSABP B-31, a randomized trial comparing doxorubicin and cyclophosphamide followed by paclitaxel (ACP) with ACP plus trastuzumab as adjuvant therapy for patients with node-positive, human epidermal growth factor receptor 2–positive breast cancer. J Clin Oncol. 2012;30(31):3792.
106. Tolaney SM, Tarantino P, Graham N, Tayob N, Parè L, Villacampa G, et al. Adjuvant paclitaxel and trastuzumab for node-negative, HER2-positive breast cancer: final 10-year analysis of the open-label, single-arm, phase 2 APT trial. Lancet Oncol. 2023;24(3):273–85.
107. Gianni L, Pienkowski T, Im Y-H, Roman L, Tseng L-M, Liu M-C, et al. Efficacy and safety of neoadjuvant pertuzumab and trastuzumab in women with locally advanced, inflammatory, or early HER2-positive breast cancer (NeoSphere): a randomised multicentre, open-label, phase 2 trial. Lancet Oncol. 2012;13(1):25–32.
108. Von Minckwitz G, Huang C-S, Mano MS, Loibl S, Mamounas EP, Untch M, et al. Trastuzumab emtansine for residual invasive HER2-positive breast cancer. N Engl J Med. 2019;380(7):617–28.
109. Martin M, Holmes FA, Ejlertsen B, Delaloge S, Moy B, Iwata H, et al. Neratinib after trastuzumab-based adjuvant therapy in HER2-positive breast cancer (ExteNET): 5-year analysis of a randomised, double-blind, placebo-controlled, phase 3 trial. Lancet Oncol. 2017;18(12):1688–700.
110. Masuda N, Lee S-J, Ohtani S, Im Y-H, Lee E-S, Yokota I, et al. Adjuvant capecitabine for breast cancer after preoperative chemotherapy. N Engl J Med. 2017;376(22):2147–59.
111. Schmid P, Cortes J, Dent R, Pusztai L, McArthur H, Kümmel S, et al. Event-free survival with pembrolizumab in early triple-negative breast cancer. N Engl J Med. 2022;386(6):556–67.
112. Gennari A, André F, Barrios C, Cortes J, de Azambuja E, DeMichele A, et al. ESMO clinical practice guideline for the diagnosis, staging and treatment of patients with metastatic breast cancer☆. Ann Oncol. 2021;32(12):1475–95.
113. Biganzoli L, Battisti NML, Wildiers H, McCartney A, Colloca G, Kunkler IH, et al. Updated recommendations regarding the management of older patients with breast cancer: a joint paper from the European Society of Breast Cancer Specialists (EUSOMA) and the International Society of Geriatric Oncology (SIOG). Lancet Oncol. 2021;22(7):e327–e40.
114. Lipton A, Fizazi K, Stopeck AT, Henry DH, Brown JE, Yardley DA, et al. Superiority of denosumab to zoledronic acid for prevention of skeletal-related events: a combined analysis of 3 pivotal, randomised, phase 3 trials. Eur J Cancer. 2012;48(16):3082–92.
115. Finn RS, Martin M, Rugo HS, Jones S, Im S-A, Gelmon K, et al. Palbociclib and letrozole in advanced breast cancer. N Engl J Med. 2016;375(20):1925–36.
116. Hortobagyi GN, Stemmer SM, Burris HA, Yap Y-S, Sonke GS, Paluch-Shimon S, et al. Ribociclib as first-line therapy for HR-positive, advanced breast cancer. N Engl J Med. 2016;375(18):1738–48.
117. Goetz MP, Toi M, Campone M, Sohn J, Paluch-Shimon S, Huober J, et al. MONARCH 3: abemaciclib as initial therapy for advanced breast cancer. J Clin Oncol. 2017;35(32):3638–46.
118. Tripathy D, Im S-A, Colleoni M, Franke F, Bardia A, Harbeck N, et al. Ribociclib plus endocrine therapy for premenopausal women with hormone-receptor-positive, advanced breast cancer (MONALEESA-7): a randomised phase 3 trial. Lancet Oncol. 2018;19(7):904–15.
119. Im S-A, Lu Y-S, Bardia A, Harbeck N, Colleoni M, Franke F, et al. Overall survival with ribociclib plus endocrine therapy in breast cancer. N Engl J Med. 2019;381(4):307–16.
120. Cristofanilli M, Turner NC, Bondarenko I, Ro J, Im S-A, Masuda N, et al. Fulvestrant plus palbociclib versus fulvestrant plus placebo for treatment of hormone-receptor-positive, HER2-negative metastatic breast cancer that progressed on previous endocrine therapy (PALOMA-3): final analysis of

the multicentre, double-blind, phase 3 randomised controlled trial. Lancet Oncol. 2016;17(4):425–39.
121. Sledge GW, Toi M, Neven P, Sohn J, Inoue K, Pivot X, et al. The effect of abemaciclib plus fulvestrant on overall survival in hormone receptor–positive, ERBB2-negative breast cancer that progressed on endocrine therapy—MONARCH 2: a randomized clinical trial. JAMA Oncol. 2020;6(1):116–24.
122. Slamon DJ, Neven P, Chia S, Fasching PA, De Laurentiis M, Im S-A, et al. Overall survival with ribociclib plus fulvestrant in advanced breast cancer. N Engl J Med. 2020;382(6):514–24.
123. Turner NC, Slamon DJ, Ro J, Bondarenko I, Im S-A, Masuda N, et al. Overall survival with palbociclib and fulvestrant in advanced breast cancer. N Engl J Med. 2018;379(20):1926–36.
124. André F, Ciruelos E, Rubovszky G, Campone M, Loibl S, Rugo HS, et al. Alpelisib for PIK3CA-mutated, hormone receptor–positive advanced breast cancer. N Engl J Med. 2019;380(20):1929–40.
125. Rugo HS, Lerebours F, Ciruelos E, Drullinsky P, Ruiz-Borrego M, Neven P, et al. Alpelisib plus fulvestrant in PIK3CA-mutated, hormone receptor-positive advanced breast cancer after a CDK4/6 inhibitor (BYLieve): one cohort of a phase 2, multicentre, open-label, non-comparative study. Lancet Oncol. 2021;22(4):489–98.
126. Baselga J, Campone M, Piccart M, Burris HA III, Rugo HS, Sahmoud T, et al. Everolimus in postmenopausal hormone-receptor–positive advanced breast cancer. N Engl J Med. 2012;366(6):520–9.
127. Piccart M, Hortobagyi GN, Campone M, Pritchard K, Lebrun F, Ito Y, et al. Everolimus plus exemestane for hormone-receptor-positive, human epidermal growth factor receptor-2-negative advanced breast cancer: overall survival results from BOLERO-2. Ann Oncol. 2014;25(12):2357–62.
128. Baselga J, Cortés J, Kim S-B, Im S-A, Hegg R, Im Y-H, et al. Pertuzumab plus trastuzumab plus docetaxel for metastatic breast cancer. N Engl J Med. 2012;366(2):109–19.
129. Rimawi M, Ferrero J-M, de la Haba-Rodriguez J, Poole C, De Placido S, Osborne CK, et al. First-line trastuzumab plus an aromatase inhibitor, with or without pertuzumab, in human epidermal growth factor receptor 2–positive and hormone receptor–positive metastatic or locally advanced breast cancer (PERTAIN): a randomized, open-label phase II trial. J Clin Oncol. 2018;36(28):2826–35.
130. Verma S, Miles D, Gianni L, Krop IE, Welslau M, Baselga J, et al. Trastuzumab emtansine for HER2-positive advanced breast cancer. N Engl J Med. 2012;367(19):1783–91.
131. Cortés J, Kim S, Chung W, editors. Trastuzumab deruxtecan (T-DXd) vs trastuzumab emtansine (T-DM1) in patients with HER2+ metastatic breast cancer: results of the randomized phase III DESTINY-Breast03 study. ESMO Congress; 2021.
132. Lin NU, Borges V, Anders C, Murthy RK, Paplomata E, Hamilton E, et al. Intracranial efficacy and survival with tucatinib plus trastuzumab and capecitabine for previously treated HER2-positive breast cancer with brain metastases in the HER2CLIMB trial. J Clin Oncol. 2020;38(23):2610.
133. Cortes J, Cescon DW, Rugo HS, Nowecki Z, Im S-A, Yusof MM, et al. Pembrolizumab plus chemotherapy versus placebo plus chemotherapy for previously untreated locally recurrent inoperable or metastatic triple-negative breast cancer (KEYNOTE-355): a randomised, placebo-controlled, double-blind, phase 3 clinical trial. Lancet. 2020;396(10265):1817–28.
134. Tutt A, Tovey H, Cheang MCU, Kernaghan S, Kilburn L, Gazinska P, et al. Carboplatin in BRCA1/2-mutated and triple-negative breast cancer BRCAness subgroups: the TNT trial. Nat Med. 2018;24(5):628–37.
135. Robson M, Im S-A, Senkus E, Xu B, Domchek SM, Masuda N, et al. Olaparib for metastatic breast cancer in patients with a germline BRCA mutation. N Engl J Med. 2017;377(6):523–33.
136. Bardia A, Messersmith W, Kio E, Berlin J, Vahdat L, Masters G, et al. Sacituzumab govitecan, a Trop-2-directed antibody-drug conjugate, for patients with epithelial cancer: final safety and efficacy results from the phase I/II IMMU-132-01 basket trial. Ann Oncol. 2021;32(6):746–56.

2 Breast Cancer Surgery: Special Focus on Preventive Strategies in Breast Cancer Related Lymphedema

Ömer Cennet and Ali Konan

2.1 Introduction

Surgery has been the mainstay of treatment for breast cancer. It is often the only effective treatment method for early-stage breast cancer. At the same time, surgery is vital for the accurate diagnosis, staging, and treatment of patients with breast cancer. Many landmark studies published in recent years have led to the transition from more radical options such as radical mastectomy to breast-conserving surgery (BCS). Similarly, the axillary approach has changed over the years due to significant morbidities such as the risk of breast cancer-related lymphedema (BCRL), impaired shoulder mobility, and arm sensation. Traditionally, axillary lymph node dissection (ALND) is performed in all patients regardless of nodal status, yet studies have established sentinel lymph node biopsy (SLNB) has been the optimal standard for surgical evaluation of the axillary region. Despite recent efforts to reduce and minimize the risks of breast and axillary surgery, BCRL remains a feared chronic sequela of surgical treatment of breast cancer. In light of new data on the risk of BCRL, some prevention strategies and treatment modalities are available.

Ö. Cennet (✉) · A. Konan
General Surgery Department, Faculty of Medicine, Hacettepe University, Altındağ, Ankara, Turkey
e-mail: omer.cennet@hacettepe.edu.tr; akonan@hacettepe.edu.tr

2.2 Diagnosis

To diagnose breast cancer, further imaging methods (USG, mammography) are used in suspected cases after a detailed history and physical examination. Many breast cancers can be detected by the patient or the physician before they become palpable on clinical examination prior to mammography screening. In case of suspicious findings (calcifications, structural distortion, or spiculated mass), a core needle biopsy should be performed for tissue diagnosis. If malignancy is detected, the obtained information (in situ vs. invasive, ductal vs. lobular, hormonal status, and molecular pattern) helps guide decisions regarding surgery as well as other treatments. Once malignancy has been diagnosed, in addition to mammography, other imaging modalities may be used including ultrasound of the breast and axilla, and in some cases (dense breast, suspicious findings, etc.) breast magnetic resonance imaging (MRI). The stage is assigned based on clinical prognostic staging according to the American Joint Committee on Cancer (AJCC) or anatomic staging (TNM), which reflects the biology of the tumor and the expected prognosis. Molecular features of tumors provide further characterization, providing additional information on prognosis and specific treatment options (Table 2.1). Patients with clinical stage III breast cancer (disease confined to the breast and axilla) and those with

Y. Bakar, A. Tuğral (eds.), *Managing Side Effects of Breast Cancer Treatment*,
https://doi.org/10.1007/978-3-031-75480-7_2

Table 2.1 Molecular subtypes of breast cancer

Subtype	Distinctive characteristics
Luminal A (ER+, PR+, HER2−, Ki67 < 14)	Good prognosis, hormonal therapy
Luminal B (ER+, PR+, HER2−, Ki67 > 14)	Higher grade, lower estrogen, hormonal therapy
HER2 enriched (ER+, PR+, HER2+)	Anti-HER agents, node positivity
Triple negative (ER−, PR−, HER2−	Poor prognosis, BRCA mutation, chemotherapy

suspicious signs/symptoms that might be associated with possible metastatic disease should undergo a thorax-abdominal computed tomography (CT) scan and bone scan or positron emission tomography (PET-CT) to evaluate distant metastatic disease.

2.3 Surgical Options

When discussing surgical options with patients, the localization of the tumor, the size of the tumor, the size and ptosis of the breast, the patient's expectations, comorbidities, etc. should be taken into consideration.

The treatment of breast cancer has undergone major changes over the years. It has evolved from Halsted's radical mastectomy, in which the pectoral muscle is removed, and all axillary lymph nodes dissected, which can cause significant morbidity, to simple excision of the tumor with a millimeter-safe margin.

The surgeon should discuss the pros and cons of all surgical options with patients who are planned initially for surgery (clinical stage I–II). However, it should be emphasized here that the long-term survival and prognosis of patients with mastectomy or breast-conserving surgery and radiotherapy are similar [1]. It should also be noted that the decision to initiate chemotherapy, hormonotherapy, and anti-HER treatment is not related to the choice of surgery but to the characteristics of the tumor. However, local recurrence is slightly higher in the lumpectomy and radiotherapy group than in the mastectomy group (5–8% vs. 2%) [2].

Mastectomy should be considered in multicentric tumors and patients who have a positive history of prior radiotherapy to the chest wall. However, in the light of recent clinical trials, with current advances in the diagnosis and management of patients with multicentric ipsilateral breast cancer, including high-quality digital imaging and continuously improving systemic therapy and radiation therapy, local recurrence rates are acceptably low and similar to those seen in patients with unifocal breast cancer [3].

Other conditions that may affect the decision-making process include family history and genetic predisposition. Detailed questioning of family history is very important in patients with breast cancer. In general, women diagnosed with breast cancer before the age of 65, patients older than 65 years with triple-negative cancer, or if they are of Ashkenazi Jewish ancestry, and all men diagnosed with breast cancer should be referred for genetic counseling [4]. A more aggressive risk-reducing surgical approach such as bilateral mastectomy may be preferred in women classified as high-risk patients.

2.4 Breast-Conserving Surgery

Breast-conserving surgery (lumpectomy, partial mastectomy, tumorectomy—often used synonymously) is the removal of the cancerous area with a safe margin while preserving as much normal breast tissue as possible. If the lesion can be palpated, this area is removed through an appropriate incision. For the best cosmetic outcomes, incisions following the circumareolar, inframammary fold, and langer's lines can be used. For deep and small lesions that cannot be palpated, localization methods can be used. The most commonly used technique is the removal of the lesion by marking it with the help of a guidewire (Fig. 2.1). Radionuclide labeling (ROLL), intraoperative ultrasound, and new wireless technologies are also available to aid tumor localization [5, 6].

Evaluation of the surgical margin is important in BCS. "No ink on tumor" in invasive tumors and 2 mm in ductal carcinoma in situ (DCIS) are

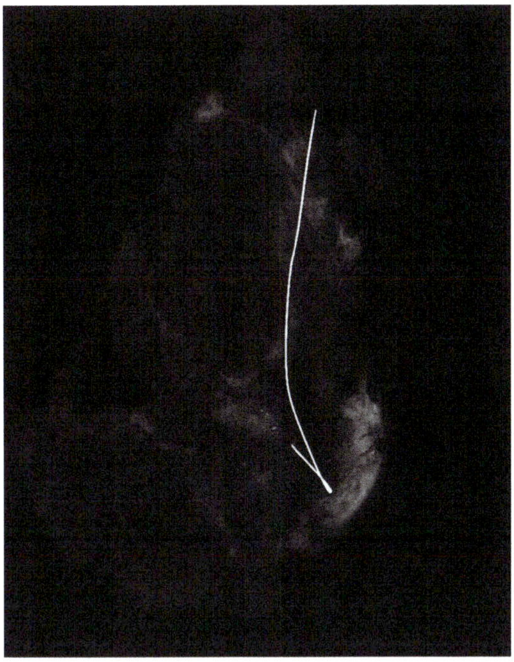

Fig. 2.1 Specimen mammography image after marking the suspicious area with guidewire

considered as safe surgical margins [7, 8]. It has been shown that a wider surgical margin does not reduce local recurrence. Positive surgical margins are associated with increased local recurrence. Re-excision rates due to positive surgical margins are around 20%. There are some approaches to reduce this rate [9]. These include intraoperative specimen radiography and ultrasound, frozen section, imprint cytology, and cavity shaving. All these procedures have reduced the rate of border positivity and reoperation [10–12].

2.5 Oncoplastic Techniques in Breast Surgery

Although BCS is considered the standard approach in the treatment of breast cancer, sometimes it may not have cosmetically satisfactory results (Fig. 2.2). Oncoplastic breast surgery aims to improve cosmetics by locally excising the tumor with a variety of plastic surgery techniques without compromising oncological principles. All indications for BCS are also suitable for oncoplastic breast surgery. These techniques

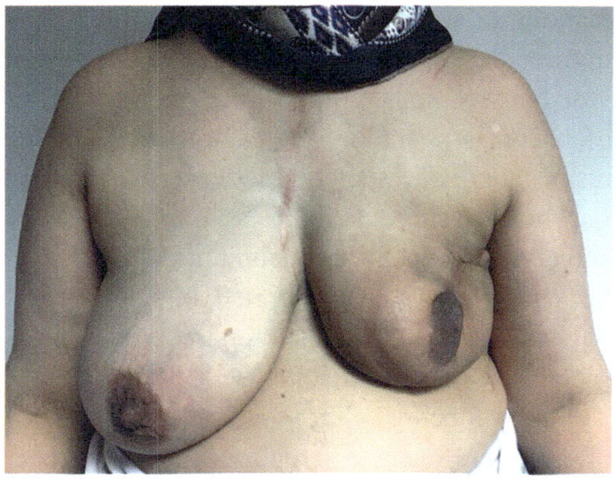

Fig. 2.2 Cosmetically unsatisfactory appearance after breast-conserving surgery

are especially suitable for patients with large tumors, small breast volumes, multicentric/multifocal tumors, and patients with more than 20% breast volume removed, which may result in poor cosmetic results. In addition, it is also suitable for tumor locations such as upper inner quadrants, and central region (areola invasion) where removal of even a small volume may lead to poor cosmetic appearance. Patients with macromastia requiring bilateral reduction are also suitable for oncoplastic reduction.

Oncoplastic breast surgery has some oncologic and cosmetic contraindications. It should not be performed in patients where a tumor-free margin cannot be achieved or where the expected cosmetic results cannot be achieved due to the structure of the breast. BCS is also not suitable for inflammatory breast carcinomas. Caution should also be exercised in patients with a history of previous radiotherapy, heavy smoking, uncontrolled diabetes, and obesity, as these may increase complications.

Oncoplastic surgery has many supposed advantages. Integrating oncoplastic techniques into cancer surgery may improve oncological safety and reduce the risk of tumor recurrence due to wider resection margins [13]. However, it should be noted that in case of a positive surgical margin, the tumor cavity may be in different positions than expected. Therefore, re-excision should be performed by the surgeon who performed the first operation. In addition, since the tumor bed will change during resection, the marking of all tumor walls is a facilitating situation for the radiation oncologist in order to provide boost radiotherapy [14]. Another advantage of oncoplastic surgery is it improves cosmetic results. In BCS, sometimes the desired results may not be achieved (Fig. 2.2). In many studies, surgery with oncoplastic techniques was found to be superior in patient-reported outcomes [15]. Patients have been shown to report better psychosocial health, "satisfaction with breasts" and "sexual wellbeing".

There are many different oncoplastic surgery techniques. They are generally divided into volume replacement and volume displacement techniques. There are also level 1–2–3 oncoplastic techniques and their definitions [16]. When deciding between these techniques, many factors such as the surgeon's experience, the patient's expectation, the symmetry of the opposite breast, the ptosis of the breast, and the location of the mass according to the quadrants are important. For example, in a patient with macromastia and a mass invading the nipple-areola, excellent cosmetic results can be obtained by planning a new areola with an inferior pedicle, therapeutic reduction, and symmetrization to the opposite breast (Fig. 2.3). Various techniques such as lateral mammaplasty, batwing mammoplasty, grisotti flap mastopexy, and Goldilocks mastectomy have been described according to different tumor localizations. The use of chest wall perforator-based flaps for volume replacement has also become widespread [17]. However, one of the issues to be considered here is the fact that onco-

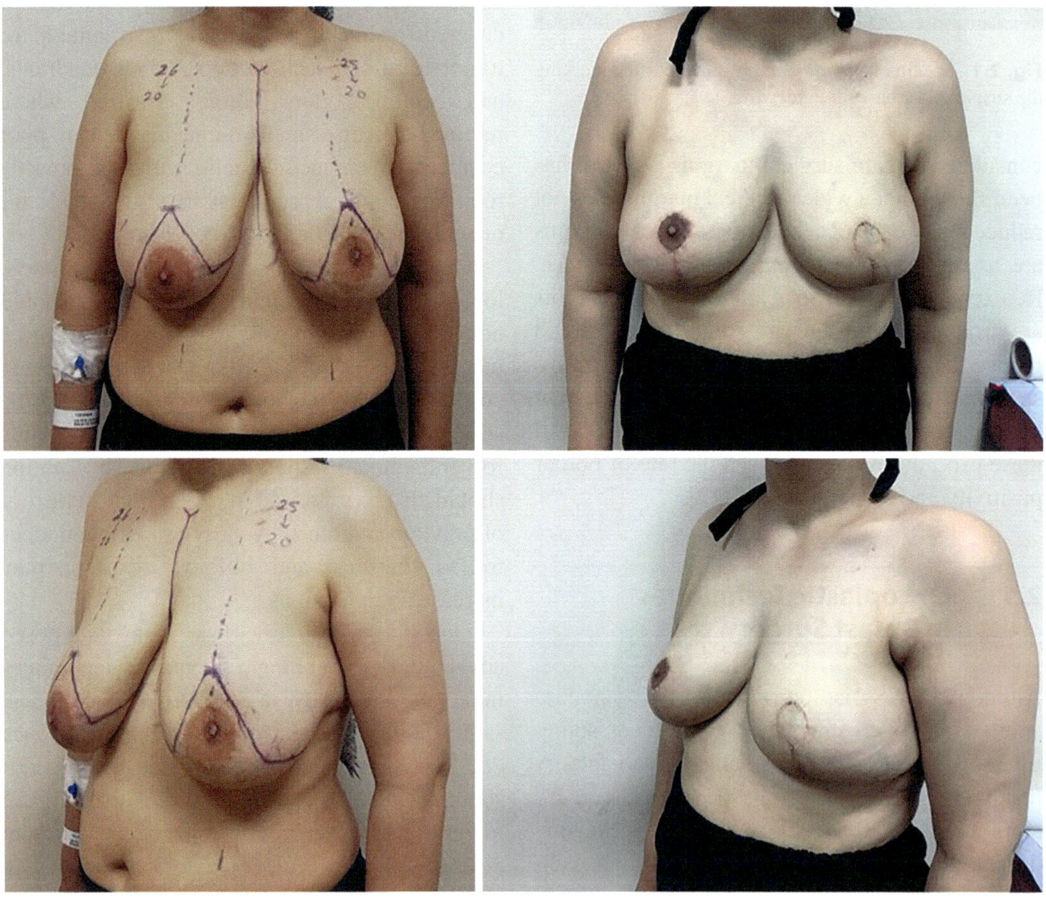

Fig. 2.3 Before and after oncoplastic reduction of a patient with macromastia and tumor invading the left nipple. Note the recession of the left nipple

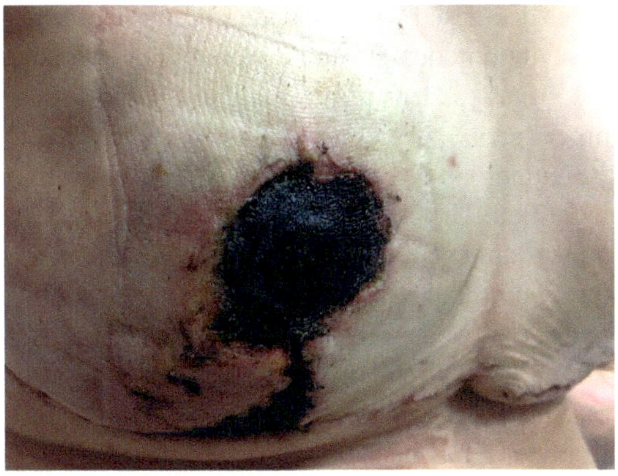

Fig. 2.4 Complete necrosis of the nipple

plastic surgeries are more complex procedures [18]. It should be noted that patients are prone to additional complications, which can cause delayed oncologic treatments specifically in unsuitable patients and inexperienced centers (Fig. 2.4).

2.6 Mastectomy

Mastectomy is the removal of all breast tissue within anatomic boundaries. The anatomic borders of the breast are the clavicle, latissimus dorsi muscle, inframammarian fold, and sternum. If no reconstruction is performed, it is called a simple mastectomy. The breast tissue, breast skin, and nipple are removed through an elliptical incision or an incision that can be modified according to the localization of the tumor. The skin is closed, leaving skin with sufficient tension. Sometimes inflammatory breast carcinoma or tumors that have invaded the breast skin can be closed by skin grafting due to excessively tight skin. If simple mastectomy is performed with level I–II axillary dissection, it is called modified radical mastectomy and is usually performed in the case of positive axillary lymph nodes. Radical mastectomy with removal of the pectoral major muscle is rarely performed in the current era only in cases of pectoral muscle invasion.

Simultaneous reconstruction can be performed during mastectomy. If the breast skin is preserved, it is called skin-sparing mastectomy, and if the nipple and areola are preserved, it is called nipple areola-sparing mastectomy. In these cases, a small elliptical incision, horizontal incision, inverted drop-shaped incision, inframammarian fold incision, or lateral incision can be applied. In cases where the nipple is preserved, taking biopsies from different quadrants behind the nipple for the subareolar margin is an appropriate approach to leave no tumor behind. It is also important to evaluate areola and skin flap viability in cases where reconstruction is performed. For this purpose, the assessment of viability with indocyanine blue has been frequently used recently (Fig. 2.5) [19].

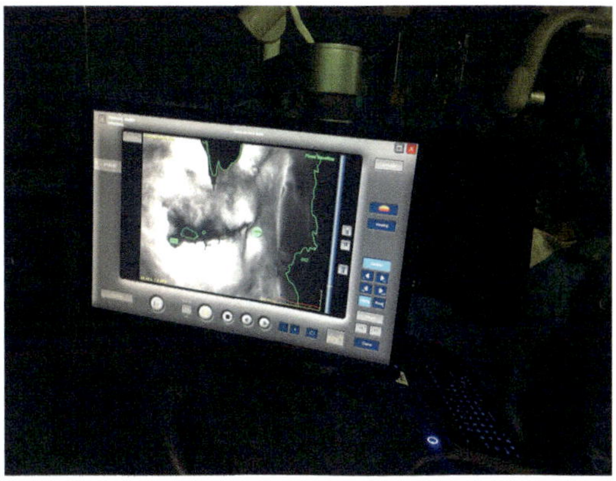

Fig. 2.5 Evaluation of flaps during mastectomy and prosthesis placement with indocyanine green

2.7 Surgical Management of Axilla—Axillary Staging

Assessing the status of the axillary lymph node is very important for both treatment decisions and prognosis. Nowadays, axillary dissection has become less frequent due to possible morbidities. The sentinel lymph node is the standard procedure in patients with clinically negative axilla. The sentinel lymph node procedure can be performed with blue dye and/or radiotracer (Fig. 2.6). In some cases, axillary dissection may not be performed even in patients with positive sentinel lymph nodes. According to the Z0011 study, no difference was found in terms of survival and regional recurrence in patients with T1

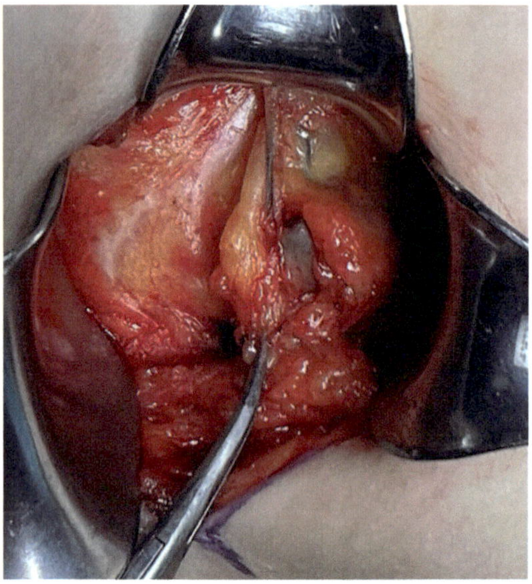

Fig. 2.6 Identification of the sentinel lymph node and lymphatic duct after blue dye injection

and T2 tumors in patients with one or two positive sentinel lymph nodes [20]. The importance of adjuvant radiotherapy for local control without the need for axillary dissection is emphasized here.

In clinical node-positive patients, a needle biopsy can be performed under US guidance. If metastasis is detected in the biopsy, level I and II axillary dissection may be performed in cases where surgery is the first step. However, in this case, neoadjuvant treatment is usually decided. Depending on the response after neoadjuvant treatment, the axilla is re-evaluated, and it is decided to perform SLNB or axillary dissection.

2.8 Prevention of Breast Cancer Related Lymphedema

With the improved prognosis in breast cancer care, treatment has focused on the quality-of-life parameters of patients with breast cancer. BCRL is still the most common and feared complication of breast cancer treatment. BCRL negatively affects patients physically and psychologically, leading to loss of strength in the affected arm. BCRL can be seen in 30% after ALND. Although it has decreased with the widespread use of sentinel lymph nodes, it can be seen at a rate close to 5% even after only sentinel lymph node procedures.

Numerous risk factors for BCRL have been identified. The extent of axilla-directed surgery is the prominent risk factor for BCRL. There is a direct correlation between the number of lymph nodes removed and the risk of BCRL. Irradiation of regional lymph nodes is another important risk-increasing condition. Regional lymph node irradiation has been found to be associated with an approximately twofold increased risk of BCRL compared to radiotherapy to the breast and chest wall alone [21]. In addition, late-stage breast cancer, obesity, certain chemotherapy regimens (e.g., taxane-based), and certain races (black women) are associated with an increased risk of BCRL.

There are many approaches to prevent BCRL. The most commonly used options include exercise and compression therapy. There are also some preventive interventions during surgery involving the axilla. If all measures fail, some surgeries have been used as a "last resort" when BCRL occurs.

Interventions that can be performed for BCRL can basically be divided into two preventive procedures during surgery for the axilla and surgeries that can be performed after the development of BCRL. Preventive procedures include sentinel lymph node application instead of axillary dissection and de-escalation from axillary dissection. Axillary dissection may be omitted, especially in patients over 70 years of age [22].

The principle of axillary reverse mapping hypothesized that the lymphatics draining the arm (in reverse) could be identified and protected from injury, thus reducing the risk of BCRL during axillary surgery. In the axillary reverse mapping technique, different tracers are given to the arm and breast (e.g., radiotracer to the breast and blue dye to the arm). In this way, lymphatics from the arm are recognized and protected. The disadvantage of this technique is the presence of crossover lymph nodes between axillary and arm lymphatics. In this case, removal of the crossover lymph nodes and reanastomosis of their lymphatic ducts is recommended [23]. A meta-analysis of 5 randomized controlled trials showed a significant reduction in BCRL in the axillary reverse mapping group compared to the standard group [24].

The LYMPHA procedure is another preventive intervention. This technique involves the identification of the lymphatics from the arm with blue dye and lymphovascular anastomosis under the microscope. The risk of BCRL is reduced with this technique [25]. However, this procedure increases the duration of surgery and requires microscopic surgical skills.

2.9 Conclusion

Surgery is a key element in the multidisciplinary management of patients diagnosed with breast cancer. Over time, the integration of surgical techniques with advances in radiation and systemic therapies has allowed for less invasive surgical procedures (e.g. breast-conserving surgery). This has resulted in reduced surgical morbidity for patients and overall improved outcomes and survival. Breast cancer-related lymphedema is a condition whose management requires a combination of surgical and conservative treatments. Further research is needed in the diagnosis and treatment of lymphedema.

References

1. Fisher B, Anderson S. Conservative surgery for the management of invasive and noninvasive carcinoma of the breast: NSABP trials. World J Surg. 1994;18(1):63–9.
2. Fisher B, Anderson S, Bryant J, Margolese RG, Deutsch M, Fisher ER, et al. Twenty-year follow-up of a randomized trial comparing total mastectomy, lumpectomy, and lumpectomy plus irradiation for the treatment of invasive breast cancer. N Engl J Med. 2002;347(16):1233–41.
3. Boughey JC, Rosenkranz KM, Ballman KV, McCall L, Haffty BG, Cuttino LW, et al. Local recurrence after breast-conserving therapy in patients with multiple ipsilateral breast cancer: results from ACOSOG Z11102 (Alliance). J Clin Oncol. 2023;41(17):3184–93.
4. Bedrosian I, Somerfield MR, Achatz MI, Boughey JC, Curigliano G, Friedman S, et al. Germline testing in patients with breast cancer: ASCO–Society of Surgical Oncology guideline. J Clin Oncol. 2024;42:584.
5. Sarlos D, Frey L, Haueisen H, Landmann G, Kots L, Schaer G. Radioguided occult lesion localization (ROLL) for treatment and diagnosis of malignant and premalignant breast lesions combined with sentinel node biopsy: a prospective clinical trial with 100 patients. Eur J Surg Oncol. 2009;35(4):403–8.
6. Nguyen CL, Cui R, Zhou M, Ali F, Easwaralingam N, Chan B, et al. Cost-effectiveness of radar localisation versus wire localisation for wide local excision of non-palpable breast cancer. Ann Surg Oncol. 2024;1-10:3916.
7. Morrow M, Van Zee KJ, Solin LJ, Houssami N, Chavez-MacGregor M, Harris JR, et al. Society of Surgical Oncology–American Society for Radiation Oncology–American Society of Clinical Oncology consensus guideline on margins for breast-conserving surgery with whole-breast irradiation in ductal carcinoma in situ. Ann Surg Oncol. 2016;23:3801–10.
8. Moran MS, Schnitt SJ, Giuliano AE, Harris JR, Khan SA, Horton J, et al. Society of Surgical Oncology–American Society for Radiation Oncology consensus guideline on margins for breast-conserving surgery with whole-breast irradiation in stages I and II invasive breast cancer. Int J Radiat Oncol Biol Phys. 2014;88(3):553–64.
9. Rossou C, Alampritis G, Patel B. Reducing re-excision rates in breast conserving surgery with margin probe: systematic review. Br J Surg. 2024;111(1):znad335.
10. Bathla L, Harris A, Davey M, Sharma P, Silva E. High resolution intra-operative two-dimensional specimen mammography and its impact on second operation for re-excision of positive margins at final pathology after breast conservation surgery. Am J Surg. 2011;202(4):387–94.
11. Chagpar AB, Killelea BK, Tsangaris TN, Butler M, Stavris K, Li F, et al. A randomized, controlled trial of cavity shave margins in breast cancer. N Engl J Med. 2015;373(6):503–10.
12. Esbona K, Li Z, Wilke LG. Intraoperative imprint cytology and frozen section pathology for margin assessment in breast conservation surgery: a systematic review. Ann Surg Oncol. 2012;19:3236–45.
13. Clough KB, Lewis JS, Couturaud B, Fitoussi A, Nos C, Falcou M-C. Oncoplastic techniques allow extensive resections for breast-conserving therapy of breast carcinomas. Ann Surg. 2003;237(1):26–34.
14. Riina MD, Rashad R, Cohen S, Brownlee Z, Sioshansi S, Hepel J, et al. The effectiveness of intraoperative clip placement in improving radiation therapy boost targeting after oncoplastic surgery. Pract Radiat Oncol. 2020;10(5):e348–e56.
15. Rose M, Svensson H, Handler J, Hoyer U, Ringberg A, Manjer J. Patient-reported outcome after oncoplastic breast surgery compared with conventional breast-conserving surgery in breast cancer. Breast Cancer Res Treat. 2020;180:247–56.

16. Armstrong K, Maxwell J. Oncoplastic surgery for breast cancer: global perspectives and trends. J Surg Oncol. 2023;128(6):967–71.
17. Agrawal SK, Mahajan S, Ahmed R, Shruti N, Sharma A. Chest wall perforator flap partial breast reconstruction: a retrospective analysis of surgical, cosmetic and survival outcome. Ecancermedicalscience. 2024;18:18.
18. Losken A, Hart AM, Dutton JW, Broecker JS, Styblo TM, Carlson GW. The expanded use of autoaugmentation techniques in oncoplastic breast surgery. Plast Reconstr Surg. 2018;141(1):10–9.
19. Kim J, Han MW, Hong KY. Prospective clinical trial for predicting mastectomy skin flap necrosis with Indocyanine green angiography in implant-based Prepectoral breast reconstruction. Aesthetic Plast Surg. 2024:1–8.
20. Giuliano AE, Ballman KV, McCall L, Beitsch PD, Brennan MB, Kelemen PR, et al. Effect of axillary dissection vs no axillary dissection on 10-year overall survival among women with invasive breast cancer and sentinel node metastasis: the ACOSOG Z0011 (Alliance) randomized clinical trial. JAMA. 2017;318(10):918–26.
21. Shaitelman SF, Chiang Y-J, Griffin KD, DeSnyder SM, Smith BD, Schaverien MV, et al. Radiation therapy targets and the risk of breast cancer-related lymphedema: a systematic review and network meta-analysis. Breast Cancer Res Treat. 2017;162:201–15.
22. Hughes KS, Schnaper LA, Bellon JR, Cirrincione CT, Berry DA, McCormick B, et al. Lumpectomy plus tamoxifen with or without irradiation in women age 70 years or older with early breast cancer: long-term follow-up of CALGB 9343. J Clin Oncol. 2013;31(19):2382.
23. Tummel E, Ochoa D, Korourian S, Betzold R, Adkins L, McCarthy M, et al. Does axillary reverse mapping prevent lymphedema after lymphadenectomy? Ann Surg. 2017;265(5):987–92.
24. Wijaya WA, Peng J, He Y, Chen J, Cen Y. Clinical application of axillary reverse mapping in patients with breast cancer: a systematic review and meta-analysis. Breast. 2020;53:189–200.
25. Feldman S, Bansil H, Ascherman J, Grant R, Borden B, Henderson P, et al. Single institution experience with lymphatic microsurgical preventive healing approach (LYMPHA) for the primary prevention of lymphedema. Ann Surg Oncol. 2015;22:3296–301.

3 Oncological Treatment of Breast Cancer

Fatma Pinar Açar

3.1 Oncological Treatment of Nonmetastatic Breast Cancer

3.1.1 Neoadjuvant Treatment

Neoadjuvant chemotherapy (NACT) is a systemic treatment administered before breast surgery. This treatment facilitates downstaging of the tumor, allowing for less invasive breast and axillary surgery [1]. Through the application of NACT, numerous patients are afforded the option of breast-conserving surgery. For some, it can circumvent the necessity for axillary dissection, thus protecting patients from potential major post-surgical morbidities [2]. Furthermore, it enables the in vivo assessment of the response to preoperative treatment, identifying high-risk patients who require adjuvant therapy and thereby pinpointing those who need more intensive treatment [3]. Early Breast Cancer Trialists' Collaborative Group compared neoadjuvant and adjuvant treatment approaches and observed a higher frequency of breast-conserving surgery (66% vs. 49%). Still, there was no difference in distant metastasis (38% vs. 34% at 15 years) or mortality (34% vs. 34% at 15 years) [4]. However, patients with a pathological complete response (pCR) have a better prognosis compared with residual disease. This situation is particularly evident in triple-negative and HER2-positive breast cancers, where a complete pathological response is observed [5]. When planning for NACT, a comprehensive evaluation should be conducted, considering the tumor's histological subtype, stage, receptor status, HER2 expression, and other characteristics [3].

Indications for neoadjuvant chemotherapy can be summarized as follows:

In locally advanced breast cancer (T3, T4, stage 3 disease) regardless of subtype, NACT application is recommended [6].

In early-stage breast cancer, stages 1 or 2, where the primary tumor is large relative to breast size and patients prefer breast conservation, or in cases where cN+ disease is expected to be pN0, NACT can be preferred. Given its potential to inform adjuvant therapy in the presence of residual disease, it is advisable for patients with HER2-positive and triple-negative breast cancer (TNBC), particularly those with ≥cT2 or ≥cN1, and even in cases of cT1c and cN0 [3].

Before initiating neoadjuvant therapy, it is recommended to place radiopaque clips in the tumor area to guide subsequent surgical intervention and allow for pathological assessment if the patient shows a complete pathological response. Similarly, the placement of radiopaque clips in pathological lymph nodes in the axillary region is

F. P. Açar (✉)
Department of Medical Oncology, Ege University Faculty of Medicine Hospital, İzmir, Turkey

Y. Bakar, A. Tuğral (eds.), *Managing Side Effects of Breast Cancer Treatment*,
https://doi.org/10.1007/978-3-031-75480-7_3

advised, contributing to the effective execution of targeted axillary surgery [7].

3.1.1.1 Neoadjuvant Systemic Therapy for HER2-Positive Disease

In HER2-positive disease, neoadjuvant systemic therapy is implemented by combining chemotherapy regimens with anti-HER2 agents. Following the observed efficacy of trastuzumab in adjuvant systemic therapy, it has also been incorporated into neoadjuvant treatments. It is summarized in Table 3.1.

Anti-HER2 Treatment Trastuzumab is the first anti-HER2 therapy approved in 1998 for the treatment of metastatic breast cancer (MBC). In patients with metastatic disease, initiating treatment that targets the HER2 significantly enhances survival rates, marking a substantial advancement over chemotherapy outcomes. Following its demonstrated effectiveness in metastatic disease, the addition of trastuzumab during NACT has been shown in numerous studies to improve pCR rates and event-free survival (EFS) [8, 9].

Table 3.1 Preoperative/adjuvant treatment options

Her2-positive breast cancer preferred regimens
TCH (docetaxel/carboplatin/trastuzumab)
TCHP (docetaxel/carboplatin/trastuzumab/pertuzumab)
AC (antracycline/cyclophosphamide) followed by taxane + trastuzumab+/− pertuzumab
Paclitaxel + trastuzumab
Residual disease after preoperative therapy: Ado-trastuzumab emtansine (TDM-1)
Her2 negative breast cancer preoperative/adjuvant therapy prescribed regimens
Dose-dense AC (doxorubicin/cyclophosphamide) followed by taxane (weekly paclitaxel, dose-dense paclitaxel every 2 weeks, docetaxel every 3 weeks are options)
TC (docetaxel and cyclophosphamide)
High-risk TNBC: Preoperative pembrolizumab + carboplatin + paclitaxel, followed by preoperative pembrolizumab + cyclophosphamide + doxorubicin or epirubicin, followed by adjuvant pembrolizumab
TNBC and residual disease after preoperative therapy: Capecitabine
Germline BRCA1/2 mutations; adjuvant olaparib in high-risk patients

Trastuzumab plays a crucial part in treating cancer, yet it may lead to adverse effects like cardiotoxicity. This condition primarily presents as a silent reduction in the left ventricular ejection fraction (LVEF) and, in rarer cases, as overt heart failure. Differing from the cardiotoxicity caused by anthracyclines, the cardiotoxic effects associated with trastuzumab do not seem to depend on the total dose received. These effects are usually reversible upon stopping the medication and are often manageable upon recovery. Using anthracyclines concurrently with trastuzumab increases the risk of heart failure, and therefore, should be avoided. Optimal monitoring for trastuzumab-related cardiotoxicity has not been defined. In the adjuvant setting, cardiac function should be evaluated at baseline and then at 3, 6, 9, and 12 months. Upon initiating therapy for metastatic disease LVEF is typically monitored at baseline and then only in the presence of symptoms. In both adjuvant and metastatic treatment settings, patient symptoms and physical examination at every visit are also assessed for signs of cardiotoxicity [10].

The strong response obtained from the combined use of trastuzumab with chemotherapy has led to the addition of another anti-HER agent, pertuzumab, to the treatment regimen. Studies have shown that adding pertuzumab to neoadjuvant chemotherapy along with trastuzumab improves pCR compared with the trastuzumab alone arm. Considering these findings, the addition of pertuzumab to NACT has become a routine practice for early-stage HER2-positive breast cancers that are T2 or larger, N1 or larger, and locally advanced and inflammatory HER2-positive breast cancers [11].

Chemotherapy Backbone Historically, the initial NACT trials conducted in HER2-positive diseases predominantly involved anthracycline-based regimens and were accepted as the standard treatment [12]. However, considering the accompanying comorbidities of diseases and the toxicity caused by chemotherapy, research has gradually shifted toward exploring anthracycline-free alternative chemotherapy regimens. In the TRAIN 2 study, chemotherapy regimens with and without anthracyclines were compared. The study found similar rates of pCR, EFS, and overall survival (OS) in both treatment arms. However, the anthracycline-free regimen had a significantly higher tolerability compared with the anthracycline-containing regimen. Notably, the anthracycline-containing treatment group observed more frequent cases of decreased LVEF and febrile neutropenia. Trastuzumab, carboplatin, and taxane combination (TCH+/−P), which is as effective as anthracycline-based regimens but causes less toxicity, has become the preferred regimen in neoadjuvant chemotherapy for HER2-positive diseases [13]. Based on a study evaluating adjuvant paclitaxel and trastuzumab, neoadjuvant therapy with paclitaxel and trastuzumab can be applied in node-negative and low-risk, early-stage HER2-positive breast cancers. Nevertheless, it has not become a standard regimen [14].

3.1.1.2 Neoadjuvant Systemic Therapy for HER2-Negative Disease

The fundamental treatment options for HER2-negative disease include an anthracycline-based regimen of anthracycline and cyclophosphamide (AC) followed by taxane administration and an anthracycline-free regimen of docetaxel plus cyclophosphamide (TC) [15]. According to the Anthracycline in Breast Cancer (ABC) study, when comparing anthracycline-based therapy with TC, the invasive DFS rates were 91% and 88%, respectively. Subgroup analyses revealed that the addition of anthracycline therapy particularly provided a significant benefit in hormone-positive breast cancer with four or more positive lymph nodes and in node-positive TNBC patients. Consequently, anthracycline-based treatments have become the standard for patients with suitable cardiac conditions and without significant comorbidities. However, the TC combination has emerged as an important alternative for fragile patients with high cardiac comorbidities and those with mid-to-low-risk disease [16].

For Stage 2–3 TNBC tumors, studies have shown that adding carboplatin to taxane therapy following AC treatment increases pCR and improves (DFS) [17, 18]. With the increasing use of immunotherapy in oncological treatments, studies have been conducted on the benefits of adding immunotherapy to chemotherapy. The KEYNOTE-522 study demonstrated that adding pembrolizumab to the taxane–carboplatin regimen following anthracycline–cyclophosphamide, along with its use in the adjuvant setting for a total treatment duration of 1 year, improved EFS by 34% regardless of programmed death ligand 1 PD-L1 levels [19].

3.1.2 Adjuvant Treatment

Adjuvant therapy is a treatment applied after breast cancer surgery to decrease the likelihood of disease recurrence. When selecting adjuvant therapy, several factors must be considered. This encompasses factors such as disease recurrence risk, hormonal status, HER2 status, lymph node involvement, stage of disease, age of the patient, and any existing comorbid conditions.

3.1.2.1 Adjuvant Systemic Therapy for Hormone Receptor-Positive Disease

Endocrine therapy is commonly included in adjuvant treatment strategies. It significantly decreases the likelihood of systemic recurrence and mortality in females diagnosed with HR-positive breast cancer. This reduction is observed irrespective of the patient's age, menopausal status, extent of nodal involvement, tumor dimensions, HER2 status, or prior chemotherapy. Therefore, for all individuals diagnosed with HR-positive breast cancer, adjuvant endocrine therapy is advised. The spectrum of endocrine treatments encompasses tamoxifen, aromatase inhibitors (AIs), and ovarian function suppression (OFS).

Tamoxifen, acting as a selective estrogen receptor modulator, blocks estrogen from binding to ER, proving effective for women regardless of menopausal status. These properties make it highly beneficial for the treatment of breast cancer. Meta-analysis results, the recurrence rates in HR-positive women completing 1, 2, or 5 years of adjuvant tamoxifen decreased by 21%,

29%, and 47%, respectively. Correspondingly, the durations of tamoxifen administration for 1, 2, or 5 years yielded mortality reductions of 12%, 17%, and 26%, respectively. These findings underscore the significance of adjuvant tamoxifen in the management of HR-positive breast cancer [20]. Standard tamoxifen therapy spans 5 years, yet the ATLAS and aTTOM studies have explored the benefits of extending tamoxifen treatment from 5 to 10 years, demonstrating a decrease in both recurrence and mortality rates. Nevertheless, prolonged tamoxifen usage elevates the risks of pulmonary embolism and endometrial cancer. While these outcomes affirm the benefits of extended tamoxifen therapy, the potential adverse effects necessitate careful consideration, particularly in early-stage patients with a minimal risk of recurrence [21, 22]. In male breast cancers, due to insufficient data on AIs in adjuvant hormone therapy, tamoxifen is primarily preferred [23].

AIs reduce estrogen production by inhibiting the enzyme that converts androgens to estrogens in peripheral tissues. They are not sufficient on their own in premenopausal or perimenopausal women because they do not adequately suppress estradiol production in the ovaries. Therefore, they should not be used in these patients without concurrent suppression of ovarian function. Within the class of aromatase inhibitors there exist both nonsteroidal inhibitors such as anastrozole and letrozole and the steroidal inhibitor exemestane; these three drugs have similar efficacy levels and side effect profiles [20].

AIs stand as the preferred choice of adjuvant endocrine therapy for HR-positive breast cancer in postmenopausal women [24]. In clinical trials that included postmenopausal patients, comparing the use of AIs with tamoxifen for breast cancer treatment, AIs were found to be significantly beneficial for patients when compared to tamoxifen. Specifically, treatment with AIs, when compared to tamoxifen, was associated with a reduced risk of breast cancer recurrence by approximately 36% during the first year and by about 20% between the second and fourth years. After completing the 5-year treatment period, no additional impact on recurrence rates was observed. Moreover, treatment with AIs resulted in a lower rate of breast cancer mortality over a 10-year period compared to those treated with tamoxifen [25]. AI treatment is typically set for a duration of 5 years. While AIs are typically used for 5 years, many studies have also examined extending adjuvant therapy with AIs to 10 years. Together, this data suggests a minor enhancement in DFS for patients who pursued aromatase inhibitor therapy after concluding an initial AI regimen, with a significant contribution from the prevention of contralateral breast cancer [26, 27].

Studies examining treatments that start with tamoxifen and then switch to aromatase inhibitors or vice versa are also available. The BIG 1–98 study compared letrozole and tamoxifen monotherapies and their sequential use in breast cancer treatment. Although letrozole demonstrated better outcomes than tamoxifen by reducing breast cancer recurrence and mortality, there was no significant difference in OS or DFS between sequential treatment and letrozole monotherapy. The efficacy of letrozole and tamoxifen against contralateral breast cancer has varied. In the early years, the aromatase inhibitor letrozole was preferred over tamoxifen; however, after several disease-free years, switching to tamoxifen has been found to be as effective as continuing AI treatment [28].

OFS in the adjuvant treatment of hormone receptor-positive breast cancer was explored by the SOFT and TEXT studies, examining its effects in combination with exemestane or tamoxifen. The long-term results showed that adding ovarian function suppression to either exemestane or tamoxifen treatment improved DFS and reduced rates of distant recurrence compared with tamoxifen alone. This benefit was particularly pronounced in women who had undergone chemotherapy or were under the age of 35, suggesting that in patients at high risk of recurrence, adding ovarian function suppression to adjuvant therapy is recommended [29].

Adjuvant Chemotherapy for Hormone Receptor-Positive Disease The decision-making process for chemotherapy in HR-positive HER2-negative breast cancer is based on clinical features, such as age and menopausal status, as well as clinicopathological factors, including tumor size, grade, lymph node involvement, and quantitative measurements of estrogen receptor (ER), progesterone receptor (PR), HER2, and Ki67, which contribute to the intrinsic subtypes characteristics. However, advanced genomic tests, such as gene expression profiling, have improved the ability to identify patients who may benefit from adjuvant chemotherapy more precisely [30]. Oncotype DX is based on gene expression analysis and is used to determine the benefit of adjuvant chemotherapy [31]. Adjuvant chemotherapies used in HR-positive HER 2-negative breast cancer are summarized in Table 3.2.

Cyclin-Dependent Kinase (CDK) 4/6 Inhibitors in Adjuvant Therapy In the management of HR-positive MBC, the integration of CDK4/6 inhibitors with AIshas demonstrated efficacy in extending progression-free survival (PFS). This subject will receive a more comprehensive discussion in the metastatic segment of the text. In light of such findings, clinical investigations have been pursued to assess the potential benefits of incorporating CDK4/6 inhibitors into endocrine therapy for localized breast cancer. However, outcomes from the PENELOPE-B and PALLAS studies did not affirm the advantage of palbociclib in an adjuvant context [32, 33]. Conversely, the MonarchE study revealed that the addition of abemaciclib to adjuvant endocrine therapy for a duration of 2 years resulted in a 6.4% improvement in invasive disease-free survival (IDFS) among patients with high-risk HR-positive HER2-negative breast cancer. This patient cohort includes those with four or more positive lymph nodes, one to three positive lymph nodes with a tumor size of 5 cm, or a grade 3 tumor. Reflecting these outcomes, abemaciclib has received approval for a two-year adjuvant treatment regimen within this specific patient population [34]. Meanwhile, the NATALEE study evaluating adjuvant ribociclib has not yet concluded [35].

Table 3.2 Systemic chemotherapy for HR-positive or -negative and Her2-negative breast cancer

Single agent options	Combination regimen options
Anthracyclines: Doxorubicin and liposomal doxorubicin	Gemcitabine/carboplatin or paclitaxel
Taxanes: Paclitaxel and docetaxel	Docetaxel/capecitabine
Antimetabolites: Capecitabine and gemcitabine	AC (antracycline/ cyclophosphamide)
Microtubule inhibitors: Vinorelbine and eribulin	CMF (cyclophosphamide/ methotrexate/fluorouracil)

3.1.2.2 Adjuvant Systemic Therapy for Triple-Negative Breast Cancer

Despite being characterized by high recurrence rates and short survival times, TNBC is more sensitive to chemotherapy than other breast cancer subtypes [36].

For the group not receiving NACT, adjuvant chemotherapy was observed to improve survival in cases of tumor size larger than 0.5 cm or, irrespective of tumor size, in cases with lymph node-positive cancer [37]. The treatment regimens used in adjuvant therapy are explained in the section on neoadjuvant therapy.

For the group that received NACT, the choice of post-neoadjuvant chemotherapy treatment is tailored according to the pathological response of the disease. The use of adjuvant capecitabine has shown a survival benefit in TNBC patients with residual disease; thus, eight cycles of capecitabine are recommended for this group with residual disease after NACT [38]. Additionally, in patients who receive pembrolizumab as part of neoadjuvant treatment, the therapy should be completed for a total duration of 1 year, including the adjuvant phase [19].

Adjuvant PARP Inhibitor Treatments for HER2-Negative Disease The OlympiA study investigated the efficacy of PARP inhibitors in patients with germline BRCA1/BRCA2 mutated HER2-negative breast cancer. It was found that adding 1 year of adjuvant olaparib in patients with high-risk TNBC (those with lymph node-positive disease or a primary tumor larger than 2 cm in node-negative disease, patients with pathological residual tumor in the primary tumor or lymph nodes after NACT) and in patients with high-risk HR-positive disease (those initially have of 4 or more lymph nodes and those not achieving a pCR after NACT with a CPS + EG score > 3) increased the 3-year IDFS from 77.1% to 86% [39].

3.1.2.3 Adjuvant Systemic Therapy for HER2-Positive Disease

Anti-HER2-targeted therapies play an important role in the management of HER2-positive breast cancer. These therapies are effective during both NACT and adjuvant therapy stages. In Stage 2 and Stage 3 HER2-positive breast cancer cases, the administration of neoadjuvant therapy has been mentioned in the previous section. However, in patients with node-negative tumors and tumor size smaller than 2 cm, direct surgical intervention may be preferred without the need for NACT. The choice of adjuvant therapy depends on whether the patient has received neoadjuvant therapy and their response to this treatment.

For patients who have received NACT, the determination of subsequent adjuvant therapy is contingent upon the degree of pathological response observed. For those achieving a pCR following neoadjuvant therapy, adjuvant trastuzumab is recommended to be continued for a total duration of 1 year. Treatment regimens shorter than 1 year have not demonstrated equivalent efficacy, nor has extending adjuvant therapy beyond 1 year been shown to confer additional benefits [40, 41]. The AFFINITY trial was designed to explore the efficacy of incorporating pertuzumab into adjuvant trastuzumab therapy for HER2-positive cancer. Findings from this trial indicate that the inclusion of pertuzumab is especially advantageous for patients with lymph node-positive disease, yielding an improvement in 3-year DFS from 83% to 88% [42].

For patients who do not achieve pCR after NACT, i.e., those with residual disease, 1 year of adjuvant ado-Trastuzumab Emtansine (TDM-1) therapy is recommended. It has been shown that administering TDM-1 to patients with residual disease in the breast or lymph nodes reduces recurrence rates and disease-related mortality compared with trastuzumab treatment [43].

Patients who did not receive NACT: The regimens described in the neoadjuvant therapy section form the basis of the adjuvant treatment options. However, in patients with node-negative tumors and tumors smaller than 2 cm, weekly paclitaxel and trastuzumab adjuvant therapy may be sufficient [44].

3.2 Oncological Management of Metastatic Breast Cancer

Although MBC is often not curable, the objective of systemic treatment is to manage the tumor load, reduce symptoms for enhanced quality of life, and prolong survival [45]. In the treatment of metastatic breast cancer, a personalized approach is adopted based on the biological structure of the tumor and clinical data. As in the management of early-stage breast cancer, a detailed evaluation of biological markers, such as ER, PR, and HER2, as well as a comprehensive assessment of the patient's previous treatment processes, symptoms, and functional status, is required. Patients with MBC are directed to comprehensive systemic medical treatments, including chemotherapy, endocrine therapy, targeted therapy, and local treatments for oligometastatic situations [46].

In metastatic breast cancer, the most common sites of metastasis are the lymph nodes, bones, lungs, chest wall, and liver. Patients with HR-positive cancer have a higher incidence of bone metastases, whereas lung metastases are more common in TNBC. In addition, the likelihood of brain metastases is higher in HER2-positive and TNBC than in the HR-positive subtype, highlighting significant differences in the distribution of metastases according to the subtype of MBC. Therefore, treatment planning and follow-up strategies must be personalized according to these biological and clinical characteristics [47]. Because of the vital importance of tumor type in disease management, a biopsy of the metastatic lesion is recommended in appropriate patients. This procedure not only confirms the diagnosis of MBC but also allows for reassessing receptor status [48].

3.2.1 Systemic Therapy for Metastatic Triple-Negative Breast Cancer

Treatment of TNBC faces significant challenges due to the absence of targetable proteins, leading to cytotoxic chemotherapy remaining the standard of care for this cancer type for many years. However, with recent developments, the treatment landscape has evolved to include PARP inhibitors for those harboring BRCA mutations, immune checkpoint inhibitors for individuals with elevated PDL-1 CPS, and fam-trastuzumab deruxtecan for the management of patients characterized as Her2 Low [49–51].

Cytotoxic chemotherapy used for the treatment of metastatic TNBC encompasses a variety of drug classes. The selection of these treatments is based on extensive clinical experience, randomized clinical trial outcomes, and the toxicity profiles of the drugs [52, 53]. Chemotherapies such as anthracyclines and taxanes are generally considered fundamental agents. However, orally administered antimetabolites such as capecitabine, due to their favorable toxicity profile, are among the preferred options, especially in cases resistant to anthracyclines and taxanes. Eribulin has shown antitumor activity in situations resistant to anthracyclines and taxanes. Treatment options also include single-agent chemotherapies such as gemcitabine, vinorelbine, and ixabepilone, which offer effective alternatives for patients who have been exposed to previous treatments [54]. In particular, platinum salts that induce DNA damage, such as cisplatin and carboplatin, are prioritized in the management of TNBC, distinctively from other histological types [55].

Combined chemotherapy may be recommended for the treatment of MBC in patients with visceral spread or rapidly progressing disease. Although this strategy offers higher response rates than single-agent therapy, its impact on OS has not been demonstrated and is associated with an increased risk of toxicity.

Sequential single-agent therapy is generally considered standard; however, there is insufficient information in the literature regarding the specific order of drugs to be preferred after anthracycline and taxane. This situation necessitates the customization of treatment options based on patient characteristics, disease progression rate, and potential side effects, thereby determining the most suitable treatment strategy for each individual [56]. Chemotherapies used in the treatment of metastatic breast cancer are summarized in Table 3.1.

The benefit of adding immune checkpoint inhibitors to chemotherapy regimens was demonstrated by the KEYNOTE-355 study. In patients with metastatic or inoperable recurrent TNBC, the addition of pembrolizumab to various chemotherapy regimens (nab-paclitaxel, paclitaxel, or gemcitabine/carboplatin) in the group with a PDL-1 CPS ≥ 10 showed an increase in median PFS from 5.6 to 9.7 months and OS from 16.1 to 23.0 months. Following these results, the combination of pembrolizumab and chemotherapy has established its place as a first-line treatment in patients with a PDL-1 CPS ≥ 10 [57].

Later line options: For patients with germline BRCA1/BRCA2 mutations and HER2-negative advanced breast cancer, treatment strategies have demonstrated the efficacy of the PARP inhibitors olaparib and talazoparib through the OlympiAD and EMBRACA trials. These therapies have become an option for individuals experiencing disease progression after first-line chemotherapy [58, 59].

Sacituzumab govitecan, a Trop-2-targeted antibody–drug conjugate, represents an alternative for subsequent lines of treatment. Trop-2 is a cell surface antigen extensively present in various tumor types, notably in breast cancer. The mechanism of this therapeutic agent involves coupling a Trop-2-specific antibody with SN-38, which is the active component of irinotecan. SN-38 acts as a topoisomerase I inhibitor, leading to DNA damage within tumor cells and ultimately causing their death. Clinical investigations involving patients with TNBC who had either not responded to or had recurred following at least two prior chemotherapy regimens have evaluated the effectiveness of sacituzumab govitecan. The outcomes demonstrate superior OS and PFS for sacituzumab govitecan compared to treatments selected by clinicians (OS: 12.1 months versus 6.7 months; PFS: 5.6 months versus 1.7 months). Nevertheless, the incidence of serious adverse effects, including diarrhea, anemia, and febrile neutropenia, was higher among patients treated with sacituzumab govitecan [60].

For Her2 Low disease, which is defined as either immunohistochemistry (IHC) 1+ or IHC 2+ and FISH test negative, the efficacy of anti-Her2 therapies has been explored. The DESTINY-Breast04 study demonstrated the effectiveness of another antibody–drug conjugate, fam-trastuzumab deruxtecan (T-Dxd), in patients with previously treated metastatic HER2-low breast cancer. T-Dxd significantly extended PFS and OS compared with the physician's choice of chemotherapy. Approximately 11% of the patients in the study had HR-negative disease, and T-Dxd was found to provide benefit in both HR-positive and HR-negative subgroups compared with chemotherapy [61]. The treatment options for triple-negative breast cancer are summarized in Table 3.3.

3.2.2 Systemic Treatment of HER2-Positive Metastatic Breast Cancer

The use of HER2-targeted therapy has significantly improved the survival rates of patients, making the application of HER2-targeted treatments recommended in both first-line and subsequent treatment phases [62]. In metastatic HER2-positive breast cancer, the effectiveness of adding a second HER2 agent to chemotherapy and trastuzumab was assessed in the Cleopatra study. This study demonstrated that adding pertuzumab to trastuzumab and docetaxel treatment in patients with HER2-positive MBC improved PFS by 6.1 months and OS by 16.3 months. Following this study, the combination of docetaxel, trastuzumab, and pertuzumab became the preferred first-choice combination. Although docetaxel was used in the Cleopatra study, other taxanes, such as paclitaxel or Nab-Paclitaxel, are equally effective. This treatment is recommended for at least 4–6 months or until the best response is achieved, whereas HER2-targeted therapy is advised to continue until disease progression. For patients experiencing relapse after adjuvant therapy, treatment decisions are based on the interval since the last treatment. For patients who have not received treatment for over 6 months, a regimen combining docetaxel, trastuzumab, and pertuzumab is suggested, whereas those who have completed trastuzumab-based adjuvant therapy in the past 6 months are recommended to pursue second-line therapy options [63].

Later line options include TDM-1, the combination of lapatinib and capecitabine, T-DXd, and the combination of tucatinib, capecitabine, and trastuzumab for patients who have developed resistance to trastuzumab and pertuzumab treatment. The EMILIA study demonstrated that T-DM1 improved PFS and decreased mortality with fewer side effects compared to the combination of lapatinib and capecitabine in patients previously treated with trastuzumab and taxanes [64]. The TH3RESA study underscored the effectiveness of T-DM1 over physician-selected treatments in patients with extensive prior treat-

Table 3.3 Triple-negative breast cancer treatment options

Settings	Biomarker	Regimen
First line	PD-L1 CPS ≥10	Pembrolizumab + chemotherapy
	PD-L1 CPS <10 and germline BRCA1/2 mutation	PARPi (olaparib, talazoparib) Platinum (cisplatin or carboplatin)
Second line	Germline BRC1/2 mutation	PARPi (olaparib, talazoparib)
	No germline BRCA1/2 mutation and HER2 IHC1+ or 2+/FISH negative	Fam-trastuzumab deruxtecan
	Any	Sacituzumab govitecan
		Systemic chemotherapy
Third line and beyond	MSI-H, NTRK, RET, TMB-H	Targeted agents

ment histories [65]. Further, the HER2CLIMB explored the addition of tucatinib to the treatment regimen of capecitabine and trastuzumab for patients who had previously received trastuzumab, pertuzumab, and T-DM1. This study observed enhancements in both PFS and OS, along with a significant decrease in the progression of intracranial metastases in breast cancer patients. To date, no research has directly compared the efficacy of T-DM1 with the combined use of tucatinib, capecitabine, and trastuzumab [66]. T-DxD is an antibody–drug complex containing a monoclonal antibody targeting HER2-positive cells, a cleavable tetrapeptide linker transporting the antibody to cancer cells, and a cytotoxic topoisomerase I inhibitor. The DESTINY-Breast03 trial indicated improvements in OS rates while reporting similar side effect profiles between groups. Despite a higher risk of interstitial lung disease or pneumonitis in patients treated with T-Dxd, these side effects are manageable, making it a preferred choice for second-line treatment. Neratinib and margetuximab are also later-line HER2 treatment options [67].

3.2.3 Systemic Treatment for Metastatic Hormone Receptor-Positive Breast Cancer: Endocrine Therapy

In metastatic HR-positive breast cancer, endocrine therapy is often the first-line treatment. However, chemotherapy may be employed for rapid disease progression or in patients at risk of organ failure because of its quicker onset of action. The choice of initial endocrine therapy depends on factors such as the patient's menopausal status, the type of endocrine therapy used for adjuvant treatment, and the time interval between this therapy and disease recurrence. Primary treatment options include AIs, tamoxifen, fulvestrant, and CDK4/6 inhibitors [68].

CDK4/6 inhibitors have revolutionized the treatment of HR-positive/HER2-negative MBC. The three agents in this group, palbociclib, ribociclib, and abemaciclib, when used in combination with endocrine therapy, improved PFS. Palbociclib was the first to be approved in 2015, following observed improvements in PFS in the PALOMA-1 trial [69]. Subsequently, ribociclib and abemaciclib were approved based on similar PFS improvements in phase 3 trials. Ribociclib, particularly in the MONALEESA-2 trial, showed statistically significant improvement in OS when used in combination with letrozole in postmenopausal women [70]. Abemaciclib in the MONARCH-3 trial improved PFS and objective response rate (ORR) when used as first-line therapy with AIs. These findings have made the combination of an AI and a CDK4/6 inhibitor the standard of care for the first-line treatment of metastatic, HR-positive/HER2-negative breast cancer [71]. Patients with endocrine-sensitive disease (i.e., those who relapse 12 months after completing endocrine therapy) may receive a CDK4/6 inhibitor with an AI or fulvestrant. Patients with endocrine-resistant disease (i.e., progression of disease while on or within 12 months after completing an AI) should be treated with a CDK4/6 inhibitor along with fulvestrant. For patients who cannot use a CDK4/6 inhibitor due to comorbidities and/or nonaggressive low-burden disease [72]. AIs or fulvestrant alone are effective agents. Studies have shown fulvestrant to be superior to AIs [73].

For patients experiencing progression after treatment with a CDK4/6 inhibitor, next-generation sequencing (NGS) is recommended to evaluate for actionable mutations. Options for patients with a BRCA mutation include olaparib or talazoparib. For patients with a PIK3CA mutation, alpelisib along with fulvestrant or an aromatase inhibitor is an option. In the presence of mutations in the PIK3CA, AKT1, or PTEN genes, the combination of capivasertib and fulvestrant, and in cases with an ESR1 mutation, elacestrant has shown effectiveness. Everolimus and exemestane are also considered treatment options. Chemotherapy remains an option for patients not suitable for these treatments [68]. Effective chemotherapy options for MBC are described in the TNBC section.

References

1. Gralow JR, Burstein HJ, Wood W, et al. Preoperative therapy in invasive breast cancer: pathologic assessment and systemic therapy issues in operable disease. J Clin Oncol. 2008;26:814–9.
2. Mougalian SS, Soulos PR, Killelea BK, Lannin DR, Abu-Khalaf MM, Digiovanna MP, Sanft TB, Pusztai L, Gross CP, Chagpar AB. Use of neoadjuvant chemotherapy for patients with stage I to III breast cancer in the United States. Cancer. 2015;121:2544–52.
3. Korde LA, Somerfield MR, Carey LA, et al. Neoadjuvant chemotherapy, endocrine therapy, and targeted therapy for breast cancer: ASCO guideline. J Clin Oncol. 2021;39:1485–505.
4. Asselain B, Barlow W, Bartlett J, et al. Long-term outcomes for neoadjuvant versus adjuvant chemotherapy in early breast cancer: a meta-analysis of individual patient data from ten randomised trials. Lancet Oncol. 2018;19:27–39.
5. Cortazar P, Zhang L, Untch M, et al. Pathological complete response and long-term clinical benefit in breast cancer: the CTNeoBC pooled analysis. Lancet. 2014;384:164–72.
6. Wolmark N, Wang J, Mamounas E, Bryant J, Fisher B. Preoperative chemotherapy in patients with operable breast cancer: nine-year results from National Surgical Adjuvant Breast and bowel project B-18. J Natl Cancer Inst Monogr. 2001;96–102.
7. Caudle AS, Yang WT, Krishnamurthy S, et al. Improved axillary evaluation following neoadjuvant therapy for patients with node-positive breast cancer using selective evaluation of clipped nodes: implementation of targeted axillary dissection. J Clin Oncol. 2016;34:1072–8.
8. Gianni L, Eiermann W, Semiglazov V, et al. Neoadjuvant and adjuvant trastuzumab in patients with HER2-positive locally advanced breast cancer (NOAH): follow-up of a randomised controlled superiority trial with a parallel HER2-negative cohort. Lancet Oncol. 2014;15:640–7.
9. Gianni L, Eiermann W, Semiglazov V, et al. Neoadjuvant chemotherapy with trastuzumab followed by adjuvant trastuzumab versus neoadjuvant chemotherapy alone, in patients with HER2-positive locally advanced breast cancer (the NOAH trial): a randomised controlled superiority trial with a parallel HER2-negative cohort. Lancet. 2010;375:377–84.
10. Ewer SM, Ewer MS. Cardiotoxicity profile of trastuzumab. Drug Saf. 2008;31:459–67.
11. Gianni L, Pienkowski T, Im YH, et al. 5-year analysis of neoadjuvant pertuzumab and trastuzumab in patients with locally advanced, inflammatory, or early-stage HER2-positive breast cancer (NeoSphere): a multicentre, open-label, phase 2 randomised trial. Lancet Oncol. 2016;17:791–800.
12. Takada M, Toi M. Neoadjuvant treatment for HER2-positive breast cancer. Chin Clin Oncol. 2020;9:32. https://doi.org/10.21037/CCO-20-123.
13. van Ramshorst MS, van der Voort A, van Werkhoven ED, et al. Neoadjuvant chemotherapy with or without anthracyclines in the presence of dual HER2 blockade for HER2-positive breast cancer (TRAIN-2): a multicentre, open-label, randomised, phase 3 trial. Lancet Oncol. 2018;19:1630–40.
14. Tolaney SM, Tarantino P, Graham N, et al. Adjuvant paclitaxel and trastuzumab for node-negative, HER2-positive breast cancer: final 10-year analysis of the open-label, single-arm, phase 2 APT trial. Lancet Oncol. 2023;24:273–85.
15. Citron ML, Berry DA, Cirrincione C, et al. Randomized trial of dose-dense versus conventionally scheduled and sequential versus concurrent combination chemotherapy as postoperative adjuvant treatment of node-positive primary breast cancer: first report of intergroup trial C9741/cancer and leukemia group B trial 9741. J Clin Oncol. 2003;21:1431–9.
16. Blum JL, Flynn PJ, Yothers G, et al. Anthracyclines in early breast cancer: the ABC trials-USOR 06-090, NSABP B-46-I/USOR 07132, and NSABP B-49 (NRG oncology). J Clin Oncol. 2017;35:2647–55.
17. Geyer CE, Sikov WM, Huober J, et al. Long-term efficacy and safety of addition of carboplatin with or without veliparib to standard neoadjuvant chemotherapy in triple-negative breast cancer: 4-year follow-up data from BrighTNess, a randomized phase III trial. Ann Oncol. 2022;33:384–94.
18. Untch M, Schneeweiss A, Salat C, et al. Long-term survival analysis of the randomized phase II trial investigating the addition of carboplatin to neoadjuvant therapy for triple-negative (TNBC) and HER2-positive early breast cancer (GeparSixto). Ann Oncol. 2017;28:v49.
19. Schmid P, Cortes J, Dent R, et al. Event-free survival with Pembrolizumab in early triple-negative breast cancer. N Engl J Med. 2022;386:556–67.
20. Huppert LA, Gumusay O, Idossa D, Rugo HS. Systemic therapy for hormone receptor-positive/human epidermal growth factor receptor 2-negative early stage and metastatic breast cancer. CA Cancer J Clin. 2023;73:480–515.
21. Gray RG, Rea D, Handley K, et al. aTTom: Long-term effects of continuing adjuvant tamoxifen to 10 years versus stopping at 5 years in 6,953 women with early breast cancer. J Clin Oncol. 2013;31:5–5. https://doi.org/10.1200/jco.2013.31.18_suppl5.
22. Davies C, Pan H, Godwin J, et al. Long-term effects of continuing adjuvant tamoxifen to 10 years versus stopping at 5 years after diagnosis of oestrogen receptor-positive breast cancer: ATLAS, a randomised trial. Lancet. 2013;381:805–16.
23. Eggemann H, Ignatov A, Smith BJ, Altmann U, Von Minckwitz G, Röhl FW, Jahn M, Costa SD. Adjuvant therapy with tamoxifen compared to aromatase inhibitors for 257 male breast cancer patients. Breast Cancer Res Treat. 2013;137:465–70.
24. Chung CT, Carlson RW. The role of aromatase inhibitors in early breast cancer. Curr Treat Options Oncol. 2003;4:133–40.

25. Bradley R, Burrett J, Clarke M, et al. Aromatase inhibitors versus tamoxifen in early breast cancer: patient-level meta-analysis of the randomised trials. Lancet. 2015;386:1341–52.
26. Goss PE, Ingle JN, Pritchard KI, et al. Extending aromatase-inhibitor adjuvant therapy to 10 years. N Engl J Med. 2016;375:209–19.
27. Mamounas EP, Bandos H, Lembersky BC, et al. Use of letrozole after aromatase inhibitor-based therapy in postmenopausal breast cancer (NRG oncology/NSABP B-42): a randomised, double-blind, placebo-controlled, phase 3 trial. Lancet Oncol. 2019;20:88–99.
28. Ruhstaller T, Giobbie-Hurder A, Colleoni M, et al. Adjuvant Letrozole and tamoxifen alone or sequentially for postmenopausal women with hormone receptor-positive breast cancer: long-term follow-up of the BIG 1-98 trial. J Clin Oncol. 2019;37:105–14.
29. Pagani O, Walley BA, Fleming GF, et al. Adjuvant Exemestane with ovarian suppression in premenopausal breast cancer: long-term follow-up of the combined TEXT and SOFT trials. J Clin Oncol. 2023;41:1376.
30. Zhang S, Fitzsimmons KC, Hurvitz SA. Oncotype DX recurrence score in premenopausal women. Ther Adv Med Oncol. 2022;14:17588359221081077. https://doi.org/10.1177/17588359221081077.
31. Jacobs F, Gaudio M, Benvenuti C, De Sanctis R, Santoro A, Zambelli A. Controversies and opportunities in the clinical daily use of the 21-gene assay for prognostication and prediction of chemotherapy benefit in HR+/HER2− early breast cancer. Cancers (Basel). 2022;15:148. https://doi.org/10.3390/CANCERS15010148.
32. Loibl S, Marmé F, Martin M, et al. Palbociclib for residual high-risk invasive HR-positive and HER2-negative early breast cancer-the Penelope-B trial. J Clin Oncol. 2021;39:1518–30.
33. Gnant M, Dueck AC, Frantal S, et al. Adjuvant Palbociclib for early breast cancer: the PALLAS trial results (ABCSG-42/AFT-05/BIG-14-03). J Clin Oncol. 2022;40:282–93.
34. Johnston SRD, Toi M, O'Shaughnessy J, et al. Abemaciclib plus endocrine therapy for hormone receptor-positive, HER2-negative, node-positive, high-risk early breast cancer (monarchE): results from a preplanned interim analysis of a randomised, open-label, phase 3 trial. Lancet Oncol. 2023;24:77–90.
35. Slamon DJ, Fasching PA, Hurvitz S, et al. Rationale and trial design of NATALEE: a phase III trial of adjuvant ribociclib + endocrine therapy versus endocrine therapy alone in patients with HR+/HER2- early breast cancer. Ther Adv Med Oncol. 2023;15:17588359231178125. https://doi.org/10.1177/17588359231178125.
36. Marra A, Curigliano G. Adjuvant and neoadjuvant treatment of triple-negative breast cancer with chemotherapy. Cancer J. 2021;27:41–9.
37. An X, Lei X, Huang R, et al. Adjuvant chemotherapy for small, lymph node-negative, triple-negative breast cancer: a single-center study and a meta-analysis of the published literature. Cancer. 2020;126(Suppl 16):3837–46.
38. Masuda N, Lee S-J, Ohtani S, et al. Adjuvant Capecitabine for breast cancer after preoperative chemotherapy. N Engl J Med. 2017;376:2147–59.
39. Geyer CE, Garber JE, Gelber RD, et al. Overall survival in the OlympiA phase III trial of adjuvant olaparib in patients with germline pathogenic variants in BRCA1/2 and high-risk, early breast cancer. Ann Oncol. 2022;33:1250–68.
40. Piccart-Gebhart MJ, Procter M, Leyland-Jones B, et al. Trastuzumab after adjuvant chemotherapy in HER2-positive breast cancer. N Engl J Med. 2005;353:1659–72.
41. Pivot X, Romieu G, Debled M, et al. 6 months versus 12 months of adjuvant trastuzumab for patients with HER2-positive early breast cancer (PHARE): a randomised phase 3 trial. Lancet Oncol. 2013;14:741–8.
42. von Minckwitz G, Procter M, de Azambuja E, et al. Adjuvant Pertuzumab and Trastuzumab in early HER2-positive breast cancer. N Engl J Med. 2017;377:122–31.
43. von Minckwitz G, Huang C-S, Mano MS, et al. Trastuzumab Emtansine for residual invasive HER2-positive breast cancer. N Engl J Med. 2019;380:617–28.
44. Tolaney SM, Barry WT, Dang CT, et al. Adjuvant paclitaxel and trastuzumab for node-negative, HER2-positive breast cancer. N Engl J Med. 2015;372:134–41.
45. Mauri D, Polyzos NP, Salanti G, Pavlidis N, Ioannidis JPA. Multiple-treatments meta-analysis of chemotherapy and targeted therapies in advanced breast cancer. J Natl Cancer Inst. 2008;100:1780–91.
46. Beslija S, Bonneterre J, Burstein HJ, et al. Third consensus on medical treatment of metastatic breast cancer. Ann Oncol. 2009;20:1771–85.
47. Kennecke H, Yerushalmi R, Woods R, Cheang MCU, Voduc D, Speers CH, Nielsen TO, Gelmon K. Metastatic behavior of breast cancer subtypes. J Clin Oncol. 2010;28:3271–7.
48. Arslan C, Sari E, Aksoy S, Altundag K. Variation in hormone receptor and HER-2 status between primary and metastatic breast cancer: review of the literature. Expert Opin Ther Targets. 2011;15:21–30.
49. Leon-Ferre RA, Goetz MP. Advances in systemic therapies for triple negative breast cancer. BMJ. 2023;381:e071674. https://doi.org/10.1136/BMJ-2022-071674.
50. Karim AM, Eun Kwon J, Ali T, Jang J, Ullah I, Lee YG, Park DW, Park J, Jeang JW, Kang SC. Triple-negative breast cancer: epidemiology, molecular mechanisms, and modern vaccine-based treatment strategies. Biochem Pharmacol. 2023;212:115545. https://doi.org/10.1016/J.BCP.2023.115545.
51. Gonzalez-Angulo AM, Timms KM, Liu S, et al. Incidence and outcome of BRCA mutations in unselected patients with triple receptor-negative breast cancer. Clin Cancer Res. 2011;17:1082–9.

52. Mayer EL, Burstein HJ. Chemotherapy for metastatic breast cancer. Hematol Oncol Clin North Am. 2007;21:257–72.
53. Geels P, Eisenhauer E, Bezjak A, Zee B, Day A. Palliative effect of chemotherapy: objective tumor response is associated with symptom improvement in patients with metastatic breast cancer. J Clin Oncol. 2000;18:2395–405.
54. Twelves C, Jove M, Gombos A, Awada A. Cytotoxic chemotherapy: still the mainstay of clinical practice for all subtypes metastatic breast cancer. Crit Rev Oncol Hematol. 2016;100:74–87.
55. Tutt A, Tovey H, Cheang MCU, et al. Carboplatin in BRCA1/2-mutated and triple-negative breast cancer BRCAness subgroups: the TNT trial. Nat Med. 2018;24:628–37.
56. Carrick S, Parker S, Thornton CE, Ghersi D, Simes J, Wilcken N. Single agent versus combination chemotherapy for metastatic breast cancer. Cochrane Database Syst Rev. 2009;2009:CD003372. https://doi.org/10.1002/14651858.CD003372.PUB3.
57. Cortes J, Rugo HS, Cescon DW, et al. Pembrolizumab plus chemotherapy in advanced triple-negative breast cancer. N Engl J Med. 2022;387:217–26.
58. Robson M, Im S-A, Senkus E, et al. Olaparib for metastatic breast cancer in patients with a germline BRCA mutation. N Engl J Med. 2017;377:523–33.
59. Litton JK, Rugo HS, Ettl J, et al. Talazoparib in patients with advanced breast cancer and a germline BRCA mutation. N Engl J Med. 2018;379:753–63.
60. Bardia A, Hurvitz SA, Tolaney SM, et al. Sacituzumab Govitecan in metastatic triple-negative breast cancer. N Engl J Med. 2021;384:1529–41.
61. Modi S, Jacot W, Yamashita T, et al. Trastuzumab Deruxtecan in previously treated HER2-low advanced breast cancer. N Engl J Med. 2022;387:9–20.
62. Balduzzi S, Mantarro S, Guarneri V, Tagliabue L, Pistotti V, Moja L, D'Amico R. Trastuzumab-containing regimens for metastatic breast cancer. Cochrane Database Syst Rev. 2014;2014:CD006242. https://doi.org/10.1002/14651858.CD006242.PUB2.
63. Swain SM, Miles D, Kim SB, et al. Pertuzumab, trastuzumab, and docetaxel for HER2-positive metastatic breast cancer (CLEOPATRA): end-of-study results from a double-blind, randomised, placebo-controlled, phase 3 study. Lancet Oncol. 2020;21:519–30.
64. Diéras V, Miles D, Verma S, et al. Trastuzumab emtansine versus capecitabine plus lapatinib in patients with previously treated HER2-positive advanced breast cancer (EMILIA): a descriptive analysis of final overall survival results from a randomised, open-label, phase 3 trial. Lancet Oncol. 2017;18:732–42.
65. Krop IE, Kim SB, Martin AG, LoRusso PM, Ferrero JM, Badovinac-Crnjevic T, Hoersch S, Smitt M, Wildiers H. Trastuzumab emtansine versus treatment of physician's choice in patients with previously treated HER2-positive metastatic breast cancer (TH3RESA): final overall survival results from a randomised open-label phase 3 trial. Lancet Oncol. 2017;18:743–54.
66. Lin NU, Borges V, Anders C, et al. Intracranial efficacy and survival with Tucatinib plus Trastuzumab and Capecitabine for previously treated HER2-positive breast cancer with brain metastases in the HER2CLIMB trial. J Clin Oncol. 2020;38:2610–9.
67. Hurvitz SA, Hegg R, Chung WP, et al. Trastuzumab deruxtecan versus trastuzumab emtansine in patients with HER2-positive metastatic breast cancer: updated results from DESTINY-Breast03, a randomised, open-label, phase 3 trial. Lancet. 2023;401:105–17.
68. Burstein HJ, Somerfield MR, Barton DL, et al. Endocrine treatment and targeted therapy for hormone receptor-positive, human epidermal growth factor receptor 2-negative metastatic breast cancer: ASCO guideline update. J Clin Oncol. 2021;39:3959–77.
69. Finn RS, Boer K, Bondarenko I, et al. Overall survival results from the randomized phase 2 study of palbociclib in combination with letrozole versus letrozole alone for first-line treatment of ER+/HER2- advanced breast cancer (PALOMA-1, TRIO-18). Breast Cancer Res Treat. 2020;183:419–28.
70. Hortobagyi GN, Stemmer SM, Burris HA, et al. Overall survival with Ribociclib plus Letrozole in advanced breast cancer. N Engl J Med. 2022;386:942–50.
71. Goetz MP, Toi M, Campone M, et al. MONARCH 3: Abemaciclib as initial therapy for advanced breast cancer. J Clin Oncol. 2017;35:3638–46.
72. André F, Ciruelos E, Rubovszky G, et al. Alpelisib for PIK3CA-mutated, hormone receptor-positive advanced breast cancer. N Engl J Med. 2019;380:1929–40.
73. Robertson JFR, Bondarenko IM, Trishkina E, et al. Fulvestrant 500 mg versus anastrozole 1 mg for hormone receptor-positive advanced breast cancer (FALCON): an international, randomised, double-blind, phase 3 trial. Lancet. 2016;388:2997–3005.

4 Radiation Treatment in Breast Cancer

Çağlayan Selenge Bedük Esen and Ferah Yıldız

4.1 Role of Radiotherapy in the Case of Adjuvant Therapy in Breast Cancer

Breast cancer treatment typically begins with surgery followed by adjuvant chemotherapy (CT) and/or radiotherapy (RT) in patients with early-stage disease who are suitable for surgery at the time of diagnosis. The major advantage of adjuvant therapies in breast-conserving surgery (BC) is to provide early access to curative local treatment and more accurate pathological staging, particularly for patients who may be resistant to CT. While whole breast irradiation (WBI) is routinely recommended in patients with breast-conserving surgery (BCS), postmastectomy radiotherapy (PMRT) is performed for selected patients after mastectomy. Although survival rates are similar in studies comparing BCS and RT with mastectomy, cosmetic outcomes are better, and quality of life is higher with BCS followed by RT [1–3]. A meta-analysis conducted by the Early Breast Cancer Trialists' Collaborative Group (EBCTCG) showed that adjuvant RT in patients undergoing BCS reduced the 10-year local-regional recurrence (LRR) rates from 35% to 19% and decreased 15-year breast cancer-related mortality from 25.2% to 21.4%. This effect was observed in both LN-positive and LN-negative cases [4]. While BCS plus RT is preferred as a surgical approach in early-stage disease and cases with good response to neoadjuvant CT, factors such as multicentric disease, large tumor size, diffuse calcifications on imaging, history of radiation therapy, pregnancy, scleroderma, or positive surgical margins despite re-excision may necessitate mastectomy, either due to medical necessity or patient preference. However, the recent ACOSOG Z1102 prospective phase 2 study revealed that patients with multiple ipsilateral BC could also be good candidates for BCS in case the multiple tumors encompass only two quadrants of the breast [5]. The cosmetic outcome data for 216 eligible women who completed therapy in that study was evaluated separately and of the 136 patients who completed the survey 2 years postoperatively, 70.6% felt the result was good or excellent, while only 3.7% of women felt the result was poor [6]. Today, adjuvant RT after BCS is considered mandatory in early-stage disease both in cases with ductal carcinoma in situ (DCIS) or invasive cancer. Postmastectomy RT on the other hand is recommended only in patients with high risk for LRR as tumor size larger than 5 cm or margins <1 mm or having LN metastasis [7].

Ç. S. Bedük Esen · F. Yıldız (✉)
Department of Radiation Oncology, Hacettepe University Faculty of Medicine, Ankara, Turkey

Y. Bakar, A. Tuğral (eds.), *Managing Side Effects of Breast Cancer Treatment*,
https://doi.org/10.1007/978-3-031-75480-7_4

4.2 Neoadjuvant Therapy in Breast Cancer and the Role of Radiotherapy

Neoadjuvant treatments such as CT and/or hormone therapy in nonmetastatic BC allow for shrinking tumor volume and facilitate local treatment in patients who are not suitable for surgery at the time of diagnosis. Additionally, neoadjuvant therapy enables BCS in patients who are not suitable for BCS at the time of diagnosis and reduces the ALND rate, which leads to decreased morbidity in the presence of limited axillary disease. Other advantages of neoadjuvant therapy are preventing micrometastases, reducing the risk of recurrence, and predicting the response to adjuvant therapies. Today, neoadjuvant therapy is considered as standard treatment approach for Her-2 positive, triple-negative, and locally advanced BC. The presence and extent of residual disease after neoadjuvant therapy are significant prognostic factors for recurrence [8–10]. Survival rates are higher in patients achieving a pathological complete response (pCR) after neoadjuvant therapy than those without a pCR [11]. It was shown that adjuvant trastuzumab-emtansin and capecitabine increased disease-free survival (DFS) rates when there was no pCR in Her-2-positive and triple-negative cases, respectively [12, 13]. In the recent meta-analysis from Early Breast Cancer Trialists' Collaborative Group, it was shown that the oncological outcomes of the patients with neoadjuvant CT (NACT) were similar to the ones who were treated with adjuvant CT [14]. However, BCS and pathological LN negativity rates were higher in patients with neoadjuvant than those receiving adjuvant CT, and higher survival rates were shown in cases developing pCR after NACT [8, 9, 14].

The striking clinical and pathological response rates after NACT led to the idea of decreasing the ALND rate and replacing it with the SLNB procedure in order to reduce axillary morbidity in recent years. In the ACOSOG Z1071 trial, among women with cN1 breast cancer receiving NACT and who had 2 or more LNs examined in SLNB, the false-negative rate was found to be 12.6% [15]. However, placement of clips on suspicious LNs before NACT and removal of ≥3 LNs with SLNB using a dual method (blue dye and radiotracer) resulted in false-negative rates of less than 5% [15]. Today, it is shown that ALND can be avoided in approximately 40% of clinically node-negative (cN0) patients after neoadjuvant treatment [16, 17]. Currently, in cN0 cases after NACT, regional nodal irradiation (RNI) or ALND is recommended when SLNB reveals metastasis; however, ALND remains the standard approach in cases with suspicious positive clinical metastatic LNs (cN+) after NACT. The ongoing study, "Alliance A11202" trial, is comparing completion ALND or RNI only in cases with positive sentinel LNs after NACT in T1–3, N1 cases.

Whole breast irradiation (WBI) is recommended for all cases undergoing BCS, regardless of pathological response after NACT. The decision of PMRT is mainly based on pathological axillary LN metastasis and residual tumor size in addition to the clinical stage at diagnosis after NACT. Buchholz et al. showed that the rate of LRR was increased up to 27% in patients with cT3–4 and/or LN-positive disease who underwent NACT and mastectomy without PMRT and the authors also demonstrated that clinical disease stage IIIB or above, pathological ≥4 LN metastases, or >2 cm residual tumor size, and nonuse of tamoxifen increased LRR rates [18]. In another study, patients who received NACT and PMRT were compared with those who did not receive PMRT, and PMRT was found to reduce the 10-year LRR rates even in cases with achieved pCR. The LRR rates were 11% with PMRT vs. 22% without PMRT in that study, and patients who presented with clinically advanced stage III or IV disease but subsequently achieved a pCR after NACT still had higher rates of LRR (10-year rates of LRR were 3% and 33% with and without PMRT, respectively) [19]. However, a pivotal randomized study, the "NSABP B-51/RTOG 1304" trial presented in the recent San Antonio Breast Cancer Symposium, revealed opposite findings [20]. That study enrolled 1641 patients diagnosed with LN–positive, nonmetastatic BC whose LNs were found to be cancer-free after NACT and who had undergone either mastectomy or BCS. Patients were randomly assigned 1:1 to either the "no RNI" arm (observation after mastectomy or WBI after BCS) or the "RNI" arm (chest wall irradiation plus RNI after mastectomy, or WBI plus RNI after BCS). Within a follow-up time of 5 years, patients in both arms had similar outcomes whether they received adjuvant RNI or not: 91.8% of patients in the no RNI arm and 92.7% of those in the RNI arm were free of invasive BC recurrences. Distant recurrence and overall survival (OS) rates were also similar between the arms, with 93.4% of patients in each arm were free of distant recurrence. However, all patients accrued in that randomized study had cT1–3, N1 disease before NACT which did not represent true locally advanced BC. The follow-up time was only 5 years, and the number of events in both arms was quite low.

Today, PMRT is still recommended in patients with cT3–4 or clinical stage III disease before NACT and triple-negative disease, regardless of NACT response, and in cases with T2N1 disease where pCR was not achieved, especially in cases with LN metastasis after NACT. Additionally, according to the international St. Gallen consensus guidelines, the addition of RNI to WBI is recommended in the presence of residual nodal disease and clinical stage III disease at diagnosis [21]. In patients with stage II BC who achieve a pCR after neoadjuvant treatment, RNI is still recommended in the presence of high-risk factors such as young age (<40), grade 3 histology, and triple-negative disease [21].

4.3 The Radiotherapy Volumes and Fractionation in Early Breast Cancer After BCS

In breast cancer RT, WBI is recommended as a standard procedure following BCS, and PMRT is applied when there are risk factors for LRR. WBI encompasses the entire breast contour, and the chest wall and lymphatics are contoured following contouring atlases established by RTOG, ESTRO, and NRG Oncology groups [22] (Fig. 4.1).

Currently, treatment planning is performed using advanced technology such as forward-planning intensity-modulated radiation therapy (FP-IMRT), inverse-planning intensity-modulated radiation therapy (IP-IMRT), or volumetric arc therapy (VART) (Fig. 4.2).

In WBI, a total dose of 45–50 Gray (Gy) is traditionally delivered in 25–28 fractions with 1.8–2 Gy per fraction. However, hypofractionated radiotherapy (HFRT) schedules administered over 1–5 weeks, it has been recently developed to shorten the treatment duration and to improve patient compliance. Effective local control is possible with HFRT schedules since in vitro studies have shown an α/β ratio between 3.4 and 4, indicating the sensitivity of BC cells to radiation. Additionally, the total cost decreases due to the shortened treatment duration. Schedules with fraction doses of less than 4 Gy are termed "moderate" hypofractionation schedules. Prospective studies comparing moderate HFRT with conventional schedules (CFRT) have typically included patients with early-stage

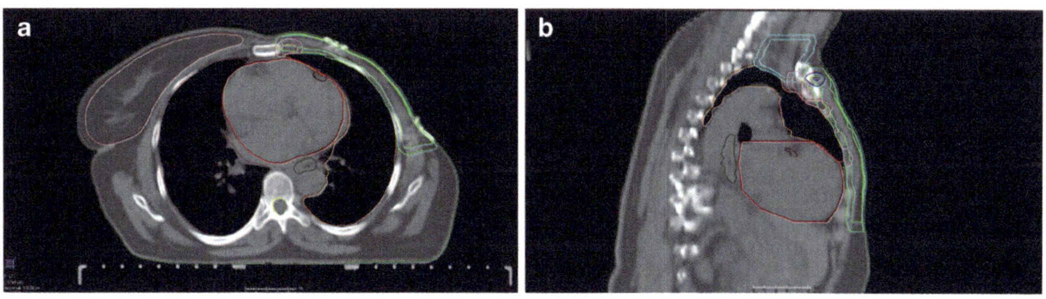

Fig. 4.1 The incision scars are marked with contrast material on the chest wall, supraclavicular fossa, level 3 axilla, and internal mammary lymphatic area contouring. (**a**) Axial section. (**b**) Sagittal section

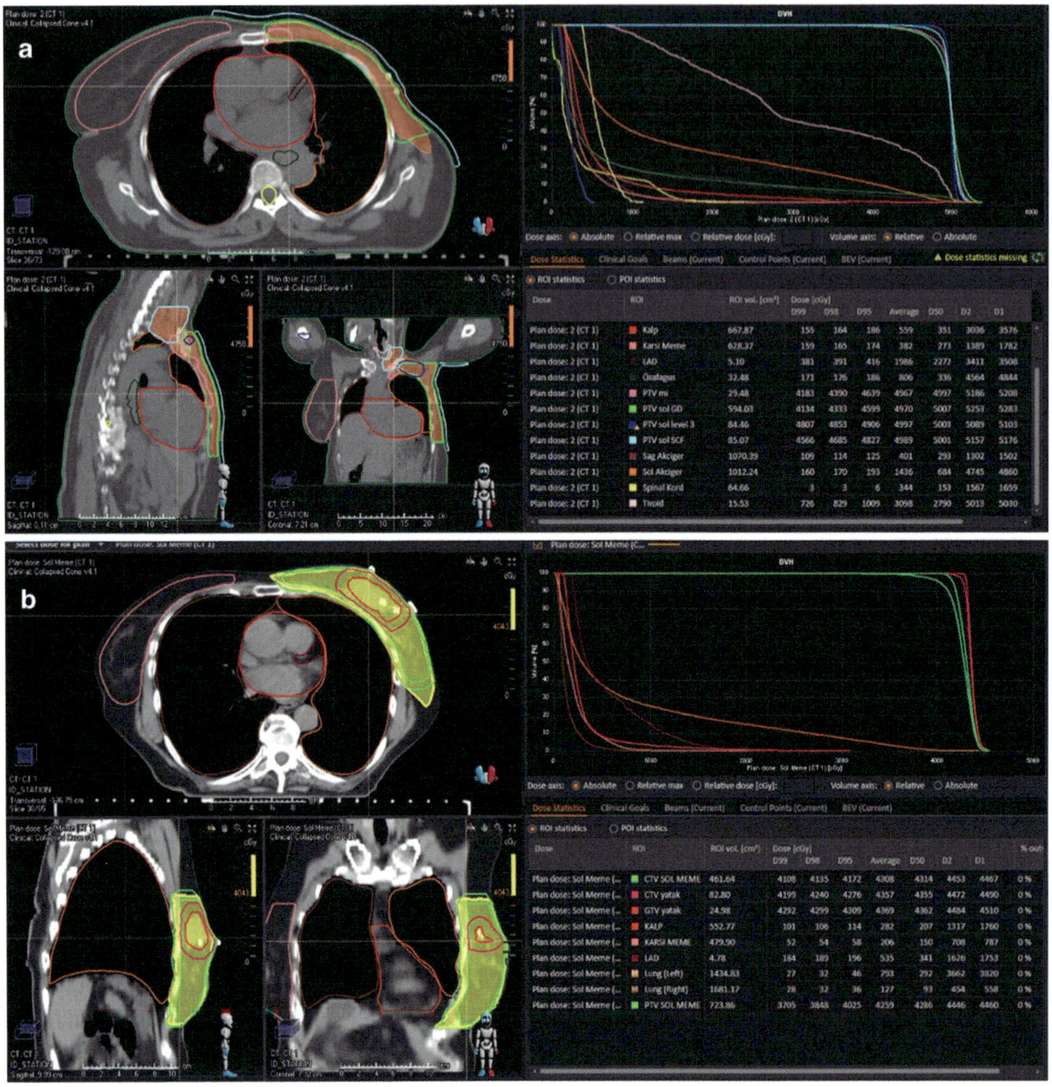

Fig. 4.2 (**a**) Treatment plan of a patient receiving radiotherapy targeting the chest wall, supraclavicular fossa, level 3 axilla, and internal mammary lymphatic region. The area shaded in orange represents the volume receiving 95% of the prescribed dose. On the right, the doses received by the target and critical organs are shown. (**b**) Treatment plan of a patient diagnosed with early-stage breast cancer receiving hypofractionated radiotherapy targeting only the breast. The area shaded in yellow represents the volume receiving 95% of the prescribed dose. On the right, the doses received by the target and critical organs are shown

BC. Despite similar rates of local control and late toxicity rates between hypofractionation and conventional schedules were reported, hypofractionation was associated with lower rates of acute toxicity compared to conventional ones [23–25]. The most frequently used fraction doses in moderate hypofractionation schedules range from 2.66 to 3.3 Gy/fraction, with a total treatment duration of 3 weeks if RT is administered daily on weekdays and of 5 weeks when a schedule of 2–3 fractions per week is applied. In routine practice, moderate hypofractionation schedules are predominantly used in women over 50 years of age since in the phase III trials comparing moderate hypofractionation schedule with conventional fractionation, patients ≤40 years old accounted for only 6% of all cases. In a recent meta-analysis, hypofractionated WBI was deemed safe, but it was emphasized that there was insufficient data for patients under 40 years old, those who received NACT, and those requiring lymphatic irradiation [26]. However, pooled analysis from randomized trials did not show any adverse effect of age, grade, type of surgery, lymph node status, or chemotherapy administration on local control in hypofractionated schedules [26]. Current guidelines strongly recommend HFRT for all early-stage BC patients who undergo BCS and do not require lymphatic radiation [27]. Patients who need RNI are not recommended to be treated with HFRT in routine practice due to the concern of late toxicity.

If the fraction dose of WBI exceeds 5 Gy, it is called ultrahypofractionation. In the FAST trial, 5 fractions of 5.7–6.0 Gy applied once a week were compared to 25 fractions of 2.0 Gy, and in the FAST-Forward trial, 26–27 Gy in 5.2–5.4 Gy per fraction delivered in just 1 week was compared to moderately hypofractionated WBI [28, 29]. Although acute toxicity and local control rates were similar in experimental arms, an increase in late toxicity was observed in schedules administering 27 Gy with 5.4 Gy/fr in 1 week or 30 Gy with 6 Gy/fr in 5 weeks [28, 29]. In light of this information, ultrahypofractionated WBI may be an option for elderly and fragile patients with low survival expectations.

4.4 Application of Radiotherapy Boost Dose to Tumor Bed Following WBI

The traditional approach involves delivering an additional dose of 10–16 Gy to the tumor bed following WBI. The RT boost dose to the tumor bed does not contribute to OS but reduces the rates of local recurrence (LR) and risk of mastectomy [30, 31]. In the EORTC 'Boost vs No Boost' trial involving 5318 patients, LR rates were significantly lower (12% vs. 16.4%) in patients receiving a boost dose to the tumor bed than those receiving only WBI during 20 years of follow-up [30]. The benefit of administering a boost dose to the tumor bed has been most evident in cases with accompanying DCIS, high-grade tumors, and patients ≤50 years old [30, 32]. Administering an additional dose to the tumor bed reduces the 20-year rates of in-breast recurrence from 31% to 15%, especially in patients with DCIS under 50 years old [33]. Again in the BIG 3–07/TROG 07.01 randomized, factorial, multicenter phase 3 trial, it was shown that a boost dose of 16 Gy in eight fractions to the tumor bed after WBI lowered the 5-year LRR from 7·3% to 2·9%, resulting in 4% fewer salvage mastectomies compared with the no-boost group in patients with non-low risk DCIS [34].

Still, there is no consensus in the literature regarding indications of RT boost to the tumor bed. According to the recommendations of the Groupe Europeen de Curietherapie (GEC)-ESTRO Breast Cancer Working Group, RT boost dose may not be applied to patients who are ≥50 years old, have ≤3 cm unicentric/unifocal tumors, have surgical margins ≥2 mm, are hormone receptor-positive, negative for lymphovascular invasion (LVI), and do not have LN metastasis. However, it is recommended to administer an RT boost dose to all other cases [35]. The ASTRO guideline suggests administering RT boost dose to patients who are ≤50 years old, aged 51–70 years, have high-grade tumors, and positive surgical margins, while it may not be recommended for patients who are >70 years old, have grade 1–2 tumors, with surgical margins ≥2 mm, and positive hormone receptors [27]. In applications of RT boost dose to the tumor bed, a safety margin of 1–2 cm is given to the tumor bed, and a total of 10–16 Gy is administered with a fraction dose of 2–2.5 Gy. Nowadays, RT boosts to the tumor bed with a simultaneous integrated boost (SIB) technique can be preferred due to its shortening of treatment duration, similar local control, and cosmetic outcomes [36, 37]. The tumor bed is determined postoperatively with the help of postoperative seroma and clips (Fig. 4.3).

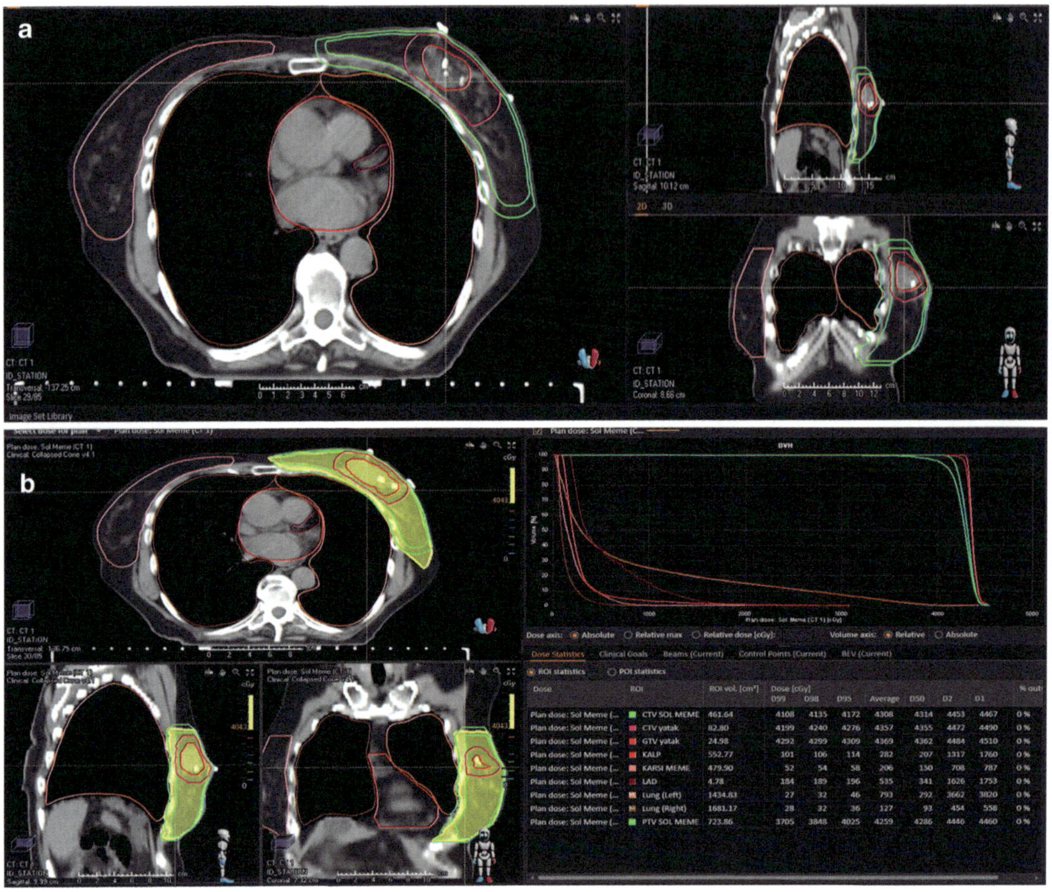

Fig. 4.3 (**a**) The tumor bed of the patient undergoing radiation therapy has been delineated using postoperative seroma and surgical clips. (**b**) Treatment plan of the patient receiving hypofractionated radiation therapy directed at the breast. The area shaded in yellow represents the volume receiving 95% of the prescribed dose. On the right, the doses received by the target and critical organs are shown

4.5 Partial Breast Irradiation in Early Stage Breast Cancer

In early-stage breast cancer, the concept of delivering RT to smaller areas than WBI called partial breast irradiation (PBI) came into the practice due to observation of residual disease and recurrences frequently within 1–1.5 cm vicinity of the tumor bed after BCS [38]. In PBI, treatment is administered with higher fraction doses and shorter durations, providing only the tumor bed with broader safety margins. PBI can be delivered through external RT, interstitial brachytherapy (BRT), intracavitary BRT, or intraoperative RT (IORT). The most commonly used technique is external RT, which can be applied using 3-dimensional conformal RT, intensity-modulated RT, or proton beam techniques. Its main advantages include being a non-invasive procedure, requiring less expertise, and allowing for treatment based on final pathology results in the postoperative period. Interstitial BRT is an invasive method and can only be applied in a limited number of centers due to the risk of infection and the expertise required. IORT is the most controversial technique [39, 40]. There are two prospective studies evaluating the efficacy of IORT within the context of PBI. The ELIOT study used electron beams, while the TARGIT study used low-energy X-rays. A common feature of both studies is the administration of a high dose of RT in a single fraction to the tumor bed immediately after surgical excision before the patient leaves the operating room. The long-term results of these two studies have shown that the LR rates with IORT were higher than with WBI [39, 40]. ASTRO guidelines currently do not recommend both forms of IORT alone, unless part of a clinical trial [41, 42].

When WBI was compared with PBI, early and medium-term local control and survival were generally similar with appropriate patient selection, but cosmetic outcomes were better with PBI [41, 43–45]. However, the 10-year results of the NSABP-B39/RTOG 0413 study, where patient selection criteria were broader and included cases with 1–3 LN metastases, showed that local control and recurrence-free survival were lower in the PBI arm [43–46]. Current ASTRO guidelines for accelerated PBI established "appropriate" patient criteria based on the results of studies in the literature, suggesting that accelerated PBI can be performed in invasive cancer cases without NACT, with T1N0 ductal tumor, ER-positive, no LVI, and extensive intraductal component, with surgical margins ≥2 mm, and ≤2.5 cm low-grade, mammography-diagnosed DCIS cases with at least 3 mm surgical margins [47].

4.6 Postmastectomy Radiotherapy

The purpose of PMRT after upfront surgery is to increase locoregional control in high-risk patients and reduce cancer-related deaths. An individual patient data (IPD) based meta-analysis by the EBCTCG showed that PMRT reduced 20-year BC-related mortality in LN-positive patients, and this effect continued in patients with 1–3 LN-positive disease who received effective chemotherapy or tamoxifen, but it did not have an impact on LRR or BC-related mortality in LN-negative patients [48]. One of the major concerns with PMRT is cardiac mortality; however, retrospective analysis of studies conducted by the Danish Breast Cancer Group (DBCG) showed that rates of ischemic heart disease, acute myocardial infarction, and cardiac death were similar between patients who did and those who did not receive PMRT [49]. In light of these findings, PMRT is routinely recommended for patients with T3–4 tumors, ≥4 LN metastases, positive surgical margins, or dermal fascia involvement in patients treated with upfront surgery and adjuvant systemic treatment [7]. However, the EBCTCG meta-analysis showed that PMRT also increased locoregional control and reduced BC-related deaths in the presence of 1–3 LN metastases [48]. Therefore, NCCN guidelines also recommend PMRT for patients with 1–3 LN metastases as having a high level of evidence [7].

PMRT is generally applied with conventional fractionation as 45–50.4 Gy in 1.8–2 Gy per fraction. Until now, HFRT has not been used in routine practice due to the concern about late toxicity in these patients, especially in patients who need RNI or RT after breast reconstruction. The recent randomized trial of fractionation after breast reconstruction (FABREC) sought to compare quality-of-life (QOL) and clinical outcomes of HFRT vs. CFRT in the setting of immediate prosthetic reconstruction between 3/2018 and 11/2021, 400 patients at 18 centers with stage 0–III BC and immediate placement of tissue expander or implant after mastectomy were randomized 1:1 to HFRT or CFRT. Respective doses in the two arms were 42.56 Gy/16 fractions to the chest wall, with or without axillary/supraclavicular LN radiation as 39.9 Gy/15 fractions and 50 Gy in 25 fractions to the chest wall and 46–50 Gy to axillary/supraclavicular LNs, respectively. Within a median follow-up of 31.8 months, physical well-being and overall toxicity profile were comparable between HF and CF-PMRT, and HFRT was even associated with better 6-month QOL in some domains among younger patients [50].

4.7 Lymph Node Evaluation and Treatment

The axillary LN status is the most important prognostic factor in patients with BC. SLNB has replaced ALND in cN0 patients, and ALND is not recommended to avoid increasing morbidity in patients with negative SLNB. Although the standard approach is ALND in patients with positive SLNB, there is an increasing trend in using RT instead of ALND to reduce surgical lymphedema, especially in low-risk patients. The treatment approach in SLNB-positive patients depends on the size of the metastasis in the LN. Metastatic foci ≤0.2 mm or <200 mm are classified as isolated tumor cells (ITC), 0.2–2 mm as micrometastases, and >2 mm as macrometastases. ALND is not recommended due to the lack of contribution to staging and the increased risk of lymphedema in patients with ITC or micrometastases [7]. The randomized phase III IBCSG 23-01 study investigated the role of ALND in early-stage BC patients who underwent BCS and had micrometastases detected in SLNB. Adjuvant RT was applied in 98% of cases after BCS in that study, and it was found that LR rates were very low, and no difference could be observed in DFS and OS rates in patients who underwent SLNB alone compared to cases where ALND was performed [51]. In the ACOSOG Z0011 study comparing completion of ALND and observation in patients with ≤2 positive LNs (micro or macrometastases) detected in SLNB, additional LN metastasis was found in 27.4% of patients who underwent ALND [52]. In this study, 89% of patients received WBI, and among those who received RT, a great portion of levels I and II axilla was included in the high tangential field in 50% of patients, and off-protocol RNI was applied in 19% of patients [53]. No difference was found in LRR and survival rates between the two arms in that study.

In the phase III EORTC 10981–22,023 AMAROS study, which investigated the effects of ALND or lymphatic RT on local-regional control and survival after SLNB, 1425 patients with SLNB-positive, T1–2, cN0 BC were randomized to ALND or lymphatic RT. With a 10-year follow-up, axillary recurrence rates were found to be very low in both arms, and no significant differences were observed between DFS and OS rates [54]. The most significant result of the AMAROS study was the significantly lower rate of lymphedema in patients who received lymphatic RT instead of ALND. The risk of lymphedema was significantly higher (24.5% vs. 11.9%) in patients who underwent ALND compared to those who received lymphatic RT [54]. In a similar OTOASOR study, comparing ALND and RNI (axillary and supraclavicular fossa (SCF) in patients with cT ≤3 cm and cN0 BC, an additional LN metastasis was detected in 38.5% of cases in the ALND group; however, there were no significant differences in terms of axillary failure and survival rates between the groups [55].

In light of these data, the American Society of Clinical Oncology (ASCO) considers WBI sufficient instead of ALND for patients with low-risk T1–2 tumors who have 1–2 LN metastases detected in SLNB since the axilla can incidentally be irradiated with WBI [55]. In the NCCN 2024 guidelines, the decision for RNI is left to the radiation oncologist's discretion for patients with 1–3 LN metastases detected in SLNB, who have not received NACT, have undergone a mastectomy, and WBI is planned [7]. ASCO recommends adding RNI to WBI regardless of whether SLNB or ALND is performed in the presence of additional risk such as being <50 years old, having internal/central tumor location, grade 3 histology, ER-negative, Her-2 positive disease, and in the presence of LVI. For patients with ≥3 LNs or 1–2 LN metastases in SLNB who refuse WBI, ASCO recommends ALND [56].

4.8 Regional Nodal Irradiation: The Volumes

The most common sites of LRR after mastectomy are the chest wall followed by SCF and level III axilla in patients who do not undergo PMRT [57, 58]. Therefore, it is recommended that the target volume should include the chest wall, SCF, and undissected axillary level or levels +/− internal mammary chain for patients who have pT3–4 and LN+ tumors especially when there is more than 3 LN metastasis (Fig. 4.4). In cases with pathological LN (−) tumors detected by either SLNB or ALND but with margin positivity or close surgical margin or fascia involvement but without other risk factors can be treated with chest wall irradiation or chest wall irradiation+reconstructed breast only.

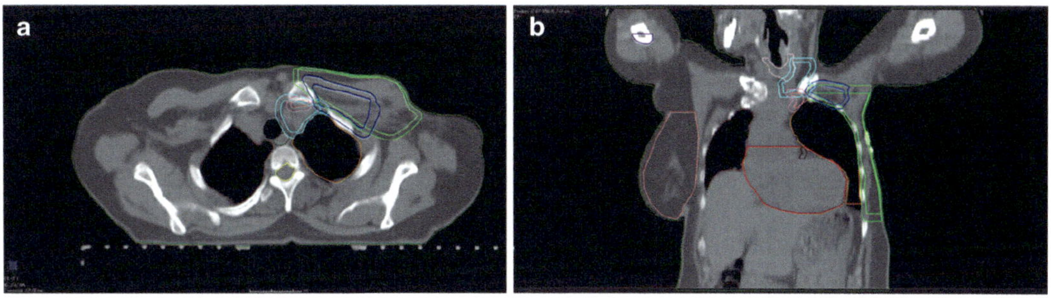

Fig. 4.4 Delineation of the chest wall, supraclavicular fossa, level 3 axilla, and internal mammary lymphatic area. (**a**) Axial section. (**b**) Coronal section

The decision to include internal mammary lymphatics in the RNI field is often left to the discretion of the radiation oncologist [59–61]. Additionally to the chest wall irradiation, RNI is still strongly recommended in the presence of 1–3 LN metastases in the axilla [7, 49]. However, the decision for indication of RT and field selection in the presence of favorable prognostic factors is left again to the discretion of the radiation oncologist. Additionally, RNI is recommended for cases with positive SLNB where ALND is not feasible or where ALND (<10 LN) is insufficient [7].

There are two prospective randomized trials investigating the outcomes of adding RNI to WBI [61, 62]. The first of these studies, the MA.20 trial, randomized nodal-positive or high-risk nodal-negative patients to WBI or WBI plus RNI including axilla-SCF and internal mammary lymphatics after BCS and systemic therapy [61]. While there was no difference in OS at a median 10-year follow-up, DFS was significantly higher in patients who received RNI. In a similar Phase III trial, the EORTC 22922 study, which accrued 4004 patients with stage I-III BC or tumors located centrally or in the inner quadrant, showed a significant decrease in BC mortality and any recurrence rates in patients who received RNI, similar to the MA.20 trial, while again no difference in OS was observed [62]. Another important finding of this study was the low toxicity rates with RNI and no increase in cardiac mortality or morbidity. Currently, studies are ongoing to determine the risk of LRR using molecular biological markers and to perform RT accordingly. The results of the TAILOR-RT study, which investigates the contribution of RNI in low-risk LN-positive or T3N0 cases, will clarify the role of RNI in early-stage cases. The current guidelines recommend WBI as the standard approach for pN0 cases after BCS; however, RNI is recommended in cases with adverse prognostic factors such as central-medial tumor location or pT3 tumor or pT2 tumor + grade 3 histology, substantial LVI, or estrogen receptor (ER) negativity [49]. While RNI is routinely recommended in cases with ≥4 positive LN metastases after BCS, it is highly recommended in cases with 1–3 LN metastases as in cases with mastectomy.

While undissected axillary levels and supraclavicular lymphatics are routinely included in the RNI field, irradiation of the internal mammary (IM) lymphatics remains controversial [60–64]. The risk of metastasis to IM lymphatics depends on the location, size of the tumor, and the extent of axillary involvement. Randomized MA.20, EORTC 22922, and non-randomized DBCG-IMN studies conducted in early-stage BC patients have shown the benefit of including IM and SCF lymphatics in the RNI field to survival [63, 64]. In the DBCG-IMN study, IM irradiation was found to reduce BC-related deaths, and this benefit was more evident in patients with LN-positive, medial/central tumor location, and particularly in cases with ≥4 LN metastases regardless of tumor localization [63]. The 15-year results of the same study revealed that IM irradiation significantly increased OS and reduced rates of distant recurrence and BC-related deaths [65]. Additionally, IM irradiation was shown not to increase the risk of cardiac death in the same study. A meta-analysis has demonstrated that RNI increases OS, DFS, and distant metastasis-free survival [66]. Based on these findings, IM irradiation is recommended in patients with T3-T4 and/or N2/−3 disease or LN-positive with medial/central tumors.

The role of RNI after NACT is still a matter of debate. Traditionally, the addition of RNI to WBI/chest wall irradiation has been recommended regardless of NACT response due to the high risk of LRR in patients with residual nodal disease after NACT or diagnosed with inflammatory BC, or presenting with clinical stage III disease [58, 67]. Additionally, NCCN guidelines recommend RNI in patients with stage II disease who achieve a pCR to NACT but with high-risk features as<50 years old, grade 3, and triple-negative histology [7]. However, the recently presented "NSABP B-51/RTOG 1304" trial which investigated the role of RNI in cases with no metastasis in LNs after NACT [20] revealed that the addition of RNI did not bring oncological outcome benefits in terms of invasive BC recurrence or distant recurrence. The mature results of this trial were not ready yet and the low number of recurrences in both arms is a matter of debate.

4.9 Radiotherapy-Related Side Effects in Breast Cancer Treatment

The survival rates are increasing in parallel to the advancements in BC treatment. Consequently, the prevention of adverse effects of the treatment became crucial. Though RT-related toxicity rates are decreasing with modern RT techniques, lymphedema, brachial plexopathy, cardiac morbidity, RT-related pneumonitis, severe radiodermatitis, and secondary cancers are still the most frightening side effects in patients in long-term follow-up [68]. Esophagitis is usually seen 2–3 weeks after the beginning of the treatment and improves within 3–4 weeks after the end of the treatment. The risk of esophagitis is approximately 5–20% if the mean esophageal dose is kept below 34 Gy [69]. Cardiac toxicity is another dose-limiting factor in the planning of BC treatment. Since studies demonstrated that the risk of cardiac toxicity increased by 7.4% per Gy of the mean heart dose, heart-sparing RT is recommended in BC patients [70]. Acute pericarditis is the most frequently seen acute cardiac toxicity and the risk of pericarditis significantly decreases with the mean heart dose of 5 Gy. It is recommended that the mean heart dose should be kept below 8 Gy in patients with left-sided tumors [71]. Reducing the risk of RT-related coronary artery disease and pulmonary toxicity in long-term follow-up is of the utmost importance. It is recommended that the mean left anterior descending artery dose, the mean ipsilateral lung dose, and V20 Gy should be kept below 20 Gy, 20 Gy, and 28–30%, respectively [69].

The other concern regarding breast cancer management is the risk of RT-related secondary cancers. A report from the SEER database showed that patients who received RT have higher rates of RT-induced secondary cancers than those who did not receive RT [72]. Furthermore, a systematic review showed that the risk of RT-related secondary cancer increases in volumes receiving ≥1 Gy [73]. In light of these findings, late adverse effects that may occur should be carefully assessed while deciding on RT volumes and doses.

References

1. Blichert-Toft M, Nielsen M, During M, et al. Long-term results of breast conserving surgery vs. mastectomy for early stage invasive breast cancer: 20-year follow-up of the Danish randomized DBCG-82TM protocol. Acta Oncol. 2008;47(4):672–81.
2. Litiere S, Werutsky G, Fentiman IS, et al. Breast conserving therapy versus mastectomy for stage I-II breast cancer: 20 year follow-up of the EORTC 10801 phase 3 randomised trial. Lancet Oncol. 2012;13(4):412–9.
3. Fisher B, Jeong JH, Anderson S, Bryant J, Fisher ER, Wolmark N. Twenty-five-year follow-up of a randomized trial comparing radical mastectomy, total mastectomy, and total mastectomy followed by irradiation. N Engl J Med. 2002;347(8):567–75.
4. Early Breast Cancer Trialists' Collaborative Group, Darby S, McGale P, et al. Effect of radiotherapy after breast-conserving surgery on 10-year recurrence and

15-year breast cancer death: meta-analysis of individual patient data for 10,801 women in 17 randomised trials. Lancet. 2011;378(9804):1707–16.
5. Boughey JC, Rosenkranz KM, Ballman KV, et al. Local recurrence after breast-conserving therapy in patients with multiple ipsilateral breast cancer: results from ACOSOG Z11102 (Alliance). J Clin Oncol. 2023;41(17):3184–93.
6. Rosenkranz KM, Ballman K, McCall L, et al. Cosmetic outcomes following breast-conservation surgery and radiation for multiple ipsilateral breast cancer: data from the Alliance Z11102 study. Ann Surg Oncol. 2020;27(12):4650–61.
7. NCCN Clinical Practice Guidelines in Oncology (NCCN Guidelines) Breast Cancer 2024. Version 1.2024. https://www.nccn.org/professionals/physician_gls/pdf/breast.pdf. Accessed 25 Jan 2024.
8. van der Hage JA, van de Velde CJ, Julien JP, Tubiana-Hulin M, Vandervelden C, Duchateau L. Preoperative chemotherapy in primary operable breast cancer: results from the European Organization for Research and Treatment of Cancer Trial 10902. J Clin Oncol. 2001;19(22):4224–37.
9. Rastogi P, Anderson SJ, Bear HD, et al. Preoperative chemotherapy: updates of National Surgical Adjuvant Breast and Bowel Project protocols B-18 and B-27. J Clin Oncol. 2008;26(5):778–85.
10. Houssami N, Macaskill P, von Minckwitz G, Marinovich ML, Mamounas E. Meta-analysis of the association of breast cancer subtype and pathologic complete response to neoadjuvant chemotherapy. Eur J Cancer. 2012;48(18):3342–54.
11. Cortazar P, Zhang L, Untch M, et al. Pathological complete response and long-term clinical benefit in breast cancer: the CTNeoBC pooled analysis. Lancet. 2014;384(9938):164–72.
12. Masuda N, Lee SJ, Ohtani S, et al. Adjuvant Capecitabine for breast cancer after preoperative chemotherapy. N Engl J Med. 2017;376(22):2147–59.
13. von Minckwitz G, Huang CS, Mano MS, et al. Trastuzumab Emtansine for residual invasive HER2-positive breast cancer. N Engl J Med. 2019;380(7):617–28.
14. Early breast cancer Trialists' Collaborative Group. Long-term outcomes for neoadjuvant versus adjuvant chemotherapy in early breast cancer: meta-analysis of individual patient data from ten randomised trials. Lancet Oncol. 2018;19(1):27–39.
15. Boughey JC, Suman VJ, Mittendorf EA, et al. Sentinel lymph node surgery after neoadjuvant chemotherapy in patients with node-positive breast cancer: the ACOSOG Z1071 (Alliance) clinical trial. JAMA. 2013;310(14):1455–61.
16. Tee SR, Devane LA, Evoy D, et al. Meta-analysis of sentinel lymph node biopsy after neoadjuvant chemotherapy in patients with initial biopsy-proven node-positive breast cancer. Br J Surg. 2018;105(12):1541–52.
17. Montagna G, Mamtani A, Knezevic A, Brogi E, Barrio AV, Morrow M. Selecting node-positive patients for axillary downstaging with neoadjuvant chemotherapy. Ann Surg Oncol. 2020;27(11):4515–22.
18. Buchholz TA, Tucker SL, Masullo L, et al. Predictors of local-regional recurrence after neoadjuvant chemotherapy and mastectomy without radiation. J Clin Oncol. 2002;20(1):17–23.
19. Huang EH, Tucker SL, Strom EA, et al. Postmastectomy radiation improves local-regional control and survival for selected patients with locally advanced breast cancer treated with neoadjuvant chemotherapy and mastectomy. J Clin Oncol. 2004;22(23):4691–9.
20. Eleftherios Mamounas HB, White J, Julian T, et al. Loco-regional irradiation in patients with biopsy-proven axillary node involvement at presentation who become pathologically node-negative after neoadjuvant chemotherapy: primary outcomes of NRG Oncology/NSABP B-51/RTOG 1304. In: San Antonio Breast Cancer Symposium; December 5–9, 2023; San Antonio, Texas; 2023. p. 84.
21. Burstein HJ, Curigliano G, Loibl S, et al. Estimating the benefits of therapy for early-stage breast cancer: the St. Gallen international consensus guidelines for the primary therapy of early breast cancer 2019. Ann Oncol. 2019;30(10):1541–57.
22. Julia White AT, Arthur D, Buchholz T, et al. Breast Cancer Atlas for Radiation Therapy Planning: Consensus Definitions. 2009. https://www.nrgoncology.org/Portals/0/Scientific%20Program/CIRO/AtlasesBreastCancerAtlas_corr.pdf?ver=2018-04-18-144201-270.
23. Haviland JS, Owen JR, Dewar JA, et al. The UK standardisation of breast radiotherapy (START) trials of radiotherapy hypofractionation for treatment of early breast cancer: 10-year follow-up results of two randomised controlled trials. Lancet Oncol. 2013;14(11):1086–94.
24. Shaitelman SF, Schlembach PJ, Arzu I, et al. Acute and short-term toxic effects of conventionally fractionated vs hypofractionated whole-breast irradiation: a randomized clinical trial. JAMA Oncol. 2015;1(7):931–41.
25. Owen JR, Ashton A, Bliss JM, et al. Effect of radiotherapy fraction size on tumour control in patients with early-stage breast cancer after local tumour excision: long-term results of a randomised trial. Lancet Oncol. 2006;7(6):467–71.
26. Budach W, Bolke E, Matuschek C. Hypofractionated radiotherapy as adjuvant treatment in early breast cancer. A review and meta-analysis of randomized controlled trials. Breast Care (Basel). 2015;10(4):240–5.
27. Smith BD, Bellon JR, Blitzblau R, et al. Radiation therapy for the whole breast: executive summary of an American Society for Radiation Oncology (ASTRO) evidence-based guideline. Pract Radiat Oncol. 2018;8(3):145–52.
28. Brunt AM, Haviland JS, Sydenham M, et al. Ten-year results of FAST: a randomized controlled trial of 5-fraction whole-breast radiotherapy for early breast cancer. J Clin Oncol. 2020;38(28):3261–72.

29. Murray Brunt A, Haviland JS, Wheatley DA, et al. Hypofractionated breast radiotherapy for 1 week versus 3 weeks (FAST-forward): 5-year efficacy and late normal tissue effects results from a multicentre, non-inferiority, randomised, phase 3 trial. Lancet. 2020;395(10237):1613–26.
30. Bartelink H, Maingon P, Poortmans P, et al. Whole-breast irradiation with or without a boost for patients treated with breast-conserving surgery for early breast cancer: 20-year follow-up of a randomised phase 3 trial. Lancet Oncol. 2015;16(1):47–56.
31. Romestaing P, Lehingue Y, Carrie C, et al. Role of a 10-Gy boost in the conservative treatment of early breast cancer: results of a randomized clinical trial in Lyon. France J Clin Oncol. 1997;15(3):963–8.
32. Kindts I, Laenen A, Depuydt T, Weltens C. Tumour bed boost radiotherapy for women after breast-conserving surgery. Cochrane Database Syst Rev. 2017;11(11):CD011987.
33. Vrieling C, van Werkhoven E, Maingon P, et al. Prognostic factors for local control in breast cancer after long-term follow-up in the EORTC boost vs no boost trial: a randomized clinical trial. JAMA Oncol. 2017;3(1):42–8.
34. Chua BH, Link EK, Kunkler IH, et al. Radiation doses and fractionation schedules in non-low-risk ductal carcinoma in situ in the breast (BIG 3-07/TROG 07.01): a randomised, factorial, multicentre, open-label, phase 3 study. Lancet. 2022;400(10350):431–40.
35. Polo A, Polgar C, Hannoun-Levi JM, et al. Risk factors and state-of-the-art indications for boost irradiation in invasive breast carcinoma. Brachytherapy. 2017;16(3):552–64.
36. Coles CE, Haviland JS, Kirby AM, et al. Dose-escalated simultaneous integrated boost radiotherapy in early breast cancer (IMPORT HIGH): a multicentre, phase 3, non-inferiority, open-label, randomised controlled trial. Lancet. 2023;401(10394):2124–37.
37. Horner-Rieber J, Forster T, Hommertgen A, et al. Intensity modulated radiation therapy (IMRT) with simultaneously integrated boost shortens treatment time and is noninferior to conventional radiation therapy followed by sequential boost in adjuvant breast cancer treatment: results of a large randomized phase III trial (IMRT-MC2 trial). Int J Radiat Oncol Biol Phys. 2021;109(5):1311–24.
38. Fisher B, Bryant J, Dignam JJ, et al. Tamoxifen, radiation therapy, or both for prevention of ipsilateral breast tumor recurrence after lumpectomy in women with invasive breast cancers of one centimeter or less. J Clin Oncol. 2002;20(20):4141–9.
39. Veronesi U, Orecchia R, Maisonneuve P, et al. Intraoperative radiotherapy versus external radiotherapy for early breast cancer (ELIOT): a randomised controlled equivalence trial. Lancet Oncol. 2013;14(13):1269–77.
40. Vaidya JS, Wenz F, Bulsara M, et al. Risk-adapted targeted intraoperative radiotherapy versus whole-breast radiotherapy for breast cancer: 5-year results for local control and overall survival from the TARGIT—a randomised trial. Lancet. 2014;383(9917):603–13.
41. Correa C, Harris EE, Leonardi MC, et al. Accelerated partial breast irradiation: executive summary for the update of an ASTRO evidence-based consensus statement. Pract Radiat Oncol. 2017;7(2):73–9.
42. Shaitelman SF, Anderson BM, Arthur DW, et al. Partial breast irradiation for patients with early-stage invasive breast cancer or ductal carcinoma in situ: an ASTRO clinical practice guideline. Pract Radiat Oncol. 2023;14:112.
43. Strnad V, Ott OJ, Hildebrandt G, et al. 5-year results of accelerated partial breast irradiation using sole interstitial multicatheter brachytherapy versus whole-breast irradiation with boost after breast-conserving surgery for low-risk invasive and in-situ carcinoma of the female breast: a randomised, phase 3, non-inferiority trial. Lancet. 2016;387(10015):229–38.
44. Coles CE, Griffin CL, Kirby AM, et al. Partial-breast radiotherapy after breast conservation surgery for patients with early breast cancer (UK IMPORT LOW trial): 5-year results from a multicentre, randomised, controlled, phase 3, non-inferiority trial. Lancet. 2017;390(10099):1048–60.
45. Whelan TJ, Julian JA, Berrang TS, et al. External beam accelerated partial breast irradiation versus whole breast irradiation after breast conserving surgery in women with ductal carcinoma in situ and node-negative breast cancer (RAPID): a randomised controlled trial. Lancet. 2019;394(10215):2165–72.
46. Vicini FA, Cecchini RS, White JR, et al. Long-term primary results of accelerated partial breast irradiation after breast-conserving surgery for early-stage breast cancer: a randomised, phase 3, equivalence trial. Lancet. 2019;394(10215):2155–64.
47. Kirby AM. Updated ASTRO guidelines on accelerated partial breast irradiation (APBI): to whom can we offer APBI outside a clinical trial? Br J Radiol. 2018;91(1085):20170565.
48. EBCTCG, McGale P, Taylor C, et al. Effect of radiotherapy after mastectomy and axillary surgery on 10-year recurrence and 20-year breast cancer mortality: meta-analysis of individual patient data for 8135 women in 22 randomised trials. Lancet. 2014;383(9935):2127–35.
49. Hojris I, Overgaard M, Christensen JJ, Overgaard J. Morbidity and mortality of ischaemic heart disease in high-risk breast-cancer patients after adjuvant postmastectomy systemic treatment with or without radiotherapy: analysis of DBCG 82b and 82c randomised trials. Radiotherapy Committee of the Danish Breast Cancer Cooperative Group. Lancet. 1999;354(9188):1425–30.
50. Wong JS, Uno H, Tramontano A, Pellegrini C, et al. Patient-reported and toxicity results from the FABREC study: a multicenter randomized trial of Hypofractionated vs. conventionally-fractionated Postmastectomy radiation therapy after implant-based reconstruction. Int J Radiat Oncol. 2023;117(4):E3–4.

51. Galimberti V, Cole BF, Viale G, et al. Axillary dissection versus no axillary dissection in patients with breast cancer and sentinel-node micrometastases (IBCSG 23-01): 10-year follow-up of a randomised, controlled phase 3 trial. Lancet Oncol. 2018;19(10):1385–93.
52. Giuliano AE, Ballman KV, McCall L, et al. Effect of axillary dissection vs no axillary dissection on 10-year overall survival among women with invasive breast cancer and sentinel node metastasis: the ACOSOG Z0011 (Alliance) randomized clinical trial. JAMA. 2017;318(10):918–26.
53. Jagsi R, Chadha M, Moni J, et al. Radiation field design in the ACOSOG Z0011 (Alliance) trial. J Clin Oncol. 2014;32(32):3600–6.
54. Bartels SAL, Donker M, Poncet C, et al. Radiotherapy or surgery of the axilla after a positive sentinel node in breast cancer: 10-year results of the randomized controlled EORTC 10981-22023 AMAROS trial. J Clin Oncol. 2023;41(12):2159–65.
55. Savolt A, Peley G, Polgar C, et al. Eight-year follow up result of the OTOASOR trial: the optimal treatment of the axilla - surgery or radiotherapy after positive sentinel lymph node biopsy in early-stage breast cancer: a randomized, single Centre, phase III, non-inferiority trial. Eur J Surg Oncol. 2017;43(4):672–9.
56. Lyman GH, Temin S, Edge SB, et al. Sentinel lymph node biopsy for patients with early-stage breast cancer: American Society of Clinical Oncology clinical practice guideline update. J Clin Oncol. 2014;32(13):1365–83.
57. Overgaard M, Nielsen HM, Tramm T, et al. Postmastectomy radiotherapy in high-risk breast cancer patients given adjuvant systemic therapy. A 30-year long-term report from the Danish Breast Cancer Cooperative Group DBCG 82bc trial. Radiother Oncol. 2022;170:4–13.
58. Strom EA, Woodward WA, Katz A, et al. Clinical investigation: regional nodal failure patterns in breast cancer patients treated with mastectomy without radiotherapy. Int J Radiat Oncol Biol Phys. 2005;63(5):1508–13.
59. Recht A, Somerfield MR, Edge SB. Postmastectomy radiotherapy: an American Society of Clinical Oncology, American Society for Radiation Oncology, and Society of Surgical Oncology focused guideline update summary. J Oncol Pract. 2016;12(12):1258–61.
60. Poortmans PM, Collette S, Kirkove C, et al. Internal mammary and medial supraclavicular irradiation in breast cancer. N Engl J Med. 2015;373(4):317–27.
61. Whelan TJ, Olivotto IA, Levine MN. Regional nodal irradiation in early-stage breast cancer. N Engl J Med. 2015;373(19):1878–9.
62. Poortmans PM, Weltens C, Fortpied C, et al. Internal mammary and medial supraclavicular lymph node chain irradiation in stage I-III breast cancer (EORTC 22922/10925): 15-year results of a randomised, phase 3 trial. Lancet Oncol. 2020;21(12):1602–10.
63. Thorsen LB, Offersen BV, Dano H, et al. DBCG-IMN: a population-based cohort study on the effect of internal mammary node irradiation in early node-positive breast cancer. J Clin Oncol. 2016;34(4):314–20.
64. Hennequin C, Bossard N, Servagi-Vernat S, et al. Ten-year survival results of a randomized trial of irradiation of internal mammary nodes after mastectomy. Int J Radiat Oncol Biol Phys. 2013;86(5):860–6.
65. Thorsen LBJ, Overgaard J, Matthiessen LW, et al. Internal mammary node irradiation in patients with node-positive early breast cancer: fifteen-year results from the Danish Breast Cancer Group Internal Mammary Node study. J Clin Oncol. 2022;40(36):4198–206.
66. Budach W, Bolke E, Kammers K, Gerber PA, Nestle-Kramling C, Matuschek C. Adjuvant radiation therapy of regional lymph nodes in breast cancer—a meta-analysis of randomized trials- an update. Radiat Oncol. 2015;10:258.
67. Recht A, Gray R, Davidson NE, et al. Locoregional failure 10 years after mastectomy and adjuvant chemotherapy with or without tamoxifen without irradiation: experience of the eastern cooperative oncology group. J Clin Oncol. 1999;17(6):1689–700.
68. Taylor C, Correa C, Duane FK, et al. Estimating the risks of breast cancer radiotherapy: evidence from modern radiation doses to the lungs and heart and from previous randomized trials. J Clin Oncol. 2017;35(15):1641–9.
69. Marks LB, Yorke ED, Jackson A, et al. Use of normal tissue complication probability models in the clinic. Int J Radiat Oncol Biol Phys. 2010;76(3 Suppl):S10–9.
70. Darby SC, Ewertz M, McGale P, et al. Risk of ischemic heart disease in women after radiotherapy for breast cancer. N Engl J Med. 2013;368(11):987–98.
71. Ma J, Li J, Xie J, Chen J, et al. Post mastectomy linac IMRT irradiation of chest wall and regional nodes: dosimetry data and acute toxicities. Radiat Oncol. 2013;8:81.
72. Burt LM, Ying J, Poppe MM, Suneja G, Gaffney DK. Risk of secondary malignancies after radiation therapy for breast cancer: comprehensive results. Breast. 2017;35:122–9.
73. Berrington de Gonzalez A, Gilbert E, Curtis R, et al. Second solid cancers after radiation therapy: a systematic review of the epidemiologic studies of the radiation dose-response relationship. Int J Radiat Oncol Biol Phys. 2013;86(2):224–33.

5 Genetic Perspective of Breast Cancer Patients: Implications for Family Members

Aslı Geçgel

5.1 Introduction

In the world, breast cancer is the most frequent cancer among women. It is a complicated ailment that is impacted by both genetic and environmental variables. It is also the main reason why people die from cancer. Women of various ages, socioeconomic statuses, and ethnic origins are impacted. Hereditary breast cancer accounts for 5–10% of cases, and germline mutations in particular genes are linked to up to 25% of hereditary cases [1]. All malignancies result from pathogenic or likely pathogenic (P/LP) mutations in specific genes involved in DNA repair and/or cell growth control, though not all of these variations are inherited genetically from a single parent. Most women with breast or ovarian cancer have a sporadic cancer rather than a hereditary cancer. Approximately 7 out of 100,000 women who undergo clinical examinations have harmful mutations in one or more genes associated with cancer [2].

Germline genetic tests include testing DNA from blood or saliva to find inherited mutations in certain genes related to the kind of cancer observed in the individual or family examination. High-penetrance mutations are linked to markedly elevated risks of cancer and frequently result in a substantial alteration in the function of the target gene product [3]. First-degree and second-degree relatives of the affected person are more likely to develop different types of cancer, according to family research. Performing genetic testing on the first family member to receive a breast or ovarian cancer diagnosis at a young age is the most effective way to identify these penetrations [4].

Germline genetic tests are very crucial for the regulation of treatment in many cancer patients such as breast, ovarian, colon, gastric, endometrium, and thyroid cancer; screening individuals who may be at hereditary risk and providing counseling to relatives of patients with these malignancies [3]. Testing was done on individuals with a significant family history of cancer up until recently, looking at a small number of genes linked to high cancer risk and certain cancer syndromes. The practical application of multigene tests, which are crucial for identifying genetic variations, has expanded with advancements in sequencing technology. It is possible to sequence numerous genes at once using next-generation sequencing (NGS) [5]. Difficulties in detecting intermediate penetrance genes and the high probability of detecting variants of uncertain significance are compelling factors in the use of these panels. A variation of unknown significance (VUS) might be a benign polymorphism with no connection to an elevated risk of cancer, or it could be a genetic alteration that could suggest a higher risk of cancer. Genetic counseling is made

A. Geçgel (✉)
Department of Medical Oncology, Ege University Faculty of Medicine Hospital, İzmir, Turkey

Y. Bakar, A. Tuğral (eds.), *Managing Side Effects of Breast Cancer Treatment*,
https://doi.org/10.1007/978-3-031-75480-7_5

more difficult by this circumstance. Retrospective analyses estimated that if a VUS was reclassified, 82.1% to 91.2% of cases were classified in the benign or possibly benign category, while 8.7% to 17.9% were upgraded from VUS to the pathogenic category [6, 7]. Multigene panel testing is now offered to most patients; however, the genes tested differ from panel to panel. Regardless of family history, it has recently been suggested that all men and women be provided multigene panel testing at the time of breast cancer diagnosis; however, this recommendation has not yet become an accepted practice.

5.2 High-Penetrance Genes

In terms of hereditary malignancies, molecular genetics advancements have led to the identification of several genes linked to inherited susceptibility to pancreatic, ovarian, and breast cancer. These genes describe the particular P/LP variation (e.g., BRCA1/2, PALB2, STK11, CDH1, PTEN, and TP53) present in people and families displaying elevated cancer risk [8]. This elevated risk of breast cancer is also linked to products of moderate penetrance genes, including BRIP1, ATM, PALB2, BARD1, CHEK2, RAD51C, and RAD51D.

Information on common high-penetrance genes that are highly linked to breast cancer will be covered in the subsections of this section.

5.2.1 BRCA Mutation

There is a correlation between several germline mutations and a higher risk of breast cancer. The most well-known genes linked to breast cancer susceptibility are BRCA1 on chromosome 17q21 and BRCA2 on chromosome 13q12 [9]. Tumor suppressors that preserve chromosomal stability through homologous recombination following double-stranded DNA breakage are protein products of the BRCA1 and BRCA2 genes [10]. According to estimates, the overall frequency of BRCA1/2 gene mutations linked to disease is 1 in 300 and 1 in 800, respectively [11].

People who have BRCA1/2 mutations are more likely to develop breast, ovarian, colon, gastric, pancreatic, and gallbladder cancers, among other cancers. Mutations in these genes are associated with autosomal dominant hereditary breast/ovarian cancer syndrome, a condition that predisposes to both breast and ovarian cancer [1]. For women with a BRCA mutation, the lifetime risks of ovarian and breast cancer are 18% to 40% and 45% to 75%, respectively [12]. While BRCA mutations account for only 5 to 10% of female instances of breast cancer (BRCA1 mutations being somewhat more frequent than BRCA2 mutations), the implications of the gene mutation on carriers are more significant. For pathogenic BRCA1 carriers, the lifetime probability of having breast cancer is 72%, and for BRCA2 carriers, it is 69% [13]. Male BRCA2 pathogenic variant carriers have a about 7% chance of developing breast cancer before the age of 80 [14].

Compared to random breast cancer, BRCA-associated breast cancer exhibits a more aggressive phenotype; triple-negative and high-grade breast cancer is more common in BRCA1-related cases, and the histological grade of BRCA2-associated breast cancer is often greater than that of random instances [1, 15, 16]. It has been suggested that the prognosis for BRCA-associated breast cancer differs from that of random breast cancer. Clinical data, however, remain debatable when it comes to the prognostic significance of BRCA mutant status. A small number of studies have demonstrated that patients with BRCA-related breast cancer have better survival rates [17–20]. Some investigations have found no difference or a worse outcome. Given the rarity of BRCA1/2 mutation carriers throughout the whole population, the research' very small sample size may help to explain this. A positive BRCA mutation does not confirm or establish a cancer diagnosis; rather, it indicates an elevated chance of developing cancer. The possibility of getting breast cancer from random or other genetic reasons does not go away with a negative BRCA test result.

Suggestions for Family Members Options including surveillance, chemoprevention, bilateral salpingo-oophorectomy (BSO), and risk-reducing mastectomy (RRM) should be chosen individually for each patient when it comes to treating breast cancer risk in these women. Early identification of breast cancer in pathogenic BRCA variant carriers has been considerably improved by starting yearly mammography and breast magnetic resonance imaging (MRI) screening (typically every 6 months) at age 25, or at an earlier age according to the earliest age of beginning in the family [9].

When compared to radiological monitoring, bilateral RRM lowers the incidence of breast cancer in individuals with BRCA mutations by more than 90% and may also show a varied increase in life expectancy [21]. It also enables the management of intense anxiety and fear of illness, which frequently jeopardize the quality of life for those who carry BRCA mutations [22]. However, nipple-sparing mastectomy and rapid reconstruction seem to be a suitable risk-reducing treatment to maximize oncological and cosmetic results and increase quality of life, should the patient and medical team decide to move forward with preventative surgery [23].

For women of reproductive age with BRCA1/2 mutations between the ages of 35 and 40, risk-reducing BSO (rrBSO) is advised due to the difficulty of early detection of ovarian or fallopian tube cancer. The National Comprehensive Cancer Center Network (NCCN) guidelines state that rrBSO can be postponed until between the ages of 40 and 45 since people with BRCA2 mutations often develop ovarian cancer 8 to 10 years later than those with BRCA1 mutations [11]. Up to 95% of ovarian cancer cases are prevented with rrBSO [24]. In the premenopausal stage, delayed oophorectomy with bilateral salpingectomy has been proposed as a substitute for rrBSO since it preserves fertility and guards against early menopause [11].

The effectiveness of chemoprevention in lowering risk is not well understood. Individuals afflicted with breast cancer and carrying BRCA1/2 P/LP mutations are at a significant risk of acquiring contralateral breast cancers. Selective estrogen receptor modulators (SERMs) and aromatase inhibitors (AIs) are two chemopreventive treatments that lower the incidence of breast cancer in high-risk individuals alone. Few information is known about tamoxifen's ability to prevent BRCA mutation carriers from developing breast cancer. It has been shown that the use of SERMs (tamoxifen, raloxifene) reduces the incidence of invasive breast cancer in postmenopausal women who are considered to be at high risk of developing breast cancer, especially ER-positive disease [25, 26]. The AIs exemestane and anastrozole have shown effective in preventing breast cancer in postmenopausal women who are most susceptible to the disease [27, 28].

A tailored interdisciplinary approach should be guarantees that appropriate psychological support, precise genetic and clinical counseling, and comprehensive knowledge of all available risk management options. Life expectancy and quality of life should be balanced when choosing clinical interventions to lower the risk of breast cancer.

5.2.2 TP53 (Li-Fraumeni Syndrome)

Germline P/LP polymorphisms in the tumor protein p53 (TP53) gene are linked to Li-Fraumeni syndrome (LFS), and bearers of this syndrome are more likely to experience numerous primary malignancies in childhood or early adulthood [11]. The tumor suppressor gene TP53, which is found on chromosome 17, produces the protein p53, which, by direct binding to DNA, is crucial for the regulation of the cell cycle and apoptosis.

One in 5000 to one in 20,000 incidences of hereditary breast cancer are thought to be influenced by it. For women carrying this mutation, the lifetime cancer risk is almost 100% [29], nonetheless, their risk is linked to more than only an increased chance of breast cancer. In addition to breast cancer, there is a significant chance of developing brain cancer, leukemias, medulloblastoma, adrenocortical malignancies, osteosarcomas, ovarian, fallopian tube, peritoneal malignancies, and associated soft tissue sarcomas [30]. For female mutation carriers, the typical age of onset is under 35, but by the time they are 60 years old, their lifetime chance of getting breast cancer is close to 50% [11]. Additionally, carriers who have already had radiation therapy are more likely to get a recurrent cancer. As a result, radiation therapy increases the incidence of radiation-induced malignancies, particularly breast cancer, in female carriers [31]. Hu C et al. TP53 P/LP variations were shown to be strongly related with ER receptor-independent HER2-positive illness in a case-control investigation of 56,480 individuals with breast cancer [32].

Suggestions for Family Members Regardless of additional risk factors, genetic testing should be pursued for other family members if there is a known TP53 P/LP mutation in the family. Family members should begin having clinical breast examinations for breast cancer at the age of 20 (or at the earliest known age of breast cancer in the family) since breast cancer has an extremely early age of beginning [11]. Recommendations for breast screening are similar to BRCA-associated hereditary breast/ovarian cancer syndrome, although screening begins at earlier ages. Beginning at age 20, annual breast MRIs with contrast (preferred) or mammograms should be performed. For women with LFS, RRM is often advised; however, some may benefit from attentive monitoring with breast MRI in lieu of this. Risk-reducing surgeries. This is a choice that should be taken patient-by-patient, considering factors such as reconstructive alternatives, age-specific degree of cancer risk, risks from other cancers, and dangers related to cancer risk reduction/preservation [11]. Given the dangers of radiation-induced cancer in this condition and radioresistance in carriers, mastectomy should typically be chosen over lumpectomy plus radiation for women with LFS who develop breast cancer [33]. In terms of rrBSO, carriers with a family history of ovarian cancer should undergo multidisciplinary evaluation [34].

5.2.3 PTEN Hamartoma Tumor Syndrome (PHTS)

The phosphatase and tensin homolog tumor suppressor gene (PTEN) germline pathogenic mutation linked to cowden syndrome falls under the spectrum of PTEN hamartoma tumor syndromes. With a 1 in 200,000 incidence, cowden syndrome is an uncommon condition [35]. The condition is inherited autosomally and is mostly linked to variations in the germline P/LP PTEN tumor suppressor gene (10q23) [9]. It is well recognized that carriers have a higher chance of developing thyroid, breast, endometrial, colon polyposis, and ovarian cancer [36]. According to earlier research, women in this patient group have a 40% to 60% greater chance of developing breast cancer, and their usual age at diagnosis ranges from 38 to 50 years. A substantial number of patients participated in a prospective trial that revealed the lifetime risk of breast cancer to be between 77% and 85% [36]. Typically, the diagnosis is made during the premenopausal stage; by the age of 50, 50% of cases are detected. Additionally, 67% of women who carry PTEN pathogenic variants are more likely to experience benign breast alterations, such as fibroadenomas, adenosis, lobular atrophy, and intraductal papillomatosis [9].

Suggestions for Family Members It is advised for people with Cowden syndrome/PHTS to have clinical breast exams every 6 months and to begin monthly breast self-examinations at the age of 18 (or 5–10 years before the age of the youngest family member who was diagnosed) [11]. Five to ten years prior to turning 30 or the age at which the first family member with breast cancer was diagnosed, annual mammograms and breast MRIs should be started. Following 75 years of age, follow-up care should be assessed individually. RRM and hysterectomy should be considered with women who have Cowden syndrome, even if there is no data about risk-reducing surgery in individuals [37]. Genetic counseling should be used to make decisions for each patient individually. Oophorectomy is not routinely indicated in people with Cowden syndrome because the risk of ovarian cancer is not increased.

5.2.4 STK11 (Peutz-Jeghers Syndrome)

Autosomal dominant Peutz-Jeghers syndrome is caused by germline serine/threonine kinase 11 (STK11) P/LP mutations on chromosome

19p13.3 (PJS). According to estimates, the prevalence of PJS is between 1 in 8300 and 1 in 280,000 individuals [38]. PJS is associated with gastrointestinal polyps, mucocutaneous pigmentation, and gastrointestinal cancers, breast cancer, nonepithelial ovarian cancers (such as Sertoli-Leydig tumors) [39]. For women with PJS, the cumulative risk of breast cancer is between 32% and 54%, and the risk rises with age [9]. The average age of diagnosis is 37 years old, with a range of 9 to 48 years old. Younger women are more likely to get diagnosed with it [40]. The majority of breast cancer cases in the research including families with STK11 PV were ER-positive and Her2 negative [41]. The absolute risk of nonepithelial ovarian cancer is 18% to 21% [42].

Suggestions for Family Members It is advised that high-risk gene carriers undergo monthly self-breast examinations beginning at age 20, mammograms and breast ultrasonography every 6–12 months, and Ca-125 testing for ovarian cancer [9]. Beginning at age 30, complementary breast MRIs should be used for early detection of breast cancer. RRM is not usually taken into account for gene carriers of intermediate risk; however, each case should be assessed separately if there is an underlying family history, a risk of breast parenchyma, or other risk factors [43].

5.2.5 CDH1 (Hereditary Diffuse Gastric Cancer)

An autosomal dominant cancer syndrome called hereditary diffuse gastric cancer (HDGC) raises the lifetime risk of diffuse-type gastric cancer with a poor clinical course. Germline P/LP variants in the Cadherin1 gene (CDH1) are associated with an increased risk of disseminated gastric cancer and breast-invasive lobular carcinoma [11]. Before the age of 40, the majority of carriers of CDH1 mutations experience cancer. The lifetime cumulative risk of developing breast cancer ranges from 39% to 52% [9].

Suggestions for Family Members It is recommended to start annual breast MRIs and mammograms at age 30. Instead, screening could start 5–10 years before the youngest person be diagnosed with breast cancer [33]. Given the lack of evidence supporting a prophylactic mastectomy's ability to improve overall survival for this syndrome, RRM ought to be taken into account in light of each patient's unique clinical circumstances. There is a lifelong risk of stomach cancer in families with CDH1 P/LP variants. Prophylactic gastrectomy is recommended for P/LP germline CDH1 carriers between the ages of 18 and 40 due to the documented high incidence of diffuse gastric cancer and the low sensitivity of endoscopy in its detection [44]. It is important to talk about the possible risks and benefits of rrBSO with carriers who have a family history of ovarian cancer, even though CDH1 PV does not seem to significantly increase the risk of ovarian cancer [43].

5.3 Intermediate-Penetrance Genes

The incidence of P/LP variants found in genes with intermediate penetrance has increased in a significant proportion of breast cancer patients due to the widespread use of multigene panel testing. As compared to high-penetrance variants, PV in these genes are more common, but they are less sensitive in identifying cancer. Information regarding common medium penetrance genes that are strongly linked to breast cancer will be covered in the subsections of this section.

5.3.1 PALB2

The Fanconi anemia gene linked to a higher risk of breast cancer is PALB2. Between 0.4% and 3% of breast cancer patients have variants of PALB2 P/LP [45]. Carriers have a lifetime risk of breast cancer ranging from 41% to 60%, with a higher risk of onset that typically happens before age 40 [46]. As more relatives are impacted by breast cancer, the risk rises accordingly. The cumulative risk of male carriers is 0.9% over a lifetime [47]. 10% of patients with PALB2 carrier breast cancer who underwent genetic testing developed contralateral breast cancer, according to one study. In addition, this study revealed that the 10-year survival rates for breast cancer patients with PALB2 carriers were 48%, BRCA1 P/LP variant carriers were 72%, and non-carriers were 75% [48]. Two large cohort studies found a strong correlation between PALB2 carriers and ER-negative breast cancer [46, 49].

Suggestions for Family Members Annual breast MRIs, tomography scans, and mammograms are advised for PALB2 P/LP carriers beginning at age 30. It is important to carefully consider the profit and loss ratio when evaluating RRM [43]. Studies have already shown that carriers of PALB2 have an increased risk of triple-negative breast cancer; however, there is no information available regarding the efficacy of hormonal chemoprevention (with tamoxifen or aromatase inhibitors) for carriers [50]. There is some evidence from certain studies linking PALB2 to an increased risk of ovarian cancer. rrBSO may be taken into consideration in carriers over 45 years of age, as a large cohort study found that the lifetime risk of ovarian cancer in PALB P/LP variant carriers was 5% [32].

5.3.2 ATM (Ataxia-Telangiectasia)

Breast cancer risk is increased by P/LP variants in the ATM (ataxia-telangiectasia mutated) gene. With the ATM P/LP variant, the cumulative lifetime risk increase for breast cancer is approximately 6% at age 50 and 33% at age 80 [51]. Evidence from studies indicates that women have a 20% to 30% lifetime risk of breast cancer [52]. Studies have found a greater association between ATM carriers with ER-positive breast cancer than with ER-negative breast cancer [32].

Suggestions for Family Members In carriers of the P/LP ATM variant, initiating yearly MRI scans at ages 30 to 35 and yearly mammograms at age 40 reduces breast cancer mortality by more than 55% [52]. The benefit of RRM in carriers is not well-documented, although each case should be assessed separately depending on risk factors like family history [53]. According to certain research, women who carry extremely rare ATM variants have a higher risk of developing contralateral breast cancer when they are exposed to radiation [54]. These are not P/LP variants, However, and a meta-analysis of five studies found that patients with heterozygous ATM P/LP variants could still receive conventional radiation therapy [55]. There is not enough evidence for rrBSO in large studies, despite the fact that ATM P/LP carriers have been found to have a slightly increased risk of ovarian cancer [56].

5.3.3 CHEK2

CHEK2 (The checkpoint kinase 2) is another gene that increases the risk of breast cancer. In patients with breast cancer, the prevalence rate of the CHEK2 P/LP variant is between 1% and 2% [45]. Women with CHEK2 P/LP variants and familial breast cancer have a cumulative lifetime risk of 20–40% for breast cancer [32]. Breast cancer risk in CHEK2 carriers has been demonstrated to be influenced by family history of the disease [57]. Research indicates that it raises the risk of carriers for every subtype of breast cancer, with the exception of triple-negative subtypes, and is most closely linked to ER-positive breast cancer [46]. Carriers have an increased risk of male breast cancer, leukemia, sarcoma, plasma cell neoplasms, gastric, prostate, kidney, thyroid, and colorectal cancer [58]. There is insufficient evidence to conclude that there is a higher risk of ovarian cancer because CHEK2 mutations are rarely found in women who have the disease [9].

Suggestions for Family Members In P/LP CHEK2 carriers, beginning yearly MRI screening between the ages of 30 and 35 lowers the death rate from breast cancer by more than 55% [52]. A breast MRI scan's initiation is contingent upon several risk factors, such as age, breast density, family history, and patient characteristics. Furthermore, starting at age 40, annual mammography is advised for carriers [52]. For those with a family history of the CHEK2 P/LP variant or other risk factors (such as atypia or a diagnosis of breast cancer), it may be reasonable to explore the option of RRM even though there is a lack of data on its benefits [43]. Given the correlation between CHEK2 mutations and the risk of ER-positive breast cancer, hormonal chemopreventive therapy may be a good option for some women who are at risk of breast cancer, though there isn't enough data to support this [46]. The risk of ovarian cancer is not markedly increased by CHEK2 pathogenic variants. Patients who have a family history of ovarian cancer should be informed about the possible risks and advantages of rrBSO.

5.3.4 NF1

The NF1 P/LP variant is the cause of neurofibromatosis type 1 (NF1), an autosomal dominantly inherited cancer syndrome. This syndrome can cause the development of café-au-lait macules, axillary and/or groin freckles, peripheral neurofibromas, optic pathway gliomas, soft tissue gliomas, and sarcomas. NF1 and breast cancer risk are significantly correlated, with a lifetime cumulative risk of 20% to 40% for breast cancer [9]. Studies reveal no increase in risk beyond age 50 and an increased risk of early-onset breast cancer, which typically occurs between the ages of 30 and 40 [59]. Breast cancer patients who were NF1 were linked to a lower 5-year survival rate; non-NF1 patients had a 5-year survival rate of 87.8%, compared to 67.9% for NF1 patients [60].

Suggestions for Family Members In carriers, annual mammography should start at age 30 [61]. When neurofibromas are present in the breast, MRI sensitivity and specificity may be affected, making it more difficult to diagnose breast cancer in carriers. Additional information is required in patients. After the ages of 30 to 50, breast MRI screening is advised [11]. RRM's benefits for carriers of NF1 P/LP variants are unknown; however, each patient's family history can be used to evaluate the procedure [43].

Mutations in the BRIP1, BARD1, RAD51C, RAD51D, DNA mismatch repair (MMR) (MLH1, MSH2, MSH6, or PMS2) genes, although less common than the above genes, are associated with an increased risk of breast cancer.

5.4 Result

It is crucial for the development of more potent cancer prevention strategies to be able to identify women at the lowest or highest ends of the risk spectrum by classifying variants in genes linked to breast cancer risk. These developments have led to important advancements in cancer treatment strategies and follow-up procedures. Genetic counseling should be offered to an individual suspected of being at risk of hereditary cancer. An individual's family history and personal history must be thoroughly examined before determining the likelihood of hereditary or familial cancer. When implementing medical and surgical options for cancer prevention, a multidisciplinary evaluation should be done. The affected individuals should be informed about the potential benefits and harms of each procedure. The increased cancer risk and possible screening methods for affected individuals should be communicated to their relatives. The availability of more cutting-edge and inventive genetic testing and treatment options may improve people's health and survival rates.

Consequently, to improve patient outcomes and prevent cancer in people who are not ill but are at risk of developing it, it is imperative to broaden the use of genetic testing and consider the findings in order to identify the best cancer risk management and treatment options.

References

1. Baretta Z, Mocellin S, Goldin E, Olopade OI, Huo D. Effect of BRCA germline mutations on breast cancer prognosis: a systematic review and meta-analysis. Medicine. 2016;95(40):e4975.
2. Kurian AW, Hughes E, Handorf EA, Gutin A, Allen B, Hartman A-R, Hall MJ. Breast and ovarian cancer penetrance estimates derived from germline multiple-gene sequencing results in women. JCO Precis Oncol. 2017;1:1–12.

3. Robson ME, Bradbury AR, Arun B, Domchek SM, Ford JM, Hampel HL, et al. American Society of Clinical Oncology policy statement update: genetic and genomic testing for cancer susceptibility. J Clin Oncol. 2015;33(31):3660–7.
4. Weitzel JN, Lagos VI, Cullinane CA, Gambol PJ, Culver JO, Blazer KR, et al. Limited family structure and BRCA gene mutation status in single cases of breast cancer. JAMA. 2007;297(23):2587–95.
5. Easton DF, Pharoah PD, Antoniou AC, Tischkowitz M, Tavtigian SV, Nathanson KL, et al. Gene-panel sequencing and the prediction of breast-cancer risk. N Engl J Med. 2015;372(23):2243–57.
6. Esterling L, Wijayatunge R, Brown K, Morris B, Hughes E, Pruss D, et al. Impact of a cancer gene variant reclassification program over a 20-year period. JCO Precis Oncol. 2020;4:944–54.
7. Mersch J, Brown N, Pirzadeh-Miller S, Mundt E, Cox HC, Brown K, et al. Prevalence of variant reclassification following hereditary cancer genetic testing. JAMA. 2018;320(12):1266–74.
8. Weitzel JN, Blazer KR, MacDonald DJ, Culver JO, Offit K. Genetics, genomics, and cancer risk assessment: state of the art and future directions in the era of personalized medicine. CA Cancer J Clin. 2011;61(5):327–59.
9. Bevers TB, Niell BL, Baker JL, Bennett DL, Bonaccio E, Camp MS, et al. NCCN guidelines® insights: breast cancer screening and diagnosis, version 1.2023: featured updates to the NCCN guidelines. J Natl Compr Canc Netw. 2023;21(9):900–9.
10. O'Donovan PJ, Livingston DM. BRCA1 and BRCA2: breast/ovarian cancer susceptibility gene products and participants in DNA double-strand break repair. Carcinogenesis. 2010;31(6):961–7.
11. Daly MB, Pal T, Maxwell KN, Churpek J, Kohlmann W, AlHilli Z, et al. NCCN guidelines® insights: genetic/familial high-risk assessment: breast, ovarian, and pancreatic, version 2.2024: featured updates to the NCCN guidelines. J Natl Compr Canc Netw. 2023;21(10):1000–10.
12. Antoniou A, Pharoah PD, Narod S, Risch HA, Eyfjord JE, Hopper JL, et al. Average risks of breast and ovarian cancer associated with BRCA1 or BRCA2 mutations detected in case series unselected for family history: a combined analysis of 22 studies. Am J Hum Genet. 2003;72(5):1117–30.
13. Zhang X, Niu J, Che T, Zhu Y, Zhang H, Qu J. Fertility preservation in BRCA mutation carriers—efficacy and safety issues: a review. Reprod Biol Endocrinol. 2020;18(1):1–13.
14. Liede A, Karlan BY, Narod SA. Cancer risks for male carriers of germline mutations in BRCA1 or BRCA2: a review of the literature. J Clin Oncol. 2004;22(4):735–42.
15. Mehta AK, Cheney EM, Hartl CA, Pantelidou C, Oliwa M, Castrillon JA, et al. Targeting immunosuppressive macrophages overcomes PARP inhibitor resistance in BRCA1-associated triple-negative breast cancer. Nat Cancer. 2021;2(1):66–82.
16. Lakhani SR, Jacquemier J, Sloane JP, Gusterson BA, Anderson TJ, van de Vijver MJ, et al. Multifactorial analysis of differences between sporadic breast cancers and cancers involving BRCA1 and BRCA2 mutations. J Natl Cancer Inst. 1998;90(15):1138–45.
17. Cortesi L, Masini C, Cirilli C, Medici V, Marchi I, Cavazzini G, et al. Favourable ten-year overall survival in a Caucasian population with high probability of hereditary breast cancer. BMC Cancer. 2010;10(1):1–9.
18. Kriege M, Seynaeve C, Meijers-Heijboer H, Collee JM, Menke-Pluymers M, Bartels C, et al. Sensitivity to first-line chemotherapy for metastatic breast cancer in BRCA1 and BRCA2 mutation carriers. J Clin Oncol. 2009;27(23):3764–71.
19. Maksimenko J, Irmejs A, Nakazawa-Miklasevica M, Melbarde-Gorkusa I, Trofimovics G, Gardovskis J, Miklasevics E. Prognostic role of BRCA1 mutation in patients with triple-negative breast cancer. Oncol Lett. 2014;7(1):278–84.
20. Gonzalez-Angulo AM, Timms KM, Liu S, Chen H, Litton JK, Potter J, et al. Incidence and outcome of BRCA mutations in unselected patients with triple receptor-negative breast cancer. Clin Cancer Res. 2011;17(5):1082–9.
21. Ludwig KK, Neuner J, Butler A, Geurts JL, Kong AL. Risk reduction and survival benefit of prophylactic surgery in BRCA mutation carriers, a systematic review. Am J Surg. 2016;212(4):660–9.
22. Alaofi RK, Nassif MO, Al-Hajeili MR. Prophylactic mastectomy for the prevention of breast cancer: review of the literature. Avicenna J Med. 2018;8(03):67–77.
23. Franceschini G, Di Leone A, Terribile D, Sanchez MA, Masetti R. Bilateral prophylactic mastectomy in BRCA mutation carriers: what surgeons need to know. Ann Ital Chir. 2019;90:1–2.
24. Manley K, Ryan N, Jenner A, Newton C, Hillard T. Counselling of path_ BRCA carriers who are considering risk-reducing oophorectomy. Post Reprod Health. 2023;29(1):42–52.
25. Cuzick J, Sestak I, Bonanni B, Costantino JP, Cummings S, DeCensi A, et al. Selective oestrogen receptor modulators in prevention of breast cancer: an updated meta-analysis of individual participant data. Lancet. 2013;381(9880):1827–34.
26. Vogel VG, Costantino JP, Wickerham DL, Cronin WM, Cecchini RS, Atkins JN, et al. Update of the national surgical adjuvant breast and bowel project study of tamoxifen and raloxifene (STAR) P-2 trial: preventing breast cancer. Cancer Prev Res. 2010;3(6):696–706.
27. Goss PE, Ingle JN, Alés-Martínez JE, Cheung AM, Chlebowski RT, Wactawski-Wende J, et al. Exemestane for breast-cancer prevention in postmenopausal women. N Engl J Med. 2011;364(25):2381–91.
28. Cuzick J, Sestak I, Forbes JF, Dowsett M, Knox J, Cawthorn S, et al. Anastrozole for prevention of breast cancer in high-risk postmenopausal women (IBIS-II): an international, double-blind, randomised placebo-controlled trial. Lancet. 2014;383(9922):1041–8.

29. Mai PL, Best AF, Peters JA, DeCastro RM, Khincha PP, Loud JT, et al. Risks of first and subsequent cancers among TP53 mutation carriers in the National Cancer Institute Li-Fraumeni syndrome cohort. Cancer. 2016;122(23):3673–81.
30. Lammens CR, Bleiker EM, Aaronson NK, Wagner A, Sijmons RH, Ausems M, et al. Regular surveillance for Li-Fraumeni syndrome: advice, adherence and perceived benefits. Fam Cancer. 2010;9:647–54.
31. Heymann S, Delaloge S, Rahal A, Caron O, Frebourg T, Barreau L, et al. Radio-induced malignancies after breast cancer postoperative radiotherapy in patients with Li-Fraumeni syndrome. Radiat Oncol. 2010;5(1):1–5.
32. Hu C, Polley EC, Yadav S, Lilyquist J, Shimelis H, Na J, et al. The contribution of germline predisposition gene mutations to clinical subtypes of invasive breast cancer from a clinical genetic testing cohort. J Natl Cancer Inst. 2020;112(12):1231–41.
33. Tung NM, Boughey JC, Pierce LJ, Robson ME, Bedrosian I, Dietz JR, et al. Management of hereditary breast cancer: American Society of Clinical Oncology, American Society for Radiation Oncology, and Society of Surgical Oncology guideline. J Clin Oncol. 2020;38(18):2080–106.
34. Armstrong DK, Alvarez RD, Bakkum-Gamez JN, Barroilhet L, Behbakht K, Berchuck A, et al. Ovarian cancer, version 2.2020, NCCN clinical practice guidelines in oncology. J Natl Compr Canc Netw. 2021;19(2):191–226.
35. Pilarski R, Eng C. Will the real Cowden syndrome please stand up (again)? Expanding mutational and clinical spectra of the PTEN hamartoma tumour syndrome. J Med Genet. 2004;41(5):323–6.
36. Cummings S, Alfonso A, Hughes E, Kucera M, Mabey B, Singh N, Eng C. Cancer risk associated with PTEN pathogenic variants identified using multigene hereditary cancer panel testing. JCO Precis Oncol. 2023;7:e2200415.
37. Takayama T, Muguruma N, Igarashi M, Ohsumi S, Oka S, Kakuta F, et al. Clinical guidelines for diagnosis and Management of Cowden Syndrome/PTEN hamartoma tumor syndrome in children and adults-secondary publication. J Anus Rectum Colon. 2023;7(4):284–300.
38. Kopacova M, Tacheci I, Rejchrt S, Bures J. Peutz-Jeghers syndrome: diagnostic and therapeutic approach. World J Gastroenterol. 2009;15(43):5397.
39. Hearle N, Schumacher V, Menko FH, Olschwang S, Boardman LA, Gille JJ, et al. Frequency and spectrum of cancers in the Peutz-Jeghers syndrome. Clin Cancer Res. 2006;12(10):3209–15.
40. Beggs A, Latchford AR, Vasen HF, Moslein G, Alonso A, Aretz S, et al. Peutz–Jeghers syndrome: a systematic review and recommendations for management. Gut. 2010;59(7):975–86.
41. Lipsa A, Kowtal P, Sarin R. Novel germline STK11 variants and breast cancer phenotype identified in an Indian cohort of Peutz–Jeghers syndrome. Hum Mol Genet. 2019;28(11):1885–93.
42. Giardiello FM, Brensinger JD, Tersmette AC, Goodman SN, Petersen GM, Booker SV, et al. Very high risk of cancer in familial Peutz–Jeghers syndrome. Gastroenterology. 2000;119(6):1447–53.
43. Foretová L, Navrátilová M, Svoboda M, Vašíčková P, Sťahlová EH, Házová J, et al. Recommendations for preventive Care for women with rare genetic cause of breast and ovarian cancer. Klin Onkol. 2019;32(Supplementum2):6–13.
44. Jacobs MF, Dust H, Koeppe E, Wong S, Mulholland M, Choi E-Y, et al. Outcomes of endoscopic surveillance in individuals with genetic predisposition to hereditary diffuse gastric cancer. Gastroenterology. 2019;157(1):87–96.
45. Couch FJ, Shimelis H, Hu C, Hart SN, Polley EC, Na J, et al. Associations between cancer predisposition testing panel genes and breast cancer. JAMA Oncol. 2017;3(9):1190–6.
46. Consortium BCA. Breast cancer risk genes—association analysis in more than 113,000 women. N Engl J Med. 2021;384(5):428–39.
47. Yang X, Leslie G, Doroszuk A, Schneider S, Allen J, Decker B, et al. Cancer risks associated with germline PALB2 pathogenic variants: an international study of 524 families. J Clin Oncol. 2020;38(7):674.
48. Cybulski C, Kluźniak W, Huzarski T, Wokołorczyk D, Kashyap A, Jakubowska A, et al. Clinical outcomes in women with breast cancer and a PALB2 mutation: a prospective cohort analysis. Lancet Oncol. 2015;16(6):638–44.
49. Hu C, Hart SN, Gnanaolivu R, Huang H, Lee KY, Na J, et al. A population-based study of genes previously implicated in breast cancer. N Engl J Med. 2021;384(5):440–51.
50. Couch FJ, Hart SN, Sharma P, Toland AE, Wang X, Miron P, et al. Inherited mutations in 17 breast cancer susceptibility genes among a large triple-negative breast cancer cohort unselected for family history of breast cancer. J Clin Oncol. 2015;33(4):304.
51. Marabelli M, Cheng SC, Parmigiani G. Penetrance of ATM gene mutations in breast cancer: a meta-analysis of different measures of risk. Genet Epidemiol. 2016;40(5):425–31.
52. Lowry KP, Geuzinge HA, Stout NK, Alagoz O, Hampton J, Kerlikowske K, et al. Breast cancer screening strategies for women with ATM, CHEK2, and PALB2 pathogenic variants: a comparative modeling analysis. JAMA Oncol. 2022;8(4):587–96.
53. Tung N, Domchek SM, Stadler Z, Nathanson KL, Couch F, Garber JE, et al. Counselling framework for moderate-penetrance cancer-susceptibility mutations. Nat Rev Clin Oncol. 2016;13(9):581–8.
54. Bernstein JL, Haile RW, Stovall M, Boice JD Jr, Shore RE, Langholz B, et al. Radiation exposure, the ATM gene, and contralateral breast cancer in the women's environmental cancer and radiation epidemiology study. J Natl Cancer Inst. 2010;102(7):475–83.
55. van Os NJ, Roeleveld N, Weemaes CM, Jongmans MC, Janssens G, Taylor AMR, et al. Health risks for ataxia-telangiectasia mutated heterozygotes: a sys-

tematic review, meta-analysis and evidence-based guideline. Clin Genet. 2016;90(2):105–17.
56. Domchek SM, Robson ME. Update on genetic testing in gynecologic cancer. J Clin Oncol. 2019;37(27):2501.
57. Cybulski C, Wokołorczyk D, Jakubowska A, Huzarski T, Byrski T, Gronwald J, et al. Risk of breast cancer in women with a CHEK2 mutation with and without a family history of breast cancer. J Clin Oncol. 2011;29(28):3747–52.
58. Näslund-Koch C, Nordestgaard BG, Bojesen SE. Increased risk for other cancers in addition to breast cancer for CHEK2* 1100delC heterozygotes estimated from the Copenhagen general population study. J Clin Oncol. 2016;34(11):1208–16.
59. Sharif S, Moran A, Huson S, Iddenden R, Shenton A, Howard E, Evans G. Women with neurofibromatosis 1 (nf1) are at a moderately increased risk of developing breast cancer and should be considered for early screening. J Med Genet. 2007;44:481.
60. Uusitalo E, Rantanen M, Kallionpää RA, Pöyhönen M, Leppävirta J, Ylä-Outinen H, et al. Distinctive cancer associations in patients with neurofibromatosis type 1. J Clin Oncol. 2016;34(17):1978–86.
61. Yip C-H, Newman LA. American Society of Clinical Oncology, American Society for Radiation Oncology, and Society of Surgical Oncology guideline for management of hereditary breast cancer. JAMA Surg. 2021;156(3):284–5.

6 Immunotherapy for Breast Cancer Survivors: Implications for Clinical Practice

Merve Özkan

6.1 Introduction

Immunotherapy is transforming the treatment of numerous solid cancers, and preliminary findings show that PD-1/PD-L1 antagonists are effective in a small proportion of metastatic breast cancer patients. If the tumor is triple negative, PD-L1 positive, and/or has a larger amount of tumor-infiltrating leukocytes, clinical activity appears to be more likely [1]. The goal of immunotherapy research is to develop treatment combinations that convert non-responders into responders while also overcoming acquired resistance to immunotherapy [2, 3]. Some of the goals for clinical development are to find biomarkers that can accurately predict how well a person will respond to monoimmunotherapy, to find the best combinations of immunotherapy, and to help choose the best treatment for people with advanced disease. The field of clinical trials will be greatly improved by smart trials that look into reasonable combinations of immunotherapy treatments and biomarkers. This will also make immunotherapy available to more breast cancer patients [1].

Anthracycline and taxane-based chemotherapy have been the primary neo-adjuvant systemic treatment for early TNBC for many years [4]. Despite the fact that immunogenic tumors are not typically associated with breast cancer, the high level of tumor-infiltrating lymphocytes (TILs) is recognized as a favorable predictive marker in early TNBC [5]. ICI targeting PD-1 and PD-L1 is currently widely used as a first-line treatment for advanced TNBC [5]. Several randomized phase II–III trials have shown that adding ICI to NACT improves pCR and EFS in early TNBC patients, establishing a new standard of care. Importantly, ICI dramatically increases EFS even in patients who do not exhibit a fully achieved pCR [6].

6.1.1 The Immune System Plays a Dualistic Function

The immune system is active in the genesis, progression, and control of breast cancer [7]. Immunoediting defines the dynamic connections between breast cancers and host immunity [8]. Acute inflammation early in breast carcinogenesis activates innate immunity, causing tumor cell death as well as the development of dendritic cells (DC), which trigger the tumor-specific T-cell response. At this stage, either immune-driven rejection of early malignancies or tumor cell variety selection to dodge immunological responses occur. In the long run, acute inflammation gives rise to chronic inflammation, which creates an extensive tumor microenvironment (TME) consisting of immune cells and stromal cells that promote immune evasion and tumor

M. Özkan (✉)
Department of Medical Oncology, Izmir Katip Celebi University Faculty of Medicine Hospital,
Izmir, Turkey

Y. Bakar, A. Tuğral (eds.), *Managing Side Effects of Breast Cancer Treatment*,
https://doi.org/10.1007/978-3-031-75480-7_6

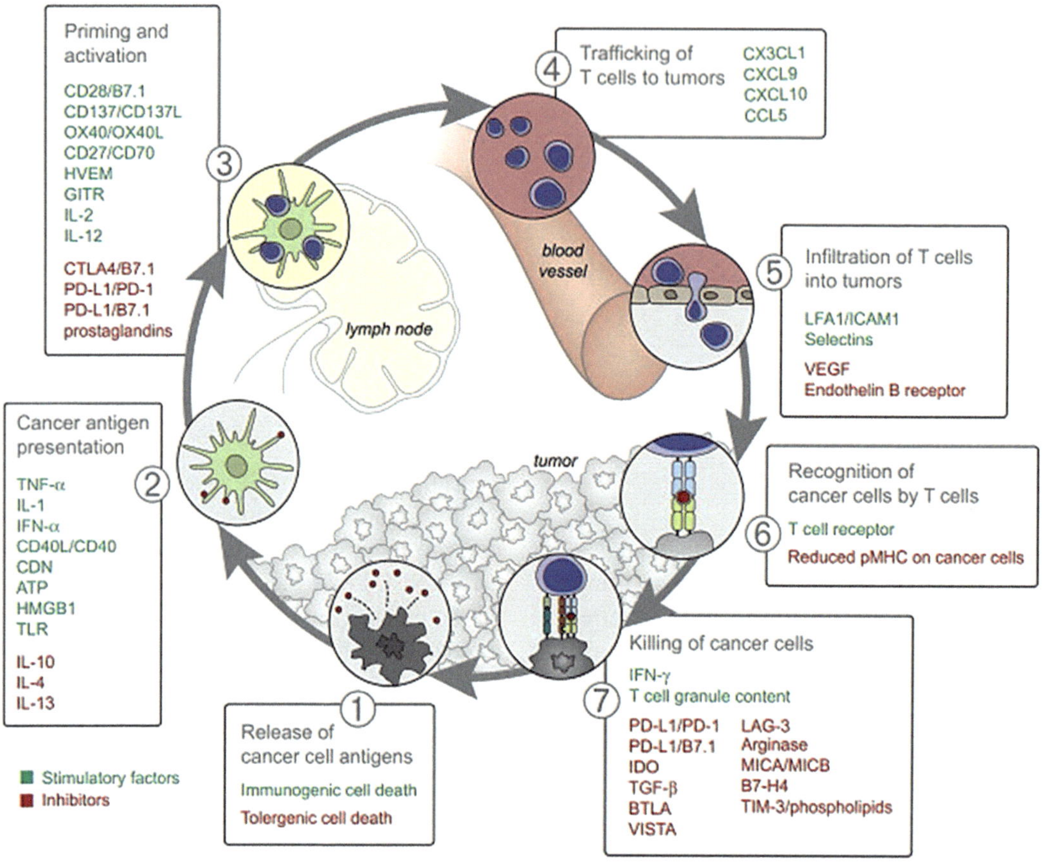

Fig. 6.1 The cancer-immunity cycle: factors that enhance immunity are depicted in green, while those that regulate the process by reducing immunological activity and preventing autoimmunity are shown in red [15]

progression [9, 10]. Throughout this transition, various immune cell types experience the activation of suppressive metabolic pathways [11–14]. These forces work together to create a powerful immune suppression network within the breast TME [12, 14].

The successful progression of the cancer immunity cycle relies on the precise coordination of various factors that either promote or hinder its different stages (Fig. 6.1). Through the elimination of the cancer cell, there is an increase in the production of tumor-associated antigen (step 1), which leads to a greater and more powerful response in subsequent cycles [15]. There are several potential scenarios that could occur. Tumor antigens may not be recognized, leading to confusion between antigens and foreign substances by DCs and T cells. This could trigger T regulatory cell responses instead of the desired effector responses. Additionally, T cells may struggle to connect with tumors or enter the tumor site. Possibly most significantly, tumor microenvironmental factors may inhibit the production of effector lymphocytes [16].

6.2 Clinical Immunomarkers for Breast Cancer

Understanding breast cancer requires a thorough analysis. There are three primary subtypes of breast cancer that have significant clinical implications: luminal, human epidermal growth factor receptor-2+ (HER-2+), and triple negative. These subtypes require distinct treatment approaches [17]. A greater likelihood of PD-L1 expression in the TME is observed in HER-2+ breast cancers and TNBCs as opposed to luminal breast cancers [18]. A higher ratio of CD8+ T-cells to Tregs has also been associated with an increased incidence of pCR after NACT [19].

6.2.1 CTLA-4 Inhibitors in Breast Cancer

CTLA-4 binds to CD80/CD86 and provides negative feedback to CD28 co-stimulation, thereby restricting T-cell activation during immunological priming, which is rapidly increased following T-cell activation [20]. This helps to keep immunity under control. In the clinic, two humanized monoclonal antibodies (mAbs) are available that are specific for CTLA-4. Tremelimumab, an anti-CTLA-4 medication, is presently undergoing research across all forms of tumors [21]. Its dual objective is to enhance systemic and local immunity. Patients diagnosed with breast cancer who get neoadjuvant immune checkpoint blockade have the potential to trigger antitumor responses [22].

6.2.2 PD-1/PD-L1 Inhibitors in Breast Cancer

CTLA-4 interacts with CD80/CD86 and plays a role in regulating CD28 costimulation, which helps control the growth of T cells during the initial stage of the rapidly enhancing immune response [20]. Humanized mAbs targeting PD-L1 (avelumab and atezolizumab) and PD-1 (pembrolizumab) are effective in treating metastatic breast cancer. The side effects linked to the use of these medications for breast cancer are typical for this kind of treatment [23].

6.2.2.1 Pembrolizumab

The inclusion of pembrolizumab alongside chemotherapy resulted in a notable improvement in the objective response rate for individuals with a PD-L1 Combined Positive Score (CPS) $\geq$10, as compared to chemotherapy alone [24]. The keynote-355 study reported adverse events, regardless of severity, in 96% of the 562 patients who received pembrolizumab-chemotherapy and 95% of the 281 patients who were given placebo-chemotherapy. The most frequently documented side effects included anemia, neutropenia, and nausea [24]. Immune-mediated adverse events occurred more frequently in pembrolizumab-chemotherapy patients than in placebo individuals. Increased thyroid problems and adrenal dysfunction were treatment-emergent side effects [25]. In the pembrolizumab-chemotherapy group, a severe skin reaction (2%) was the only immune-associated reaction of grade 3 or higher observed in at least ten patients. On the other hand, no such adverse events were reported in the placebo-chemotherapy group. Thyroiditis had a low occurrence rate, with 1% of those undergoing treatment in the pembrolizumab-chemotherapy group being affected, compared to 0% in the placebo-chemotherapy group. No deaths were reported as a result of immune-triggered adverse events [24].

6.2.2.2 Avelumab

Avelumab targets PD-L1 and is a human Ig-G1 monoclonal antibody [26]. Avelumab suppresses PD-L1-PD-1 interactions while leaving the PD-L2-PD-1 pathway intact. The phase Ia/Ib JAVELIN research tested Avelumab in a variety of tumor types. Phase Ib of this study involved 168 patients in an expansion cohort focused on breast cancer. All patients, regardless of their disease subtype or PD-L1 expression, were included in the study. More than half of the patients had received three or more rounds of treatment for metastatic disease. All breast cancer subtypes showed responses, with TNBC showing the highest sensitivity [26, 27].

6.3 Immunotherapy-Related Toxicities and Management

6.3.1 Dermatological Adverse Event(s)

The most frequently observed immune-related adverse event associated with ICI treatment is dermatologic toxicity. Inflammatory skin issues often appear within the first two cycles of treatment (or within a few weeks) [28–30]. Ipilimumab consistently shows a higher incidence of dermatologic adverse effects across all grades, when compared to PD-1/PD-L1 inhibitors [29, 31]. High-grade dermatological irAEs are similar across ICI classes, with ipilimumab and PD-1/PD-L1 inhibitors accounting for 1–3%. In general, anti-PD-1/PD-L1 and CTLA-4 inhibitory medications induced more frequent, severe, and early-onset dermatological damage [32]. The most typical manifestation is a maculopapular rash, which can be seen with or without pruritus. Patients undergoing ICI treatment may experience symptoms such as eczematous, allergic, and psoriasiform manifestations and bullous dermatitis [32, 33]. Alopecia and hair repigmentation have also been documented [34]. Most dermatological irAEs are typically mild and can be effectively managed with proper care, allowing for continued use of ICI treatment. On rare occasions, there have been reports of major cutaneous actions, such as Stevens-Johnson syndrome, toxic epidermal necrolysis, drug rash with eosinophilia, and systemic symptoms. Although significant problems often necessitate hospitalization, resolution was possible through systemic immunosuppressive medication and ICI cessation [32, 33].

The flattened macules and elevated papules characterize a maculopapular rash. It is referred to as morbilliform rash and is one of the most prevalent cutaneous adverse events. It typically affects the upper trunk, spreads upward, and may be accompanied by pruritus. Oral antihistamines and topical emollients are advised [35]. A topical corticosteroid of moderate potency should be used to treat a mild (G1) maculopapular rash while ICI therapy is in progress. For moderate rashes (G2), utilize topical corticosteroids of high potency or prednisone at a rate of 0.5–1 mg/kg/day. Suspension of immunotherapy and administration of high-potency topical steroids and 0.5–1 mg/kg/day prednisone are recommended for the management of severe rashes (G3/4). Urgent dermatological consultation is advised; inpatient care can be considered. Once symptoms are reduced to <G1 and only topical therapies are needed, reinitiation of immunotherapy should be considered. Bullous dermatitis, like other blistering skin responses, is distinguished by dermatitis and fluid-filled bullae. It is recommended to hold immunotherapy until the bullous dermatitis is resolved. Topical corticosteroids with high potency (G1) or prednisone/methylprednisolone (G2) at 0.5–1 mg/kg/day are recommended. Hospitalization and withdrawal of immunotherapy are essential for serious or life-threatening bullous dermatitis, as well as all cases of SJS/TEN [36].

6.3.2 Gastrointestinal Adverse Event(s)

6.3.2.1 Immunotherapy-Induced Diarrhea

The occurrence of diarrhea with immunotherapies such as nivolumab, pembrolizumab, and ipilimumab is dose dependent [37]. Ipilimumab causes diarrhea in around 30% of individuals, but PD-1 blockade causes diarrhea less commonly. Patients undergoing immunotherapy should be educated on the potentially fatal side effects of severe colitis and the importance of reporting symptoms promptly [37]. Checkpoint inhibitor-induced diarrhea is treated differently than other kinds of diarrhea, frequently needing corticosteroids [38]. Loperamide, an inhibitory drug on diarrhea, should be taken with caution since it may hide underlying autoimmune illnesses. For severe cases, high-dose intravenous corticosteroids (prednisone or methylprednisolone 1–2 mg/kg daily) and infliximab (5 mg/kg every 2 weeks) should be provided [39].

6.3.2.2 Immunotherapy-Induced Colitis

There are several factors that could potentially influence the development of ICI-induced colitis. There may be a connection between the reduction of regulatory T-cells in the intestines, an inherited trait like a CTLA-4 polymorphism, or changes in the gut microbiota and the pathophysiology. The breakdown of gastrointestinal mucosal immunity can lead to an increase in baseline microbial antibodies and fecal calprotectin (FC); however, none of these markers can accurately predict the onset of ICI-induced colitis [40]. Retrospectively, immunotherapy treatment has been linked to an increase in the risk of inflammatory bowel disease (IBD) by 41% [41, 42]. Patients receiving ipilimumab appear to have an increased risk of getting ICI-induced colitis when nonsteroidal anti-inflammatory medications are utilized [40]. The incidence of diarrhea and colitis varies according to the ICI regimen, dosage, and tumor type. The incidence of all-grade diarrhea is 35–40% with anti-CTLA-4, 11–17% with anti-PD1, and 32% with a combination of the two. The rate of colitis was reported as 8.4–11.3% with anti-CTLA-4, 0.3–3.4% with anti-PD-1, and 14% with the combined use, respectively [41]. Although enterocolitis is the most common symptom observed in patients undergoing anti-CTLA-4 therapy, instances of enteric neuropathy accompanied by severe constipation and microscopic colitis have also been documented in this subset of patients [43].

The histopathological inflammation patterns are characterized by acute colitis, chronic colitis, and microscopic colitis; however, some patients have a combination of these characteristic features of distinct inflammatory changes. The most frequent pattern of inflammation is acute colitis, which is distinguished by an increase in cryptitis, crypt abscesses, and crypt epithelium cell apoptosis accompanied by crypt atrophy/dropout, as well as cryptitis and cryptitis in the lamina propria. Different types of inflammation include diffuse, irregular, and focal [44].

Supportive care is suggested for patients suffering from grade 1 diarrhea. Treating symptoms involves implementing dietary modifications, such as adopting a low-fiber diet and using loperamide. In cases of mild diarrhea, the administration of ICIs can be maintained without any stoppage or delay in treatment. All instances of grade 3 and 4 diarrhea, as well as grade 2 diarrhea accompanied by fever, tachycardia, and dehydration, should be advised to undergo hospitalization. It would be worthwhile to focus on patient education to detect early signs of diarrhea and/or colitis. It is important to promote the reporting of any changes in bowel habits by patients. It is important to customize this strategy for each patient and consider the practical capabilities of each center [39]. Based on the literature, it is supported to use systemic corticosteroids like oral prednisone 1–2 mg/kg/day or an equivalent dose of methylprednisolone as the initial treatment for ICI-induced colitis [45]. In a retrospective investigation of 117 diarrhea patients, Wang et al. found that 68% of patients required systemic corticosteroid therapy. Initiating corticosteroids within 5 days of ICI-induced diarrhea resulted in faster symptom remission compared to the initiation of endoscopic examination [39, 45]. Corticosteroids are usually the primary option for the treatment of gastrointestinal irAEs. Early evaluation of steroid response (as defined as clinical response to grade 1 diarrhea) is recommended, following a period of 2–3 days. Once a preliminary clinical improvement is observed in grade 1 diarrhea, the administration of systemic steroids should gradually be reduced for a minimum of 4–6 weeks. Diarrhea and colitis symptoms generally improve in approximately 50% of patients who respond well to corticosteroid treatment [46, 47]. In retrospective studies of patients with ICI-related enterocolitis, corticosteroid treatment alleviated symptoms in roughly 40–60% of cases [45, 48]. However, an updated retrospective study reported that patients were diagnosed with greater infection rates among those treated with long-term steroids (>30 days). Prolonged use of corticosteroids without infliximab was related to a higher infection risk compared to short-duration steroids with infliximab, implying that non-steroid immunosuppressive medication may result in better outcomes in earlier settings [47]. Endoscopy demonstrated that colonic ulcerations were more prevalent in steroid-refractory subjects. Case reports show that infliximab effectively treats Ipilimumab-associated severe, steroid-resistant colitis [48, 49]. Vedolizumab has demonstrated its efficacy in treating enterocolitis that is associated with immune checkpoint inhibitors, as well as cases where patients are dependent on steroids or do not respond to steroid treatment. This has been observed in various case series and reports [50]. Inflammation of the small intestines and colon, which are resistant to infliximab may respond favorably well to vedolizumab [51, 52].

6.3.3 Hepatic Toxicity

While immune-related hepatotoxicity is less prevalent than diarrhea or colitis, it is a thoroughly documented adverse effect induced by ICIs. While it is generally mild, in rare instances, it can become severe or even catastrophic. Asymptomatic alanine transaminase (ALT) and aspartate transaminase (AST) elevations are the most frequently encountered adverse effects in the liver [53]. The estimated aggregate incidence of immune-related hepatotoxicity for ipilimumab is 3–9%, while for PD-1/PD-L1 inhibitors it ranges from 0.7% to 1.8% [54]. The utilization of combination therapy is correlated with a significantly elevated prevalence of hepatotoxicity in patients who encounter any grade and high-grade hepatotoxicity, as 29% and 17%, respectively [54, 55]. Although the median time of onset is 5–6 weeks after treatment initiation, irAEs can manifest months later [56, 57]. Although drug-induced hepatitis and autoimmune hepatitis may manifest similarly and be difficult to differentiate, their histological and imaging characteristics frequently serve to do so [58, 59]. Recent research has identified the unique histological patterns that are linked to hepatitis when PD-1/PD-L1 blockade is utilized as opposed to CTLA-4 [57]. Corticosteroids are the most commonly used therapy in studies of ICI-mediated hepatotoxicity. In many cases, reinitiation of corticosteroids following taper is required due to deteriorating liver results [54, 57]. Acute persistent hepatitis that did not respond to corticosteroid therapy has been managed with mycophenolate [54, 60, 61]. Another study found that cyclosporine could be used as a second immunosuppressant in the treatment of steroid-refractory hepatotoxicity [62]. Due to concerns about liver toxicity, Infliximab should not be used in this context, even though it has not been evaluated in this regard. Tacrolimus may also be an effective treatment for ICI-associated hepatitis that is resistant to standard treatment, according to case report data [63, 64].

Treatment advice is split based on the presence of high bilirubin. The treatment of transaminitis without high bilirubin is graded according to the extent to which enzymes surpass the upper limit of normal (ULN). In cases of mild transaminitis (G1), treatment can be maintained while closely monitoring transaminase levels. Consider delaying immunotherapy due to troubling test value patterns. Patients with moderate transaminitis (G2) should stop immunotherapy and undergo liver function tests (LFT) every 3–5 days. Initial treatment with prednisone consists of a daily dose of 0.5–1 mg/kg. Moderate or critical transaminitis (G3/4) necessitates the permanent cessation of ICI medication, a hepatology consultation, and LFT monitoring every 1–2 days. It is recommended to provide intensive therapy for G4 transaminitis and hospitalization for G3. If no contraindications exist, a liver biopsy may be considered. Start prednisone at 1–2 mg/kg/day (G3) or 2 mg/kg/day (G4). It may be beneficial to investigate the addition of mycophenolate mofetil (MMF) for patients who have persistent catastrophic hepatitis, even after undergoing 3 days of high-dose steroid treatment [36]. Patients with high G2 transaminases and bilirubin levels higher than 1.5 ULN (but not Gilbert syndrome) should not have the same treatment as people with high-grade hepatitis who do not have higher bilirubin levels. It is advised to stop immunotherapy permanently and prescribe prednisone at a dose of 2 mg/kg each day. LFTs should be monitored daily, and consultation with a hepatologist is recommended. For refractory instances after 3 days, MMF can be used in addition to steroids. All corticosteroid-treated hepatitis cases should be tapered when liver tests improve or return to ≤G1. It is advisable to continue to taper the dose over at least 1 month, with re-escalation as needed for recovering enzyme levels. For G2 hepatitis without increased bilirubin, physicians can restart immunotherapy if liver enzymes return to normal and prednisone (or equivalent) is decreased to ≤10 mg daily. After experiencing high-grade (G3/4) irAEs, the challenge of re-implementation of immunotherapy should be avoided [36].

6.3.4 Pancreatic Toxicity

Increased amylase and/or lipase can occur after ICI therapy, while usually seen as asymptomatic. The significance of asymptomatic increases is unknown, although discontinuing therapy based solely on these findings is not typically indicated [65, 66]. Although uncommon, acute pancreatitis has been reported in individuals on ICIs, and radiological signs of immune-related pancreatitis have been identified [59, 67, 68]. There have been reports of recurring pancreatitis following the resumption of PD-1 inhibitors after a pause for the first irAE [69]. Hospitalization, intensive resuscitation with fluids, and pain management should be provided similarly for acute pancreatitis symptoms. If clinical examination and/or imaging results indicate moderate/severe acute pancreatitis, gastroenterology consultation and immunosuppression are recommended. For mild (G2) pancreatitis, immunotherapy should be ceased, and methylprednisolone/prednisone at 0.5–1 mg/kg/day should be initiated. For severe (G3/4) pancreatitis, termination of ICI medication permanently and administering 1–2 mg/kg/day of corticosteroid [36].

6.3.5 Endocrine Toxicity

Endocrine gland autoimmunity caused by ICI has resulted in thyroid, pituitary, adrenal, and pancreatic dysfunction. Sznol et al. and Byun et al. explored the mechanisms underlying ICI-mediated endocrinopathies [70, 71]. Diagnosing endocrine toxicity can be difficult because many symptoms are similar to those of other acute diseases or underlying malignancies. Furthermore, physicians must determine whether to adapt treatment and whether the etiology of endocrine dysfunction is central (i.e., pituitary) or primary (e.g., adrenal or thyroid) accordingly [70, 71]. Because of the potential complexity, endocrinology professionals have a crucial role in managing these irAEs, especially in severe or complex cases. Different ICI regimens have been associated with various patterns of endocrine disruption. Ipilimumab causes hypophysitis, but PD-1/PD-L1 inhibitors are more likely to cause thyroid dysfunction. A very small number of people also have other endocrine irAEs, like primary adrenal failure and type 1 diabetes. Overall, combined ICI therapy was linked to a higher incidence of endocrinopathy [71, 72]. A 2018 meta-analysis investigated the occurrence of endocrine dysfunction in 38 randomized trials involving a total of 7551 patients who were administered either monotherapy or a combination of ICIs. The incidence of hypothyroidism with ipilimumab was initially 3.8%, but when combined with therapy, this rate significantly increased to 13.2%. There was a notable increase in the risk of hypothyroidism with PD-1 inhibitors when compared to ipilimumab [72]. Regular monitoring every 4–6 weeks is recommended for individuals with thyroid problems. The duration can be prolonged to a maximum of 4 months in those with normal thyroid function or those who continue to show no symptoms. In the presence of aberrant findings, it is recommended to evaluate the level of total T3. For subclinical hypothyroidism, which is defined as increased TSH with normal free T4, maintaining regular monitoring and initiation of immunotherapy are recommended. If TSH levels are beyond 10 mIU/L, levothyroxine might be prescribed. Primary hypothyroidism is defined by increased TSH values (>10 mIU/L) and low free T4 levels in conjunction with clinical symptoms. In this case, providing thyroid supplements and considering an endocrine consultation is necessary. Before beginning thyroid replacement therapy, testing the cortisol levels to rule out concomitant adrenal insufficiency is needed. In the case of hypophysitis-induced TSH deficiency, considering the free T4 levels for thyroid replacement [36, 70]. Thyrotoxicosis, characterized by suppressed TSH (<0.01 mIU/L) and elevated free T4 and/or total triiodothyronine (T3), can cause symptoms when free T4 levels are high. If symptoms persist (e.g., palpitations, anxiety, insomnia), seek an endocrine consultation, and propranolol should be prescribed to treat symptoms until they resolve [36, 70, 73].

Hypophysitis can cause acute symptoms such as headaches, photophobia, dizziness, nausea/emesis, fever, anorexia, visual field deficiencies, and extreme exhaustion [74]. Weight loss and exhaustion are examples of chronic complaints. Hypophysitis testing should include ACTH, cortisol, FSH, LH, TSH, free T4, testosterone in men, and estrogen in premenopausal women. Immunotherapy should be ceased in the case of acute, symptomatic hypophysitis, and methylprednisolone/prednisone should be initiated until resolution of acute symptoms, which typically takes 1–2 weeks. The steroids should then be tapered fast to physiological replacement levels as the patient improves. Resuming ICI therapy is considered once the symptoms of mass effect have disappeared [36, 74].

Permanent insulin-dependent diabetes is a result of the autoimmune destruction of the pancreatic islet cells. DM typically manifests after approximately 4–5 cycles of immunotherapy, although it may present earlier when using a combination therapy of anti-PD(L)1 and anti-CTLA-4 [75]. Hyperglycemia can be seen in people who have recently developed high blood sugar or have a history of type II diabetes, possibly as a result of corticosteroids. Continuing immunotherapy involves conducting blood glucose testing after each dose. It is advised to make diet and lifestyle changes and consider taking medications as recommended by the institution [75, 76].

6.3.6 Pulmonary Toxicity

Immunorelated (IR)-pulmonary toxicities include IR-interstitial lung disease (IR-ILD), IR-pneumonitis, and rarer types such as IR-bronchiolitis and IR-lung sarcoidosis [76]. The term IR-ILD or IR-pneumonitis refers to a local or extensive inflammatory process of the lung parenchyma [76]. ICI therapy can lead to the development of pneumonia [76–78]. Unlike the majority of other irAEs, ipilimumab monotherapy shows a lower incidence of pneumonitis than PD-1/PD-L1 inhibitors, which were reported to be associated with lower rates of less than 1% [79, 80]. Although the duration to commencement of irAE varies, the median period from starting treatment is 2.5 months, with combination therapy often causing faster onset than monotherapy [76, 77, 81].

Diagnosing IR-ILD in cancer patients can be challenging as it is often complicated by pre-existing inflammatory lung disease, chemotherapy-induced chronic obstructive pulmonary disease, radiation therapy, infections, or drug-induced pneumonia [82]. Although the precise risk factors for IR-ILD are unknown, smokers and those with lung cancer who already have chronic lung conditions like COPD may be more susceptible to more severe pneumonitis [83]. Five potential subtypes of IR-ILD have been identified based on their radiological characteristics: interstitial, hypersensitivity, cryptogenic organizing pneumonia, ground-glass opacities, and pneumonitis if not specified otherwise. The imaging findings mirror the classification of interstitial pneumonia according to the guidelines of the American Thoracic Society and European Respiratory Society [84]. Asymptomatic mild pneumonitis (G1) is limited to one lobe or less than 25% of the lung parenchyma. The presence of new or increasing symptoms such as lack of breath, cough, chest ache, and fever indicates moderate pneumonitis (G2). Severe pneumonitis (G3) affects each lobe of the lung or more than half of the parenchyma. Usually, the symptoms restrict activities of daily living (ADLs) related to self-care. Life-threatening (G4) pneumonitis is characterized by severe respiratory impairment [76]. Dyspnea should provoke a comprehensive clinical work-up, including the elimination of viral pneumonia, tumor development, pulmonary embolism, cardiac diseases, and pleural carcinomatosis or effusion [76]. Consideration should be given to bronchoalveolar lavage for determining infection or tumor infiltration, as well as sputum, blood, and urine culture investigations for infection if it is clinically indicated [76]. For mild to severe pneumonitis (G1), it is indicated to consider ceasing immunotherapy and monitoring symptoms with repeated imagings in 4 weeks or sooner via a chest CT if symptoms increase. Reevaluation of mild pneumonitis, including a physical examination and pulse oximetry both at rest and when walking in 1–2 weeks is recommended. For moderate pneumonitis (G2), see a pulmonologist and request an infectious workup that includes a nasal swab for suspected viral infections as well as sputum, blood, and urine culture. Bronchoscopy with bronchoalveolar lavage can be performed to rule out infection and malignant pulmonary infiltration. Repeated chest CT imaging should be considered in 3–4 weeks [36]. If the infection has not yet been completely ruled out, think about using empiric antibiotics. Methylprednisone/prednisolone at a dose of 1–2 mg/kg every day should be started. Every 3–7 days, perform a physical examination and use pulse oximetry. Corticosteroids should be used until symptoms improve to <G1 level, then tapered over 4–6 weeks [36]. Planning a moderate reduction of corticosteroids over ≥6 weeks after assessing the response within 48 h is recommended. If no improvement is seen after 48 h of treatment, consider further immunosuppression with infliximab, MMF, or IVIG [36]. When radiographical signs of improvement appear, immunotherapy may be resumed for mild pneumonitis. After G2 irAE, rechallenge can be considered if pneumonitis resolves to <G1 and no steroid is required [36]. If there is no improvement within 72 h after corticosteroid use, other options include tocilizumab (8 mg/kg, every 2 weeks) and infliximab (5 mg/kg, every 2 weeks) [85–87], and IVIG (2 g/kg over 2–5 days) [88]. Other alternatives include MMF (1 g twice daily) and cyclophosphamide [82, 88].

6.3.7 Additional Immune-Related Toxicities

It was reported that 10% of cancer patients have rheumatic and musculoskeletal adverse events during ICI therapy [89]. The expected incidence of neurological irAEs is 1–5% [90]. Symptoms of encephalitis, myasthenia gravis, or serious polyradiculopathy such as Guillain-Barre syndrome (GBS) during immunotherapy associated with a low threshold for hospitalization yet may require immediate attention, for a fast work-up and monitoring for severe and/or fatal manifestations [90]. ICIs can lead to a range of cardiovascular complications, including heart failure, non-inflammatory left ventricular dysfunction, myocarditis, pericarditis, vasculitis, severe coronary conduction disease (such as complete heart block), and atrial and ventricular arrhythmias. Another potential complication is Takotsubo syndrome, along with other cardiovascular toxicities [91]. Patients with moderate, clinically uncomplicated IR myocarditis are advised to engage in a multidisciplinary team discussion prior to resuming ICI treatment. Treatment for uncomplicated IR pericarditis typically involves the use of oral prednisolone and colchicine (500 mg twice daily). Treatment for IR pericarditis complicated by moderate or severe pericardial effusion involves the administration of 1000 mg intravenous methylprednisone and colchicine (500 mg twice daily). In urgent cases, percutaneous pericardiocentesis is necessary for large pericardial effusions with tamponade physiology [76, 92]. The prevalence of IR-renal dysfunction ranges from 2% to 7%, with anti-PD(L1), anti-CTLA-4 combined therapy accounting for 5% [93]. Hematological toxicity caused by IR-major side effects is uncommon (less than 5%), but it can result in substantial mortality [94, 95]. For optimal treatment, it is recommended to incorporate blood replacement and growth factor support alongside IV (methyl)prednisolone 1 mg/kg as the initial approach. Anti-IL-6R treatment could also be used. Eltrombopag may be considered for IVIG- and CS-refractory IR-thrombocytopenia in conjunction with a consultant hematologist [96]. Although IR-ocular toxicity is uncommon (<1%), it might pose a risk to vision deficiencies if not detected and treated promptly. The time to onset varies; however, it can occur shortly after starting ICI medication. Clinical manifestations include dry, itchy, or watery eyes, discomfort, and alterations in vision, such as fuzzy or double vision [97, 98]. The degree of IR-ocular damage determines how it is treated; mild uveitis, for instance, frequently responds well to local treatments like topical corticosteroids. In cases of more severe IR-ocular toxicities, notably orbital myopathies, ICI therapy should be terminated and systemic CSs delivered, with second-line immunosuppressants should be implemented as needed in CS-refractory situations. Subsequent continuation of ICI therapy should be approached cautiously, taking into account the individualized benefits and risk factors [97]. For suspected cases of IR-ocular toxicity, it is crucial to seek immediate examination from an ophthalmologist to ensure accurate diagnosis and timely treatment [76]. To make a long story short, any side effects particular to each unit should be reviewed with the department's specialist.

6.4 Immunotherapy for Older Adults in Cancer

Although immunotherapy achievements are pleasant for many cancer patients, they also create new problems in older persons with cancer. Older persons, particularly frail older adults, continue to be underrepresented in cancer trials. Given the lower toxicity profile of ICI, certain fragile older patients with cancer who may not have previously been provided cancer-directed therapy may now be considered for ICI treatment. Aging is also related to immune system alterations, which may have an impact on immunotherapy outcomes in older persons. As a result, it is critical to assess available data on ICI efficacy and toxicity in older persons with cancer, as well as to recognize the limits of current research [99]. While a comprehensive meta-analysis of clinical trials involving PD-L1 inhibitors revealed similar effectiveness in both older and younger adults, a significant drawback of these seminal ICI trials was that they failed to include vulnerable or fragile older adults [100]. The majority of these trials excluded patients with organ failure or an Eastern Cooperative Oncology Group (ECOG) performance status ≥ 2, limiting their generalizability to more fragile older persons treated for cancer in clinical practice. A few modest retrospective studies that assessed ICI effectiveness in older persons outside of clinical trials reported no difference in OS by age [101, 102].

Incorporating a geriatric evaluation throughout cancer treatment may reduce the risk of developing major adverse effects. A geriatric evaluation can thoroughly identify impairments or vulnerabilities in functional status, emotions, mental capacities, polypharmacy, various medical problems, and social interaction, which can then be addressed before and during ICI treatment. To avoid and detect probable adverse effects in older people, a full medical record, physical evaluation, and laboratory tests are essential before ICI initiation, as well as close monitoring during therapy. Early treatment of low-grade adverse effects may help older people avoid acquiring severe adverse effects, which are more likely to cause morbidity and mortality for older people than younger ones. Ideally, any treatment approach for adverse effects in older persons should consider their prior comorbidities. Corticosteroids are the primary treatment for adverse effects, particularly in patients with grade 2 or higher toxicities [44]. However, older persons are more prone to suffer from chronic conditions like diabetes or osteoporosis, which can worsen with steroid medication [103]. Older persons with diabetes may require more frequent glucose testing and may need to temporarily increase their diabetic drug regimen until corticosteroids can be stopped. Corticosteroids are also more likely to cause delirium in older persons; therefore, older patients and their caregivers should be counseled ahead of time about the signs of changing mental status. Patients who have refractory adverse effects may require longer courses of corticosteroids or other immunosuppressive treatments. Older persons are at higher risk of opportunistic infections and may need antibiotic prophylaxis [44, 104].

6.5 Conclusion

While immunotherapy generally has fewer adverse effects compared to chemotherapy, there are rare instances where these side effects can result in death. Therefore, it is imperative to continuously follow patients undergoing immunotherapy treatment and carefully document and evaluate any new symptoms during each visit. While corticosteroids are the primary method of managing immunological adverse effects, immunosuppressive medications can also be employed progressively. We suggest conducting a collaborative assessment of the specific organ toxicity with the appropriate professional in the field.

References

1. Emens LA. Breast cancer immunotherapy: facts and hopes. Clin Cancer Res. 2018;24(3):511–20.
2. Mittendorf EA, Zhang H, Barrios CH, Saji S, Jung KH, Hegg R, et al. Neoadjuvant atezolizumab in combination with sequential nab-paclitaxel and anthracycline-based chemotherapy versus placebo and chemotherapy in patients with early-stage triple-negative breast cancer (IMpassion031): a randomised, double-blind, phase 3 trial. Lancet. 2020;396(10257):1090–100.
3. Schmid P, Cortes J, Pusztai L, McArthur H, Kümmel S, Bergh J, et al. Pembrolizumab for early triple-negative breast cancer. N Engl J Med. 2020;382(9):810–21.
4. Loi S, Sirtaine N, Piette F, Salgado R, Viale G, Van Eenoo F, et al. Prognostic and predictive value of tumor-infiltrating lymphocytes in a phase III randomized adjuvant breast cancer trial in node-positive breast cancer comparing the addition of docetaxel to doxorubicin with doxorubicin-based chemotherapy: BIG 02-98. J Clin Oncol. 2013;31(7):860–7.
5. Loi S, Drubay D, Adams S, Pruneri G, Francis PA, Lacroix-Triki M, et al. Tumor-infiltrating lymphocytes and prognosis: a pooled individual patient analysis of early-stage triple-negative breast cancers. J Clin Oncol. 2019;37(7):559–69.
6. Downs-Canner S, Mittendorf EA. Preoperative immunotherapy combined with chemotherapy for triple-negative breast cancer: perspective on the KEYNOTE-522 study. Ann Surg Oncol. 2023;30(6):3166–9.
7. Emens LA. Breast cancer immunobiology driving immunotherapy: vaccines and immune checkpoint blockade. Expert Rev Anticancer Ther. 2012;12(12):1597–611.
8. Smyth MJ, Dunn GP, Schreiber RD. Cancer immunosurveillance and immunoediting: the roles of immunity in suppressing tumor development and shaping tumor immunogenicity. Adv Immunol. 2006;90:1–50.
9. Coussens LM, Pollard JW. Leukocytes in mammary development and cancer. Cold Spring Harb Perspect Biol. 2011;3(3):a003285.
10. DeNardo DG, Coussens LM. Inflammation and breast cancer. Balancing immune response: crosstalk between adaptive and innate immune cells during breast cancer progression. Breast Cancer Res. 2007;9(4):212.
11. Allard B, Beavis PA, Darcy PK, Stagg J. Immunosuppressive activities of adenosine in cancer. Curr Opin Pharmacol. 2016;29:7–16.
12. Ho PC, Kaech SM. Reenergizing T cell anti-tumor immunity by harnessing immunometabolic checkpoints and machineries. Curr Opin Immunol. 2017;46:38–44.
13. DeNardo DG, Barreto JB, Andreu P, Vasquez L, Tawfik D, Kolhatkar N, et al. CD4+ T cells regulate pulmonary metastasis of mammary carcinomas by enhancing protumor properties of macrophages. Cancer Cell. 2009;16(2):91–102.
14. Ribas A. Adaptive immune resistance: how cancer protects from immune attack. Cancer Discov. 2015;5(9):915–9.
15. Chen DS, Mellman I. Oncology meets immunology: the cancer-immunity cycle. Immunity. 2013;39(1):1–10.
16. Motz GT, Coukos G. Deciphering and reversing tumor immune suppression. Immunity. 2013;39(1):61–73.
17. Gradishar WJ, Moran MS, Abraham J, Abramson V, Aft R, Agnese D, et al. NCCN guidelines® insights: breast cancer, version 4.2023. J Natl Compr Cancer Netw. 2023;21(6):594–608.
18. Li X, Li M, Lian Z, Zhu H, Kong L, Wang P, et al. Prognostic role of programmed death ligand-1 expression in breast cancer: a systematic review and meta-analysis. Target Oncol. 2016;11(6):753–61.
19. Asano Y, Kashiwagi S, Goto W, Kurata K, Noda S, Takashima T, et al. Tumour-infiltrating CD8 to FOXP3 lymphocyte ratio in predicting treatment responses to neoadjuvant chemotherapy of aggressive breast cancer. Br J Surg. 2016;103(7):845–54.
20. Pardoll DM. The blockade of immune checkpoints in cancer immunotherapy. Nat Rev Cancer. 2012;12(4):252–64.
21. Vonderheide RH, LoRusso PM, Khalil M, Gartner EM, Khaira D, Soulieres D, et al. Tremelimumab in combination with exemestane in patients with advanced breast cancer and treatment-associated modulation of inducible costimulator expression on patient T cells. Clin Cancer Res. 2010;16(13):3485–94.
22. Nguyen VP, Campbell KM, Nowicki TS, Elumalai N, Medina E, Baselga-Carretero I, et al. A pilot study of neoadjuvant nivolumab, ipilimumab, and

intralesional oncolytic virotherapy for HER2-negative breast cancer. Cancer Res Commun. 2023;3(8):1628–37.
23. Emens LA, Kok M, Ojalvo LS. Targeting the programmed cell death-1 pathway in breast and ovarian cancer. Curr Opin Obstet Gynecol. 2016;28(2):142–7.
24. Cortes J, Cescon DW, Rugo HS, Nowecki Z, Im SA, Yusof MM, et al. Pembrolizumab plus chemotherapy versus placebo plus chemotherapy for previously untreated locally recurrent inoperable or metastatic triple-negative breast cancer (KEYNOTE-355): a randomised, placebo-controlled, double-blind, phase 3 clinical trial. Lancet. 2020;396(10265):1817–28.
25. Schmid P, Park YH, Muñoz-Couselo E, Kim SB, Sohn J, Im SA, et al. Pembrolizumab (pembro) + chemotherapy (chemo) as neoadjuvant treatment for triple negative breast cancer (TNBC): preliminary results from KEYNOTE-173. J Clin Oncol. 2017;35(15 Suppl):556.
26. Gulley JL, Rajan A, Spigel DR, Iannotti N, Chandler J, Wong DJL, et al. Avelumab for patients with previously treated metastatic or recurrent non-small-cell lung cancer (JAVELIN Solid Tumor): dose-expansion cohort of a multicentre, open-label, phase 1b trial. Lancet Oncol. 2017;18(5):599–610.
27. Heery CR, O'Sullivan-Coyne G, Madan RA, Cordes L, Rajan A, Rauckhorst M, et al. Avelumab for metastatic or locally advanced previously treated solid tumours (JAVELIN Solid Tumor): a phase 1a, multicohort, dose-escalation trial. Lancet Oncol. 2017;18(5):587–98.
28. Belum VR, Benhuri B, Postow MA, Hellmann MD, Lesokhin AM, Segal NH, et al. Characterisation and management of dermatologic adverse events to agents targeting the PD-1 receptor. Eur J Cancer. 2016;60:12–25.
29. Weber JS, Kähler KC, Hauschild A. Management of immune-related adverse events and kinetics of response with ipilimumab. J Clin Oncol. 2012;30(21):2691–7.
30. De Velasco G, Je Y, Bossé D, Awad MM, Ott PA, Moreira RB, et al. Comprehensive meta-analysis of key immune-related adverse events from CTLA-4 and PD-1/PD-L1 inhibitors in cancer patients. Cancer Immunol Res. 2017;5(4):312–8.
31. Lacouture ME, Wolchok JD, Yosipovitch G, Kähler KC, Busam KJ, Hauschild A. Ipilimumab in patients with cancer and the management of dermatologic adverse events. J Am Acad Dermatol. 2014;71(1):161–9.
32. Sibaud V. Dermatologic reactions to immune checkpoint inhibitors: skin toxicities and immunotherapy. Am J Clin Dermatol. 2018;19(3):345–61.
33. Naidoo J, Schindler K, Querfeld C, Busam K, Cunningham J, Page DB, et al. Autoimmune bullous skin disorders with immune checkpoint inhibitors targeting PD-1 and PD-L1. Cancer Immunol Res. 2016;4(5):383–9.
34. Zarbo A, Belum VR, Sibaud V, Oudard S, Postow MA, Hsieh JJ, et al. Immune-related alopecia (areata and universalis) in cancer patients receiving immune checkpoint inhibitors. Br J Dermatol. 2017;176(6):1649–52.
35. Geisler AN, Phillips GS, Barrios DM, Wu J, Leung DYM, Moy AP, et al. Immune checkpoint inhibitor-related dermatologic adverse events. J Am Acad Dermatol. 2020;83(5):1255–68.
36. Thompson JA, Schneider BJ, Brahmer J, Achufusi A, Armand P, Berkenstock MK, et al. Management of immunotherapy-related toxicities, version 1.2022, NCCN clinical practice guidelines in oncology. J Natl Compr Cancer Netw. 2022;20(4):387–405.
37. Kourie HR, Klastersky J. Immune checkpoint inhibitors side effects and management. Immunotherapy. 2016;8(7):799–807.
38. Yanai S, Nakamura S, Matsumoto T. Nivolumab-induced colitis treated by infliximab. Clin Gastroenterol Hepatol. 2017;15(4):e80–1.
39. Thompson JA, Schneider BJ, Brahmer J, Andrews S, Armand P, Bhatia S, et al. NCCN guidelines insights: management of immunotherapy-related toxicities, version 1.2020. J Natl Compr Cancer Netw. 2020;18(3):230–41.
40. Marthey L, Mateus C, Mussini C, Nachury M, Nancey S, Grange F, et al. Cancer immunotherapy with anti-CTLA-4 monoclonal antibodies induces an inflammatory bowel disease. J Crohns Colitis. 2016;10(4):395–401.
41. Meserve J, Facciorusso A, Holmer AK, Annese V, Sandborn WJ, Singh S. Systematic review with meta-analysis: safety and tolerability of immune checkpoint inhibitors in patients with pre-existing inflammatory bowel diseases. Aliment Pharmacol Ther. 2021;53(3):374–82.
42. Abu-Sbeih H, Faleck DM, Ricciuti B, Mendelsohn RB, Naqash AR, Cohen JV, et al. Immune checkpoint inhibitor therapy in patients with preexisting inflammatory bowel disease. J Clin Oncol. 2020;38(6):576–83.
43. Collins M, Soularue E, Marthey L, Carbonnel F. Management of patients with immune checkpoint inhibitor-induced enterocolitis: a systematic review. Clin Gastroenterol Hepatol. 2020;18(6):1393–1403.e1.
44. Brahmer JR, Lacchetti C, Schneider BJ, Atkins MB, Brassil KJ, Caterino JM, et al. Management of immune-related adverse events in patients treated with immune checkpoint inhibitor therapy: American Society of Clinical Oncology Clinical Practice Guideline. J Clin Oncol. 2018;36(17):1714–68.
45. Geukes Foppen MH, Rozeman EA, van Wilpe S, Postma C, Snaebjornsson P, van Thienen JV, et al. Immune checkpoint inhibition-related colitis: symptoms, endoscopic features, histology and response to management. ESMO Open. 2018;3(1):e000278.
46. Mooradian MJ, Wang DY, Coromilas A, Lumish M, Chen T, Giobbie-Hurder A, et al. Mucosal inflam-

mation predicts response to systemic steroids in immune checkpoint inhibitor colitis. J Immunother Cancer. 2020;8(1):e000451.
47. Wang Y, Abu-Sbeih H, Mao E, Ali N, Ali FS, Qiao W, et al. Immune-checkpoint inhibitor-induced diarrhea and colitis in patients with advanced malignancies: retrospective review at MD Anderson. J Immunother Cancer. 2018;6(1):37.
48. Jain A, Lipson EJ, Sharfman WH, Brant SR, Lazarev MG. Colonic ulcerations may predict steroid-refractory course in patients with ipilimumab-mediated enterocolitis. World J Gastroenterol. 2017;23(11):2023–8.
49. Wang Y, Abu-Sbeih H, Mao E, Ali N, Qiao W, Trinh VA, et al. Endoscopic and histologic features of immune checkpoint inhibitor-related colitis. Inflamm Bowel Dis. 2018;24(8):1695–705.
50. Bergqvist V, Hertervig E, Gedeon P, Kopljar M, Griph H, Kinhult S, et al. Vedolizumab treatment for immune checkpoint inhibitor-induced enterocolitis. Cancer Immunol Immunother. 2017;66(5):581–92.
51. Diana P, Mankongpaisarnrung C, Atkins MB, Zeck JC, Charabaty A. Emerging role of vedolizumab in managing refractory immune checkpoint inhibitor-induced enteritis. ACG Case Rep J. 2018;5:e17.
52. Hsieh AHC, Ferman M, Brown MP, Andrews JM. Vedolizumab: a novel treatment for ipilimumab-induced colitis. BMJ Case Rep. 2016;2016:bcr2016216641.
53. Naidoo J, Page DB, Li BT, Connell LC, Schindler K, Lacouture ME, et al. Toxicities of the anti-PD-1 and anti-PD-L1 immune checkpoint antibodies. Ann Oncol. 2015;26(12):2375–91.
54. Suzman DL, Pelosof L, Rosenberg A, Avigan MI. Hepatotoxicity of immune checkpoint inhibitors: an evolving picture of risk associated with a vital class of immunotherapy agents. Liver Int. 2018;38(6):976–87.
55. Sznol M, Ferrucci PF, Hogg D, Atkins MB, Wolter P, Guidoboni M, et al. Pooled analysis safety profile of nivolumab and ipilimumab combination therapy in patients with advanced melanoma. J Clin Oncol. 2017;35(34):3815–22.
56. Ziemer M, Koukoulioti E, Beyer S, Simon JC, Berg T. Managing immune checkpoint-inhibitor-induced severe autoimmune-like hepatitis by liver-directed topical steroids. J Hepatol. 2017;66(3):657–9.
57. De Martin E, Michot JM, Papouin B, Champiat S, Mateus C, Lambotte O, et al. Characterization of liver injury induced by cancer immunotherapy using immune checkpoint inhibitors. J Hepatol. 2018;68(6):1181–90.
58. Alessandrino F, Tirumani SH, Krajewski KM, Shinagare AB, Jagannathan JP, Ramaiya NH, et al. Imaging of hepatic toxicity of systemic therapy in a tertiary cancer centre: chemotherapy, haematopoietic stem cell transplantation, molecular targeted therapies, and immune checkpoint inhibitors. Clin Radiol. 2017;72(7):521–33.
59. Cramer P, Bresalier RS. Gastrointestinal and hepatic complications of immune checkpoint inhibitors. Curr Gastroenterol Rep. 2017;19(1):3.
60. Tripathi A, Kaymakcalan MD, LeBoeuf NR, Harshman LC. Programmed cell death-1 pathway inhibitors in genitourinary malignancies: specific side-effects and their management. Curr Opin Urol. 2016;26(6):548–55.
61. Chmiel KD, Suan D, Liddle C, Nankivell B, Ibrahim R, Bautista C, et al. Resolution of severe ipilimumab-induced hepatitis after antithymocyte globulin therapy. J Clin Oncol. 2011;29(9):e237–40.
62. Huffman BM, Kottschade LA, Kamath PS, Markovic SN. Hepatotoxicity after immune checkpoint inhibitor therapy in melanoma: natural progression and management. Am J Clin Oncol. 2018;41(8):760–5.
63. Grover S, Rahma OE, Hashemi N, Lim RM. Gastrointestinal and hepatic toxicities of checkpoint inhibitors: algorithms for management. Am Soc Clin Oncol Educ Book. 2018;38:13–9.
64. Spänkuch I, Gassenmaier M, Tampouri I, Noor S, Forschner A, Garbe C, et al. Severe hepatitis under combined immunotherapy: resolution under corticosteroids plus anti-thymocyte immunoglobulins. Eur J Cancer. 2017;81:203–5.
65. Postow MA. Managing immune checkpoint-blocking antibody side effects. Am Soc Clin Oncol Educ Book. 2015:76–83.
66. Kumar V, Chaudhary N, Garg M, Floudas CS, Soni P, Chandra AB. Current diagnosis and management of immune related adverse events (irAEs) induced by immune checkpoint inhibitor therapy. Front Pharmacol. 2017;8:49.
67. Hofmann L, Forschner A, Loquai C, Goldinger SM, Zimmer L, Ugurel S, et al. Cutaneous, gastrointestinal, hepatic, endocrine, and renal side-effects of anti-PD-1 therapy. Eur J Cancer. 2016;60:190–209.
68. Widmann G, Nguyen VA, Plaickner J, Jaschke W. Imaging features of toxicities by immune checkpoint inhibitors in cancer therapy. Curr Radiol Rep. 2016;5(11):59.
69. Pollack MH, Betof A, Dearden H, Rapazzo K, Valentine I, Brohl AS, et al. Safety of resuming anti-PD-1 in patients with immune-related adverse events (irAEs) during combined anti-CTLA-4 and anti-PD1 in metastatic melanoma. Ann Oncol. 2018;29(1):250–5.
70. Sznol M, Postow MA, Davies MJ, Pavlick AC, Plimack ER, Shaheen M, et al. Endocrine-related adverse events associated with immune checkpoint blockade and expert insights on their management. Cancer Treat Rev. 2017;58:70–6.
71. Byun DJ, Wolchok JD, Rosenberg LM, Girotra M. Cancer immunotherapy—immune checkpoint blockade and associated endocrinopathies. Nat Rev Endocrinol. 2017;13(4):195–207.
72. Barroso-Sousa R, Barry WT, Garrido-Castro AC, Hodi FS, Min L, Krop IE, et al. Incidence of endocrine dysfunction following the use of different immune checkpoint inhibitor regimens: a sys-

tematic review and meta-analysis. JAMA Oncol. 2018;4(2):173–82.
73. Brancatella A, Viola N, Brogioni S, Montanelli L, Sardella C, Vitti P, et al. Graves' disease induced by immune checkpoint inhibitors: a case report and review of the literature. Eur Thyroid J. 2019;8(4):192–5.
74. Faje A, Reynolds K, Zubiri L, Lawrence D, Cohen JV, Sullivan RJ, et al. Hypophysitis secondary to nivolumab and pembrolizumab is a clinical entity distinct from ipilimumab-associated hypophysitis. Eur J Endocrinol. 2019;181(3):211–9.
75. de Filette JMK, Pen JJ, Decoster L, Vissers T, Bravenboer B, Van der Auwera BJ, et al. Immune checkpoint inhibitors and type 1 diabetes mellitus: a case report and systematic review. Eur J Endocrinol. 2019;181(3):363–74.
76. Haanen J, Obeid M, Spain L, Carbonnel F, Wang Y, Robert C, et al. Management of toxicities from immunotherapy: ESMO clinical practice guideline for diagnosis, treatment and follow-up. Ann Oncol. 2022;33(12):1217–38.
77. Naidoo J, Wang X, Woo KM, Iyriboz T, Halpenny D, Cunningham J, et al. Pneumonitis in patients treated with anti-programmed death-1/programmed death ligand 1 therapy. J Clin Oncol. 2017;35(7):709–17.
78. Nishino M, Giobbie-Hurder A, Hatabu H, Ramaiya NH, Hodi FS. Incidence of programmed cell death 1 inhibitor-related pneumonitis in patients with advanced cancer: a systematic review and meta-analysis. JAMA Oncol. 2016;2(12):1607–16.
79. Hodi FS, O'Day SJ, McDermott DF, Weber RW, Sosman JA, Haanen JB, et al. Improved survival with ipilimumab in patients with metastatic melanoma. N Engl J Med. 2010;363(8):711–23.
80. Wolchok JD, Neyns B, Linette G, Negrier S, Lutzky J, Thomas L, et al. Ipilimumab monotherapy in patients with pretreated advanced melanoma: a randomised, double-blind, multicentre, phase 2, dose-ranging study. Lancet Oncol. 2010;11(2):155–64.
81. Chuzi S, Tavora F, Cruz M, Costa R, Chae YK, Carneiro BA, et al. Clinical features, diagnostic challenges, and management strategies in checkpoint inhibitor-related pneumonitis. Cancer Manag Res. 2017;9:207–13.
82. Delaunay M, Prévot G, Collot S, Guilleminault L, Didier A, Mazières J. Management of pulmonary toxicity associated with immune checkpoint inhibitors. Eur Respir Rev. 2019;28(154):190012.
83. Suresh K, Voong KR, Shankar B, Forde PM, Ettinger DS, Marrone KA, et al. Pneumonitis in non-small cell lung cancer patients receiving immune checkpoint immunotherapy: incidence and risk factors. J Thorac Oncol. 2018;13(12):1930–9.
84. Travis WD, Costabel U, Hansell DM, King TE, Lynch DA, Nicholson AG, et al. An official American Thoracic Society/European Respiratory Society statement: update of the international multidisciplinary classification of the idiopathic interstitial pneumonias. Am J Respir Crit Care Med. 2013;188(6):733–48.
85. Cooksley T, Marshall W, Gupta A. Early infliximab in life-threatening immune-mediated pneumonitis. QJM. 2019;112(12):929–30.
86. Sawai Y, Katsuya Y, Shinozaki-Ushiku A, Iwasaki A, Fukayama M, Watanabe K, et al. Rapid temporal improvement of pembrolizumab-induced pneumonitis using the anti-TNF-α antibody infliximab. Drug Discov Ther. 2019;13(3):164–7.
87. Stroud CR, Hegde A, Cherry C, Naqash AR, Sharma N, Addepalli S, et al. Tocilizumab for the management of immune mediated adverse events secondary to PD-1 blockade. J Oncol Pharm Pract. 2019;25(3):551–7.
88. Petri CR, Patell R, Batalini F, Rangachari D, Hallowell RW. Severe pulmonary toxicity from immune checkpoint inhibitor treated successfully with intravenous immunoglobulin: case report and review of the literature. Respir Med Case Rep. 2019;27:100834.
89. Calabrese LH, Calabrese C, Cappelli LC. Rheumatic immune-related adverse events from cancer immunotherapy. Nat Rev Rheumatol. 2018;14(10):569–79.
90. Haugh AM, Probasco JC, Johnson DB. Neurologic complications of immune checkpoint inhibitors. Expert Opin Drug Saf. 2020;19(4):479–88.
91. Lyon AR, Yousaf N, Battisti NML, Moslehi J, Larkin J. Immune checkpoint inhibitors and cardiovascular toxicity. Lancet Oncol. 2018;19(9):e447–58.
92. McDonagh TA, Metra M, Adamo M, Gardner RS, Baumbach A, Böhm M, et al. 2021 ESC Guidelines for the diagnosis and treatment of acute and chronic heart failure. Eur Heart J. 2021;42(36):3599–726.
93. Seethapathy H, Zhao S, Chute DF, Zubiri L, Oppong Y, Strohbehn I, et al. The incidence, causes, and risk factors of acute kidney injury in patients receiving immune checkpoint inhibitors. Clin J Am Soc Nephrol. 2019;14(12):1692–700.
94. Kramer R, Zaremba A, Moreira A, Ugurel S, Johnson DB, Hassel JC, et al. Hematological immune related adverse events after treatment with immune checkpoint inhibitors. Eur J Cancer. 2021;147:170–81.
95. Delanoy N, Michot JM, Comont T, Kramkimel N, Lazarovici J, Dupont R, et al. Haematological immune-related adverse events induced by anti-PD-1 or anti-PD-L1 immunotherapy: a descriptive observational study. Lancet Haematol. 2019;6(1):e48–57.
96. Özdemir BC, Latifyan S, Perreau M, Fenwick C, Alberio L, Waeber G, et al. Cytokine-directed therapy with tocilizumab for immune checkpoint inhibitor-related hemophagocytic lymphohistiocytosis. Ann Oncol. 2020;31(12):1775–8.
97. Fang T, Maberley DA, Etminan M. Ocular adverse events with immune checkpoint inhibitors. J Curr Ophthalmol. 2019;31(3):319–22.
98. Bitton K, Michot JM, Barreau E, Lambotte O, Haigh O, Marabelle A, et al. Prevalence and clinical patterns of ocular complications associated with

anti-PD-1/PD-L1 anticancer immunotherapy. Am J Ophthalmol. 2019;202:109–17.
99. Presley CJ, Gomes F, Burd CE, Kanesvaran R, Wong ML. Immunotherapy in older adults with cancer. J Clin Oncol. 2021;39(19):2115–27.
100. Elias R, Giobbie-Hurder A, McCleary NJ, Ott P, Hodi FS, Rahma O. Efficacy of PD-1 & PD-L1 inhibitors in older adults: a meta-analysis. J Immunother Cancer. 2018;6(1):26.
101. Baxi S, Yang A, Gennarelli RL, Khan N, Wang Z, Boyce L, et al. Immune-related adverse events for anti-PD-1 and anti-PD-L1 drugs: systematic review and meta-analysis. BMJ. 2018;360:k793.
102. Sattar J, Kartolo A, Hopman WM, Lakoff JM, Baetz T. The efficacy and toxicity of immune checkpoint inhibitors in a real-world older patient population. J Geriatr Oncol. 2019;10(3):411–4.
103. Manzo C, Serra-Mestres J, Castagna A, Isetta M. Behavioral, psychiatric, and cognitive adverse events in older persons treated with glucocorticoids. Medicines (Basel). 2018;5(3):82.
104. Kyi C, Hellmann MD, Wolchok JD, Chapman PB, Postow MA. Opportunistic infections in patients treated with immunotherapy for cancer. J Immunother Cancer. 2014;2:19.

7 Hormone Therapy and Oral Medications in Breast Cancer

Cigdem Dinckal and Murat Akyol

7.1 Introduction

In patients with hormone receptor (HR) positive early breast cancer (eBC), endocrine therapy (ET) is one of the adjuvant therapies used to lower the risk of recurrence and death. Also, anti-estrogen therapy is a crucial part of treating HR positive breast cancer in advanced stages. Treatment for early-stage and advanced-stage BC expressing the estrogen receptor (ER) and/or progesterone receptor (PR) must include anti-estrogen medication that targets the estrogen-mediated signaling system [1]. By definition, 80% of all breast tumors express ER and/or PR, making them susceptible to treatments known as "ET" that target the estrogen signaling system [2]. Despite its proven efficacy, ET has side effects, which can persist over time even if low grade, and may deteriorate the quality of life of patients undergoing ET. This might result in early treatment termination and poor therapeutic adherence, which would worsen survival results. Therefore, side effect management should be a part of the treatment of breast cancer patients receiving ET [3].

Estrogen is a steroid hormone by nature. The most important natural estrogens include E1, E2, and estriol (E3). In the pre-menopausal period, estrogen biosynthesis in women occurs in the granulose cells of mature follicles in the ovaries. During pregnancy, estrogen synthesis also occurs from the placenta. The mechanism of active estrogen synthesis from steroid sulfate is defined as "intracrine estrogen synthesis." This synthesis of estrogens occurs especially in peripheral tissues such as skin, muscle, fat, bone, and mammary glands, catalyzed by the aromatase enzyme [4]. It is accepted that intracrine estrogen synthesis in the peripheral tissue plays an important role in constituting 75% of the total estrogen formation in premenopausal women and nearly 100% in postmenopausal women [4]. Before menopause, estrogen and progesterone formation occur in the ovary. These hormones are controlled by the hypothalamus via gonadotropin-releasing hormone (GnRH) and by follicle-stimulating hormone (FSH) and luteinizing hormone (LH) from the anterior pituitary lobe. The interruption of the premenopausal and postmenopausal hormonal axis with hormonal treatment is schematized (Fig. 7.1).

Aromatase transforms androgens produced by the breast, ovaries, adrenal glands, adipose tissue, and other tissues into estrogens. The ER dimerizes and translocates to the nucleus after binding

C. Dinckal (✉)
Department of Medical Oncology, Izmir Katip Celebi University Ataturk Training and Research Hospital, Izmir, Turkey

M. Akyol
Department of Medical Oncology, Izmir Bakircay University Cigli Training and Research Hospital, Izmir, Turkey

Y. Bakar, A. Tuğral (eds.), *Managing Side Effects of Breast Cancer Treatment*,
https://doi.org/10.1007/978-3-031-75480-7_7

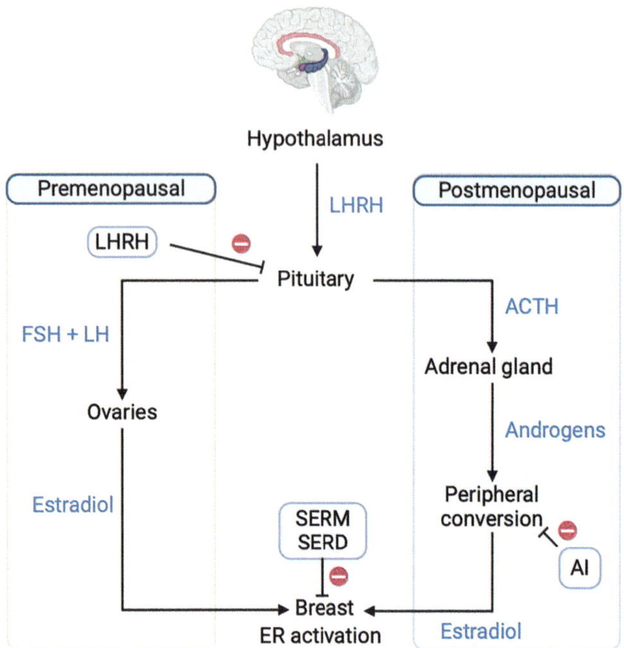

Fig. 7.1 Hormonal treatment for ER positive breast cancer. (Created with Biorender.com). Postmenapausal pathway: ACTH, adrenocorticotropic hormone; ER, estrogen receptor. Premenapausal pathway: FSH, follicle stimulating hormone; LH, luteinizing hormone; ER, estrogen receptor. Pathway blockers: AI, aromatase inhibitor; LHRHa, luteinizing hormone releasing hormone agonist; SERD, selective estrogen receptor degrader; SERM, selective estrogen receptor modulator

to estrogen. There, it binds to coactivators (CoA) to create an ER complex that is transcriptionally active [2]. The ER, a steroid hormone nuclear receptor, is composed of the transcriptional activation function domains 1 (AF1) and 2 (AF2), the ligand-binding domain (LBD), and the DNA-binding domain (DBD). Through its DBD or interactions with other transcription factors, activated ER can interact with estrogen-responsive regions within the DNA [5]. The ER functions as a transcription factor activated by estrogen binding and plays a role in regulating numerous genes implicated in tumor formation [6].

The mainstays of antiestrogen therapy include fulvestrant (SERD), tamoxifen (SERM), and anastrozole, letrozole, exemestane (AIs). Since its FDA approval, tamoxifen remains the most important part of the treatment of HR-positive BC. Effective targeted medicines, including CDK4/6 inhibitors and PI3K/Akt/mTOR signaling pathway inhibitors, have been developed by studying the molecular biology of estrogen-positive BC. However, research on new hormonal treatments (including SERD) to overcome endocrine resistance in HR-positive breast cancer continues rapidly [7].

Over the course of their treatment, many patients become resistant to hormone therapy. The primary mechanism of resistance, constitutive receptor activation in the absence of ligand, is caused by mutations that appear in the estrogen receptor gene (ESR1). As hormone therapy is used as the first line of treatment for metastatic BC, ESR1 mutations may not be present in these patients. However, as hormone therapy resistance develops, liquid biopsy can discover these mutations more frequently. Numerous other genetic changes are linked to resistance in addition to ESR1 mutations [6].

For high-risk ER positive eBC, the aim is to reduce short- and long-term recurrence risk through a locally controlled system and treatment with surgery, radiation, and ET. Despite these interventions, clinical trials, such as targeting receptor alpha (ERα) of novel oral receptors for ER positive disease, are ongoing due to the risk of relapse [8].

Anti-estrogen treatments are covered in this chapter, some of which were created to circumvent prevalent endocrine resistance mechanisms. Among the latest generation of medications are proteolysis targeting chimeras (PROTACs), selective estrogen receptor covalent antagonists (SERCAs), selective estrogen receptor modulators (SERMs), selective estrogen receptor degraders (SERDs), and complete estrogen receptor antagonists (CERANs). These medications are being assessed in early and metastatic settings and are in different phases of drug development [9].

We give a summary of the many classes of hormone therapy that are currently being developed for use in clinical practice as well as the newer forms of treatment. This section aims to give a summary of the evidence that is currently available about the mechanisms of action of ET and a review of the adverse effects associated with ET.

7.2 Selective Estrogen Receptor Modulators (SERMs)

Tamoxifen and raloxifene are examples of SERMs that competitively limit the binding of estrogen to the ER. Interactions between ER dimers bound to SERM and the chromatin at estrogen response elements exist. Nonetheless, corepressors (CoR), which suppress ER transcriptional activity in the breast, are linked to SERM-bound ER dimers [10].

A class of nonsteroidal drugs known as SERMs has antiestrogen effects (antagonism) on certain tissues (e.g., breast or uterus) and estrogen-like actions (agonism) on other tissues (e.g., bone, skin, heart, or vaginal epithelium). These drugs can have varied therapeutic effects, indications, and unfavorable side effects depending on the tissue specificity and balance of the agonist and antagonist activities. Therapy or prevention of postmenopausal osteoporosis (raloxifene, bazedoxifene), therapy or prevention of BC (tamoxifen, toremifene, raloxifene), and relief of menopausal symptoms (ospemifene) are common indications for SERMS [11]. SERM drugs are classified according to their chemical groups together with their side effects in Table 7.1 [12].

Tamoxifen was the first hormone treatment to be discovered. Since the FDA approved it in the late 1970s, it has been the gold standard for treating BC and is credited with saving many lives all over the world. Tamoxifen is sometimes called an antiestrogen therapy since it blocks the effects of estrogen in breast tissue. It can also mimic the effects of estrogen in other tissues, including the bone and uterus, which could account for certain significant negative effects associated with long-term use. A woman who has surgery for early-stage, invasive breast cancer is more likely to live a longer life if the tamoxifen is prescribed. Adjuvant therapy is usually taken for a minimum of 5 years and can be given after surgery. Also, tamoxifen can help limit the spread of the disease. More than that, tamoxifen is a chemopreventive drug that may be helpful for women who are more likely to develop breast cancer [13].

Antiestrogen medications differ in how they affect different tissues and compete with estrogen for ER binding. In other tissues, they can mimic the effects of estrogen binding and exhibit agonistic action, but in the breast, they function as antagonists by recruiting transcriptional corepressors to prevent ER-dependent transcription. Because menopause naturally lowers estrogen levels, SERMs are the most frequently used medications by premenopausal women [12].

Table 7.1 Common adverse events and the chemical structures of various SERM classes

Pharmacological group	Generic group	Adverse events
Triphenylethylene	Tamoxifen	Endometrial stimulation, hot flushes
	Clomifene	Hot flushes
	Toremifene	Endometrial stimulation, hot flushes
	Ospemiphene	Endometrial stimulation, vaginal maturation
Other nonsteroidal compounds	Raloxifene	Endometrial stimulation, hot flushes
Naphthalenes	Lasofoxifene	Endometrial stimulation, vaginal maturation, hot flush
Findoles	Basedoxifene	Hot flushes

Tamoxifen is a nonsteroidal anti-estrogen drug frequently used in the treatment of ER+ BC. It has a partial estrogen agonist effect. Resistance is the main problem in ET. Response to tamoxifen is often limited in time, indicating that individuals may eventually become resistant to the drug. Despite the great success of ET combined with tamoxifen, therapeutic resistance occurs in 20–30% of patients. More than 50% of individuals with ER+ BC respond to the drug tamoxifen, but metastatic phase reports indicate that 40% of patients receiving tamoxifen as adjuvant therapy eventually relapse and die from the disease [14].

A number of pathways, including genetic and epigenetic variables, are responsible for the development of resistance to ET. Mutations in the ESR1 gene have been linked to acquired resistance from chronic exposure to ET with anti-estrogens, which is one of the key pathways leading to tamoxifen resistance. The reduction of ER expression and the emergence of treatment resistance are caused by certain point mutations in ESR1 that are linked to resistance. When hormone stimulation is absent, these alterations lead to further tumor growth and proliferation [14].

Regarding the side effects of SERM drugs, although constitutional symptoms are common in patients taking tamoxifen, caution should be exercised in terms of rare significant side effects.

The mode of action of tamoxifen involves acting as a competitive antagonist of the alpha-estrogen receptor in breast tissue while exhibiting agonistic properties in endometrial tissue, the extent of which depends on dosage and duration. The impact of the beta-estrogen receptor in the endometrium clarifies the heightened occurrence of endometrial pathologies such as hyperplasia, atypia, or malignancy. Prolonged exposure, particularly in postmenopausal women with pre-existing uterine conditions, escalates the risk of associated uterine malignancies. Hence, regular gynecological examinations for patients are crucial due to the potential risk of endometrial cancer [15].

Additional drugs in the SERM class include toremifene, which is structurally very similar to tamoxifen and has similar efficacy and safety profiles, and raloxifene, a second-generation SERM that is approved for reducing the risk of invasive BC in postmenopausal women but it is not used as a therapy. Because of its actions on the bone, raloxifene can prevent bone loss, and it is licensed for the treatment and prevention of postmenopausal osteoporosis [11].

Lasofoxifene is a next generation nonsteroidal SERM originally developed to treat vulvovaginal atrophy and osteoporosis because of its ability to mimic estrogen in the bone. It binds to the ER with a similar potency as estrogen and causes a conformational change that prevents the recruitment of cofactors. It is effective in inhibiting lung and liver metastasis in ESR1-mutant models. Lasofoxifene is being evaluated in a phase II trial in comparison with fulvestrant for the treatment of postmenopausal and premenopausal women with locally advanced or metastatic ER-positive BC and an ESR1 mutation, whose disease has progressed after treatment with the standard-of-care therapy (AI plus CDK4/6 inhibitor) [16]. The most common side effects of lasofoxifene are fatigue, nausea, arthralgias, and hot flashes [9].

Bazedoxifene is a third-generation nonsteroidal SERM that functions as an agonist in the bone (it is approved in Europe for the treatment of osteoporosis) but can also induce ER degradation in the reproductive system and is therefore considered a SERM/SERD hybrid. Bazedoxifene has shown activity in tamoxifen-resistant preclinical models and against mutant ESR1 in combination with the CDK4/6 inhibitor palbociclib. This combination is currently being evaluated in patients with ER+, endocrine-resistant metastatic BC [17].

7.3 Aromatase Inhibitors (AIs)

Aromatase inhibitors (AIs), which were first approved in the 1990s, work by inhibiting the enzyme that is responsible for producing estrogen. They are used in postmenopausal women to prevent residual synthesis of estrogen in extra-ovarian tissues (adrenal glands and adipose tissue). Some premenopausal women with ER+ BC may also benefit from treatment with an AI if their ovarian function is compromised. When treating early-stage ER+ BC, tamoxifen has more detrimental side effects than AIs [18].

By preventing the aromatization of androgens to estrogens, nonsteroidal, reversible AIs like letrozole or anastrozole and steroidal, irreversible AIs like exemestane prevent the synthesis of estrogen [19] (Table 7.2).

For postmenopausal ER+ BC patients, AIs represent one of the main therapeutic alternatives. By inhibiting the aromatase enzyme, which changes androgen hormone into trace levels of estrogen, AIs prevent postmenopausal women from producing estrogen. Worldwide, all clinical stages of breast cancer are treated with AIs such as letrozole, exemestane, and anastrozole. While exemestane is a steroidal AI, anastrozole and letrozole are nonsteroidal AIs. While it has been demonstrated that these three substances can reduce total plasma and tissue estrogen levels by more than 90%, research indicates that letrozole is among the nonsteroidal substances with the highest potency. When a patient develops resistance to the initial treatment, these AIs can be utilized in a sequential manner to treat metastatic BC and perhaps elicit new responses. For instance, if a patient with metastatic breast cancer relapses after receiving initial treatment with a nonsteroidal AI (letrozole or anastrozole), they may benefit from a steroidal AI (exemestane). There is, nevertheless, little data regarding the advantages of utilizing a nonsteroidal AI following a steroid AI [14].

The following are examples of common adverse responses (10% incidence): uterine atrophy, sexual dysfunction, asthenia, joint disorders like arthralgia or arthritis, osteoporosis, fractures, bone pain, back pain, dry vagina, dyspareunia, thromboembolic events, heart attacks and cerebrovascular events, insomnia, nausea, and hot flashes. Especially in the post-menopausal period, one should be very careful in terms of osteoporosis, and patients should have a baseline bone mineral density test (DEXA) before initiating the treatment [20].

Classical anti-estrogen treatments that we have tried to summarize so far; the drug class, pharmacokinetics, toxicities, and doses are summarized in Table 7.3 [21].

Table 7.2 Classification of aromatase inhibitors

Drug generation	Tip1 steroidal inhibitor	Tip2 nonsteroidal inhibitor
First	None	Aminoglutethimide
Second	Formestan	Fadrazole, rogletimide
Third	Exemestane	Anastrozole, letrozole, vorozole

Table 7.3 Classic anti-estrogen therapies

Drug	Drug class	Pharmacokinetics	Toxicity	Dosage
Tamoxifen	Nonsteroidal antiestrogen; cytostatic actions on malignant cells that are both estrogen-dependent and -independent	Both tamoxifen and its metabolite are not present in the bile or urine. Its oral bioavailability is good. It has a half-life of approximately 7 days after being metabolized in the liver	Generally, well tolerated. The most common constitutional symptoms are hot flushes, sweating, mood swings, and weight gain. Other symptoms are nausea, vomiting, diarrhea, and constipation. Menstrual abnormalities such as heavy vaginal bleeding, myelosuppression, retinopathy, and venous thromboembolism are rare	10 mg PO BID or 20 mg QD
Letrozole	Nonsteroidal aromatase inhibitor	With a daily dosage, about 100% absorption, a 2-day half-life, and steady state plasma levels reached in 4–6 weeks	Well tolerated. Hot flushes, exhaustion, muscle aches, and nausea are rare. Urticaria, indigestion, and weight fluctuation are uncommon	2.5 mg PO QD
Fulvestrant	Binds to ER, leading to degradation and loss of ER from the cell	Peak plasma levels in 7 days, CYP3A4 metabolism, half-life of 40 days	Hot flushes, peripheral edema, nausea, vomiting	500 mg intramuscular days 1, 15, 29, first month, then every month after that
Exemestane	Steroidal aromatase inhibitor	The quantity of exemestane absorbed from the GI tract rises after a fatty meal. Cytochrome p450 3A4 is responsible for the liver's metabolism of exemestane	Hot flashes or sporadic flushing, headaches, moderate nausea, exhaustion, vomiting, and dyspnea	25 mg PO QD

Adapted from: Abeloff Textbook Cancer Pharmacology, Chapter 25, Part I: Science and Clinical Oncology

7.4 Luteinizing Hormone-Releasing Hormone Agonists (LHRHa)

The cornerstones of treatment for both early-stage and advanced HR-positive (HR+) BC include chemotherapy and endocrine treatments. The advantages of combining ovarian function suppression (OFS) with ET in premenopausal women with HR+ malignancies have been discussed. As such, the accepted standard of care for ET in the adjuvant situation has been tamoxifen monotherapy for many years. However, recent research has shown that OFS plus tamoxifen or AIs can considerably improve survival compared to tamoxifen alone in certain premenopausal patients. FSH and LH are released from the pituitary, and prolonged suppression of this process is achieved by LHRHa, such as goserelin, triptorelin, and leuprorelin, to produce OFS. Consequently, this inhibits the synthesis and release of estradiol, an ovarian hormone that promotes the growth, survival, and multiplication of cancer cells [3].

The quality of life of patients is significantly impacted by the numerous negative symptoms of LHRHa, including osteopenia, metabolic syndrome, loss of muscular mass, heat flushes, and sexual dysfunction. Therefore, it is important to evaluate patients at routine intervals with comprehensive biochemistry and to follow them up in terms of bone health [22]. Practical information

Table 7.4 Luteinizing hormone releasing-hormone agonists

Drug	Drug class	Pharmacokinetics	Toxicity	Dosage
Leuprolide acetate, leuprorelin acetate	With prolonged exposure, GnRH agonists paradoxically block the pituitary gland's secretion of gonadotropins. This prevents a sharp decrease in gonadal hormones and also the growth of hormone-dependent tumors	Once administered subcutaneously, the medication is absorbed. While the drug's depot form absorbs slowly over days, the injectable solution absorbs over hours. The medication has a 3-h half-life in serum	Hot flashes, impotence, gynecomastia, breast tenderness, decreased libido, amenorrhea, atrophic vaginitis, elevated cholesterol, vomiting, constipation or diarrhea, hepatitis, rash, depression, emotional disorder, rare cardiac toxicity	Leuprorelin acetate corresponding to 7.5, 22.5, and 45 mg leuprorelin, respectively, is contained in SC or IM depot injections (1, 3, 6 monthly)
Goserelin acetate	LHRH pituitary-gonadal pressures cause withdrawal of steroid hormones from relevant tissues	The drug's depot is progressively released over 28 days after SC injection into adipose tissue, peaking at 12–15 days. The medicine is almost entirely eliminated through the urinary system, with an elimination half-life of 4 h	Amenorrhea, gynecomastia, impotence, hot flashes, decreased libido, and breakthrough vaginal bleeding	3.6 mg SC every 28 days or 10.8 mg SC every 3 months

Adapted from: Abeloff Textbook Cancer Pharmacology, Chapter 25, part I: Science and Clinical Oncology

and side effects regarding the use of LHRHa are summarized in Table 7.4 [21].

7.5 Selective Estrogen Receptor Downregulators (SERDs)

Pure ER antagonists are defined as SERDs, like fulvestrant. Recently, the diminished capacity of ER bound to SERDs to translocate to the nucleus was suggested as the cause of the inhibitory impact of SERDs. Moreover, the ER-SERD complex is not able to create an open chromatin conformation that would aid in ER-regulated gene transcription. The deterioration of SERD-bound ER results from reduced mobility [23]. These materials cling to the ER, stopping it from migrating into the nucleus and weakening and destabilizing it in the process. Fulvestrant is the first approved SERD. Later, its application was broadened to encompass first-line care for cancer patients who had not previously received ET and were either progressed or metastatic. Fulvestrant was first licensed to treat postmenopausal patients with metastatic disease who had been resistant to prior ET. Unlike tamoxifen, fulvestrant does not have estrogen-like actions in the uterus [23].

Fulvestrant functions as an ER antagonist by binding to, blocking, and degrading ER and suppressing ER transcriptional activity. Unlike tamoxifen, fulvestrant is an ER positive regulator with little cytotoxicity. As a result, it has a stronger effect than tamoxifen. Fulvestrant can only be administered as an intramuscular injection, which limits the dose that can be delivered and makes the administration less practical. However, the main advantages of this class of agents are that they can be administered orally and have better absorption and higher potency.

Furthermore, oral SERDs demonstrated activity in preclinical models of ESR1 mutation, which exhibited resistance to fulvestrant. Patients

Table 7.5 Typical side effects of new oral SERDs

SERDs	Daily monotherapy dose (mg)	Common adverse events
Elacestrant	400	Nausea, exhaustion, vomiting, loss of appetite, and arthralgia
Giredestrant	30	Exhaustion, arthritis, back discomfort, nausea, diarrhea, coughing, constipation
Camizestrant	75	Bradycardia, nausea, exhaustion, dizziness, vomiting, asthenia, and visual abnormalities
Imlunestrant	400	Constipation, headache, arthralgia, diarrhea, nausea, and urinary tract infection
Rintodestrant	800	Exhaustion, hot flushes, nausea, diarrhea, and vomiting

with the ESR1 mutant tumors, severely pretreated ER-positive, HER2 negative metastatic BC, and patients who had progressed on CDK4/6 inhibitor and/or fulvestrant therapy have all responded to oral SERDs. Phase III trials are testing the following five oral SERDs: Elacestrant, Amcenestrant, Giredestrant, Camizestrant, and Imlunestrant. The FDA approved Elacestrant as the first oral SERD in 2023 [24].

Overall, the oral SERDs have been well tolerated; fatigue and nausea are the most common class-related adverse effects in the grade 1–2 range. Certain SERDs also showed hot flushes and arthritis, which are typical side effects of AIs. The most common gastrointestinal side effects of elacestrant include nausea, vomiting, and dyspepsia; however, with the tablet formulation, these side effects were half as common as with the capsule form [23]. Since new oral SERDs have just entered practice and are still in the clinical research phase, awareness about their side effects is important. These new SERDs may also have unique side effects. A summary of common adverse events is presented in Table 7.5.

7.6 Selective Estrogen Receptor Covalent Antagonists (SERCAs)

This class of compounds covalently inactivates both wild type and mutant ER by targeting an amino acid residue that is conserved in both and promotes a conformational change that represses the transcription of estrogen target genes. The oral H3B-6545 is a first-in-class agent described that confirmed its increased antitumor activity compared to fulvestrant in mouse models carrying both wild-type and mutant ER. H3B-6545 is being investigated in phase I trials in locally advanced and metastatic BC as a monotherapy and in combination with CDK4/6 inhibitors [25]. The most common side effects of H3B-6545 are nausea, fatigue, diarrhea, decrease in GFR, anemia, lymphopenia, increase in ALT and AST, bilirubin, creatinine, and asymptomatic sinus bradycardia [9].

7.7 Complete Estrogen Receptor Antagonists (CERANs)

ER contains two domains that can activate gene transcription. Research has shown that tamoxifen is a partial ER antagonist because it only blocks one of the two activating domains. The oral small molecule OP-1250 represents a pioneering complete ER antagonist, capable of deactivating both wild type and mutant ER domains, as evidenced by its efficacy in preclinical investigations. Notably, OP-1250 exhibits no agonistic effects in the uterus, thus mitigating concerns regarding heightened susceptibility to endometrial cancer [26]. The most frequent adverse reactions of OP-1250 include neutropenia, nausea, constipation, headache, exhaustion, vomiting, and maculopapular rash [9].

7.8 Proteolysis-Targeting Chimeras (PROTACs)

ER ligands and a ligand that acts as a substrate for the E3 ubiquitin ligase complex combine to form heterobifunctional molecules known as proteolysis targeting chimeras, or PROTACs. Once PROTACs attach to ER, they attract the E3 ubiquitin ligase complex, which polyubiquitylates ER and designates it for breakdown by proteases [27]. These agents exploit the body's protein degradation machinery to degrade oncogenic proteins. They bind to the ER and recruit the E3 ubiquitin ligase, which targets the receptor for rapid and complete degradation, affording complete antagonistic activity. ARV-471 is a first-in-class PROTAC currently in phase II trial for testing as a single agent and in combination with CDK-4/6 inhibition in patients with locally advanced or metastatic BC [28]. AST rise, weariness, nausea, and vomiting are the most frequent side effects of ARV-471 [9].

7.9 Conclusion

Anti-estrogen therapy plays a crucial role in treating both early and advanced-stage HR-positive BC. Despite the availability of several endocrine therapies for ER positive BC, their therapeutic efficacy is hampered by drug resistance. ESR1 mutations commonly underlie resistance to endocrine therapy. While fulvestrant, a first-generation SERD, shows promise against ESR1 mutant cancers, its efficacy is limited by poor absorption and the need for intramuscular injection, hindering optimal dosage delivery. The emergence of next-generation drugs, including orally administered SERMs, SERDs, and innovative agents such as CERANs, PROTACs, and SERCAs, is being explored at various stages of drug development, both in the early and metastatic phases (Fig. 7.2).

Although ET has advantages, there are often negative side effects as well. Various endocrine-related side effects, such as vasomotor symptoms, musculoskeletal problems, menopause, fatigue, psychological disorders, ocular toxicity, metabolic changes, and bone density loss, are frequently seen by breast cancer patients undergoing ET. Vasomotor symptoms, which can appear as hot flashes and/or night sweats, are the most common adverse effect among these, affecting up to 95% of premenopausal persons and 30% of postmenopausal patients getting adjuvant ET for eBC [29]. Sometimes the side effects lead to people stopping their treatment, which lowers their quality of life. Table 7.6 lists the most common side effects associated with ET. It is possible to manage these adverse effects with pharmaceutical and non-pharmacological methods, such as cognitive behavioral therapy and lifestyle modifications [3].

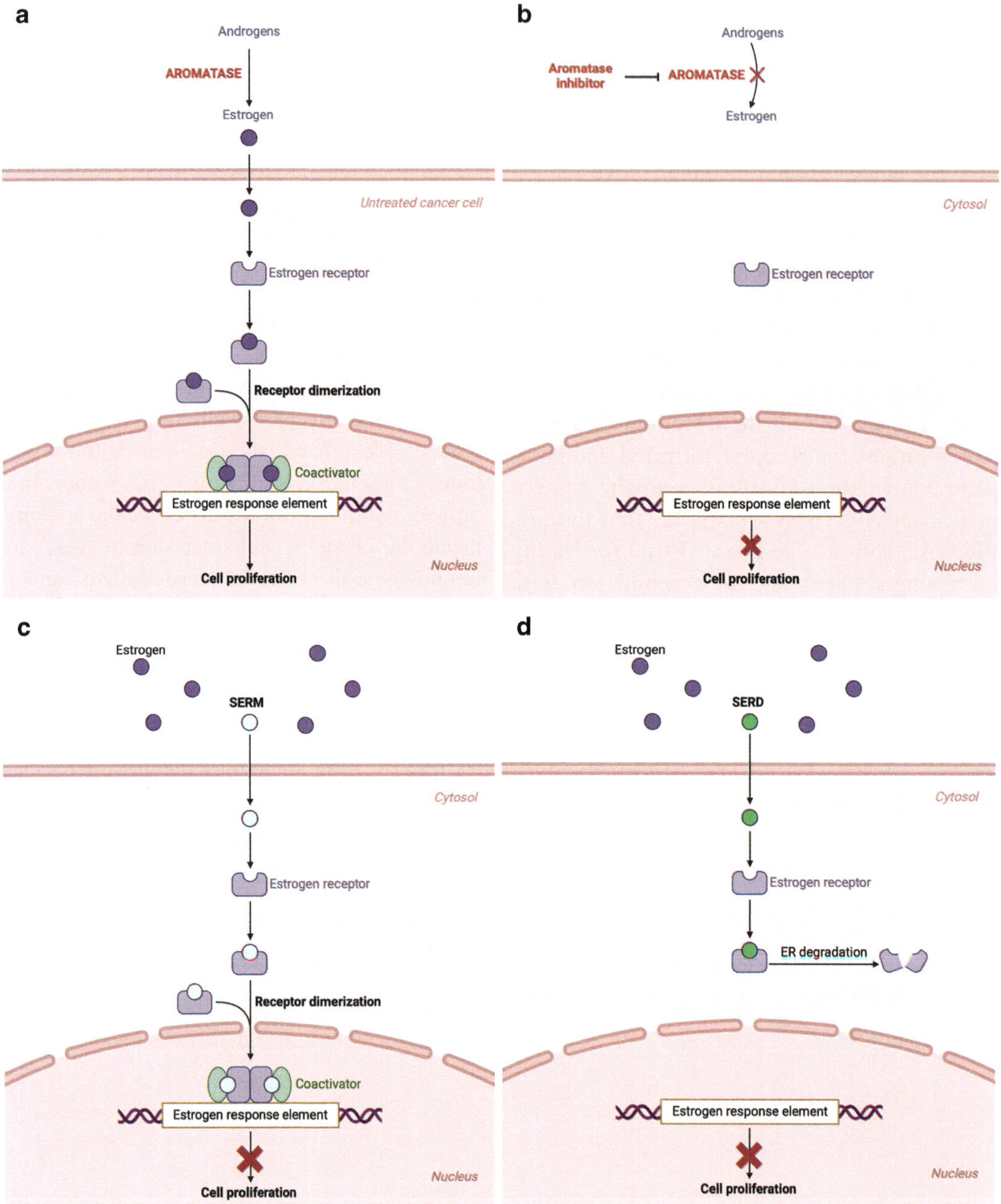

Fig. 7.2 Mechanism of action of endocrine therapies. (**a**) The estrogen receptor's dimerization and intranuclear localization are made possible by an activating conformational shift that is induced when estrogen binds to its ligand binding domain. By interacting with estrogenresponsive components, an activated estrogen receptor can facilitate gene transcription, which promotes cell survival and growth. (**b**) By blocking aromatase, which changes androgens into estrogens, aromatase inhibitors prevent the generation of estrogen. (**c**) SERMs competitively block estrogen from binding to the estrogen receptor. (**d**) Pure estrogen receptor antagonists are known as SERDs. In order to enable transcription of genes controlled by the estrogen receptor (ER), the SERD-estrogen receptor complex is unable to go into the nucleus or adopt an open chromatin shape. After that, the SERD-ER complex is broken down by proteasomes. (**e**) Bifunctional molecules known as PROTACs are made up of two ligands: one that attaches to the ER and the other to the E3 ubiquitin ligase. The connection triggers the ubiquitin-proteasome complex to ubiquitinate and degrade the target protein. (**f**) CERANs block both transcriptional activation domains of the ER (AF1 and AF2) via nuclear receptor corepressors to inactivate AF1 and directly inhibit AF2. (**g**) SERCAs inactivate the ER and limit gene transcription by covalently attaching to a cysteine residue on the ER. (Created with Biorender.com)

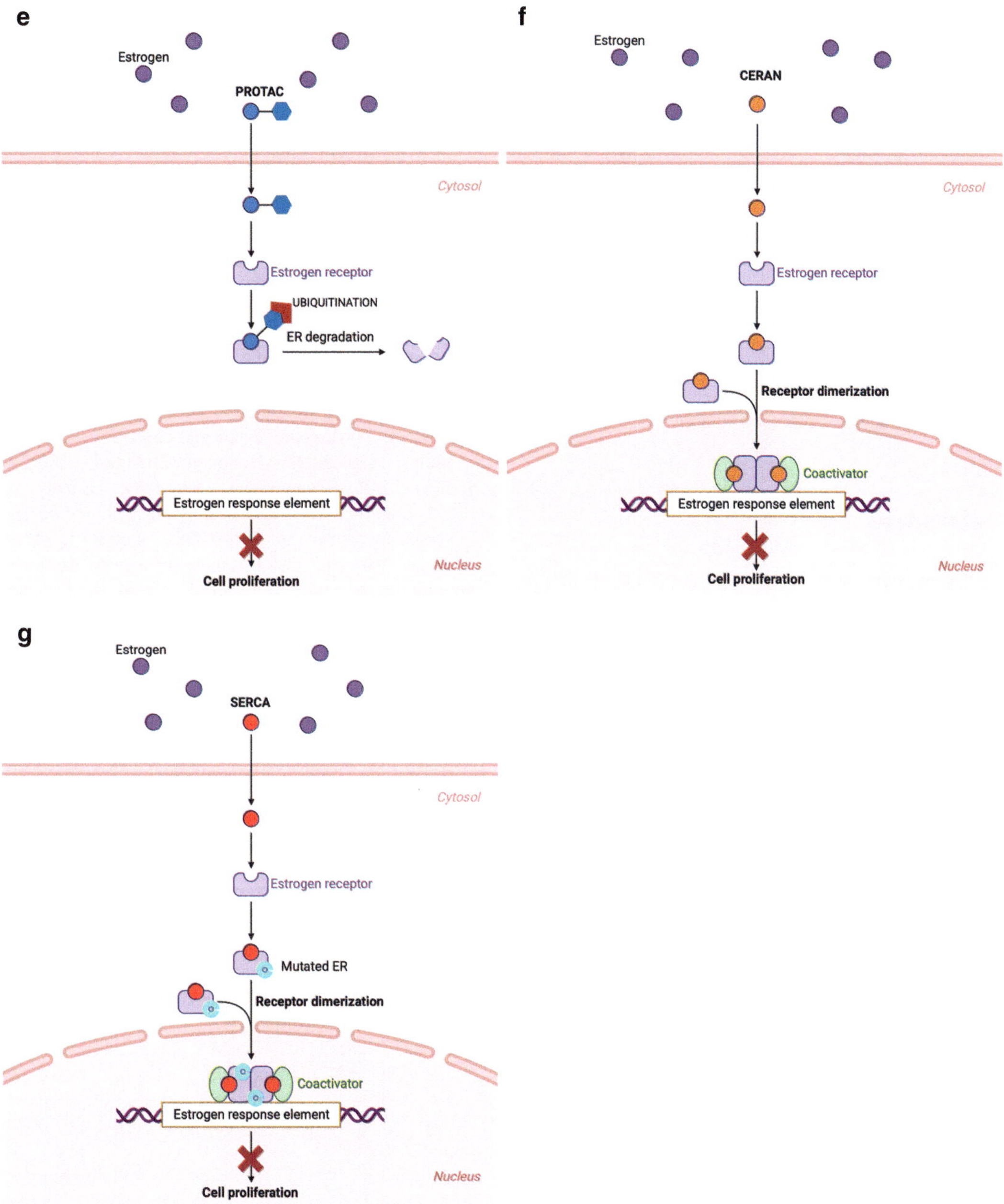

Fig. 7.2 (continued)

Table 7.6 Side effects of major endocrine therapy in patients with breast cancer

Major endocrine therapy side effects	Incidence %
Vasomotor symptoms	>95%
Musculoskeletal issues	>46%
Metabolic disorders	~20%
Menopause	25–55%
Fertility impairment	NA
Osteopenia/osteoporosis	NA
Alopecia	2.5–9%
Fatigue	60%
Insomnia	50%
Psychosomatic disorders	~30%
Ocular toxicity	~30%

ET endocrine therapy, *NA* not available

References

1. Burstein HJ, Somerfield MR, Barton DL, Dorris A, Fallowfield LJ, Jain D, et al. Endocrine treatment and targeted therapy for hormone receptor-positive, human epidermal growth factor receptor 2-negative metastatic breast cancer: ASCO guideline update. J Clin Oncol. 2021;39(35):3959–77.
2. Hanker AB, Sudhan DR, Arteaga CL. Overcoming endocrine resistance in breast cancer. Cancer Cell. 2020;37(4):496–513.
3. Cucciniello L, Garufi G, Di Rienzo R, Martinelli C, Pavone G, Giuliano M, et al. Estrogen deprivation effects of endocrine therapy in breast cancer patients: incidence, management and outcome. Cancer Treat Rev. 2023;120:102624.
4. Sasano H, Suzuki T, Nakata T, Moriya T. New development in intracrinology of breast carcinoma. Breast Cancer. 2006;13(2):129–36.
5. Heldring N, Pike A, Andersson S, Matthews J, Cheng G, Hartman J, et al. Estrogen receptors: how do they signal and what are their targets. Physiol Rev. 2007;87(3):905–31.
6. Hartkopf AD, Grischke EM, Brucker SY. Endocrine-resistant breast cancer: mechanisms and treatment. Breast Care (Basel). 2020;15(4):347–54.
7. Raheem F, Karikalan SA, Batalini F, El Masry A, Mina L. Metastatic ER+ breast cancer: mechanisms of resistance and future therapeutic approaches. Int J Mol Sci. 2023;24(22):16198.
8. Brett JO, Mayer EL. New developments in systemic management for high-risk early-stage hormone-receptor-positive, HER2-negative breast cancer. Curr Treat Options Oncol. 2023;24(6):594–610.
9. Patel R, Klein P, Tiersten A, Sparano JA. An emerging generation of endocrine therapies in breast cancer: a clinical perspective. NPJ Breast Cancer. 2023;9(1):20.
10. Liu JH. Selective estrogen receptor modulators (SERMS): keys to understanding their function. Menopause. 2020;27(10):1171–6.
11. Selective estrogen receptor modulators. LiverTox: clinical and research information on drug-induced liver injury, Bethesda, MD; 2012.
12. Patel HK, Bihani T. Selective estrogen receptor modulators (SERMs) and selective estrogen receptor degraders (SERDs) in cancer treatment. Pharmacol Ther. 2018;186:1–24.
13. Cosman F, Lindsay R. Selective estrogen receptor modulators: clinical spectrum. Endocr Rev. 1999;20(3):418–34.
14. Luque-Bolivar A, Perez-Mora E, Villegas VE, Rondon-Lagos M. Resistance and overcoming resistance in breast cancer. Breast Cancer (Dove Med Press). 2020;12:211–29.
15. Ghanavati M, Khorshidi Y, Shadnoush M, Akbari ME, Ardehali SH, Chavarri-Guerra Y, et al. Tamoxifen use and risk of endometrial cancer in breast cancer patients: a systematic review and dose-response meta-analysis. Cancer Rep (Hoboken). 2023;6(4):e1806.
16. Goetz MP, Bagegni NA, Batist G, Brufsky A, Cristofanilli MA, Damodaran S, et al. Lasofoxifene versus fulvestrant for ER+/HER2- metastatic breast cancer with an ESR1 mutation: results from the randomized, phase II ELAINE 1 trial. Ann Oncol. 2023;34(12):1141–51.
17. Wardell SE, Ellis MJ, Alley HM, Eisele K, VanArsdale T, Dann SG, et al. Efficacy of SERD/SERM hybrid-CDK4/6 inhibitor combinations in models of endocrine therapy-resistant breast cancer. Clin Cancer Res. 2015;21(22):5121–30.
18. Avvaru SP, Noolvi MN, Aminbhavi TM, Chkraborty S, Dash A, Shukla SS. Aromatase inhibitors evolution as potential class of drugs in the treatment of post-menopausal breast cancer women. Mini Rev Med Chem. 2018;18(7):609–21.
19. Chumsri S, Howes T, Bao T, Sabnis G, Brodie A. Aromatase, aromatase inhibitors, and breast cancer. J Steroid Biochem Mol Biol. 2011;125(1–2):13–22.
20. Nabholtz JM. Long-term safety of aromatase inhibitors in the treatment of breast cancer. Ther Clin Risk Manag. 2008;4(1):189–204.
21. Collins JM. 25—Cancer pharmacology. In: Niederhuber JE, Armitage JO, Kastan MB, Doroshow JH, Tepper JE, editors. Abeloff's clinical oncology (sixth edition). Philadelphia: Elsevier; 2020. p. 411–9.e44.
22. Walker LM, Tran S, Robinson JW. Luteinizing hormone—releasing hormone agonists: a quick reference for prevalence rates of potential adverse effects. Clin Genitourin Cancer. 2013;11(4):375–84.
23. Downton T, Zhou F, Segara D, Jeselsohn R, Lim E. Oral selective estrogen receptor degraders (SERDs) in breast cancer: advances, challenges, and current status. Drug Des Devel Ther. 2022;16:2933–48.
24. Gombos A, Goncalves A, Curigliano G, Bartsch R, Kyte JA, Ignatiadis M, et al. How I treat endocrine-dependent metastatic breast cancer. ESMO Open. 2023;8(2):100882.
25. Furman C, Puyang X, Zhang Z, Wu ZJ, Banka D, Aithal KB, et al. Covalent ERalpha antagonist H3B-6545 demonstrates encouraging preclinical activity

in therapy-resistant breast cancer. Mol Cancer Ther. 2022;21(6):890–902.
26. Ferraro E, Walsh EM, Tao JJ, Chandarlapaty S, Jhaveri K. Accelerating drug development in breast cancer: new frontiers for ER inhibition. Cancer Treat Rev. 2022;109:102432.
27. Liu Z, Hu M, Yang Y, Du C, Zhou H, Liu C, et al. An overview of PROTACs: a promising drug discovery paradigm. Mol Biomed. 2022;3(1):46.
28. Bekes M, Langley DR, Crews CM. PROTAC targeted protein degraders: the past is prologue. Nat Rev Drug Discov. 2022;21(3):181–200.
29. Cole KM, Clemons M, Alzahrani M, Liu M, Larocque G, MacDonald F, et al. Vasomotor symptoms in early breast cancer—a "real world" exploration of the patient experience. Support Care Cancer. 2022;30(5):4437–46.

Part II

Common Problems in Breast Cancer Survivorship and Management

8 Breast Cancer-Related Lymphedema: From Description to Management

Yeşim Bakar

8.1 Breast Cancer-Related Lymphedema

Breast cancer-related lymphedema (BCRL) stands out as a particularly dreaded complication arising from breast cancer treatment [1, 2]. For many breast cancer survivors, BCRL imposes a lifelong burden, while nearly all individuals who have survived breast cancer are at risk indefinitely. Regrettably, BCRL defies easy solutions; it cannot be cured and becomes increasingly evident in advanced stages, making it quite challenging [3]. Its enduring effects extend beyond the physical realm, manifesting in symptoms like arm swelling, pain, and reduced function, which often necessitate the adoption of compensatory movement strategies [4]. Moreover, BCRL significantly diminishes quality of life, disrupts psychosocial interactions, and affects emotional well-being [5, 6]. Additionally, BCRL imposes substantial financial strains on patients, caregivers, third-party payers, and society [7] (Picture 8.1).

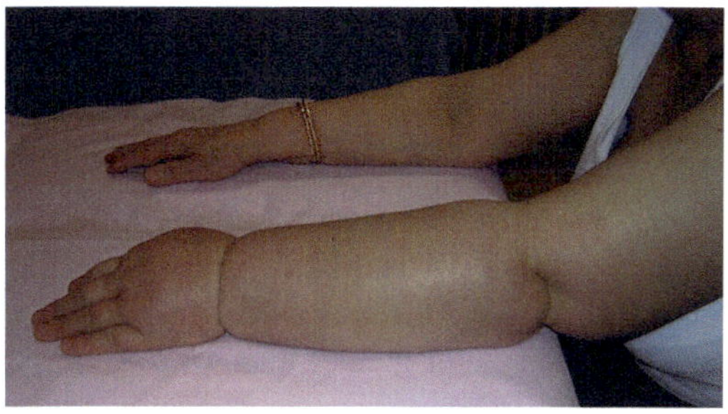

Picture 8.1 Breast cancer-related lymphedema

8.2 Risk Factors for Breast Cancer-Related Lymphedema

8.2.1 Axillary Surgery

Risk factors for BCRL are varied and complex; however, axillary surgery is emerging as the most significant contributor. The incidence of BCRL is challenging to ascertain due to the delayed onset of symptoms following breast cancer treatment [8].

Axillary lymph node dissection (ALND) is associated with a higher risk of BCRL compared to sentinel lymph node biopsy (SLNB) [8–11]. The removal of a greater number of lymph nodes is consistently identified as a risk factor for BCRL. However, recent advancements in breast cancer clinical trials have focused on reducing the intensity of locoregional therapy, particularly in the axillary region [9, 12, 13]. While the primary outcomes of these trials typically relate to survival or local recurrence, many also include

Y. Bakar (✉)
Institute of Postgraduate Education,
Izmir Bakircay University, Izmir, Turkey
e-mail: yesim.bakar@bakircay.edu.tr

Y. Bakar, A. Tuğral (eds.), *Managing Side Effects of Breast Cancer Treatment*,
https://doi.org/10.1007/978-3-031-75480-7_8

secondary objectives related to BCRL. Notably, the risk of BCRL following SLNB ranges between 3% and 8% [8–10]. The data series from the single institution corroborates the significance of axillary surgery as a risk factor for BCRL. Seven thousand six hundred seventeen patients were observed over a median follow-up of 60 months, and BCRL was found at a rate of 3% in patients who underwent SLNB [14]. Similarly, another study reported BCRL at a rate of 3.4% in SLNB-negative patients [15].

Regarding ALND, several trials have documented that the risk of BCRL is ranging from 13% to 60%. Most studies utilize a relative volume change (RVC) of greater than 10% as a diagnostic threshold for BCRL [8–11, 13]. However, it is crucial to note that the length of follow-up and diverse criteria for diagnosis can significantly influence the relatively highly varied incidence rates. For instance, researchers defined BCRL as a volume change of greater than 15%, and they found that BCRL was apparent in only 5% of patients who underwent ALND, with noticeable progressive swelling changes observed over 5 years. However, upon expanding the definition to encompass any form of swelling, 26% of ALND patients were classified as experiencing BCRL. These findings underscore the importance of careful interpretation when comparing the incidence of BCRL across studies, considering variations in follow-up duration and diagnostic criteria [16].

In a prospective trial, all patients underwent ALND, with 87% of them also receiving additional radiation therapy [9]. After a median follow-up of 3 years, significant proportions of women showed symptoms of arm swelling (37.8%), measured BCRL exceeding 10% (58.4%), and experienced an RVC in the ipsilateral arm greater than 20% (36.9%). Notably, in this study, BCRL was not confirmed through clinical examination, and it remains unclear whether those who conducted the measurements received any training to minimize interrater variability. Additional studies have also recognized a correlation between ALND and regional lymph node radiation (RLNR), albeit with lower BCRL rates ranging from 31.2% to 38.7%.

Despite these lower rates compared to ALND or RLNR alone, they still suggest the cumulative impact of multimodal regional nodal therapies on BCRL development. These findings highlight the importance of considering the combined effects of different treatment modalities, such as ALND and RLNR, in understanding the risk of BCRL. Additionally, ensuring standardized assessment methods and rigorous training for those performing measurements are essential for accurate evaluation and interpretation of the incidence of BCRL in clinical trials and practice [17].

8.2.2 Regional Lymph Node Radiation

Regional lymph node radiation (RLNR) has gained attention due to positive findings from trials [18, 19]. Warren et al. [20] conducted an evaluation involving 1476 patients and found that administering radiation to the supraclavicular field, regardless of whether a posterior axillary boost was given, significantly elevated the risk of BCRL. This underscores the importance of considering the impact of RLNR on BCRL development, particularly in patients with positive lymph nodes or those at high risk for recurrence.

Naoum et al. [21] conducted a prospective observation in 1811 patients, revealing that the risk of BCRL primarily hinges on the extent of axillary surgery. They categorized patients based on the extent of axillary surgery with or without RLNR. Their findings demonstrated that the cumulative incidences of BCRL at 5 years varied significantly across different surgical groups: SLNB alone (7.7%), SLNB plus RLNR (10.8%), ALND alone (29%), and ALND plus RLNR (38.7%).

Multivariable analysis indicated no significant disparity in BCRL risk between SLNB groups and ALND groups, irrespective of RLNR use. However, both ALND groups exhibited higher BCRL risks compared to those who underwent SLNB. Such evidence underscores the potential benefits of strategic modifications in surgical approaches to minimize the risk of BCRL while maintaining effective local control of breast cancer [11, 13].

8.2.3 Body Mass Index

Having a body mass index (BMI) of ≥30 kg/m^2 at the time of breast cancer diagnosis is identified as an independent risk factor for BCRL [22]. In a randomized study involving overweight breast cancer survivors with BCRL, the effects of weight loss were investigated. Participants were divided into groups receiving weight loss interventions, either alone or combined with home-based exercise. Despite significant weight loss observed in both groups, amounting to 27.37% and 28.06% of baseline weight, weight loss did not result in improved BCRL outcomes. These outcomes were evaluated based on clinical assessment, symptom severity, frequency of BCRL exacerbations, incidence of cellulitis, and changes in limb volume. These findings underscore the complexity of BCRL management and suggest that weight loss alone may not be sufficient to alleviate symptoms of BCRL or reduce the risk of complications [23].

Furthermore, the exact impact of weight fluctuation following surgery on BCRL requires further investigation to provide more comprehensive guidance for patient education and management strategies.

8.2.4 Cellulitis

Cellulitis is recognized as a well-established risk factor for BCRL. It can exacerbate the existing BCRL and contribute to a cycle of recurrent cellulitis and BCRL flare-ups. However, the precise pathophysiological relationship between cellulitis and BCRL remains unclear [24–26] (Picture 8.2).

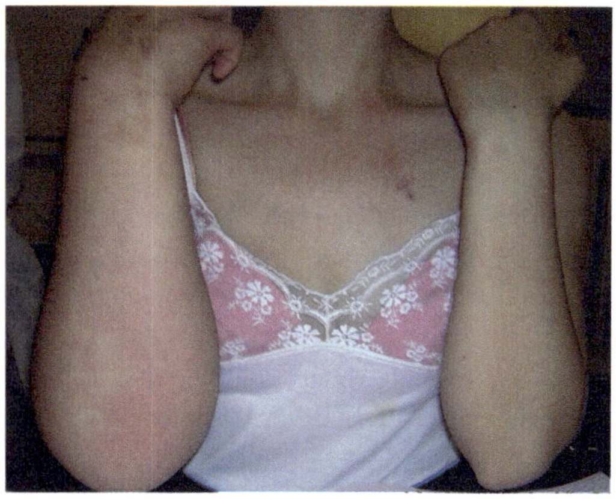

Picture 8.2 Right arm cellulitis

8.2.5 Low-Level Limb Volume Changes

Low-level limb volume changes following breast cancer surgery have been identified as precursors to the progression of BCRL [27, 28]. Studies have shown that even slight increases in arm volume, referred to as RVC can indicate an increased risk of developing BCRL. For example, the research observed that patients who experienced RVC increases of 3% to >5% from baseline within 3 months after surgery or increases of 5% to >10% from baseline at any point after surgery were more likely to progress to BCRL (defined as RVC ≥10%) [29]. Similarly, another study demonstrated similar findings in patients who underwent the removal of ≥5 lymph nodes and experienced arm swelling at 6- or 12-months post-surgery [28].

These findings highlight the importance of monitoring even minor changes in limb volume following breast cancer surgery, as they can serve as early indicators of BCRL development. Early detection and intervention based on such changes may help mitigate the progression of BCRL and improve patient outcomes.

8.3 The Onset of Breast Cancer-Related Lymphedema

In a cohort of 2171 prospectively screened women, the onset of BCRL was found to peak between 12 and 30 months after surgery. However, the onset of BCRL is varied and depends on the type of treatment received. Early-onset BCRL, defined as occurring within 12 months postoperatively, was significantly associated with ALND but not with RLNR. Conversely, late-onset BCRL, occurring more than 12 months postoperatively, was associated with both RLNR and ALND. Specifically, the highest risk of the onset of BCRL was observed at different time intervals depending on the treatment group: 6–12 months in the ALND group without RLNR, 18–24 months in the ALND plus RLNR group, and 36–48 months in the SLNB plus RLNR group. Understanding the onset of BCRL is crucial for screening practices and for patient education. This knowledge can help healthcare providers tailor surveillance protocols and provide timely interventions to mitigate the impact of BCRL on clinical outcomes [30].

8.4 The Screening of Breast Cancer-Related Lymphedema

There is an increasing consensus and backing for the adoption of a forward-looking screening framework aimed at promptly diagnosing and halting the advancement of BCRL. This approach emphasizes the utilization of objective metrics, symptom evaluation, and clinical examinations to identify BCRL at its latent/preclinical stages and intervene accordingly [31, 32].

8.4.1 Preoperative Baseline Measurement

A critical aspect of managing BCRL is the establishment of objective limb measurements at baseline and regular follow-up intervals [29, 31, 33]. Without baseline measurements, there might be a risk of incorrect diagnoses of BCRL due to the existing natural arm asymmetry. In a cohort study with 1028 patients, it was shown that a significant proportion of patients had preoperative arm asymmetry of ≥5% (28.3%) and ≥10% (2.9%). Substituting a postoperative pseudo-baseline for a true preoperative baseline measurement led to misdiagnosis in 40–50% of patients in the same cohort. These findings underscore the importance of conducting accurate preoperative baseline measurements to establish a reference point for comparison during follow-up assessments. Failure to do so can result in misdiagnosis and inappropriate management of BCRL. Therefore, ensuring the availability of baseline measurements is crucial for optimizing diagnostic accuracy and guiding effective treatment strategies for BCRL [34].

8.4.2 Relative Volume Change (RVC)

In diagnosing BCRL, it is crucial to consider volume changes in the affected limb compared to a preoperative baseline volume since the changes in volume can also be accounted for weight fluctuations [35]. For patients who have undergone unilateral surgery, the contralateral arm can serve as a control for comparison. However, for patients who have undergone bilateral surgery and lack a control arm, a weight-adjusted change (WAC) equation has been developed. The WAC equation allows for adjustments based on weight fluctuations relative to baseline, ensuring accurate assessments of limb volume changes. Formulas for determining RVC and the WAC equation are provided in Table 8.1 [36]. By incorporating these calculations into BCRL diagnosis, healthcare providers can effectively monitor and assess changes in limb volume over time, facilitating early detection and intervention for BCRL when necessary.

Table 8.1 Formulas for calculating breast cancer-related lymphedema volume changes in patients with and without an unaffected control limb [36]

Unilateral at-risk limb	Bilateral at-risk limbs
Relative volume change (RVC)	Weight-adjusted change (WAC)
RVC = ((A2 × U1)/(U2 × A1)) − 1	WAC = ((A2 × W1)/(W2 × A1)) − 1
A1 = volume of the affected limb at baseline	A1 = volume of the affected limb at baseline
A2 = volume of the affected limb at a given time point	A2 = volume of the affected limb at a given time point
U1 = volume of the unaffected limb at baseline	W1: Body weight at baseline
U2 = volume of the unaffected limb at a given time point	W2: Body weight at a given time point

This approach enhances the accuracy of BCRL diagnosis and enables tailored treatment strategies to optimize patient outcomes [37].

8.4.3 The Definition of Breast Cancer-Related Lymphedema

Breast cancer-related lymphedema (BCRL) is typically defined as an RVC or WAC of 10% or more, occurring more than 3 months after breast surgery. While an RVC or WAC of 10% is commonly regarded as the diagnostic threshold warranting intervention, certain studies have suggested improved treatment efficacy even at RVC levels as low as 3%. However, it is important to note that these studies lacked a control group not receiving treatment, potentially influencing the interpretation of their findings [32].

In the past, diagnosing BCRL relied on detecting a volume increase of 200 mL or a circumference increase of 2 cm in the at-risk arm, which is more prone to measurement error since this approach overlooks baseline arm volume and typical weight fluctuations. In a study, an absolute volume increase of ≥200 mL corresponded to RVC ranging from 2.9% to 15.7%, depending on the preoperative arm volume. Similarly, defining BCRL as a 2-cm increase in the affected arm relative to baseline resulted in RVC ranging from 6.0% to 9.8% [35].

8.4.4 Objective Diagnostic Methods Used in Breast Cancer-Related Lymphedema

The absence of standardized measurement protocols has greatly impeded research efforts in BCRL. Various methods for gathering objective data have been reported, each offering distinct advantages and drawbacks (Table 8.2) [38].

Table 8.2 Comparison of different diagnostic tools for the diagnosis of breast cancer-related lymphedema [38]

Method features	Outcome	Advantages	Disadvantages
Circumference measurement	• Circumferential differences using tape measurer	• Simple and economical • Can be used to monitor BCRL progression	• Not precise • Moderate inter- and intra-rater variability
Water displacement	• Water overflow	• Reliable and validated • Includes hand	• Hygienic concerns • No swelling localization information • Contraindicated in case of open wounds
Perometry	• IR scanning with the calculation of multiple limb area volumes	• Rapid measurement • Can measure bilateral BCRL • Can localize swelling • Can detect a 3% limb volume change • Can measure the torso with some models	• Expensive • Equipment not available everywhere • Difficulty with reliable hand measurement • Positioning can be problematic
Bioimpedance spectroscopy	• Impedance ratio between limbs • Calculates L-Dex ratio	• Rapid, non-invasive testing • Repeatable results • Early detection is possible	• Expensive • Limited interpretations in case of bilateral limb involvement • Limited to arm and leg use

(continued)

Table 8.2 (continued)

Method features	Outcome	Advantages	Disadvantages
Tissue dielectric constant	• Localized skin tissue water	• Hand-held probe • Easily performed • Available to use wherever it is needed • Non-invasive • Superior ability to detect pre-clinical BCRL	• Requires special equipment • Sensitive but not specific • Results can be affected by different conditions and skin
3D laser scanning	• Real-time digital 3D image	• Sensitive to small variations in arm volume	• Expensive • Difficulties in determining the arm reference point • Uncertain reliability
Computed tomography	• Skin thickening • Honeycombing • Fat lobules	• Objective volume measurement	• Expensive • Exposure to radiation • Need trained personnel
Lymphoscintigraphy	• Axillary/elbow lymph nodes • Lymphatic ducts • Dermal backflow	• Has been the gold standard for the diagnosis of lymphedema • Shows the severity of lymphatic obstruction • Shows deep lymph flow	• Protocol is not standardized • Poor image quality • Little subdermal lymphatic information
ICG Lymphography	• Superficial lymphatic ducts • Dermal backflow	• Detailed visualization • Intra-operative measurement • No radiation exposure	• Limited to lymphatics ~2.0 cm into subcutaneous tissue • Is not available everywhere • Technically demanding
MR Lymphangiography	• Lymphatics • Fat deposition • Muscle compartments • Precise limb volume	• Gives information on lymphatic function • No radiation exposure	• Expensive • Not available everywhere • Technically demanding

BCRL: breast cancer-related lymphedema; ICG: indocyanine green; IR: infrared; L-Dex: lymphedema index; MR: magnetic resonance

Published with permission from MDPI (Source: [38], an open access article distributed under the terms and conditions of the Creative Commons Attribution (CC BY) license

8.5 Severity of Breast Cancer-Related Lymphedema

Understanding the various stages of lymphedema is crucial, as its severity ranges from soft, pitting edema (Picture 8.3) to irreversible non-pitting edema with fatty and fibrotic deposition. Several classifications and staging systems, which rely on clinical and imaging findings, have been proposed in the medical literature to aid in this understanding.

The International Society of Lymphology (ISL) classification, which is widely used for staging the severity of lymphedema, divides it into three stages [29]:

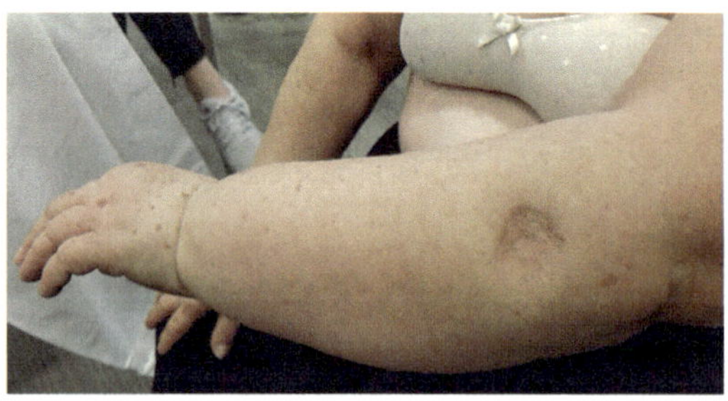

Picture 8.3 Pitting edema

1 Stage 0 (latent or sub-clinical lymphedema): This stage is characterized by injured lymphatic channels with impaired lymph transport but without measurable swelling or edema.

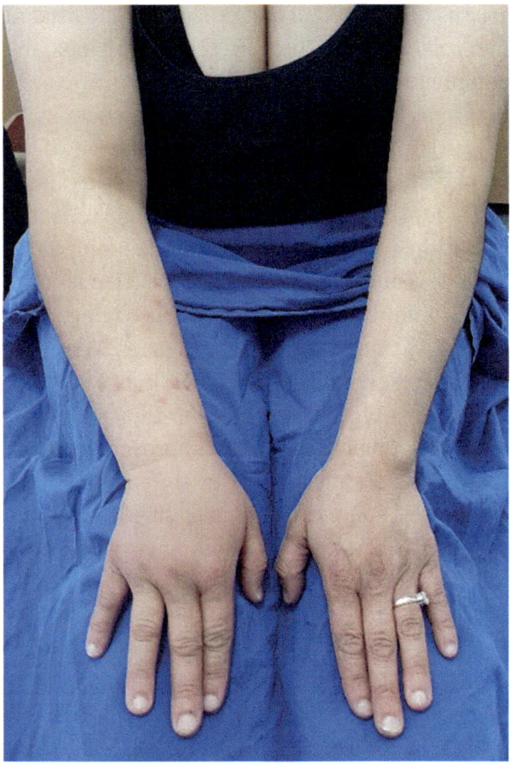

Picture 8.4 Stage I BCRL

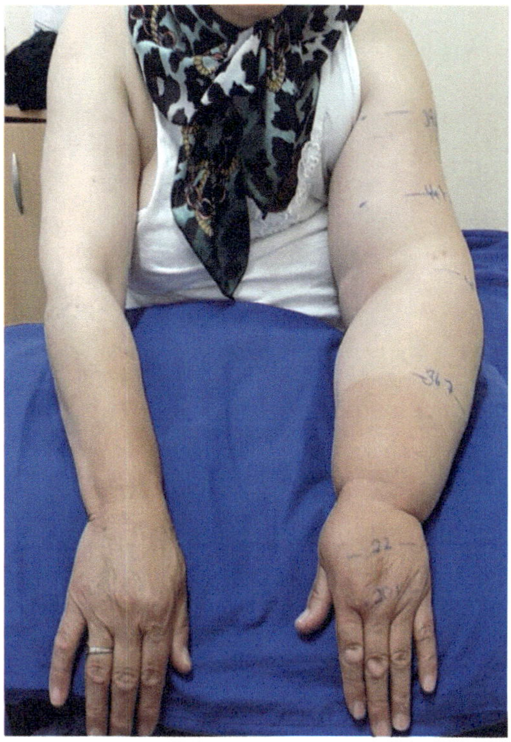

Picture 8.5 Stage II BCRL

2 Stage I (spontaneously reversible lymphedema): Patients in this stage exhibit measurable swelling and pitting of the skin due to lymph fluid accumulation. Swelling decreases with limb elevation or the use of compression garments (Picture 8.4).
3 Stage II (spontaneously irreversible lymphedema): At this stage, significant adipose tissue deposition and accumulation of protein-rich fluid hinder the effectiveness of limb elevation or compression garments in reducing symptoms. In late Stage II, the limb may exhibit increased fat and fibrosis (Picture 8.5).
4 Stage III (lymphostatic elephantiasis): This is the most advanced stage, characterized by severe swelling, excessive fat deposition, fibrosis, and significant skin changes such as acanthosis or hyperkeratosis (Picture 8.6).

Other classification systems are also available as follows: Campisi, Arm Dermal Backflow, MD Anderson, Cheng's Lymphedema grading, and Taiwan Lymphoscintigraphy Staging [38].

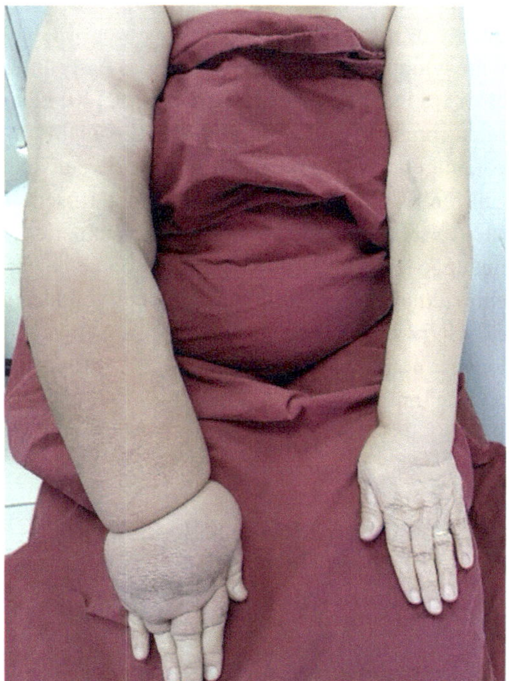

Picture 8.6 Stage III BCRL

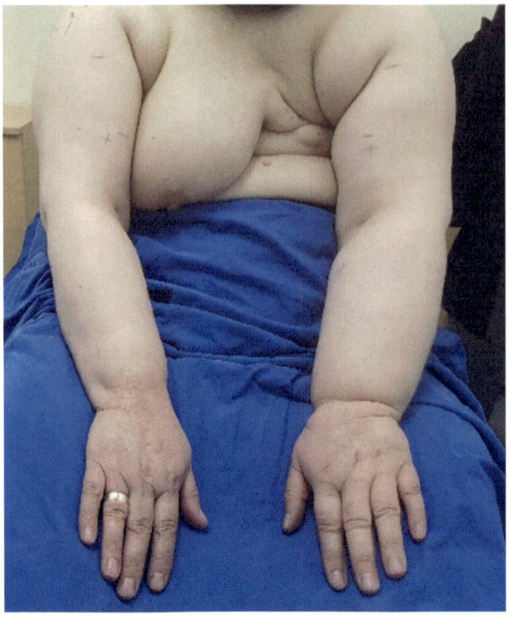

Picture 8.7 Breast cancer-related lymphedema

8.6 Symptoms Related to Breast Cancer-Related Lymphedema

Patients affected by BCRL often report a lower quality of life compared to those without BCRL, with symptoms potentially serving as early indicators of its onset [39, 40]. Armer et al. [40] identified predictive factors for BCRL, including patient reports of "heaviness in the past year" and "current swelling." Additionally, Fu and Rosedale [41] observed that patients described experiencing up to ten symptoms daily, which could be categorized into four psychosocial themes: enduring ongoing discomfort, facing unforeseen challenges, grappling with changes in identity, and feeling limited in daily life activities [39] (Picture 8.7).

8.7 Management of Breast Cancer-Related Lymphedema

Complex decongestive therapy (CDT) remains the gold standard for the treatment of early-stage BCRL. CDT is a comprehensive program integrating various therapeutic methods including manual lymphatic drainage (MLD), bandaging, compression garments, exercise, and self-care. It is primarily utilized for treating moderate to severe lymphedema, specifically for stages II and III [42] (Picture 8.8). CDT comprises two phases: reduction and maintenance. During the reduction phase, the primary goal is to reduce limb volume and alleviate symptoms using CDT. This involves MLD, multilayer compression bandaging, exercise, skincare, and patient education. Typically spanning several days per week over several weeks, this phase aims to achieve maximal volume reduction and symptom improvement. Once these goals are met, the focus shifts to maintaining limb volume and managing symptoms. Maintenance entails transitioning from multilayer bandaging to compression garments, incorporating self-MLD, continuing with exercise, and maintaining skincare routines [17].

CDT remains the established benchmark for addressing early-stage BCRL [43]. Systematic analysis conducted by Lasinski et al. [44] underscored the robust evidence supporting the efficacy of CDT as the optimal clinical approach to BCRL.

8.7.1 Manual Lymph Drainage

Manual lymph drainage (MLD) is a form of specific massage modality wherein therapists apply gentle, rhythmic pumping motions combined with directed stretching of the skin to the affected area. By doing so, MLD stimulates lymphatic contractility, thereby improving lymphatic drainage [45]. MLD is recognized as a treatment option for lymphedema universally.

Despite its widespread use, the evidence regarding the effectiveness of MLD on lymphedema is inconsistent. Nine systematic reviews, including four meta-analyses, attempted to determine the effect of MLD on lymphedema, yielding mixed results. Some studies suggested that adding MLD to standard therapy could enhance the volume reduction. A systematic review revealed that MLD was deemed safe and, when combined with compression bandages, could

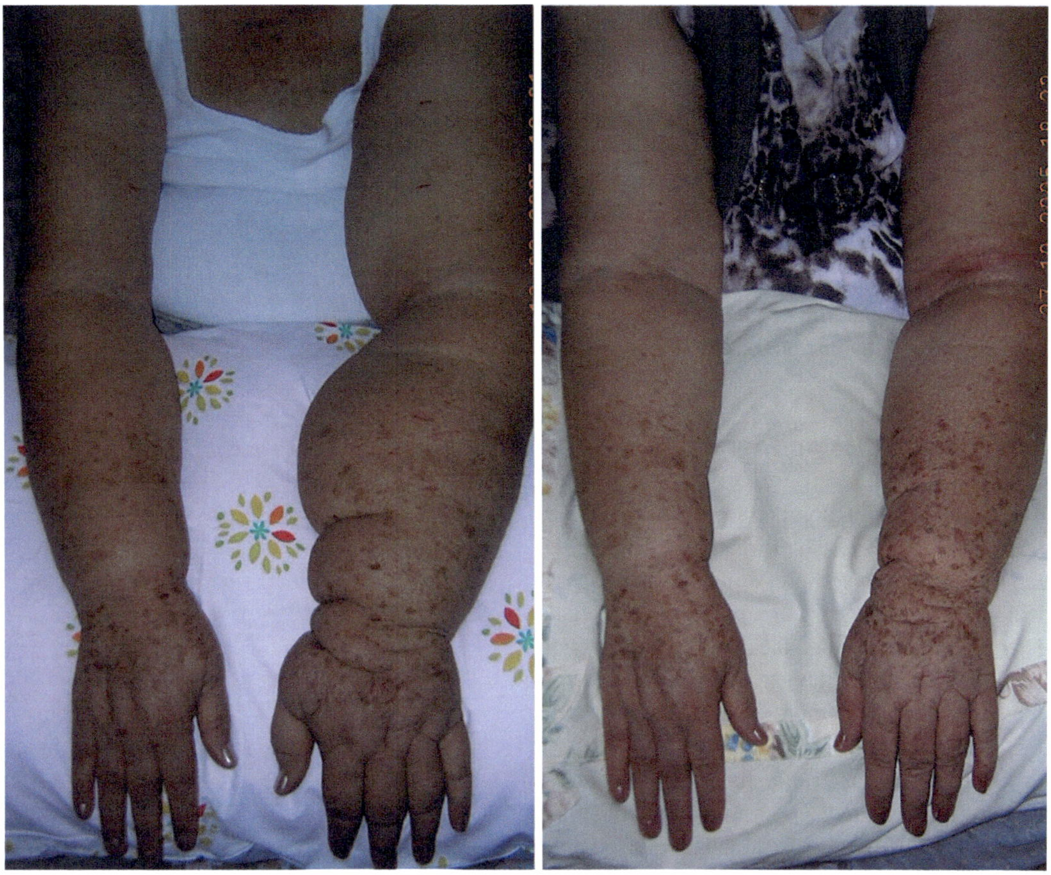

Picture 8.8 Before and after complex decongestive therapy

potentially offer additional advantages in reducing swelling for BCRL compared to using compression bandages alone. This effect was particularly notable for patients with mild-to-moderate BCRL severity [46]. However, other meta-analyses failed to find a significant improvement in BCRL with MLD. Partial improvement was observed in specific subgroups, including patients under 60 years old, those having mild lymphedema (Stage I), individuals receiving more than 20 MLD sessions, and those undergoing CDT for over 1 month. A recently developed method involves incorporating indocyanine green (ICG) imaging during MLD to visualize alternative lymphatic pathways, enabling the integration of personalized adjustments to therapy. While no trials have yet compared the effectiveness of this approach, it holds the potential to offer additional benefits in the management of BCRL [47].

Based on current literature, it may not be advisable to routinely recommend MLD to patients with BCRL, as its effectiveness appears to be limited. Larger trials with more rigorous study protocols are necessary to reach a definitive conclusion regarding the efficacy of this treatment option.

8.7.2 Skin Care

Skincare constitutes a fundamental aspect of CDT. Breaks in the skin can create opportunities for bacteria to infiltrate, leading to potentially severe infections due to compromised local immunity in a lymphedematous limb. Common skin conditions associated with lymphedema include dry/flaky skin, dermatitis (eczema), hyperkeratosis, papillomatosis, skin folds, folliculitis, cellulitis (erysipelas), fungal infections, and lymphorrhoea. Approximately 70% of cellulitis/erysipelas cases stem from minor injuries like cuts, insect bites, burns, interdigital mycosis, and radiation ulcers. To mitigate the risk of fungal or bacterial colonization, meticulous hygiene and proactive skin care are indispensable [48].

Throughout the course of their lymphedema journey, it is crucial to consistently monitor patients' understanding of the benefits of skincare and their adherence to instructions.

8.7.3 Compression Therapy

The application of compression therapy varies depending on the phase of treatment. During the reduction phase, compression is administered using a multilayer compression bandage. However, in the maintenance phase, compression is achieved through the use of compression garments. Multilayer compression bandaging using low-stretch bandages is a cornerstone of CDT and has demonstrated effectiveness in reducing lymphedema volume. This bandaging technique, performed repetitively by trained therapists, typically requires 15–20 sessions, each lasting 45–60 min over 3–6 weeks to achieve maximum volume reduction. The optimal pressure exerted by the bandaging is still under investigation (Picture 8.9).

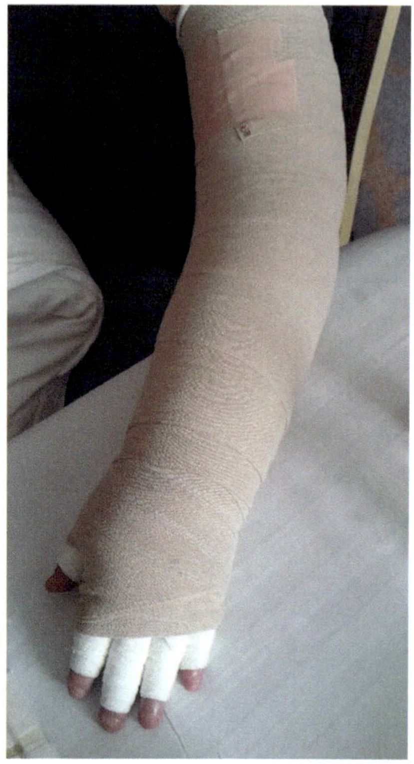

Picture 8.9 Multilayer compression bandage

Nonelastic compression Velcro wraps may offer advantages over multilayer bandaging in terms of ease of application and efficacy for reducing lymphedema volume. Unlike multilayer bandaging, which is typically applied only by therapists during the intensive treatment phase, Velcro wraps can be utilized by both therapists and patients during the maintenance phase of the treatment [49].

Compression garments are integral parts during the maintenance phase of therapy to uphold the outcomes of intensive edema reduction and prevent lymphedema progression. Preceding the prescription of these garments, multilayer bandage application is primarily employed in the intensive treatment phase. Subsequently, well-fitted compression garments are typically worn during daytime hours of upright activity and can be supplemented with additional nocturnal garments as needed. Many prefer custom-made flat-knit garments due to their ability to maintain fit without rolling or causing tourniquet effects, especially in cases of limb distortion. However, the availability of financial support for these expensive garments varies widely, often influencing the choice of the final garment design. Proper fitting of compression garments is crucial, as they provide graded compression, with the highest pressure typically applied at the distal part of the extremity [50] (Picture 8.10).

The effectiveness of compression garments in preventing upper extremity lymphedema in breast cancer patients has been explored in research [51]. Paramanandam et al. [52] investigated the prophylactic use of compression garments to mitigate arm edema in women at high

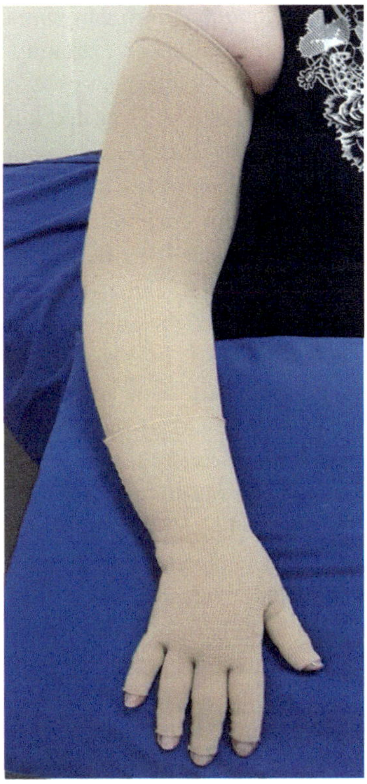

Picture 8.10 Compression garment

risk for BRCL. In their phase III trial, 307 women who had undergone ALND were randomized to receive or not receive compression garments. Those who received the intervention wore compression garments postoperatively until 3 months after completion of adjuvant treatments. Results showed that women in the compression garment group experienced delayed onset and lower rates of lymphedema. At the 1-year mark, the incidence of arm swelling was 42% for women using compression sleeves compared to 52%. The study concluded that prophylactic compression garments reduced and delayed arm swelling in high-risk breast cancer patients following surgery.

The combination of compression bandages with a compression garment has been shown to notably decrease the volume of the swollen limb in comparison to using a compression garment alone [45]. Compression therapy alone may be adequate to halt the progression of swelling in patients with subclinical BCRL and could even reduce limb volume with or without MLD in those with BCRL. However, advanced BCRL usually requires CDT [53].

Intermittent pneumatic compression (IPC) has been employed in the treatment of BCRL since the 1950s. These pumps and their associated devices are applied to the limb, exerting pressure gradients as they inflate and deflate, resembling the action of MLD performed by a certified lymphedema therapist. However, the effectiveness of IPC in improving BCRL outcomes remains uncertain. It is not recommended as a first-line or stand-alone BCRL treatment [54].

8.7.4 Exercise

Exercise has become increasingly recognized as a vital recommendation for survivors of breast cancer following treatment [55]. Schmitz et al. [56, 57] compared twice-per-week weightlifting to standard care in breast cancer survivors at risk for or with BCRL. Their findings revealed that a carefully structured, facility-based weightlifting program led to a 35% reduction in BCRL. Participants with BCRL who engaged in the weightlifting program experienced reduced symptoms compared to those in the control group. The study's findings indicated that a personalized, supervised, and gradually progressive aerobic and resistance exercise program did not trigger or intensify BCRL.

While CDT remains the primary treatment for BCRL, its effectiveness is further enhanced when combined with additional therapies. This combined approach yields more substantial improvements in arm volume, upper arm function, BCRL symptoms, and overall quality of life. However, it is important to note that augmenting CDT with supplementary therapies necessitates the involvement of interdisciplinary teams, may involve intrusive procedures, and can lead to increased expenses [58].

8.8 Prevention

8.8.1 Precautionary Measures

The National Lymphedema Network (NLN) has issued precautionary recommendations aimed at reducing the risk of BCRL. These guidelines advise on skin care, avoiding blood pressure cuffs, venipuncture, and trauma, as well as wearing compression garments during air travel [59]. However, despite their intention to mitigate risk, adherence to these guidelines has not been proven to reduce the incidence of BCRL [25, 26, 60].

In a study involving 632 patients who were prospectively screened, Ferguson et al. [25] found no association between arm volume increase and activities such as blood pressure readings, blood draws, or air travel. Similar results were reported in another study involving 327 patients who underwent bilateral breast cancer surgery [60]. Additionally, other research has indicated that activities such as air travel, arm trauma, medical procedures, and arm use did not increase the risk of BCRL in women who had more than five lymph nodes removed [61].

The American Society of Breast Surgeons recommends that, within the framework of an early detection/surveillance program incorporating baseline and follow-up assessments, many risk-reducing behaviors are not routinely supported. Specifically, using the ipsilateral arm for intravenous (IV) lines or blood pressure measurements is not contraindicated, according to their guidelines [62]. This recommendation aligns with the International Society of Lymphology (ISL) stance [29]. However, there is currently no universal consensus on precautionary measures due to the evolving nature of this issue.

8.8.2 Surgery for the Prevention of Lymphedema

There is growing attention to prophylactic surgical methods employed during initial axillary surgery to prevent BCRL. One such technique is axillary reverse mapping (ARM), which operates on the hypothesis that injecting blue dye into the volar aspect of the upper arm can map the lymphatic drainage of the upper extremity. During surgery, the surgeon then endeavors to safeguard the identified blue lymphatics or nodes [63].

A systematic review, encompassing eight studies, each including at least 50 patients who underwent ARM in conjunction with either SLNB or ALND, revealed that BCRL occurred in 0–6% of patients who underwent ARM plus SLNB and 5.9–24% of patients who underwent ARM plus ALND [64]. In a recent prospective trial, 107 patients requiring ALND were randomly assigned to undergo ARM or not. After 24 months of follow-up, no significant difference in objective BCRL rates was observed between the ALND group (32.3%) and the ARM plus ALND group (23.5%; $p = 0.43$). However, patients who underwent both ARM and ALND reported significantly less symptomatic BCRL than those who underwent ALND alone (6.1% vs. 26.7%, respectively; $p = 0.025$) [65].

Yuan et al. [66] aimed to enhance the ARM technique and upper extremity nodal identification and preservation principles with their novel approach, termed the Identification and Preservation of Arm and Lymphatic (DEPART) technique. In this method, after identifying the ARM node, it was intraoperatively injected to map and consequently safeguard the next echelon of lymph nodes involved in upper extremity lymphatic drainage. Demonstrating the feasibility of their technique, they subsequently randomly assigned 1354 patients requiring ALND to undergo either DEPART plus ALND or ALND alone. Overall, a higher proportion of patients undergoing ALND alone developed BCRL, defined as an RVC of more than 10%, compared to those undergoing DEPART plus ALND (15.3% vs. 3.3%, respectively; $p < 0.001$). ARM nodes were not identified in 17% of patients and contained metastases in 6.8% of cases.

Another innovative technique, the Lymphatic Microsurgical Preventative Healing Approach (LYMPHA), aims to preserve lymphatic flow into the venous system by employing microsurgical methods to reposition transacted axillary lymphatics into a nearby vein with a competent valve. While fewer patient series have been published to validate this procedure, limited data suggest its potential value. In the initial publication by Boccardo et al. [67], BCRL was reported in 30% of patients who underwent ALND without LYMPHA, whereas only 4% of patients who underwent LYMPHA experienced BCRL. More recently, Feldman et al. [68] observed a higher incidence of BCRL in standard ALND patients (50%) compared to LYMPHA patients (12.5%). Consequently, further investigation into the role of LYMPHA is warranted.

8.9 Surgical Management of Breast Cancer-Related Lymphedema

Advancements in microsurgical skills and technology have revitalized discussions surrounding surgical interventions for symptomatic and progressive BCRL. These interventions are broadly categorized as reductive (involving the removal of fibrotic lymphatic tissue) or reconstructive (involving the reestablishment of lymphatic flow through re-anastomosis of lymphatic vessels to veins, other lymphatics, or lymph node transfer). Suction-assisted protein lipectomy, a contemporary reductive technique, has demonstrated effectiveness in removing nearly 100% of excess limb volume in advanced stages of BCRL. However, it necessitates strict adherence to lifelong compression therapy to sustain volume reductions since it does not improve lymphatic function. Reconstructive techniques, on the other hand, aim to restore lymphatic flow and are typically more effective in earlier stages of BCRL (stage I or II) where some level of residual lymphatic function exists [69]. However, emerging data on these techniques are heterogeneous regarding indications, benefits, follow-up, and outcomes, making standardized implementation challenging. Nevertheless, it is evident that patients considered for these surgical interventions should undergo assessment by a multidisciplinary team with expertise in BCRL and postoperative care. Surgery should be viewed as part of a multimodal treatment approach of BCRL [62].

8.10 The Future of Breast Cancer-Related Lymphedema

Exciting advancements in contemporary science propose alternative inherent risk factors for BCRL, particularly genetic predisposition and biomarker identification. It is speculated that individual genetic variations may account for why only a portion of patients undergoing the same locoregional and systemic treatments eventually develop BCRL. Some genetic variations may confer protection against BCRL, while others may increase the risk of BCRL [70, 71].

Visser et al. [72]. have recently identified 18 genes that influence BCRL risk, contributing to our understanding of the mechanistic basis of BCRL development. Additionally, evolving data suggest that inflammatory, immunologic, and extracellular matrix modulator biomarkers may also influence the risk of BCRL. Pilot studies have shown promise for oral anti-inflammatory medications like ketoprofen in the treatment of lymphedema [17].

These findings hold the potential to complement existing clinicopathologic and treatment variables, aiding in better risk stratification or the selection of patients for therapeutic intervention in the future.

8.11 Conclusion

To enhance patient outcomes and elevate their quality of life, healthcare professionals should employ evidence-based techniques like CDT for risk reduction, prevention, and adaptation. Instead of solely relying on a single aspect of CDT to prevent or slow down the progression of BCRL, it is crucial to proactively address all facets of CDT early on. Alongside exercises and compression as preventive measures, comprehensive CDT encompasses various domains to tackle BCRL. Further research is necessary to ascertain whether CDT is more efficacious as a risk reduction behavior compared to its role as a management and treatment strategy.

References

1. Ostby PL, Armer JM, Smith K, Stewart BR. Patient perceptions of barriers to self-management of breast cancer-related lymphedema. West J Nurs Res. 2018;40:1800–17.
2. Sun F, Hall A, Tighe MP, Brunelle CL, Sayegh HE, Gillespie TC, Daniell KM, Taghian AG. Perometry versus simulated circumferential tape measurement for the detection of breast cancer-related lymphedema. Breast Cancer Res Treat. 2018;172:83–91.
3. Ridner SH, Bonner CM, Deng J, Sinclair VG. Voices from the shadows: living with lymphedema. Cancer Nurs. 2012;35:E18–26.
4. Fu MR, Axelrod D, Cleland CM, Qiu Z, Guth AA, Kleinman R, Scagliola J, Haber J. Symptom report in detecting breast cancer-related lymphedema. Breast Cancer (Dove Med Press). 2015;7:345–52.
5. Ahmed RL, Prizment A, Lazovich D, Schmitz KH, Folsom AR. Lymphedema and quality of life in breast cancer survivors: the Iowa Women's Health Study. J Clin Oncol. 2008;26:5689–96.
6. Fu MR, Kang Y. Psychosocial impact of living with cancer-related lymphedema. Semin Oncol Nurs. 2013;29:50–60.
7. De Vrieze T, Nevelsteen I, Thomis S, De Groef A, Tjalma WAA, Gebruers N, Devoogdt N. What are the economic burden and costs associated with the treatment of breast cancerrelated lymphoedema? A systematic review. Support Care Cancer. 2020;28:439–49.
8. Krag DN, Anderson SJ, Julian TB, et al. Sentinel-lymph-node resection compared with conventional axillary-lymph-node dissection in clinically node-negative patients with breast cancer: overall survival findings from the NSABP B-32 randomised phase 3 trial. Lancet Oncol. 2010;11:927–33.
9. Boughey JC, Suman VJ, Mittendorf EA, et al. Sentinel lymph node surgery after neoadjuvant chemotherapy in patients with node-positive breast cancer: the ACOSOG Z1071 (Alliance) clinical trial. JAMA. 2013;310:1455–61.
10. Galimberti V, Cole BF, Zurrida S, et al. Axillary dissection versus no axillary dissection in patients with sentinel-node micrometastases (IBCSG 23-01): a phase 3 randomised controlled trial. Lancet Oncol. 2013;14:297–305.
11. Shaitelman SF, Chiang Y-J, Griffin KD, et al. Radiation therapy targets and the risk of breast cancer-related lymphedema: a systematic review and network meta analysis. Breast Cancer Res Treat. 2017;162:201–15.
12. Giuliano AE, Hunt KK, Ballman KV, et al. Axillary dissection vs no axillary dissection in women with invasive breast cancer and sentinel node metastasis: a randomized clinical trial. JAMA. 2011;305:569–75.
13. Donker M, van Tienhoven G, Straver ME, et al. Radiotherapy or surgery of the axilla after a positive sentinel node in breast cancer (EORTC 10981-22023 AMAROS): a randomised, multicentre, open-label, phase 3 non-inferiority trial. Lancet Oncol. 2014;15:1303–10.
14. Byun HK, Chang JS, Im SH, et al. Risk of lymphedema following contemporary treatment for breast cancer: an analysis of 7617 consecutive patients from a multidisciplinary perspective. Ann Surg. 2021;274(1):170–8.
15. Belmonte R, Messaggi-Sartor M, Ferrer M, et al. Prospective study of shoulder strength, shoulder range of motion, and lymphedema in breast cancer patients from pre-surgery to 5 years after ALND or SLNB. Support Care Cancer. 2018;26:3277–87.
16. Wetzig N, Gill PG, Espinoza D, et al. Sentinel-lymph-node-based management or routine axillary clearance? Five-year outcomes of the RACS sentinel node biopsy versus axillary clearance (SNAC) 1 trial: assessment and incidence of true lymphedema. Ann Surg Oncol. 2017;24:1064–70.
17. McLaughlin SA, Brunelle CL, Taghian A. Breast cancer-related lymphedema: risk factors, screening, management, and the impact of locoregional treatment. J Clin Oncol. 2020;38(20):2341–50.
18. Poortmans P, Collette S, Struikmans H, et al. Fifteen-year results of the randomised EORTC trial 22922/10925 investigating internal mammary and medial supraclavicular (IM-MS) lymph node irradiation in stage I-III breast cancer. J Clin Oncol. 2018;36(Suppl 15; abstr 504).
19. Whelan TJ, Olivotto IA, Parulekar WR, et al. Regional nodal irradiation in early-stage breast cancer. N Engl J Med. 2015;373:307–16.
20. Warren LEG, Miller CL, Horick N, et al. The impact of radiation therapy on the risk of lymphedema after treatment for breast cancer: a prospective cohort study. Int J Radiat Oncol Biol Phys. 2014;88:565–71.
21. Naoum GE, Roberts SA, Shui AM, et al. Quantifying the impact of regional lymph node irradiation on lymphedema risk in breast cancer patients treated with SLNB or ALND: long-term results from a prospective screening trial. Int J Radiat Oncol. 2019;105:S42.
22. Jammallo LS, Miller CL, Singer M, et al. Impact of body mass index and weight fluctuation on lymphedema risk in patients treated for breast cancer. Breast Cancer Res Treat. 2013;142:59–67.
23. Schmitz KH, Troxel AB, Dean LT, et al. Effect of home-based exercise and weight loss programs on breast cancer-related lymphedema outcomes among overweight breast cancer survivors: the WISER survivor randomized clinical trial. JAMA Oncol. 2019;5(11):1605–13.
24. McLaughlin SA, Wright MJ, Morris KT, et al. Prevalence of lymphedema in women with breast cancer 5 years after sentinel lymph node biopsy or axillary dissection: objective measurements. J Clin Oncol. 2008;26:5213–9.
25. Ferguson CM, Swaroop MN, Horick N, et al. Impact of ipsilateral blood draws, injections, blood pressure measurements, and air travel on the risk of lymph-

edema for patients treated for breast cancer. J Clin Oncol. 2016;34:691–8.
26. Asdourian MS, Skolny MN, Brunelle C, et al. Precautions for breast cancer-related lymphoedema: risk from air travel, ipsilateral arm blood pressure measurements, skin puncture, extreme temperatures, and cellulitis. Lancet Oncol. 2016;17:e392–405.
27. Specht MC, Miller CL, Russell TA, et al. Defining a threshold for intervention in breast cancer-related lymphedema: what level of arm volume increase predicts progression? Breast Cancer Res Treat. 2013;140:485–94.
28. Kilbreath SL, Lee M-J, Refshauge KM, et al. Transient swelling versus lymphoedema in the first year following surgery for breast cancer. Support Care Cancer. 2013;21:2207–15.
29. International Society of Lymphology. The diagnosis and treatment of peripheral lymphedema: 2013 consensus document of the International Society of Lymphology. Lymphology. 2013;46:1–11.
30. McDuff SGR, Mina AI, Brunelle CL, et al. Timing of lymphedema after treatment for breast cancer: when are patients most at risk? Int J Radiat Oncol Biol Phys. 2019;103:62–70.
31. Brunelle C, Skolny M, Ferguson C, et al. Establishing and sustaining a prospective screening program for breast cancer-related lymphedema at the Massachusetts General Hospital: lessons learned. J Pers Med. 2015;5:153–64.
32. Stout Gergich NL, Pfalzer LA, McGarvey C, et al. Preoperative assessment enables the early diagnosis and successful treatment of lymphedema. Cancer. 2008;112:2809–19.
33. National Lymphedema Network. Position statement of the National Lymphedema Network: screening and measurement for early detection of breast cancer related lymphedema. https://lymphnet.org/position-papers.
34. Sun F, Skolny MN, Swaroop MN, et al. The need for preoperative baseline arm measurement to accurately quantify breast cancer-related lymphedema. Breast Cancer Res Treat. 2016;157:229–40.
35. Ancukiewicz M, Miller CL, Skolny MN, et al. Comparison of relative versus absolute arm size change as criteria for quantifying breast cancer-related lymphedema: the flaws in current studies and need for universal methodology. Breast Cancer Res Treat. 2012;135:145–52.
36. Miller CL, Specht MC, Horick N, et al. A novel, validated method to quantify breast cancer-related lymphedema (BCRL) following bilateral breast surgery. Lymphology. 2013;46:64–74.
37. Ancukiewicz M, Russell TA, Otoole J, et al. Standardized method for quantification of developing lymphedema in patients treated for breast cancer. Int J Radiat Oncol Biol Phys. 2011;79:1436–43.
38. Pappalardo M, Starnoni M, Franceschini G, Baccarani A, De Santis G. Breast cancer-related lymphedema: recent updates on diagnosis, severity and available treatments. J Pers Med. 2021;11(5):402.
39. Ridner SH. Quality of life and a symptom cluster associated with breast cancer treatment-related lymphedema. Support Care Cancer. 2005;13:904–11.
40. Armer JM, Radina ME, Porock D, et al. Predicting breast cancer-related lymphedema using self-reported symptoms. Nurs Res. 2003;52:370–9.
41. Fu MR, Rosedale M. Breast cancer survivors' experiences of lymphedema-related symptoms. J Pain Symptom Manag. 2009;38:849–59.
42. Cheville AL, McGarvey CL, Petrek JA, Russo SA, Taylor ME, Thiadens SR. Lymphedema management. Semin Radiat Oncol. 2003;13(3):290–301.
43. Zuther JE, Norton S. Complete decongestive therapy. Lymphedema management: the comprehensive guide for practitioners. 3rd ed. New York, NY: Thieme; 2013. p. 129–35.
44. Lasinski BB, Thrift KM, Squire D, et al. Asystematic review of the evidence for complete decongestive therapy in the treatment of lymphedema from 2004 to 2011. PM&R. 2012;4:580–1.
45. Rockson SG. Lymphedema after breast cancer treatment. N Engl J Med. 2018;379:1937–44.
46. Ezzo J, Manheimer E, McNeely ML, Howell DM, Weiss R, Johansson KI, et al. Manual lymphatic drainage for lymphedema following breast cancer treatment. Cochrane Database Syst Rev. 2015;2015:CD003475.
47. Anuszkiewicz K, Jankau J, Kur M. What do we know about treating breast-cancer-related lymphedema? Review of the current knowledge about therapeutic options. Breast Cancer. 2023;30(2):187–99.
48. Weissleder H, Schuchhardt C. Lymphedema diagnosis and therapy. 2nd ed. Koln: Viavital Verlag GmbH; 1997. p. 97.
49. McNeely ML, Campbell KL, Webster M, et al. Efficacy of night-time compression for breast cancer related lymphedema (LYNC): protocol for a multicenter, randomized controlled efficacy trial. BMC Cancer. 2016;16:601.
50. Rockson SG, Keeley V, Kilbreath S, Szuba A, Towers A. Cancer-associated secondary lymphoedema. Nat Rev Dis Primers. 2019;5(1):22.
51. Ochalek K, Gradalski T, Partsch H. Preventing early postoperative arm swelling and lymphedema manifestation by compression sleeves after axillary lymph node interventions in breast cancer patients: a randomized controlled trial. J Pain Symptom Manag. 2017;54:346–54.
52. Paramanandam VS, Dylke E, Clark GM, et al. Prophylactic use of compression sleeves reduces the incidence of arm swelling in women at high risk of breast cancer-related lymphedema: a randomized controlled trial. J Clin Oncol. 2022;40:2004–12.
53. McNeely ML, Magee DJ, Lees AW, et al. The addition of manual lymph drainage to compression therapy for breast cancer related lymphedema: a randomized controlled trial. Breast Cancer Res Treat. 2004;86:95–106.
54. Shao Y, Qi K, Zhou Q-H, et al. Intermittent pneumatic compression pump for breast cancer-related

lymphedema: a systematic review and meta-analysis of randomized controlled trials. Oncol Res Treat. 2014;37:170–4.
55. Schmitz KH, Courneya KS, Matthews C, et al. American College of Sports Medicine roundtable on exercise guidelines for cancer survivors. Med Sci Sports Exerc. 2010;42:1409–26.
56. Schmitz KH, Ahmed RL, Troxel AB, et al. Weight lifting for women at risk for breast cancer-related lymphedema: a randomized trial. JAMA. 2010;304:2699–705.
57. Schmitz KH, Ahmed RL, Troxel A, et al. Weight lifting in women with breast-cancer-related lymphedema. N Engl J Med. 2009;361:664–73.
58. Shamoun S, Ahmad M. Complete decongestive therapy effect on breast cancer related to lymphedema: a systemic review and meta-analysis of randomized controlled trials. Asian Pac J Cancer Prev. 2023;24(7):2225–38.
59. National Lymphedema Network. Lymphedema risk reduction practices. https://atlanticlymph.ca/en/wp-content/uploads/2012/09/nlnriskreduction.pdf.
60. Asdourian MS, Swaroop MN, Sayegh HE, et al. Association between precautionary behaviors and breast cancer-related lymphedema in patients undergoing bilateral surgery. J Clin Oncol. 2017;35:3934–41.
61. Kilbreath SL, Refshauge KM, Beith JM, et al. Risk factors for lymphoedema in women with breast cancer: a large prospective cohort. Breast. 2016;28:29–36.
62. McLaughlin SA, DeSnyder SM, Klimberg S, et al. Considerations for clinicians in the diagnosis, prevention, and treatment of breast cancer-related lymphedema, recommendations from an expert panel: part 2: preventive and therapeutic options. Ann Surg Oncol. 2017;24:2827–35.
63. Thompson M, Korourian S, Henry-Tillman R, et al. Axillary reverse mapping (ARM): a new concept to identify and enhance lymphatic preservation. Ann Surg Oncol. 2007;14:1890–5.
64. Ahmed M, Rubio IT, Kovacs T, et al. Systematic review of axillary reverse mapping in breast cancer. Br J Surg. 2016;103:170–8.
65. Luiten EJT, Beek MA, Rubio IT. Clinical utility of axillary reverse mapping (ARM) in an era of changing perceptions concerning axillary surgery. Eur J Surg Oncol. 2016;42:585–7.
66. Yuan Q, Wu G, Xiao SY, et al. Identification and preservation of arm lymphatic system in axillary dissection for breast cancer to reduce arm lymphedema events: a randomized clinical trial. Ann Surg Oncol. 2019;26:3446–54.
67. Boccardo FM, Casabona F, Friedman D, et al. Surgical prevention of arm lymphedema after breast cancer treatment. Ann Surg Oncol. 2011;18:2500–5.
68. Feldman S, Bansil H, Ascherman J, et al. Single institution experience with lymphatic microsurgical preventive healing approach (LYMPHA) for the primary prevention of lymphedema. Ann Surg Oncol. 2015;22:3296–301.
69. Granzow JW. Lymphedema surgery: the current state of the art. Clin Exp Metastasis. 2018;35:553–8.
70. Rockson SG. A population-based assessment of the problem of lymphatic disease. Lymphat Res Biol. 2008;6:1–2.
71. Rockson SG. Progress in the approach to lymphatic vascular malformation. Lymphat Res Biol. 2019;17:495.
72. Visser J, van Geel M, Cornelissen AJM, et al. Breast cancer-related lymphedema and genetic predisposition: a systematic review of the literature. Lymphat Res Biol. 2019;17:288–93.

Physiotherapy and Rehabilitation for Pain in Breast Cancer: From Background to Management

9

Gamze Nalan Çinar and Ceren Gürşen

9.1 Breast Cancer Treatments and Pain

Breast cancer is the most common type of malignancy in women worldwide. It begins to be seen with puberty, and its incidence increases with age [1]. According to the data from the World Health Organization (WHO), approximately 2.3 million women worldwide were diagnosed with breast cancer in 2022, and 670,000 deaths occurred due to breast cancer [1]. However, with the development of diagnostic and imaging systems and more effective treatment strategies, the number of breast cancer survivors is gradually increasing [2]. However, a significant number of breast cancer survivors may experience physical (neuropathy, fatigue syndromes, lymphedema, axillary web syndrome (AWS), limitation in range of motion, menopause, pain, etc.) and psychological symptoms (fear of death or recurrence, financial stress, changes in body image, etc.) [3]. These complications can be seen not only during treatment but also in the long term [4].

The International Association for the Study of Pain (IASP) defines pain as "an unpleasant sensory and emotional experience associated with actual or potential tissue damage" [5]. Pain is one of the most common problems in individuals undergoing cancer treatment and for cancer survivors [4]. After cancer treatment, it is usually expected that pain will decrease as tissue damage heals or the threat disappears. In some cases, pain is not a short-term problem associated with treatment but can become a chronic problem that can last for months, years, or even a lifetime. Cancer-related pain is based on identifiable tissue damage; therefore, the cancer population who suffer from pain is different from individuals with chronic pain but no history of cancer [4]. Studies show that 30–50% of patients experience pain symptoms during cancer treatment; this rate can be reached up to 70% in cases of metastasis [6]. It has also been reported that about 30% of breast cancer survivors suffer from pain even 10 years after the end of treatment [7]. A meta-analysis evaluating breast cancer-related pain (BCRP) reported that the prevalence of pain was 39% between 3 months and 1 year postoperatively, 31% between 1 and 2 years postoperatively, and 29% after the second postoperative year [8].

Studies show some sociodemographic factors (age, body mass index, education, alcohol, smoking, and parity), psychological factors, race, cancer treatments (chemotherapy, radiotherapy, and hormone therapy), type of breast surgery, tumor size, cancer stage, type of axillary intervention, lymphedema, and axillary web syndrome as risk factors for developing pain [5]. There is evidence that preexisting chronic pain conditions

G. N. Çinar (✉)
Faculty of Physiotherapy and Rehabilitation, Hacettepe University, Ankara, Turkey

C. Gürşen
Leuven University (KU Leuven), Leuven, Belgium

Y. Bakar, A. Tuğral (eds.), *Managing Side Effects of Breast Cancer Treatment*, https://doi.org/10.1007/978-3-031-75480-7_9

(migraine, low back pain, fibromyalgia syndrome, etc.) may also be a risk factor for the development of pain in patients prior to breast cancer treatment. This is thought to be related to potentially increased nociceptive input and central sensitization [9].

In terms of patient-related risk factors, the literature shows that younger age may be a risk factor for the development of BCRP. According to the results of a meta-analysis, each 10-year decrease in age is associated with a 1.36-fold increase in the odds of pain. The reasons for this may be attributed to physiological differences such as having a higher histopathological tumor grade, an excess of estrogen receptors, and a higher sensitivity of pain receptors in younger patients compared to older ones [9].

Axillary lymph node dissection (ALND) is a risk factor in the development of BCRP. A study of 475 patients followed for 1 year after mastectomy found that women who underwent ALND were 3.1 times more likely to have moderate to severe pain at rest than those who underwent lumpectomy. It is stated that the incidence of pain development is lower after sentinel lymph node biopsy (SLNB). However, node-positive patients who underwent secondary ALND after SLNB did not differ from node-positive patients who underwent single-stage axillary dissection in terms of either objective or subjective morbidity [10].

The effect of intercostobrachial nerve (ICBN) damage during breast surgery on the development of acute or chronic pain is unclear in the literature. In one study, patients undergoing ALND with breast surgery were divided into three groups according to the preservation of the ICBN: ICBN preserved, ICBN partially preserved, and ICBN damaged [11]. It was found that there was no difference in the development of pain between these three groups in the acute and chronic periods [11]. In addition to ICBN injury, any surgical procedure can cause changes in the musculoskeletal system that may cause pain. For example, during breast surgery, partial dissection of the pectoralis muscle can shorten the pectoralis muscle and reduce the range of motion of the glenohumeral joint, causing musculoskeletal dysfunction [9]. Although breast surgery can cause postmastectomy pain and/or phantom pain, the relationship between the type of surgery and the risk of pain is unclear in the literature. Some publications have reported that more invasive approaches (e.g., axillary dissection and breast reconstruction) do not cause more pain than lumpectomy. However, less invasive surgical techniques have not been proven to reduce the development of postoperative pain. Radiotherapy, chemotherapy, anxiety, depression, and pain catastrophizing are among the other risk factors for postoperative pain. Genetic predisposition also contributes to the risk of developing pain [9, 12].

Chemotherapy and/or adjuvant radiotherapy are frequently administered after breast cancer surgery. These treatments can cause neurotoxicity and neuropathic pain. Chemotherapy has been reported to cause chemotherapy-induced peripheral neuropathy (CIPN), particularly by damaging the peripheral sensory nerves. By affecting the peripheral nervous system, the function of the somatosensory processing mechanism is altered. This alteration can cause allodynia, primary and secondary hyperalgesia, and therefore pain. A meta-analysis found that people who received chemotherapy were 1.44 times more likely to develop BCRP than those who did not. Similarly, people who received hormone therapy were 1.33 times more likely to develop BCRP, and those who received radiotherapy were 1.32 times more likely than those who did not [5]. Although adjuvant radiotherapy is effective against tumor potential, it has been reported to cause delayed painful brachial and lumbosacral plexopathies, osteoradionecrosis, fractures, and in some cases secondary malignancies [5].

9.2 Pain Mechanisms in Breast Cancer Patients

Different types of pain can be seen in patients with BCRP. BCRP has been classified in the literature as nociceptive, neuropathic, nociplastic, and mixed pain. IASP defines these pain types as follows:

- *Nociceptive Pain:* Inflammatory pain that is proportional to the amount of tissue damage, resulting from noxious chemical, mechanical, or thermal stimuli and occurring with activation of nociceptors.
- *Neuropathic Pain:* Pain that occurs as a direct result of a lesion or disease affecting the somatosensory nervous system and may be accompanied by paresthesia and/or weakness.
- *Nociceptive Pain:* Pain associated with an increased response of nociceptive neurons in the central nervous system (CNS) to normal or subthreshold afferent input.
- *Mixed-Type Pain:* Regardless of the type of surgery, both peripheral and central sensitization mechanisms have been implicated in BCRP. For this reason, breast cancer patients may experience mixed-type pain, where three types of pain occur together [13].

In determining the type of pain in BCRP, the following algorithm can be used for this purpose as investigating whether the pain has neuropathic characteristics as a first step. This is done by assessing whether the lesion of the nervous system (central and peripheral) and the pain are neuroanatomically compatible with structures associated with breast cancer and related treatments. In this assessment, clinical examination findings, imaging techniques, and laboratory tests are used. If neuropathic pain is excluded, the second step is to assess the presence of nociplastic pain [13].

It has been found that neuropathic pain is the most common type of pain in BCRP. Bokhari et al. reported that 20–50% of patients experience neuropathic pain after breast cancer treatment [14]. However, it is stated that the development of neuropathic pain depends on the disease and the phase of cancer treatment, whether acute or chronic. Chemotherapy-induced neuropathic pain is reported to occur in 90% of patients receiving chemotherapy. Similarly, post-mastectomy pain syndrome (PMPS) is a type of neuropathic pain that occurs in the ipsilateral breast, pectoral region, or arm after breast surgery. PMPS is also frequently seen after ALND [15].

9.3 Physical and Psychosocial Aspects of Pain in Breast Cancer Patients

9.3.1 Physical Aspects of Pain in Breast Cancer Patients

9.3.1.1 Myofascial Pain Syndrome

Myofascial pain syndrome (MPS) is characterized by myofascial trigger points in the flexible bands of skeletal muscles in the area of the lesion and in distant areas, which can be palpated and cause regional pain. A study investigating the incidence of MPS after breast cancer surgery found that 52 of 116 patients (45%) developed MPS. Most patients with MPS in this study had active trigger points in the shoulder girdle muscles. It has been reported that MPS is frequently seen in the latissimus dorsi, serratus anterior, pectoralis major, and infraspinatus muscles after breast cancer surgery [16].

9.3.1.2 Brachial Plexopathy and Radiation Fibrosis Syndrome

Nerve damage, fibrosis, and adhesions can cause pain in the arm and trunk, reduced range of motion in joints, and reduced muscle strength and lymphatic flow in the upper extremities as a result of radiotherapy in breast cancer patients. Brachial plexopathy (BP) is a problem originating from damage to and pressure on the brachial plexus. Although BP has many causes, its incidence increases after breast surgery and radiotherapy [17]. The literature suggests that 9% of patients who receive radiotherapy to the axillary region develop BP. In addition, one study found that 6 months after mastectomy, 27.2% of patients had shoulder and/or scapulothoracic pain and a decrease in upper extremity activities [18]. However, it is reported that in any painful case, the risk of metastasis and recurrence must be excluded before making this diagnosis [19].

9.3.1.3 Postmastectomy/Postsurgical Pain Syndrome

Post-mastectomy pain syndrome (PMPS) is defined as a chronic pain condition that begins after breast cancer treatment persists beyond the recovery period (approximately 3 months) and is often characterized by neuropathic origin/pain. PMPS can cause chronic pain in the breast tissue (mastalgia), pectoral region, axillary region, and/or arm. Symptoms include hyperalgesia, paresthesia, dysesthesia, allodynia, and loss of shoulder function. It has been suggested that the development of PMPS may be more common in patients who underwent breast reconstruction along with a breast prosthesis. Various studies of PMPS have reported an incidence of pain that can range from 4% to 56%. Risk factors for PMPS include age (younger patients are at higher risk), ICBN, long thoracic and thoracodorsal nerve damage, and high BMI. ICBN damage has been found to be the most common cause of PMPS (20–50%). In PMPS following ICBN injury, paresthesia, numbness, and neuropathic pain occur in the medial part of the upper arm [20].

9.3.1.4 Chemotherapy-Induced Peripheral Neuropathy

Chemotherapy-induced peripheral neuropathy (CIPN) is the most common neurological complication caused by the neurotoxic effects of some chemotherapy drugs used to treat breast cancer. Pain in CIPN is usually described as burning, tingling, or numbness. The symptoms are usually characterized by neuropathic pain affecting the distal part of both extremities. The severity of the symptoms depends on the dose of chemotherapy exposure. Risk factors for CIPN include a history of preexisting neuropathy, age ≥60 years, and genetic polymorphisms [4].

9.3.1.5 Arthralgia Syndrome

Arthralgia is a problem characterized by pain or stiffness in a joint. Women treated for hormone-positive breast cancer, particularly postmenopausal women, are prescribed aromatase inhibitors (AI) to inhibit the aromatase enzyme that converts androgens to estrogens and to reduce plasma estrogen levels. A cross-sectional study found that arthralgia that occurred within 3 months of starting AI treatment can cause pain in 50% of women. The most commonly affected joints are the hands and ankles, fingers and toes, elbows, and knees [21].

9.3.2 Psychosocial Aspects of Pain in Breast Cancer Patients

9.3.2.1 Pain Catastrophization

Pain catastrophizing is a condition typically based on constantly thinking about the pain. The threatening dimension of the pain increases, and patients think that they cannot control the pain. It is observed that patients complaining of pain after mastectomy have higher levels of pain catastrophization, as well as somatization, anxiety, and sleep disorders. However, it is stated that hypersensitivity and catastrophizing are highest in the first 2 years after surgery [9].

9.3.2.2 Depression and Anxiety

Studies investigating the effect of pain on psychosocial symptoms after breast cancer surgery have found that depression and anxiety are the most common problems experienced by these patients [9, 22]. It has also been reported that there is a bi-directional relationship between the intensity of pain and the level of depression/anxiety. In fact, it has been found that patients with higher levels of anxiety and depression are more likely to experience chronic pain after breast surgery [23].

9.3.2.3 Sleep and Fatigue

Pain and sleep problems that develop after breast cancer are two concepts that are often evaluated together in clinical settings. Studies report that 60–99% of treated patients and 40% of cancer survivors experience sleep disturbance and fatigue. Factors affecting sleep quality include chest and neck/shoulder pain, shoulder movement limitation, and upper extremity muscle weakness. Patients with chronic pain often report difficulty falling asleep. It was also reported that sleep is interrupted several times by pain. Therefore, although the sleep duration of patients is sufficient, their sleep quality is generally low. Therefore, sleep is an important aspect that needs to be considered in chronic pain management [24].

9.3.2.4 Sexual Dysfunction

Studies indicate that changes in body image in women who have undergone breast surgery and increased sensitivity and pain in the breast and surrounding tissues due to breast cancer treatment can lead to sexual dysfunction [25].

9.4 Physiotherapy and Rehabilitation for Pain Management in Breast Cancer Patients

The key to success in rehabilitation interventions for BCRP is an accurate and specific diagnosis, supported by a detailed and comprehensive clinical assessment. Therefore, in addition to a detailed history, the assessment should include a detailed physical examination and supportive electrodiagnostic, imaging, and/or laboratory tests. Pain management should be multidisciplinary and multimodal. The most successful and most frequently consulted approach to the treatment of BCRP is physical therapy and rehabilitation [4]. The methods used to manage BCRP are explained below.

9.4.1 Patient Education

The success of treatment depends on patients having the information they need to protect and improve their health and manage their behavior accordingly. In recent years, studies on BCRP have found that patients understand pain better when the neurophysiology of pain is explained. Pain Neuroscience Education (PNE) explains the definition of pain, the differences between acute and chronic pain, normal pain neurophysiology, changes in the peripheral and central nervous system in chronic pain, factors that influence pain, and methods of coping with pain. PNE aims to promote pain-related adaptive behaviors by increasing the level of knowledge about pain. In this way, the individual can evolve from being a passive recipient of a treatment to an active participant. PNE breaks the fear-pain-tension cycle that accompanies pathological conditions. As a result, the patient's perception of pain changes through the underlying mechanism of PNE, which is characterized by understanding that the pain is not only caused by tissues and disorders. False beliefs about pain can be changed via increased participation and belief in the treatment, and thus fear and kinesiophobia are mitigated [26]. The second step in chronic pain management is graded activity training. This involves facing directly the feared activity rather than using imagery or visualization. The third step in PNE is stress management, and the fourth step is sleep hygiene. This training involves the conscious management of parameters that may affect sleep by the patient [24].

9.4.2 Manual Therapy

Manual therapy is used in breast cancer treatment to reduce myofascial dysfunction, AWS, and pain both in the early and chronic postoperative periods. Within postoperative manual therapy approaches in breast cancer treatment, active and passive joint mobilization, myofascial (skin, superficial and deep fascia, and muscles) mobilization, and soft transverse friction can be used to prevent scar tissue and adhesions in the surgical area [27].

9.4.3 Exercises

Exercise is an important part of pain management. There is a high level of evidence that exercise is effective management against complications such as lymphedema, fatigue, musculoskeletal problems, and pain that can be caused by breast cancer treatment [28]. In general, patients limit physical activity and exercise after breast cancer surgery for fear of developing lymphedema. In addition, upper extremity activity has historically been restricted after ALND and/or radiotherapy. This recommendation stems from the belief that exercise may trigger or worsen upper extremity lymphedema [29]. However, increasing levels of physical activity and exercise during and after breast cancer treatment improves patients' psychosocial and physical conditions, increases survival and quality of life, and reduces pain and kinesiophobia [28]. Studies evaluating the effectiveness of exercise for BCRP have reported that exercise programs should be started early after breast surgery [30]. It has also been reported that as exercise intensity increases, pain intensity decreases, and quality of life increases. Group exercises have been found to have a positive effect on pain and quality of life, particularly in women with severe pain-related functional disability and advanced cancer [31].

The literature suggests that aerobic exercise is the most beneficial type of exercise for reducing complications that can cause pain in people with breast cancer. Although there are no definitive recommendations about the intensity of exercise, the literature suggests that moderate-to-vigorous intensity exercise should be recommended [32]. A systematic review reported that yoga exercises performed for 20–120 min were effective in the treatment of BCRP, reducing shoulder and arm pain compared with a no-intervention control group [33]. According to the results of studies conducted on patients receiving chemotherapy and AI, the Tai Chi program, which includes rhythmic exercise and meditation approaches performed for 15–60 min, has a healing effect on the perception and severity of pain [33]. The Cochrane review found that dance and movement therapy was effective in improving pain, quality of life, somatization, and cancer-related fatigue in patients receiving breast cancer treatment [34].

9.4.4 Stress Management

Since breast cancer treatment involves coping with many physical, psychological, and social situations, psychological factors also need to be fully addressed in the management of pain. There is evidence that cognitive behavioral techniques provide moderate benefits in coping with depression, anxiety, and pain compared with patients receiving standard care after breast cancer [9]. In addition, relaxation training, music therapy, hypnotherapy, and mindfulness approaches might also be effective in coping with pain after breast cancer [9].

9.4.5 Sleep Education

The literature suggests that lifestyle interventions that promote physical activity, along with behavioral therapies such as cognitive behavioral therapy, may be effective in reducing sleep problems in breast cancer patients. In particular, yoga and mind-body based breathing and exercise have been shown to improve sleep quality in these patients. One randomized trial found that aerobic and resistance exercise also improved sleep problems in breast cancer survivors [35]. In addition, recommendations given on sleep hygiene can be effective in chronic pain management. These recommendations are as follows:

- Wake up at the same time every morning, no matter what time you go to bed.
- Go to bed at about the same time every night.
- Prepare yourself for half an hour of sleep before going to bed; make time for yourself.
- Do not lie down in bed until you are ready to sleep.
- Relaxation techniques are especially helpful if you are worried about not being able to sleep or about pain. You can benefit from relaxation techniques, breathing exercises, and meditation.
- Avoid heavy, fatty, or sweetened foods before bed.
- Cut out caffeine, coffee, coke, and chocolate 4 h before bed.
- Exercise moderately, but avoid strenuous exercise within 2–3 h of bedtime. This will increase your heart rate and body temperature, making it harder to fall asleep.
- The greater the difference between daylight and darkness, the more "melatonin" the body produces. This is a hormone that promotes sleep.
- Reduce the amount of light in your bedroom.

- Increase the amount of sunlight during the day.
- Create a quiet environment.
- When you fall asleep, your body temperature drops. Taking a hot shower in the evening will help you fall asleep [24].

9.4.6 Desensitization and Sensory Re-Education

Desensitization has been found to reduce neuropathic pain in PPMS (e.g., phantom pain or scar tissue hypersensitivity) or radiation fibrosis syndrome [9]. Desensitization techniques that can be used for this purpose include:

- *Tactile and Sensory Education*: This helps the patient regain the ability to touch and apply light pressure to the surgical area. A variety of touch techniques are used to gently move the hand over the skin, reducing skin sensitivity over time.
- *Mindfulness and Breathing Exercises*: Mindfulness and breathing exercises can help the patient cope with sensitivity in the surgical area. During these exercises, the patient is encouraged to focus and breathe deeply. Breathing exercises can also reduce stress and provide general body relaxation.
- *Tactile and Sensory Stimulation Exercises*: These exercises use sensory stimuli, such as touching the surgical site, gentle massage, or feeling different types of tissue. This can help to re-stimulate nerve endings and reduce skin sensitivity.
- *Mirror Therapy*: Mirror therapy can be used to cope with changes in body image that occur after breast surgery. The patient is encouraged to see and accept the changes in the surgical area. As a result, it can better adapt to sensory experiences.
- *Heat or Cold Therapy*: Hot or cold applications to the surgical area can reduce skin sensitivity and provide relief. Applications of heat or cold can relieve discomfort at the surgical site by reducing the sensitivity of nerve endings. This application may be preferred in the long term after surgery [36].

9.5 Conclusion

Breast cancer is the most common malignancy in women worldwide. Today, the number of breast cancer survivors is increasing. However, a significant proportion of breast cancer survivors experience physical and psychological complications. Pain is one of the most common problems experienced by individuals undergoing cancer treatment and by cancer survivors. Sociodemographic factors, psychological factors, multimodal cancer treatments (surgery, chemotherapy, radiotherapy, hormone therapy), lymphedema, and AWS have all been reported to contribute to pain. The key to successful management of BCRP is an accurate and specific diagnosis, supported by a detailed and comprehensive clinical assessment. Treatment should include pain management using a multidisciplinary and multimodal strategy. Physiotherapy and rehabilitation approaches are recommended for the management of BCRP, including patient education, pain neuroscience education, manual therapy, exercise, sleep training, stress management, desensitization, and sensory re-education.

Competing Interests The authors declare no conflict of interest.

References

1. WHO BC. https://www.who.int/news-room/fact-sheets/detail/breast-cancer.
2. Katanoda K, Matsuda T. Five-year relative survival rate of breast cancer in the USA, Europe and Japan. Jpn J Clin Oncol. 2014;44(6):611.
3. Gülören G, Doğan Y, Özgül S, Gürşen C, Çinar GN, İpekten F, Akbayrak T. Acute effects of remedial exercises with and without compression on breast-cancer-related lymphedema. Healthcare. 2023;11(22):2949.
4. Glare P. Pain in cancer survivors. Asia Pac J Clin Oncol. 2016.

5. Leysen L, Beckwee D, Nijs J, Pas R, Bilterys T, Vermeir S, Adriaenssens N. Risk factors of pain in breast cancer survivors: a systematic review and meta-analysis. Support Care Cancer. 2017;25:3607–43.
6. Goudas LC, Bloch R, Gialeli-Goudas M, Lau J, Carr DB. The epidemiology of cancer pain. Cancer Investig. 2005;23(2):182–90.
7. Forsythe LP, Alfano CM, George SM, McTiernan A, Baumgartner KB, Bernstein L, Ballard-Barbash R. Pain in long-term breast cancer survivors: the role of body mass index, physical activity, and sedentary behavior. Breast Cancer Res Treat. 2013;137:617–30.
8. Wang L, Cohen JC, Devasenapathy N, Hong BY, Kheyson S, Lu D, et al. Prevalence and intensity of persistent post-surgical pain following breast cancer surgery: a systematic review and meta-analysis of observational studies. Br J Anaesth. 2020;125(3):346–57.
9. Tait RC, Zoberi K, Ferguson M, Levenhagen K, Luebbert RA, Rowland K, et al. Persistent post-mastectomy pain: risk factors and current approaches to treatment. J Pain. 2018;19(12):1367–83.
10. Madsen AH, Haugaard K, Soerensen J, Bokmand S, Friis E, Holtveg H, et al. Arm morbidity following sentinel lymph node biopsy or axillary lymph node dissection: a study from the Danish Breast Cancer Cooperative Group. Breast. 2008;17(2):138–47.
11. Andersen KG, Aasvang E, Kroman N, Kehlet H. Intercostobrachial nerve handling and pain after axillary lymph node dissection for breast cancer. Acta Anaesthesiol Scand. 2014;58(10):1240–8.
12. Andersen KG, Duriaud HM, Jensen HE, Kroman N, Kehlet H. Predictive factors for the development of persistent pain after breast cancer surgery. Pain. 2015;156(12):2413–22.
13. Nijs J, Leysen L, Adriaenssens N, Aguilar Ferrándiz ME, Devoogdt N, Tassenoy A, et al. Pain following cancer treatment: guidelines for the clinical classification of predominant neuropathic, nociceptive and central sensitization pain. Acta Oncol. 2016;55(6):659–63.
14. Bokhari F, Sawatzky J-AV. Chronic neuropathic pain in women after breast cancer treatment. Pain Manag Nurs. 2009;10(4):197–205.
15. Leysen L, Adriaenssens N, Nijs J, Pas R, Bilterys T, Vermeir S, et al. Chronic pain in breast cancer survivors: nociceptive, neuropathic, or central sensitization pain? Pain Pract. 2019;19(2):183–95.
16. Lacomba MT, Del Moral OM, Zazo JLC, Gerwin RD, Goñí AZ. Incidence of myofascial pain syndrome in breast cancer surgery: a prospective study. Clin J Pain. 2010;26(4):320–5.
17. Jaeckle KA. Neurologic manifestations of neoplastic and radiation-induced plexopathies. Semin Neurol. 2010;30(3):254–62.
18. Fabro EAN, Bergmann A, Silva BAE, Ribeiro ACP, de Souza Abrahão K, Ferreira MGCL, et al. Post-mastectomy pain syndrome: incidence and risks. Breast. 2012;21(3):321–5.
19. Burton AW, Fanciullo GJ, Beasley RD, Fisch MJ. Chronic pain in the cancer survivor: a new frontier. Pain Med. 2007;8(2):189–98.
20. Macdonald L, Bruce J, Scott NW, Smith WCS, Chambers W. Long-term follow-up of breast cancer survivors with post-mastectomy pain syndrome. Br J Cancer. 2005;92(2):225–30.
21. Mao JJ, Stricker C, Bruner D, Xie S, Bowman MA, Farrar JT, et al. Patterns and risk factors associated with aromatase inhibitor-related arthralgia among breast cancer survivors. Cancer. 2009;115(16):3631–9.
22. Gulluoglu BM, Cingi A, Cakir T, Gercek A, Barlas A, Eti Z. Factors related to post-treatment chronic pain in breast cancer survivors: the interference of pain with life functions. Int J Fertil Womens Med. 2006;51(2):75–82.
23. Miaskowski C, Paul SM, Cooper B, West C, Levine JD, Elboim C, et al. Identification of patient subgroups and risk factors for persistent arm/shoulder pain following breast cancer surgery. Eur J Oncol Nurs. 2014;18(3):242–53.
24. Malfliet A, Leysen L, Pas R, Kuppens K, Nijs J, Van Wilgen P, et al. Modern pain neuroscience in clinical practice: applied to post-cancer, paediatric and sports-related pain. Braz J Phys Ther. 2017;21(4):225–32.
25. Paterson CL, Lengacher CA, Donovan KA, Kip KE, Tofthagen CS. Body image in younger breast cancer survivors: a systematic review. Cancer Nurs. 2016;39(1):E39–58.
26. Nijs J, Wijma AJ, Leysen L, Pas R, Willaert W, Hoelen W, et al. Explaining pain following cancer: a practical guide for clinicians. Braz J Phys Ther. 2019;23(5):367–77.
27. da Silva FP, Moreira GM, Zomkowski K, de Noronha MA, Sperandio FF. Manual therapy as treatment for chronic musculoskeletal pain in female breast cancer survivors: a systematic review and meta-analysis. J Manip Physiol Ther. 2019;42(7):503–13.
28. Cormie P, Zopf EM, Zhang X, Schmitz KH. The impact of exercise on cancer mortality, recurrence, and treatment-related adverse effects. Epidemiol Rev. 2017;39(1):71–92.
29. Cheema B, Gaul CA, Lane K, Fiatarone Singh MA. Progressive resistance training in breast cancer: a systematic review of clinical trials. Breast Cancer Res Treat. 2008;109:9–26.
30. Batdorf NJ, Lemaine V, Lovely JK, Ballman KV, Goede WJ, Martinez-Jorge J, et al. Enhanced recovery after surgery in microvascular breast reconstruction. Plast Reconstr Surg. 2015;68(3):395–402.
31. Kalter J, Buffart LM, Korstjens I, van Weert E, Brug J, Verdonck-de Leeuw IM, et al. Moderators of the effects of group-based physical exercise on cancer survivors' quality of life. Support Care Cancer. 2015;23:2623–31.
32. Brenin DR, Dietz JR, Baima J, Cheng G, Froman J, Laronga C, et al. Pain management in breast surgery: recommendations of a multidisciplinary expert

panel—the American Society of Breast Surgeons. Ann Surg Oncol. 2020;27:4588–602.
33. Behzadmehr R, Dastyar N, Moghadam MP, Abavisani M, Moradi M. Effect of complementary and alternative medicine interventions on cancer related pain among breast cancer patients: a systematic review. Complement Ther Med. 2020;49:102318.
34. Bradt J, Shim M, Goodill SW. Dance/movement therapy for improving psychological and physical outcomes in cancer patients. Cochrane Database Syst Rev. 2015;1(1):CD007103.
35. Kwak A, Jacobs J, Haggett D, Jimenez R, Peppercorn J. Evaluation and management of insomnia in women with breast cancer. Breast Cancer Res Treat. 2020;181:269–77.
36. Silver JK, Slowman LS. Breast cancer-related pain. Pain in women: a clinical guide. Berlin: Springer; 2012. p. 277–89.

10 Chemotherapy-Induced Peripheral Neuropathy (CIPN) in Breast Cancer: A Detailed View of the Burdensome Side Effect of Chemotherapy

Gözde Kaya Uçar, Melike Taş, and Alper Tuğral

10.1 Introduction

Cancer is a leading cause of both morbidity and mortality on a global scale, affecting all regions of the world [1]. Breast cancer remains to be the most prevalent form of cancer and constitutes a widespread public health concern [1]. Considering developments in early cancer diagnosis and treatment, patients have extended lifespans, leading to an increasing number of cancer survivors [2]. Existing therapeutic interventions yield significant clinical benefits for cancer patients [3]. Despite the ongoing research and advancements in cancer therapy, (neo)adjuvant chemotherapy regimens continue to be the foremost treatment options for breast cancer due to their proven efficacy on survival [4]. Chemotherapeutic agents such as taxanes (i.e., paclitaxel and docetaxel), anthracycline, platinum, and capecitabine derivatives are commonly used as systemic chemotherapy options for breast cancer patients [5].

Nevertheless, (neo)adjuvant therapies require cautiousness regarding their potential side effects and systemic toxicity on different systems and organs [3]. Breast cancer patients and survivors may experience a variety of long-term side effects during and after chemotherapy, such as fatigue, cognitive impairments, cardiotoxicity, sleep problems, and neuropathy. Chemotherapy-induced side effects are rising health concerns, as they might have the potential to diminish the quality of life of breast cancer patients [6, 7]. Chemotherapeutic agents have the potential to induce peripheral neuropathy, characterized by symptoms resulting from damage to peripheral nerves and related structures. This condition is known as chemotherapy-induced peripheral neuropathy (CIPN) [8]. CIPN affects the somatic (sensory and/or motor) and/or autonomic nervous system, and it is a debilitating adverse effect of neurotoxic chemotherapy agents [9]. Due to its prominent impact on the large sensory myelinated (Aβ) fibers or dorsal root ganglia, CIPN commonly results in sensory neuropathy. However, CIPN has the potential to impact any part of the peripheral nervous system, including motor fibers, as well as thin myelinated (Aδ) and unmyelinated (C) fibers [10].

G. Kaya Uçar · M. Taş · A. Tuğral (✉)
Faculty of Health Sciences, Department of Physical Therapy and Rehabilitation, Izmir Bakircay University, Izmir, Turkey
e-mail: gozde.kaya@bakircay.edu.tr; melike.tas@bakircay.edu.tr; alper.tugral@bakircay.edu.tr

Y. Bakar, A. Tuğral (eds.), *Managing Side Effects of Breast Cancer Treatment*,
https://doi.org/10.1007/978-3-031-75480-7_10

10.2 Incidence and Prevalence for CIPN

The epidemiological data on CIPN are somewhat conflicting owing to variations in diagnostic criteria, assessment methods, severity levels, study settings (clinical oncology, neurology), research methodologies, and timing of assessments [11]. The investigation of CIPN occurrence with a meta-analysis of 31 studies revealed that the prevalence was 68.1% within the first month post-chemotherapy, 60% at 3 months, and 30% at 6 months and beyond [12]. The epidemiology of CIPN also varies depending on the specific chemotherapy agent used. The prevalence of CIPN was found to be higher in the use of platinum-based drugs (70–100%) and taxanes (11–87%) compared to other chemotherapy agents [13]. Notable is the finding of another study that, after the conclusion of chemotherapy (mean time: 5.6 years), 58.4% of breast cancer survivors reported CIPN symptoms [14]. Cancer incidence is projected to increase further over the years. Early identification, together with increased accessibility of chemotherapy treatments, will result in more cancer patients surviving. Nevertheless, early detection and management of CIPN are critical, as a considerable proportion of these patients are susceptible to CIPN development [11].

10.3 Pathophysiology and Mechanism of CIPN

The pathophysiological processes involved in the occurrence of CIPN still need to be fully elucidated. Due to the multifactorial nature behind it, several changes at the cellular and molecular levels are commonly discussed. The alterations in cellular structures (particularly mitochondria and DNA), apoptosis, altered expression of ion channels and release of specific neurotransmitter(s), axon degeneration, changes in cell-signaling pathways, membrane remodeling, immunological responses, and inflammation that occur due to systemic neurotoxic effects of chemotherapy have a detrimental impact on neuronal and glial cells in CIPN [15–17]. The pathophysiology of CIPN shares similar mechanisms across several chemotherapy agents but also shows variation based on the specific agent [15, 18]. For specific emphasis on the taxane-induced CIPN mechanism, this specific type of drugs damage microtubules and hamper axonal transport, resulting in alterations in ion channels and increased excitability of peripheral neurons. Mitochondrial damage leads to oxidative stress, which contributes to the demyelination of peripheral neurons. Neuroinflammation, involving immune cell activation and production of proinflammatory cytokine(s), increases the nociceptor's sensitivity [19].

Notably, in contrast to the central nervous system, the peripheral nervous system lacks a structure resembling the blood–brain barrier. Consequently, antineoplastic drugs exert substantial direct toxicity on peripheral neurons. Furthermore, indirect effects, primarily attributable to inflammation, contribute to the development of CIPN [20]. Notwithstanding, the peripheral mechanism of CIPN can lead to maladaptive changes in the brain that impact CIPN [16]. Comprehending the CIPN mechanism is of the utmost importance in defining a holistic approach to prevention and treatment [9].

10.4 Risk Factors for CIPN

Identifying risk factors that contribute to the development or worsening of CIPN is crucial, as some of them may be managed. When identifying the risk factors, it might be possible to avoid the development of CIPN by implementing precautionary measures or to decrease the severity of current CIPN with appropriate treatment strategies [21, 22]. Several sociodemographic and clinical risk factors contributing to CIPN have been reported [22, 23]. The specific chemotherapy type (such as platinum drugs or taxanes) is one of the significant risk factors [23]. A combination of chemotherapy, higher doses, and multiple courses all increase the risk of CIPN [8].

In patients with breast cancer, the use of docetaxel or paclitaxel (taxanes) as chemotherapeutic agents increases the risk of CIPN [6]. Nevertheless, paclitaxel presents a higher risk for CIPN in comparison to docetaxel [24, 25]. Preexisting neuropathy is another risk factor for CIPN, especially in breast cancer patients receiving taxane-based chemotherapy [23]. The majority of patients with diabetes mellitus (DM) are at risk of developing peripheral neuropathy. The relationship between DM and CIPN risk has produced conflicting results. However, the meta-analysis study findings confirm that DM raises the incidence of CIPN and is a contributing risk factor [26]. Since DM increases the risk of CIPN, a close follow-up is essential for DM, particularly in the presence of diabetic neuropathy [26]. The main risk factor for CIPN is the use of higher doses of chemotherapy. Body surface area, or obesity, considering its effect on chemotherapy dose, is another risk factor for CIPN in breast cancer patients. As the body surface area plays a role in adjusting the chemotherapy dosage, a larger body surface area may increase the risk of CIPN [27]. The larger body surface area of obese individuals compared to those of normal weight increases the risk of CIPN by requiring the use of higher chemotherapy dosages [14, 28]. Additionally, there have been findings suggesting that normoglycemic obese individuals may develop obesity-related neuropathy in addition to an increased risk of developing DM [29]. The mechanisms underlying the association between obesity and CIPN risk require further investigation. Some other risk factors for the onset or severity of CIPN in breast cancer patients include metastatic cancer [25], older age [14], history of smoking [24], insomnia [14], poor nutritional status (such as low levels of serum albumin) [30], proinflammatory status prior to chemotherapy [31], symptom clusters of fatigue, anxiety, and depression [31], and low physical activity [21]. In addition to known risk factors for the development of CIPN, interindividual differences suggest that genetic factors might augment vulnerability [32]. The findings of a meta-analysis indicated that genetic polymorphism could potentially have a significant impact on the prediction of individual susceptibility to taxane-induced peripheral neuropathy in breast cancer [32]. CIPN risk factors in breast cancer are summarized in Fig. 10.1.

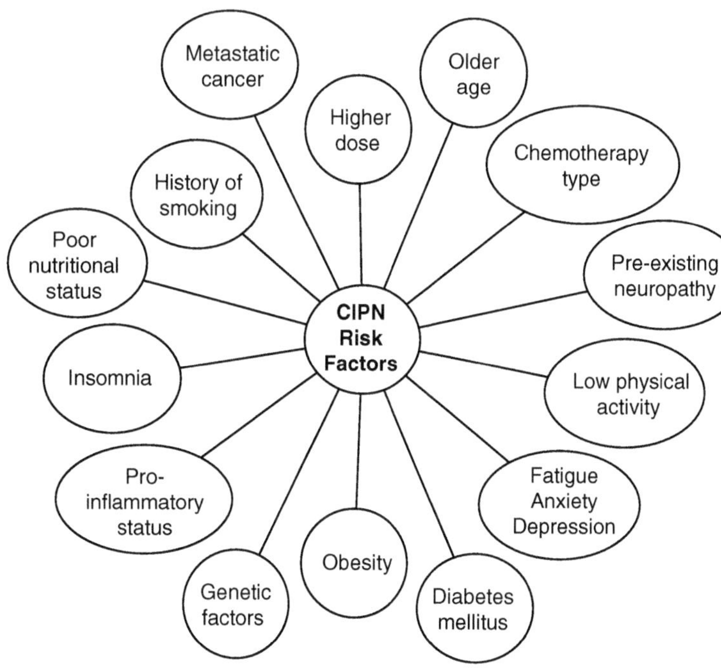

Fig. 10.1 CIPN risk factors in breast cancer

10.5 Symptoms of CIPN

CIPN symptoms are multidimensional and are affected by physiological and psychological factors [33]. CIPN symptoms may appear as motor, sensory, and autonomic changes depending on the affected nerve(s) [34]. The type of neuropathy differs depending on the chemotherapy agent used, including pure sensory (e.g., cisplatin/oxaliplatin), mixed sensory-motor (e.g., paclitaxel), or mixed sensory-motor and autonomic (e.g., vincristine) neuropathy [20].

CIPN symptoms are dose-dependent, indicating they worsen with ongoing treatment. Therefore, CIPN might cause a dose reduction or even an early cessation of chemotherapy [35]. CIPN symptoms commonly develop acutely and progress during the treatment and often resolve upon completion of chemotherapy. In some patients, CIPN may be pursued after treatment has ended, leading to chronic symptoms that impair the quality of life of patients substantially [36]. CIPN can develop, or severity can continue to worsen in many patients even after treatment has been ended, a phenomenon referred to as "coasting" [36].

CIPN symptoms manifest as the characteristic symmetric "glove and stocking" neuropathy [34]. As the severity of neuropathy rises, symptoms that initially appeared in the fingers and toes can eventually extend to the proximal extremities [37]. CIPN often presents with a sensory axonal neuropathy that primarily affects large sensory myelinated fibers (Aβ) or dorsal root ganglion [18, 38]. Since chemotherapeutic agents frequently affect sensory fibers initially, CIPN is characterized by predominantly sensory neuropathy [37]. Numbness, tingling, paresthesia, hot or cold sensitivity, neuropathic pain, allodynia, and hyperpathia are prevalent sensory symptoms [8, 34, 37]. Patients may experience a decline in vibration and proprioception senses as CIPN worsens [34].

Motor and autonomic symptoms are less common but tend to manifest later and in more advanced stages of the disease [39]. Some of the motor symptoms are muscle weakness, muscle atrophy in the distal extremity [39], diminished or absence of deep tendon reflexes [37], and difficulty in fine motor abilities, including writing, buttoning, and handling small objects [8]. Autonomic symptoms such as orthostatic hypotension, constipation, and sexual dysfunction have been reported in patients with vincristine-induced peripheral neuropathy [40].

Taxane-induced peripheral neuropathies are dose-dependent, and sensory involvement is prominent. Motor symptoms may occur with increasing doses but are less frequent. Although the coasting phenomenon is more commonly seen with platinum agents, it can also be seen with taxane-based treatments [39]. Rattanakrong et al. [41] demonstrated that women with breast cancer who underwent taxane-based chemotherapy were more likely to experience sensory neuropathy than motor neuropathy. Vincristine has the highest neurotoxicity among vinca alkaloids. Vincristine-induced neuropathy often manifests with sensory symptoms; however, motor, autonomic, and cranial nerve symptoms (such as vision and hearing dysfunctions, facial nerve, and vocal cord paralysis) can also occur [42]. The coasting phenomena is also observed in vincristine-induced peripheral neuropathy [18].

A symptom cluster is a group of at least two related symptoms that occur together [43]. Wang et al. [44] reported that sensory neuropathy symptoms were the main symptom clusters of CIPN. They also indicated that there was no identified pure motor symptom cluster, but a mixed sensory-motor neuropathy symptom cluster was observed [44]. Patients with CIPN may also experience more generalized symptoms such as sleep disturbance, pain, anxiety, depression, and fatigue. These symptoms, which may have similar underlying mechanisms, are often clustered together [45]. Understanding CIPN symptom clusters improves comprehension of the links between symptoms and their underlying causes [44].

10.6 CIPN-Associated Dysfunctions

Physical functions, psychological states, and social roles could all be negatively influenced by CIPN [46]. The symptoms associated with CIPN might result in various functional impairments. CIPN may lead to balance impairments and postural instability in individuals with breast cancer [47]. Therefore, CIPN increases the risk of falling, and it is significantly increased by motor neuropathy symptoms compared to sensory neuropathy symptoms [48, 49]. Mobility problems are a significant negative consequence of CIPN. As the severity of CIPN worsens, the degree of functional impairment increases [50]. Research has shown that individuals with CIPN are still experiencing functional decline even after completing chemotherapy. They exhibit decreased walking speed, shorter step length, and prolonged stance phase time to maintain stability [51]. Furthermore, symptoms of CIPN can interfere with both gross and fine motor skills and can lead to challenges in many daily living tasks such as dressing, cooking, performing housework, climbing stairs, walking, driving, engaging in leisure time activities, working, and participating in social interactions [46]. Consequently, functional impairments may lead to restrictions in participation and activities of daily living [46]. Additionally, it has been demonstrated that CIPN impairs the quality of sleep, emotional well-being, and quality of life, as well as functional impairments [52]. Functional impairment due to CIPN should be considered in detail while assessing and managing CIPN [53].

10.7 Diagnosis and Assessment of CIPN

Diagnosis and assessment of CIPN are crucial for understanding CIPN epidemiology, managing the condition, and monitoring [22]. However, it is challenging due to the lack of a defined gold standard criteria for the diagnosis of CIPN [9]. CIPN diagnosis mainly depends on identifying symptoms, with objective diagnostic methods focusing on the damaged nerve fibers [9]. For diagnosis, other possible causes of peripheral neuropathy besides CIPN need to be excluded. Differential diagnosis should be prioritized, especially in individuals with preexisting neuropathy or potential comorbidities [54]. It should be borne in mind that the presence of such conditions also increases the risk of developing CIPN, as previously mentioned. Medical history, neurological examination, patient-based subjective assessment methods, objective assessment methods, and composite scoring systems are used to diagnose and evaluate CIPN [9, 54, 55].

The first step in diagnosis and assessment is conducting a detailed medical history. The history includes symptoms (sensory, motor, autonomic, or combined), distribution of symptoms (symmetrical, distal) and effects of symptoms on daily living, previous treatments, examination of related risk factors (such as diabetes or other neuropathies), and the current treatment regimen (including chemotherapeutic agent, dosage, and duration). Subsequently, a neurological examination should be conducted, emphasizing sensory and motor function, reflexes, and gait function [54, 55]. The assessment of CIPN should encompass a comprehensive evaluation of sensory function, muscular strength, and physical performance, which includes evaluating balance, gait, and functional mobility [53].

Assessment should be performed pre-chemotherapy, throughout chemotherapy, and post-chemotherapy. Moreover, prior to chemotherapy, patients should be assessed for variables that increase their risk of developing CIPN. Due to the cumulative effects of chemotherapy, the risk and severity of developing CIPN rise. Therefore, patients should be assessed for the onset or progression of CIPN at each chemotherapy session throughout chemotherapy. Post-chemotherapy assessments should be maintained to assess the severity of CIPN or monitor for new CIPN-related symptom(s) caused by the coasting phenomena [56].

10.7.1 Subjective Assessment Methods

An ideal CIPN assessment tool should be specific to CIPN, capable of early diagnosis, have robust psychometric properties, be easy to use, and be validated across various chemotherapeutic agents or tumor types [22]. Patient-reported outcome measures (PROMs) are crucial tools that assess the severity of CIPN symptoms and their impact on daily activities based on the patients' perspective [57, 58]. The systematic review recommended using the European Organization for Research and Treatment of Cancer Quality of Life Chemotherapy-Induced Peripheral Neuropathy Questionnaire (EORTC QLQ-CIPN20) and Functional Assessment of Cancer Therapy/Gynecologic Oncology Group-Neurotoxicity (FACT/GOG-Ntx) for evaluating CIPN considering their robust psychometric features [58]. However, it has been underscored that many variables, including the objectives of the research and the target population, can significantly influence the selection of the most suitable PROM [58]. Besides PROMs, Common Toxicity Criteria (CTC) scales are clinician-based grading scales that include subjective evaluation based on symptoms reported by the patient. They are commonly employed for evaluating CIPN in both clinical settings and research purposes [59]. Frequently used subjective assessment methods are shown in Table 10.1.

10.7.2 Instrumental Measurement

Neurophysiological approaches offer significant advantages in providing objective information related to the underlying pathophysiology, prognosis, and severity of CIPN. They may also enable the monitoring of physiological changes before clinical symptoms appear [18]. Nerve Conduction Studies (NCS) and Quantitative Sensory Testing (QST) are commonly used objective assessment methods for the evaluation of CIPN. NCS is considered the gold standard for diagnosing and assessing CIPN. Specifically, conducting NCS on the sural nerve is valuable for assessing CIPN and identifying individuals with an increased risk of developing CIPN [10]. NCS offers an objective evaluation of the large nerve fibers [9]. One of its main advantages is its ability to distinguish between demyelination and axonopathy [60]. NCS can also help revealing the specific impacts of chemotherapy drugs on both the symptoms and pathology of CIPN. According

Table 10.1 CIPN assessment methods

Subjective assessment methods
Patients reported outcome measures
Functional Assessment of Cancer Therapy/Gynecologic Oncology Group-Neurotoxicity (FACT/GOG-NTx)
European Organization for Research and Treatment of Cancer Quality of Life Chemotherapy-Induced Peripheral Neuropathy Questionnaire (EORTC QLQ-CIPN20)
Chemotherapy-Induced Peripheral Neuropathy Rasch-Built Overall Disability Scale (CIPN-R-ODS)
Patient Neurotoxicity Questionnaire (PNQ)
Chemotherapy-induced Peripheral Neuropathy Assessment Tool (CIPNAT)
Comprehensive Assessment Scale for Chemotherapy-Induced Peripheral Neuropathy (CAS-CIPN)
Oxaliplatin-Associated Neurotoxicity Questionnaire (OANQ)
Indication for CTC Grading of Peripheral Neuropathy Questionnaire
Clinician-based grading scales-common toxicity criteria
National Cancer Institute-Common Toxicity Criteria (NCI-CTC)
NCI Common Terminology Criteria for Adverse Events (NCI-CTCAE)
World Health Organization (WHO) Neurotoxicity Scale
Eastern Cooperative Oncology Group (ECOG) Criteria
The Ajani Scale
Objective assessment methods
Nerve Conduction Studies (NCS)
Quantitative Sensory Testing (QST)
Nerve Excitability
High-Resolution Ultrasound (HRUS)
Skin Biopsy
Magnetic Resonance Imaging (MRI)
Corneal Confocal Microscopy (CCM)
Laser-Evoked Potential (LEP)-Contact Heat-Evoked Potential (CHEP)
Autonomic Testing
Magnetic Resonance Neurography (MRN)
Diffusion Tensor Imaging (DTI)
Needle Electromyography (EMG)
Microneurography
Blood molecular biomarker analysis
Composite scales
Total Neuropathy Score (TNS), TNS-reduced version (TNSr), TNS-clinical version (TNSc), TNS-reduced version short form TNSr-SF, Rasch transformed-TNSc, TNSr 5-item, Modified TNS

[10, 58, 59, 61]

to the NCSs, paclitaxel and vincristine are associated with distal predominantly sensory axonal neuropathy, and distal sensorimotor axonal neuropathy, respectively [18]. The limitation of NCS is that it provides information only about Aβ nerve fibers [10]. On the other hand, QST assesses sensory function by conducting tests that offer insights into the function of Aβ, C, and Aδ nerve fibers [10]. The QST evaluates many types of sensory impairments by assessing thresholds for pain, thermal, touch, and vibration. However, the process is time-consuming, and the outcomes of the evaluation are contingent upon the participants' subjective responses [10].

Nerve imaging techniques can offer insights into nerve structure [10]. High-resolution ultrasound (HRUS) can be used to evaluate CIPN with the advantages of being rapidly applicable and noninvasive [38]. Magnetic resonance imaging (MRI) yields information on the anatomical structure of the nerve and the dorsal root ganglia. Additionally, it can indicate whether CIPN induces alterations in the central nervous system [38]. Methods including skin biopsy and corneal confocal microscopy can assess small unmyelinated nerve fibers that NCS is unable to assess [10].

There is ongoing research into novel methods to enhance the precision of diagnosis and assessments in CIPN. Current evaluation methods continue to have limitations, and there is a significant gap in an accurate diagnosis and assessment. Blood molecular biomarker analysis has emerged as a focus area of research in the assessment of prognosis and diagnosis of CIPN [38, 61]. Neurotrophic factors such as nerve growth factor and brain-derived neurotrophic factor, small noncoding micro ribonucleic acids, neurofilament proteins, and metabolites are among the markers investigated as blood molecular biomarkers in CIPN [61]. Velasco et al. [62] determined that serum neurofilament light chain levels, which increased during chemotherapy in breast cancer patients, were in line with NCS. They indicated that the combined use of both procedures can enhance the precision of diagnosis [62]. Levels of neurotrophin-3 [63], serum osteopontin [64], and circulating microribonucleic acids (miRNAs) [65] are other promising biomarkers identified for CIPN in breast cancer. Further investigation is required on objective assessment techniques [10]. A list of the other objective methods that may be used to assess CIPN is provided in Table 10.1.

10.7.3 Composite Scales

Composite scales are evaluation tools that include objective and subjective assessments to enhance the evaluation of CIPN [66]. While composite scales offer advantages such as combining subjective and objective assessment, they are relatively intricate and time-consuming. The inclusion of instrumental evaluations may limit their applicability [66]. Total Neuropathy Score (TNS) is a composite scale that evaluates both objective (such as vibration, reflex, muscular strength, and nerve conduction studies) and subjective (patient-reported sensory, motor, or autonomic complaints) nature of CIPN [66, 67]. Because the original form was time consuming and required specialized tools, simpler versions were developed [66].

In the systematic review, the use of the FACT/GOG-Ntx and the TNS scales was recommended in evaluating CIPN based on their robust psychometric properties [68]. In another systematic review and Delphi study of 117 different CIPN assessment tools, the Patient Neurotoxicity Questionnaire (PNQ) scored highest for overall and PROM assessment, while the TNS clinical version scored highest for clinician-based assessment. Nevertheless, there is no consensus on the best method for evaluating CIPN [69]. FACT/GOG-Ntx, National Cancer Institute Common Toxicity Criteria (NCI-CTC), Common Terminology Criteria of Adverse Events (CTCAE), TNS clinical version (TNSc), EORTC-QLQ-CIPN 20, FACT-Taxane, and Chemotherapy-induced Peripheral Neuropathy Assessment Tool (CIPNAT) are some of the scales used to assess CIPN in breast cancer [3, 33, 70].

Several studies in the literature have identified weak to moderate correlations or inconsistencies between subjective and objective evaluation techniques for assessing CIPN in breast cancer. It is advised to employ both objective and subjective methods while assessing CIPN [71–73]. Zhi et al. [73] stated that PROMs and QST can be used in combination to detect CIPN symptoms and monitor treatment outcomes in breast cancer survivors. Sohn et al. [74] also recommended a comprehensive evaluation of taxane-induced peripheral neuropathy in breast cancer patients, involving a clinician-based scale, a patient-reported scale, and specialized tests to identify small nerve fiber involvement.

Algorithms or clinical practice pathways for CIPN assessment and management have also been reported [75, 76]. The clinical practice pathway for enhancing clinical decision-making underscores the need to evaluate the patient for risk factors associated with CIPN, provide education on CIPN, and conduct screening for any preexisting neuropathy before initiating treatment. Additionally, ongoing evaluations for CIPN are advised both during and following treatment [76]. To improve the CIPN evaluation and management process, it is essential that healthcare professionals increase their adherence to pertinent evidence-based decision-making algorithms to ensure standardization in the assessment and management of CIPN [53, 75].

Although many studies have been conducted on CIPN assessment techniques, the recommended measuring methods vary, and there currently needs to be an agreement on a measurement that can be considered the gold standard [77]. Studies investigating the efficacy of CIPN management approaches lack consistency in their assessment method. Thus, establishing the core assessment method is crucial for identifying effective therapeutic approaches for CIPN [57]. The standardized assessment of CIPN remains an unresolved issue. Evaluating current instruments for their psychometric qualities and determining suitable evaluation procedures for various cancer and chemotherapy agents is still necessary.

10.8 Management of CIPN

Various pharmacological and non-pharmacological agents are used in the management of CIPN. However, although there is no agent used for direct protection against CIPN in clinical use, there are different therapy approaches that mainly focus on prevention and improvement in the symptom based approach [78].

Chemotherapy agents used in cancer treatment cause changes in the excitation potential of ion channels. To repair the changes in these potentials, ion channel treatment approaches are preferred. Although many chemotherapy agents cannot cross the blood–brain barrier, some of them can rarely cross the blood–brain barrier. They cannot invade cerebral tissues and cannot cluster in these areas. On the contrary, they are known to cluster in the peripheral nervous system. They are generally found in high density in the dorsal root ganglion and nerve fiber terminals and precipitate in these areas. This accumulation is characterized by an increase in the release of transcription factor-3, which triggers axonal injury mechanisms. Myelin sheath degeneration and axonal damage, which begins with the involvement of intraepidermal nerve fibers, spread proximally. As a result, CIPN occurs, which is characterized by degeneration of peripheral nerve fibers, axons, and myelin sheaths [79].

10.8.1 Erythropoietin

Erythropoietin (EPO) is one of the preferred cytokines in treatment approaches for anemia. It is released from the adrenal glands and is associated with erythropoiesis. Recent studies have shown that EPO has neuroprotective as well as neurotrophic effects. In rat studies, it was found that EPO supports the amplitude of movement in muscle fibers by protecting healthy peripheral nerves. It is also stated that it provides protection against neuropathy caused by cisplatin by triggering peripheral myelinization [78].

Although the nerve regeneration feature of EPO constitutes a possible option for the treatment of CIPN, caution should be exercised in its use to prevent CIPN in cancer patients due to the lack of human experiments [79].

10.8.2 Glutathione

Glutathione, consisting of glutamyl-cysteinyl-glycine, reduces heavy metal accumulation caused by platinum group drugs in the dorsal root ganglion. It is thought that glutathione also provides a protective effect against neuropathy caused by cisplatin. Additionally, studies have shown that glutathione treatment does not interfere with the oncolytic activity of chemotherapy [80].

10.8.3 *N*-Acetylcysteine

It is thought that oral use of *N*-acetylcysteine, a glutathione precursor antioxidant, may reduce the symptoms of oxaliplatin-induced neuropathy, and more research is needed [79].

10.8.4 Lidocaine and Mexiletine

The working principle of lidocaine is based on the blockade of Na^+ channels. Mexiletine is an antiarrhythmic drug similar to lidocaine in its structure and working principle. Research emphasizes that lidocaine and mexylene provide successful results in the treatment of diabetic peripheral neuropathy. When the current literature is examined, animal studies have been initiated to determine the effectiveness of the treatment of CIPN. Although they have been clinically tested on a few patients, it is not yet known what effects lidocaine and mexiletine will have in the treatment of CIPN [81, 82].

10.8.5 Calcium (Ca) and Magnesium (Mg)

If CIPN is associated with oxaliplatin, treatment with Ca and Mg is preferred. It was noted that in patients treated with Ca and Mg supplementation, there was a decrease in the frequency and severity of neuropathic symptoms along with a lack of negative changes in the effectiveness of chemotherapy treatment. As a result of phase III studies, it was also reported that Ca and Mg infusions did not prevent neurotoxicity or reduce existing neurotoxicity [79]. In the randomized controlled phase III study conducted by Loprinzi et al. [83], it was noted that treatment with Ca and Mg did not show any significant difference in preventing CIPN.

10.8.6 Gabapentin and Pregabalin

Gabapentin and Pregabalin are antiepileptic drugs used in neuropathic pain management. The working principles of these drugs are based on the blockade of Ca^+ channels. There are conflicting phase III studies regarding the effectiveness of gabapentin and regabalin in the treatment of CIPN [79].

10.8.7 Menthol

Menthol is a natural compound used in neuropathic pain management. Since an increase in the severity of neuropathic pain has been determined in cases of overdose, attention should be paid to safe dosage administration [84].

10.8.8 Glutamine

It is thought that glutamine has a protective effect against peripheral neuropathy caused by paclitaxel and oxaliplatin. Additionally, it has been reported that glutamine treatment does not have any negative effect on the effectiveness of chemotherapy [78].

10.8.9 Carbamazepine/Oxcarbazepine

Carbamazepine is an antiepileptic pharmacological agent that prevents abnormal discharges from ion channels by blocking voltage-gated Na channels. Oxcarbazepine is one of the carbamazepine derivatives, and it is emphasized that it has fewer side effects and drug interactions compared to carbamazepine [78].

10.8.10 Vitamin E

The expected neuropathy effects of vitamin E, which is used as a protectant against CIPN, are not yet clear and contain contradictions. Vitamin E levels are low in cancer patients receiving cisplatin treatment. It is emphasized that the incidence of peripheral neuropathy decreases by 86% with E-vitamin supplementation applied to these patients. However, in subsequent studies, no significant difference was found between the patient group receiving vitamin E supplements and the placebo control group, neither in the incidence of peripheral neuropathy nor in the time until the onset of neuropathy [85].

Therefore, more research is needed to investigate the protective effect of vitamin E against CIPN [86].

10.8.11 Allopregnanolone

Allopregnanolone, a progesterone metabolite neurosteroid, is associated with various receptors and gates such as GABA receptors and Ca channels. Based on animal experiments, it is thought that allopregnanolone not only has neuroprotective effects but also neurogenic and analgesic effects. However, human studies have not yet provided sufficient data for the safety of the use of allopregnanolone in cancer patients [78].

10.8.12 Exercise

Recently published research highlighted that exercise provides reductions in CIPN symptoms and improvements in quality of life, pain, balance, and activity level [87].

Stretching, strengthening, yoga, balance, sensory, and aerobic exercises are well-recognized types of exercises performed in cancer patients to alleviate CIPN symptoms. Although there is no consensus among experts regarding exercise duration and frequency, there is increasing rehabilitative evidence that exercise therapy improves symptoms of CIPN [87].

In the study by Huang et al. examining exercise studies for CIPN, 15 randomized controlled studies were examined. The duration of the exercises varies between 15–60 min, and 30–60 min are generally preferred. Exercise frequency can vary from 1 application per day to 5–7 applications per day. The duration of exercise programs varies between 2 weeks and 36 weeks [87].

In 2021, 60 patients over 18 were included in Simşek et al.'s randomized controlled exercise study for CIPN, consisting of exercise therapy ($n = 30$) and control groups ($n = 30$). While routine cancer treatment and cold pack applications were applied to the patients in the control group, balance exercise combined with stretching exercise was applied to the exercise therapy group in addition to chemotherapy. The exercise frequency was applied 5 times a week and continued for 12 weeks. This study is thought to be the first study comparing the effects of cold application and exercise therapy in the management of CIPN. When results were compared after 12 weeks of application, it was found that the CIPN symptoms of cancer patients who received exercise therapy were significantly controlled compared to the control group [88].

In the randomized controlled study published by Ikio et al. [89], 39 individuals with cancer consisting of exercise therapy ($n = 19$) and control groups ($n = 20$) were included in the study. While patients in the control group received chemotherapy, the exercise therapy group received combined upper extremity strengthening training in addition to chemotherapy. Exercises were continued for 30 min, at least 3 days a week. The exercise load was applied as a "low-to-moderate" load. Ten to 20 strengthening exercises, 1–3 sets in each exercise session, were applied for 6–8 weeks. As a result of the study, the effects of the treatments received by the exercise training group and the control group on CIPN symptoms were compared. The exercise training for the management of CIPN symptoms has been emphasized as an effective non-pharmacological method in upper extremity functionality, improvement of daily living activities, and pain management [89].

In the randomized controlled study published by Gui et al. [90], researchers studied a total of 79 cancer patients (n = 51 in the exercise therapy group, n = 28 in the control group) in which an additional sensory training was implemented in the exercise group for 2 weeks. Significant improvements in pain, peripheral neurotoxicity symptoms, and functionality of the patients in the sensory training group were observed. In addition, improvements were found in walking and occupational skills, as well as sleep quality in the group receiving sensory training [90].

Based on all this information, it can be said that exercise training in the management of CIPN is seriously effective in controlling the symptoms. However, there is no consensus among experts as to which exercise is more effective or in which frequency range the exercise load should be performed. More evidence-based scientific research is needed to compare different types of exercise and different exercise loads.

10.9 Conclusion

CIPN is a side effect of chemotherapy that warrants attention owing to its effects on the quality of life of breast cancer patients, which potentially may necessitate a decrease in treatment dosage or premature cessation of therapy. Although a widely accepted measurement method for the comprehensive assessment of CIPN remains unclear, it is recommended that a combination of objective and subjective evaluation techniques be used. Systematic screening, starting with the diagnosis of breast cancer, is necessary to avoid overlooking CIPN and to assess the severity, symptoms, and related dysfunctions when CIPN is present. In the management of CIPN, both pharmacological and nonpharmacological strategies are implemented. Physical therapy approaches, especially exercise training, demonstrate promising results. Regarding the management of CIPN, emphasis should be placed on identifying standard evaluation and treatment protocols. It is recommended that the wide use of evidence-based decision-making algorithms be increased in clinical practice to manage CIPN.

References

1. Sung H, Ferlay J, Siegel RL, Laversanne M, Soerjomataram I, Jemal A, et al. Global cancer statistics 2020: GLOBOCAN estimates of incidence and mortality worldwide for 36 cancers in 185 countries. CA Cancer J Clin. 2021;71(3):209–49.
2. de Moor JS, Mariotto AB, Parry C, Alfano CM, Padgett L, Kent EE, et al. Cancer survivors in the United States: prevalence across the survivorship trajectory and implications for care. Cancer Epidemiol Biomarkers Prev. 2013;22(4):561–70.
3. Rivera DR, Ganz PA, Weyrich MS, Bandos H, Melnikow J. Chemotherapy-associated peripheral neuropathy in patients with early-stage breast cancer: a systematic review. J Natl Cancer Inst. 2018;110(2):djx140.
4. Škubník J, Pavlíčková V, Ruml T, Rimpelová S. Current perspectives on taxanes: focus on their bioactivity, delivery and combination therapy. Plants (Basel). 2021;10(3):569.
5. Kerr AJ, Dodwell D, McGale P, Holt F, Duane F, Mannu G, et al. Adjuvant and neoadjuvant breast cancer treatments: a systematic review of their effects on mortality. Cancer Treat Rev. 2022;105:102375.
6. Runowicz CD, Leach CR, Henry NL, Henry KS, Mackey HT, Cowens-Alvarado RL, et al. American Cancer Society/American Society of Clinical Oncology breast cancer survivorship care guideline. J Clin Oncol. 2016;34(6):611–35.
7. Di Nardo P, Lisanti C, Garutti M, Buriolla S, Alberti M, Mazzeo R, et al. Chemotherapy in patients with early breast cancer: clinical overview and management of long-term side effects. Expert Opin Drug Saf. 2022;21(11):1341–55.
8. Brown TJ, Sedhom R, Gupta A. Chemotherapy-induced peripheral neuropathy. JAMA Oncol. 2019;5(5):750.
9. Burgess J, Ferdousi M, Gosal D, Boon C, Matsumoto K, Marshall A, et al. Chemotherapy-induced peripheral neuropathy: epidemiology, pathomechanisms and treatment. Oncol Ther. 2021;9(2):385–450.
10. Argyriou AA, Park SB, Islam B, Tamburin S, Velasco R, Alberti P, et al. Neurophysiological, nerve imaging and other techniques to assess chemotherapy-induced peripheral neurotoxicity in the clinical and research settings. J Neurol Neurosurg Psychiatry. 2019;90(12):1361–9.
11. Cavaletti G, Alberti P, Argyriou AA, Lustberg M, Staff NP, Tamburin S. Chemotherapy-induced periph-

eral neurotoxicity: a multifaceted, still unsolved issue. J Peripher Nerv Syst. 2019;24(Suppl 2):S6–12.
12. Seretny M, Currie GL, Sena ES, Ramnarine S, Grant R, MacLeod MR, et al. Incidence, prevalence, and predictors of chemotherapy-induced peripheral neuropathy: a systematic review and meta-analysis. Pain. 2014;155(12):2461–70.
13. Banach M, Juranek JK, Zygulska AL. Chemotherapy-induced neuropathies—a growing problem for patients and health care providers. Brain Behav. 2017;7(1):e00558.
14. Bao T, Basal C, Seluzicki C, Li SQ, Seidman AD, Mao JJ. Long-term chemotherapy-induced peripheral neuropathy among breast cancer survivors: prevalence, risk factors, and fall risk. Breast Cancer Res Treat. 2016;159(2):327–33.
15. Starobova H, Vetter I. Pathophysiology of chemotherapy-induced peripheral neuropathy. Front Mol Neurosci. 2017;10:174.
16. Omran M, Belcher EK, Mohile NA, Kesler SR, Janelsins MC, Hohmann AG, et al. Review of the role of the brain in chemotherapy-induced peripheral neuropathy. Front Mol Biosci. 2021;8:693133.
17. Boyette-Davis JA, Hou S, Abdi S, Dougherty PM. An updated understanding of the mechanisms involved in chemotherapy-induced neuropathy. Pain Manag. 2018;8(5):363–75.
18. Kandula T, Farrar MA, Kiernan MC, Krishnan AV, Goldstein D, Horvath L, et al. Neurophysiological and clinical outcomes in chemotherapy-induced neuropathy in cancer. Clin Neurophysiol. 2017;128(7):1166–75.
19. Zajączkowska R, Kocot-Kępska M, Leppert W, Wrzosek A, Mika J, Wordliczek J. Mechanisms of chemotherapy-induced peripheral neuropathy. Int J Mol Sci. 2019;20(6):1451.
20. Was H, Borkowska A, Bagues A, Tu L, Liu JYH, Lu Z, et al. Mechanisms of chemotherapy-induced neurotoxicity. Front Pharmacol. 2022;13:750507.
21. Timmins HC, Mizrahi D, Li T, Kiernan MC, Goldstein D, Park SB. Metabolic and lifestyle risk factors for chemotherapy-induced peripheral neuropathy in taxane and platinum-treated patients: a systematic review. J Cancer Surviv. 2023;17(1):222–36.
22. Colvin LA. Chemotherapy-induced peripheral neuropathy: where are we now? Pain. 2019;160 Suppl 1(Suppl 1):S1–10.
23. Kerckhove N, Collin A, Condé S, Chaleteix C, Pezet D, Balayssac D. Long-term effects, pathophysiological mechanisms, and risk factors of chemotherapy-induced peripheral neuropathies: a comprehensive literature review. Front Pharmacol. 2017;8:86.
24. Engvall K, Gréen H, Fredriksson M, Åvall-Lundqvist E. Persistent neuropathy among early-stage breast cancer survivors in a population-based cohort. Br J Cancer. 2021;125(3):445–57.
25. Song SJ, Min J, Suh SY, Jung SH, Hahn HJ, Im SA, et al. Incidence of taxane-induced peripheral neuropathy receiving treatment and prescription patterns in patients with breast cancer. Support Care Cancer. 2017;25(7):2241–8.
26. Gu J, Lu H, Chen C, Gu Z, Hu M, Liu L, et al. Diabetes mellitus as a risk factor for chemotherapy-induced peripheral neuropathy: a meta-analysis. Support Care Cancer. 2021;29(12):7461–9.
27. Ghoreishi Z, Keshavarz S, Asghari Jafarabadi M, Fathifar Z, Goodman KA, Esfahani A. Risk factors for paclitaxel-induced peripheral neuropathy in patients with breast cancer. BMC Cancer. 2018;18(1):958.
28. Verbraecken J, Van de Heyning P, De Backer W, Van Gaal L. Body surface area in normal-weight, overweight, and obese adults. A comparison study. Metabolism. 2006;55(4):515–24.
29. Callaghan BC, Xia R, Reynolds E, Banerjee M, Rothberg AE, Burant CF, et al. Association between metabolic syndrome components and polyneuropathy in an obese population. JAMA Neurol. 2016;73(12):1468–76.
30. Robertson J, Raizer J, Hodges JS, Gradishar W, Allen JA. Risk factors for the development of paclitaxel-induced neuropathy in breast cancer patients. J Peripher Nerv Syst. 2018;23(2):129–33.
31. Kleckner IR, Jusko TA, Culakova E, Chung K, Kleckner AS, Asare M, et al. Longitudinal study of inflammatory, behavioral, clinical, and psychosocial risk factors for chemotherapy-induced peripheral neuropathy. Breast Cancer Res Treat. 2021;189(2):521–32.
32. Guijosa A, Freyria A, Espinosa-Fernandez JR, Estrada-Mena FJ, Armenta-Quiroga AS, Ortega-Treviño MF, et al. Pharmacogenetics of taxane-induced neurotoxicity in breast cancer: systematic review and meta-analysis. Clin Transl Sci. 2022;15(10):2403–36.
33. Kim M, Jung MS. Effects of chemotherapy-induced peripheral neuropathy in women with breast cancer: a structural equation approach with the theory of unpleasant symptoms. Cancer Nurs. 2021;44(2):145–53.
34. Flatters SJL, Dougherty PM, Colvin LA. Clinical and preclinical perspectives on chemotherapy-induced peripheral neuropathy (CIPN): a narrative review. Br J Anaesth. 2017;119(4):737–49.
35. Hershman DL, Lacchetti C, Dworkin RH, Lavoie Smith EM, Bleeker J, Cavaletti G, et al. Prevention and management of chemotherapy-induced peripheral neuropathy in survivors of adult cancers: American Society of Clinical Oncology clinical practice guideline. J Clin Oncol. 2014;32(18):1941–67.
36. Cavaletti G, Alberti P, Frigeni B, Piatti M, Susani E. Chemotherapy-induced neuropathy. Curr Treat Options Neurol. 2011;13(2):180–90.
37. Stubblefield MD, Burstein HJ, Burton AW, Custodio CM, Deng GE, Ho M, et al. NCCN task force report: management of neuropathy in cancer. J Natl Compr Cancer Netw. 2009;7(Suppl 5):S1–26.
38. Alberti P. A review of novel biomarkers and imaging techniques for assessing the severity of chemotherapy-induced peripheral neuropathy. Expert Opin Drug Metab Toxicol. 2020;16(12):1147–58.

39. Molinares D, Kurtevski S, Zhu Y. Chemotherapy-induced peripheral neuropathy: diagnosis, agents, general clinical presentation, and treatments. Curr Oncol Rep. 2023;25(11):1227–35.
40. Argyriou AA, Kyritsis AP, Makatsoris T, Kalofonos HP. Chemotherapy-induced peripheral neuropathy in adults: a comprehensive update of the literature. Cancer Manag Res. 2014;6:135–47.
41. Rattanakrong N, Siriphorn A, Boonyong S. Incidence density and factors associated with peripheral neuropathy among women with breast cancer during taxane-based chemotherapy. Sci Rep. 2022;12(1):10632.
42. Li GZ, Hu YH, Li DY, Zhang Y, Guo HL, Li YM, et al. Vincristine-induced peripheral neuropathy: a mini-review. Neurotoxicology. 2020;81:161–71.
43. Kim H-J, McGuire DB, Tulman L, Barsevick AM. Symptom clusters: concept analysis and clinical implications for cancer nursing. Cancer Nurs. 2005;28(4):270–82.
44. Wang M, Cheng HL, Lopez V, Sundar R, Yorke J, Molassiotis A. Redefining chemotherapy-induced peripheral neuropathy through symptom cluster analysis and patient-reported outcome data over time. BMC Cancer. 2019;19(1):1151.
45. Knoerl R, Chornoby Z, Smith EML. Estimating the frequency, severity, and clustering of SPADE symptoms in chronic painful chemotherapy-induced peripheral neuropathy. Pain Manag Nurs. 2018;19(4):354–65.
46. Bakitas MA. Background noise: the experience of chemotherapy-induced peripheral neuropathy. Nurs Res. 2007;56(5):323–31.
47. Kneis S, Wehrle A, Freyler K, Lehmann K, Rudolphi B, Hildenbrand B, et al. Balance impairments and neuromuscular changes in breast cancer patients with chemotherapy-induced peripheral neuropathy. Clin Neurophysiol. 2016;127(2):1481–90.
48. Autissier E. Chemotherapy-induced peripheral neuropathy: association with increased risk of falls and injuries. Clin J Oncol Nurs. 2019;23(4):405–10.
49. Gewandter JS, Fan L, Magnuson A, Mustian K, Peppone L, Heckler C, et al. Falls and functional impairments in cancer survivors with chemotherapy-induced peripheral neuropathy (CIPN): a University of Rochester CCOP study. Support Care Cancer. 2013;21(7):2059–66.
50. McCrary JM, Goldstein D, Wyld D, Henderson R, Lewis CR, Park SB. Mobility in survivors with chemotherapy-induced peripheral neuropathy and utility of the 6-min walk test. J Cancer Surviv. 2019;13(4):495–502.
51. Winters-Stone KM, Horak F, Jacobs PG, Trubowitz P, Dieckmann NF, Stoyles S, et al. Falls, functioning, and disability among women with persistent symptoms of chemotherapy-induced peripheral neuropathy. J Clin Oncol. 2017;35(23):2604–12.
52. Tofthagen CS, Cheville AL, Loprinzi CL. The physical consequences of chemotherapy-induced peripheral neuropathy. Curr Oncol Rep. 2020;22(5):50.
53. Stoller S, Capozza S, Alberti P, Lustberg M, Kleckner IR. Framework to leverage physical therapists for the assessment and treatment of chemotherapy-induced peripheral neurotoxicity (CIPN). Support Care Cancer. 2023;31(5):293.
54. Hausheer FH, Schilsky RL, Bain S, Berghorn EJ, Lieberman F. Diagnosis, management, and evaluation of chemotherapy-induced peripheral neuropathy. Semin Oncol. 2006;33(1):15–49.
55. Wasilewski A, Mohile N. Meet the expert: how I treat chemotherapy-induced peripheral neuropathy. J Geriatr Oncol. 2021;12(1):1–5.
56. Knoerl R. CE: chemotherapy-induced peripheral neuropathy. Am J Nurs. 2021;121(4):26–30.
57. Park SB, Tamburin S, Schenone A, Kleckner IR, Velasco R, Alberti P, et al. Optimal outcome measures for assessing exercise and rehabilitation approaches in chemotherapy-induced peripheral-neurotoxicity: systematic review and consensus expert opinion. Expert Rev Neurother. 2022;22(1):65–76.
58. Li T, Park SB, Battaglini E, King MT, Kiernan MC, Goldstein D, et al. Assessing chemotherapy-induced peripheral neuropathy with patient reported outcome measures: a systematic review of measurement properties and considerations for future use. Qual Life Res. 2022;31(11):3091–107.
59. Park SB, Alberti P, Kolb NA, Gewandter JS, Schenone A, Argyriou AA. Overview and critical revision of clinical assessment tools in chemotherapy-induced peripheral neurotoxicity. J Peripher Nerv Syst. 2019;24(Suppl 2):S13–25.
60. Gutiérrez-Gutiérrez G, Sereno M, Miralles A, Casado-Sáenz E, Gutiérrez-Rivas E. Chemotherapy-induced peripheral neuropathy: clinical features, diagnosis, prevention and treatment strategies. Clin Transl Oncol. 2010;12(2):81–91.
61. Meregalli C, Bonomo R, Cavaletti G, Carozzi VA. Blood molecular biomarkers for chemotherapy-induced peripheral neuropathy: from preclinical models to clinical practice. Neurosci Lett. 2021;749:135739.
62. Velasco R, Argyriou AA, Marco C, Mariotto S, Stradella A, Hernández J, et al. Serum neurofilament levels correlate with electrodiagnostic evidence of axonal loss in paclitaxel-induced peripheral neurotoxicity. J Neurol. 2023;270(1):531–7.
63. Tonyan S, Pospelova M, Krasnikova V, Fionik O, Alekseeva T, Samochernykh K, et al. Neurotrophin-3 (NT-3) as a potential biomarker of the peripheral nervous system damage following breast cancer treatment. Pathophysiology. 2023;30(2):110–22.
64. Pizzamiglio C, Ripellino P, Prandi P, Clemente N, Saggia C, Rossi V, et al. Nerve conduction, circulating osteopontin and taxane-induced neuropathy in breast cancer patients. Neurophysiol Clin. 2020;50(1):47–54.
65. Davey MG, Abbas R, Kerin EP, Casey MC, McGuire A, Waldron RM, et al. Circulating microRNAs can predict chemotherapy-induced toxicities in patients being treated for primary breast cancer. Breast Cancer Res Treat. 2023;202(1):73–81.

66. Cavaletti G, Frigeni B, Lanzani F, Mattavelli L, Susani E, Alberti P, et al. Chemotherapy-induced peripheral neurotoxicity assessment: a critical revision of the currently available tools. Eur J Cancer. 2010;46(3):479–94.
67. Cornblath DR, Chaudhry V, Carter K, Lee D, Seysedadr M, Miernicki M, et al. Total neuropathy score: validation and reliability study. Neurology. 1999;53(8):1660–4.
68. Haryani H, Fetzer SJ, Wu CL, Hsu YY. Chemotherapy-induced peripheral neuropathy assessment tools: a systematic review. Oncol Nurs Forum. 2017;44(3):E111–23.
69. McCrary JM, Goldstein D, Boyle F, Cox K, Grimison P, Kiernan MC, et al. Optimal clinical assessment strategies for chemotherapy-induced peripheral neuropathy (CIPN): a systematic review and Delphi survey. Support Care Cancer. 2017;25(11):3485–93.
70. van Haren F, van den Heuvel S, Ligtenberg M, Vissers K, Steegers M. Diagnostic tools should be used for the diagnosis of chemotherapy induced peripheral neuropathy in breast cancer patients receiving taxanes. Cancer Rep (Hoboken). 2022;5(10):e1577.
71. Saito T, Makiura D, Inoue J, Doi H, Yakushijin K, Okamura A, et al. Comparison between quantitative and subjective assessments of chemotherapy-induced peripheral neuropathy in cancer patients: a prospective cohort study. Phys Ther Res. 2020;23(2):166–71.
72. Nyrop KA, Deal AM, Reeder-Hayes KE, Shachar SS, Reeve BB, Basch E, et al. Patient-reported and clinician-reported chemotherapy-induced peripheral neuropathy in patients with early breast cancer: current clinical practice. Cancer. 2019;125(17):2945–54.
73. Zhi WI, Chen P, Kwon A, Chen C, Harte SE, Piulson L, et al. Chemotherapy-induced peripheral neuropathy (CIPN) in breast cancer survivors: a comparison of patient-reported outcomes and quantitative sensory testing. Breast Cancer Res Treat. 2019;178(3):587–95.
74. Sohn EH, Lee JS, Jung MS, Kim JR. A prospective study of taxane-induced neuropathy with breast cancer: proper assessment tool for taxane-induced neuropathy. South Asian J Cancer. 2021;10(2):58–63.
75. Knoerl R, Mazzola E, Hong F, Salehi E, McCleary N, Ligibel J, et al. Exploring the impact of a decision support algorithm to improve clinicians' chemotherapy-induced peripheral neuropathy assessment and management practices: a two-phase, longitudinal study. BMC Cancer. 2021;21(1):236.
76. Mizrahi D, Goldstein D, Kiernan MC, Robinson L, Pitiyarachchi O, McCullough S, et al. Development and consensus process for a clinical pathway for the assessment and management of chemotherapy-induced peripheral neuropathy. Support Care Cancer. 2022;30(7):5965–74.
77. Molassiotis A, Cheng HL, Lopez V, Au JSK, Chan A, Bandla A, et al. Are we mis-estimating chemotherapy-induced peripheral neuropathy? Analysis of assessment methodologies from a prospective, multinational, longitudinal cohort study of patients receiving neurotoxic chemotherapy. BMC Cancer. 2019;19(1):132.
78. Abudayyak M, Yalçin CÖ, Korkut E. Kemoterapi ile indüklenmiş periferal nöropatinin tedavisi ve önlenmesine yönelik farmakolojik yaklaşımlar. FABAD J Pharm Sci. 2018;43(2):113–27.
79. Hu LY, Mi WL, Wu GC, Wang YQ, Mao-Ying QL. Prevention and treatment for chemotherapy-induced peripheral neuropathy: therapies based on CIPN mechanisms. Curr Neuropharmacol. 2019;17(2):184–96.
80. Cascinu S, Cordella L, Del Ferro E, Fronzoni M, Catalano G. Neuroprotective effect of reduced glutathione on cisplatin-based chemotherapy in advanced gastric cancer: a randomized double-blind placebo-controlled trial. J Clin Oncol. 1995;13(1):26–32.
81. Kanai A, Segawa Y, Okamoto T, Koto M, Okamoto H. The analgesic effect of a metered-dose 8% lidocaine pump spray in posttraumatic peripheral neuropathy: a pilot study. Anesth Analg. 2009;108(3):987–91.
82. Navez ML, Monella C, Bösl I, Sommer D, Delorme C. 5% lidocaine medicated plaster for the treatment of postherpetic neuralgia: a review of the clinical safety and tolerability. Pain Ther. 2015;4(1):1–15.
83. Loprinzi CL, Qin R, Dakhil SR, Fehrenbacher L, Flynn KA, Atherton P, et al. Phase III randomized, placebo-controlled, double-blind study of intravenous calcium and magnesium to prevent oxaliplatin-induced sensory neurotoxicity (N08CB/Alliance). J Clin Oncol. 2014;32(10):997–1005.
84. Colvin LA, Johnson PR, Mitchell R, Fleetwood-Walker SM, Fallon M. From bench to bedside: a case of rapid reversal of bortezomib-induced neuropathic pain by the TRPM8 activator, menthol. J Clin Oncol. 2008;26(27):4519–20.
85. Salehi Z, Roayaei M. Effect of vitamin E on oxaliplatin-induced peripheral neuropathy prevention: a randomized controlled trial. Int J Prev Med. 2015;6:104.
86. Pace A, Giannarelli D, Galiè E, Savarese A, Carpano S, Della Giulia M, et al. Vitamin E neuroprotection for cisplatin neuropathy: a randomized, placebo-controlled trial. Neurology. 2010;74(9):762–6.
87. Huang Y, Tan T, Liu L, Yan Z, Deng Y, Li G, et al. Exercise for reducing chemotherapy-induced peripheral neuropathy: a systematic review and meta-analysis of randomized controlled trials. Front Neurol. 2023;14:1252259.
88. Şimşek NY, Demir A. Cold application and exercise on development of peripheral neuropathy during taxane chemotherapy in breast cancer patients: a randomized controlled trial. Asia Pac J Oncol Nurs. 2021;8(3):255–66.
89. Ikio Y, Sagari A, Nakashima A, Matsuda D, Sawai T, Higashi T. Efficacy of combined hand exercise intervention in patients with chemotherapy-induced peripheral neuropathy: a pilot randomized controlled trial. Support Care Cancer. 2022;30(6):4981–92.
90. Gui Q, Li D, Zhuge Y, Xu C. Efficacy of exercise rehabilitation program in relieving oxaliplatin induced peripheral neurotoxicity. Asian Pac J Cancer Prev. 2021;22(3):705–9.

11 Postural and Balance Problems in Breast Cancer Survivors and Managing Options

Mahmut Sürmeli

Breast cancer survivors (BCS) often confront a spectrum of medical, physical, and mental health challenges following breast surgery and multimodal treatments like radiotherapy (RT) and chemotherapy (CT) [1]. These interventions can result in diverse adverse effects on the musculoskeletal system, including fatigue, muscle weakness, and neuropathy, all linked to postural disorders, as well as gait and balance impairments [2–4]. Postural [5], balance and gait [2, 4] problems in BCS stand as significant challenges, exerting considerable influence on their quality of life [6] and daily functioning [7, 8].

Extensive research has shed light on the multifaceted nature of these issues, indicating a range of factors contributing to postural changes and balance impairments among BCS. Breast cancer treatments, such as CT and breast surgery mainly including mastectomy and axillary lymph node dissection (ALND) which is associated with significant morbidity, including lymphedema and reduced shoulder mobility, have been identified as pivotal elements influencing postural control and alterations [5, 8–10]. This chapter delves into the intricate interplay of factors affecting postural and balance challenges in BCS, exploring potential management options and interventions designed to enhance their overall well-being.

11.1 The Importance of Postural and Balance Disorders in Patients with Breast Cancer

Patients diagnosed with and undergoing treatment for breast cancer may develop postural abnormalities over time [8, 11, 12]. The frequency of postural changes after treatment in BCS is higher compared to healthy individuals [12]. Research indicates that individuals undergoing surgery [8] and CT [9] experience disturbances in postural control and sensory organization during quiet stance [3] and dynamic tasks [13]. For instance, taxane-based CT has been reported to cause balance disturbances, indicating the presence of postural instability [9]. Additionally, surgical techniques, especially mastectomy and ALND in breast cancer treatment, have been associated with postural changes [8, 14–16], emphasizing the need for evaluation and comparison to understand their impact [14]. Furthermore, lymphedema may exacerbate postural abnormalities and affect arm function [17].

It has been noted that increased energy expenditure for movement control due to postural and balance disorders leads to elevated levels of fatigue, thus potentially resulting in limitations in

M. Sürmeli (✉)
Faculty of Health Sciences, Department of Physical Therapy and Rehabilitation, Tokat Gaziosmanpaşa University, Tokat, Turkey
e-mail: mahmut.surmeli@gop.edu.tr

Y. Bakar, A. Tuğral (eds.), *Managing Side Effects of Breast Cancer Treatment*,
https://doi.org/10.1007/978-3-031-75480-7_11

physical function [8]. Moreover, cognitive function impairment associated with multimodal cancer treatment is highlighted as a condition that could impair daily activities, reduce quality of life, and worsen the difficulties faced due to postural and balance disorders [18]. Additionally, sleep disturbances are a common occurrence that can affect various aspects of sleep quality and potentially worsen postural and balance problems [19]. Though there is a wide variety of issues linked to postural and balance problems due to the multifaceted nature of the treatment, specific issues related to physical contributors to the postural and balance problems are tried to be explained in detail in the following text.

11.1.1 Postural Alterations

Postural abnormalities observed in BCS include various symptoms such as shoulder protraction, spinal misalignment, scapular displacement, forward head posture, increased pelvic tilt, and foot posture abnormalities [16, 20]. Research indicates that postural abnormalities arise due to conditions such as surgery [11, 12, 15, 21], muscle imbalances [6], pain [22, 23], scar tissue formation [24, 25], and avoidant posture, as well as lymphedema [26, 27]. Furthermore, spinal postural changes manifest differently in various planes [8, 21].

Recently, attention has been drawn to evaluate postural control following mastectomy in the breast cancer literature [2, 11, 12, 15, 28]. Studies often examine the effects of mastectomy on the body [12, 15, 28] and analyze the body posture of women who have undergone this procedure [5, 8, 10, 11, 14, 21]. BCS following mastectomy have been observed to exhibit disorders in the sagittal, coronal, and frontal planes of the spine, increased trunk inclination, surface rotation, and lateral deviation [8]. Moreover, postural imbalance has also been reported in patients undergoing breast-conserving therapy, independent of the type of axillary intervention, suggesting the possibility of encountering postural disorder even without extensive surgery [29]. Particularly in extensive surgeries, weaknesses, and muscle imbalances in the upper extremity between pectoralis major, serratus anterior, upper trapezius, rhomboid muscles, and latissimus dorsi may be observed, highlighting them as significant factors contributing to postural disorders [6]. These changes in spinal alignment and posture worsen the overall postural stability and balance of BCS [20, 28, 30].

Asymmetry in the Head and Neck Breast cancer treatment, especially mastectomy and adjuvant therapies, can potentially influence head and neck posture. The alterations in body alignment, muscle tone distribution, and overall postural control associated with breast cancer treatment may contribute to changes in head and neck posture [16]. Particularly an anterior tilt of the head and lateral tilt of the neck are expected to be observed following unilateral mastectomy. However, it is noteworthy that, they notably worsens over time. The observed alterations in head and neck posture in almost all patients during long-term follow-up highlight the significance of unilateral mastectomy on surrounding structures and body alignment [31].

In addition, it has been demonstrated that unilateral lymphedema is associated with these changes and is generally considered a factor that can exacerbate postural dysfunction [26]. In women with lymphedema, anteriorization of the head, rotation of the head towards the operated side, and lateral flexion are observed. Moreover, the weight of the limb affected by lymphedema is also a significant factor that can lead to retraction of the shoulder and shoulder girdle muscles, tension in cervical and neck muscles, bending rotation, and lateral flexion of the neck [26, 32].

Trunk Asymmetry and Spinal Curvatures Unilateral mastectomy surgeries lead to body asymmetry in both short [33] and long term [11] compared to pre-surgery conditions. Research confirms that unilateral mastectomy has a significant impact on the spine in the long term, aiming to compensate the weight of the missing breast. Comparing pre- and post-surgery values, a study emphasizes the importance of angular changes after surgery, highlighting the risk of scoliosis progression in patients with preexisting idiopathic scoliosis. Among patients who underwent a unilateral mastectomy, there is an increase in the spinal bending angle toward the left side for those with a right mastectomy and toward the right side for those with a left mastectomy, demonstrating an increase in Cobb angle [11]. On the other hand, in patients undergoing breast reconstruction surgery (BRS), body asymmetry is also observed compared to pre-surgery conditions. However, this ratio tends to be higher than in those who undergo mastectomy without BRS [33]. Additionally, another study has confirmed that mastectomy surgeries contribute to an increase in Cobb angle at the upper thoracic level, indicating an increase in spinal curvature. This research also suggests that this condition can be somewhat mitigated with BRS [34]. In summary, it has been observed that there is a change in the Cobb angle in the opposite direction of the mastectomy side. The significance of reconstructive breast surgeries is emphasized in balancing the altered body weight [10].

One of the most noticeable changes observed in the spine occurs in the anterior–posterior direction, especially in the thoracic and lumbar regions. Individuals who have undergone surgery exhibit greater restriction in angular values of trunk movement in the sagittal plane [8]. The presence of lymphedema exacerbates this process. These changes may contribute to the development of scoliosis, balance issues, restricted thoracic cage mobility, and potential respiratory function problems [21].

In patients with mastectomy, particularly those with increased thoracic kyphosis and lumbar lordosis, deviations in the anterior–posterior direction affect the capacity of trunk muscles to produce force regardless of the muscle group. An increase in kyphotic posture is associated with lower force–velocity values. Therefore, it is evident that changes in posture also affect the functions of trunk muscles [35]. Additionally, after mastectomy surgeries, there is a significant increase in the lumbosacral angle, lumbar lordosis, thoracic inclination angle, and thoracic kyphosis, but these increase are less pronounced in those who undergo BRS [14].

In summary, it can be said that kyphotic posture is one of the most significant spinal postures in terms of spinal changes. Furthermore, the impact of mastectomy surgeries on this process has been emphasized [14, 35], and it has been highlighted that kyphotic posture can be somewhat corrected with BRS [14]. However, it should be noted that postural changes may still occur even when external prostheses or tissue expanders are used after total mastectomy [10].

Although research has shown the contributions of mastectomy to spinal curvatures and other postural abnormalities, another important point is the presence of existing scoliosis in these patients. Evaluations before and after breast cancer surgery in a population of patients with previous scoliosis has shown that postoperative changes in the spine may be more severe in this group of patients [36].

Furthermore, it is observed that trunk lateral flexion is inclined more toward the opposite side of the surgery. In this way, the height of the scapula on the operated side also increases, which confirms the data indicating higher scapular height on the operated side [32]. Additionally, the mass of the excised breast tissue has been found to be associated with the magnitude of the change in spinal curvature in those undergoing unilateral mastectomy without breast reconstruction. Patients with large breasts who undergo unilateral mastectomy alone may present a further risk of developing an exacerbated increase in lateral deviation [36].

Asymmetry in the Shoulder and Pelvic Girdle After mastectomy, postural changes around the shoulder and pelvis also become apparent. These changes are characterized by an increase in the forward inclination angle of the trunk, higher positioning of the scapula on the affected side in the frontal plane, increased anterior pelvic tilt angle, and more abduction and elevation of the scapula, leading to shoulder protraction. These alterations, occurring alongside increased thoracic kyphosis and lumbar lordosis of the spine, disrupt the overall body alignment and balance [15]. Additionally, in the early postoperative period, due to protective posture and imbalances in body weight distribution, ipsilateral shoulder elevation and protraction are more pronounced [15], while, in the long term, contralateral shoulder elevation may also become evident [11].

Shoulder protraction is dominant on the side where mastectomy is performed. Additionally, pain contributes to protective posture in this process [16, 37]. Additionally, changes in the position of the scapulae are observed. The scapulae on the side of the operation is positioned at a higher level compared to the contralateral scapula. This may signify a change in the activation and coordination of muscles responsible for scapular stabilization [38]. A study that included a 12-month follow-up from the early postoperative period showed that approximately half of the patients developed shoulder and scapular asymmetry in the first 6 months after surgery, with the prevalence of shoulder asymmetry increasing significantly after the first month. Furthermore, while pelvic tilt was observed in only 11–13% of patients in the early postoperative period, this rate increased to 44% during the 12-month follow-up period in the same study. This emphasizes that shoulder girdle problems are prominent in the early stages, especially for patients with mastectomy, and besides an increase in shoulder girdle problems in the long term, significant pelvic tilt changes will also occur [31].

Another important factor besides the effect of the surgery is the presence of lymphedema. It has been observed that the presence of lymphedema increases the likelihood of scapular dyskinesis by altering pain sensitivity in the trapezius and deltoid muscles, affecting upper extremity functions [23]. It is noteworthy that the elevation of the scapula is characterized by whether or not upper limb lymphedema is present on the operated side [32].

Foot Following breast cancer treatment, changes in the musculoskeletal system along with comprehensive postural alterations involving the entire body could potentially lead to changes in foot posture [8]. Especially, the treatment process resulting in a change in the center of gravity will affect body alignment and postural control not only in the trunk but also encompassing the entire body [37]. Additionally, the distribution of muscle tone throughout the body, which can be affected by breast cancer and its treatment, may have implications for foot posture [28].

11.1.2 Postural Control and Balance Disturbances

Postural control and balance are closely related concepts. The term "postural control" refers to the body's ability to control both stability and orientation. This entails maintaining balance across different positions and activities, with various sensory inputs and motor responses being harmoniously in tune. On the other hand, "balance" describes the act of achieving, maintaining, or regaining a state of equilibrium during any position or activity [39]. It is a fundamental aspect of daily activities and sports performance [40]. Postural control covers a spectrum that includes static postural control, postural control involving voluntary and involuntary actions, and postural control during external perturbations [41]. These various conditions highlight the complexity of postural control mechanisms and the body's actions upon various challenges in maintaining stability [42].

Postural control, a vital component of balance, holds crucial importance in daily life, particularly for maintaining posture during activities such as walking, running, or other routine tasks. However, advanced age [43] along with various disorders and diseases [41] can lead to a decrease in postural control and balance disturbances. This process, characterized by an increased risk of falls, results in significant health risks [44].

Postural control impairment following breast cancer treatment, mainly mastectomy and CT, has been examined in various studies, and the importance of management strategies to prevent potential problems associated with balance disturbances has been emphasized [8, 12, 15, 37]. Postural stability and balance issues are observed in BCS due to various reasons such as muscle imbalances, tissue tightness, muscle weakness, pain, chemotherapy-induced peripheral neuropathy (CIPN), and lymphedema. It has been observed that balance is disrupted due to chemotherapy-related toxicity, and there is a progressive deterioration in postural control from the early stages of treatment [9]. In these patients, balance disturbances, particularly manifested in gait disturbances, also increase the risk of falls [45].

In addition to disturbances in the body's posture in the frontal, sagittal, and horizontal planes, it has been shown that sway increases under both eyes' open and closed conditions, and this increase is proportional to the amount of energy required to maintain postural balance [8]. Furthermore, a walking alteration characterized by a decrease in step length and walking speed has been observed following breast cancer treatment [46]. Additionally, balance analyses have revealed poor balance outcomes indicative of disturbances in sensorimotor organization [47].

Primarily, in survivors of breast cancer, significant decreases in the rate of center of pressure changes during reactions for maintaining balance, walking speed, and timed performance data have been demonstrated, particularly in situations where the feet are in contact with the ground, indicating a substantial impact on dynamic balance. Moreover, it has been noted that disturbances in static balance increase significantly when visual and proprioceptive stimuli are challenged [2]. Another study suggests that while significant changes may not occur in static balance in patients undergoing breast cancer treatment, dynamic balance may be more affected than static balance. It is also observed that indicators of dynamic balance based on timed performance are significantly poorer in BCS [13]. Therefore, it can be assumed that balance disturbances may be prominent, particularly in dynamic balance, following breast cancer-related conditions, but static balance may not always manifest at a significant level.

Lymphedema can also affect postural control and balance in women undergoing breast cancer treatment. It has been shown that middle-aged women with unilateral lymphedema exhibit less postural stability compared to healthy women, which may increase to the risk of falls due to the asymmetrical distribution of fluids in the upper extremities [30]. Regarding the correlation of the volume difference between extremities and balance variables, it has been reported that a rise in volume negatively affects the time spent on a task, thus efforts are made to maintain balance during dynamic tasks [48].

11.2 Factors Contributing to Posture and Balance Disorders in Breast Cancer Survivors

Posture disorders and balance issues in BCS can be linked to several factors. These include such as surgery, radiotherapy, CT, CIPN, hormonal changes, reduced joint mobility, muscle imbalances, pain, psychological disorders, reduced physical activity, older age and any preexisting musculoskeletal conditions.

11.2.1 Surgical Effects

Surgical procedures like mastectomy or breast-conserving surgery have significant effects on posture following treatment [5, 6, 8]. Depending on the type of surgery alterations in spine alignment, increased thoracic kyphosis, upper limb dysfunctions, and decreased shoulder joint angles mainly on the operated side can be seen and the contribute further to postural changes. These surgeries may also result in fibrosis, shortening of pectoral muscles, and alterations in the angle of the shoulder blade, further impacting posture [16].

11.2.2 Lymphedema

The presence of lymphedema can lead to limitations in shoulder movement in the upper limb, influencing posture [27] and balance [17]. It results in alterations in spinal alignment [21, 27] and upper limb dysfunction [49]. Swelling, discomfort, and reduced range of motion in the affected limb due to lymphedema are contributing symptoms [50].

11.2.3 Muscle Weakness and Imbalances

Surgical procedures can lead to changes in musculoskeletal structures, alterations in muscle tension distribution, and disruptions in postural control, all of which can contribute to balance impairments [15, 28]. Additionally, surgery-induced alterations in muscle strength and proprioception can affect the ability to maintain balance and stability [15]. Moreover, dissection of muscles and soft tissue structures during surgery can lead to muscle weakness in the upper limb, affecting muscle function [51] and potentially leading to postural control disorders [52].

CT has been shown to have deleterious effects on muscle size, mitochondrial structures, and muscle function [53]. The alterations in muscle size, neurogenic changes, and mitochondrial damage resulting from like systemic CT and radiotherapy can lead to long-term impacts on muscle strength [54]. Weakened muscles, including the pectoralis major, serratus anterior, upper trapezius, rhomboid muscles, and latissimus dorsi, can act as main contributors to the postural alterations.

11.2.4 Scar Tissue Formation

Surgical scars and tissue changes resulting from breast cancer treatments, such as surgery and radiotherapy, can impact the flexibility and movement of muscles and joints [22, 51]. Tissue fibrosis and protective posturing can contribute to the shortening of soft tissues in the anterior chest wall [55], including the pectoralis major and minor muscles, losing their gliding ability that is relative to the shoulder joint [55].

11.2.5 Peripheral Neuropathy

CIPN is recognized as a factor contributing to gait and balance disorders in breast cancer patients. Agents like taxanes, platinum-based drugs, and vinca alkaloids, commonly used in CT, are known to induce CIPN, causing sensory symptoms such as tingling, burning, numbness, pain, and loss of balance. The severity of these symptoms can range from bothersome to disabling, affecting motor function and causing muscle weakness in both upper and lower extremities [56]. It results in deficits in gait parameters, which may be exacerbated in challenging walking environments, potentially leading to balance issues. Furthermore, CIPN has been linked to falls and functional impairments in breast cancer patients, highlighting its impact on mobility and balance [57].

11.2.6 Joint Stiffness (Limited Shoulder Mobility)

Surgery, particularly procedures involving the axillary region, can lead to restrictions in shoulder joint mobility, resulting in stiffness and reduced range of motion [24, 25]. Axillary radiotherapy can also play a role in causing joint stiffness and reduced flexibility [24]. The impairment of movement patterns and compensatory mechanisms can be explanatory factors for postural control disturbances associated with joint stiffness or movement limitations [15].

11.2.7 Hormonal Changes

Hormonal therapy can indeed pose a risk factor for balance problems in BCS. It has been associated with musculoskeletal symptoms [54, 58]. BCS, following hormone therapy, may experience general pain, myalgia, and physical discomfort, which can affect their physical well-being [58]. In addition, it leads to disruption in force production and muscle strength [54].

11.2.8 Pain and Discomfort

Pain, discomfort [16], myofascial dysfunctions [59], and arthralgias [60] can indeed lead to posture and balance problems in BCS. Additionally, psychological factors such as pain catastrophizing can heighten emotional distress among with BCS with persistent breast pain, further exacerbating their physical discomfort [61].

11.2.9 Psychological Factors

Psychological disorders are significant posttreatment experiences of BCS, influencing various aspects of their physical and mental health, including posture and balance. Psychological distress, anxiety, and depression have been linked to impaired postural control and balance in this population [62].

11.2.10 Deconditioning

Muscle deconditioning in breast cancer patients may be driven by a decrease in overall physical activity during their treatment, leading to reduced exercise capacity and early skeletal muscle deconditioning, affecting posture and balance [63].

11.3 Managing Strategies

Approaches addressing postural deviations and balance problems emerging after breast cancer treatments should complement each other, encompassing surgical, complementary, and conservative methods. It is evident that the issues arising are not solely triggered by surgery but also by various problems such as pain, neuropathy, and lymphedema, which can lead to functional problems related to movement and balance. Therefore, fundamental approaches must include a combination of breast reconstructive surgeries, breast prostheses, exercise-based interventions, and pain management approaches based on symptom management, such as complex decongestive therapy and psychotherapy to overcome changes in mood disorders known to affect posture. Thus, the following text will try to cover the aspects of physical contributors to the potential deviations in posture and balance management strategies.

11.3.1 Breast Reconstructive Surgeries and Breast Prostheses

BRS encompass a variety of surgical techniques aimed at restoring the shape, symmetry, and appearance of the breast following mastectomy [64]. These methods can involve using autologous tissues, implants, or a combination of both, and the timing of the reconstruction can be immediate, delayed, or delayed-immediate. The primary goal of breast reconstruction in breast cancer patients is to improve body image and enhance self-esteem, thereby positively impacting the physical health, psychological well-being, and quality of life of individuals who have undergone mastectomy [65].

Research indicates that applying early or delayed BRS following mastectomy has positive effects on both physical and psychosocial health. In addition to physical effects like postural distortions, it is noted that these surgeries also enhance patients' psychological confidence and quality of life [66].

As detailed above, changes in spinal alignment, particularly in the sagittal plane, and postural distortions in areas such as the head, neck, and shoulder girdle are commonly observed. Studies on the effects of BRS highlight the importance of these surgeries not only for aesthetic purposes but also for reducing postural distortions, with reconstructions showing better postures compared to mastectomy without reconstruction. Especially, early-stage BRS following mastectomy has a corrective effect on spinal alignment, emphasizing the necessity of adding reconstruction surgeries to the options following mastectomy [67, 68]. Moreover, it is suggested that while implant or autologous BRS reduces the negative effects of spinal misalignment in the long term, autologous reconstructive surgeries may have better effects than implants. In summary, BRS stands as a significant option for achieving better physical and psychosocial outcomes following mastectomy [10].

On the other hand, besides being a frequently preferred approach, external breast prostheses are also among the options. However, it is observed that the corrective effect of external breast prostheses on posture during use is not as significant as that of reconstruction surgeries. Moreover, it has been noted that they do not have a clinically significant effect on posture and body movements, especially during functional physical activities. Therefore, their use is seen to have limited effects on body biomechanics and posture for maintaining balance. However, it is still emphasized that they should be considered among the options [37, 69].

11.3.2 Exercise and Physiotherapy

Exercise practices are essential in managing postural disorders in patients undergoing breast cancer surgery. Research has demonstrated that exercise interventions can positively impact posture, upper limb function, and quality of life in BCS. Various exercise modalities, including myofascial release, stretching, strengthening exercises, and aerobic exercise, have been shown to improve postural balance, spinal curvatures, range of motion, strength, shoulder pain, and disability in BCS [44, 59]. These exercises not only address physical impairments but also enhance overall well-being and quality of life in this patient population [70].

A comprehensive study analyzing approaches applied to patients within a 12-month period following surgery reveals a focus on increasing shoulder mobility and corrective postural exercises during the initial 2 weeks post-surgery. As weeks progress, there is an escalation in the implementation of exercises targeting shoulder girdle and thoracic region stretching. Beyond the first month, long-term regional strengthening exercises are incorporated into the programs, and in the long term, exercises aimed at enhancing physical fitness are increasingly integrated into the regimens. One significant finding from this analysis is the substantial emphasis on exercises aimed at incrementally increasing shoulder mobility and correcting posture during the initial months, with foundational exercises and other physiotherapy programs persisting in the long term [71]. Therefore, the necessity of creating a comprehensive program incorporating various types of exercises aimed at improving overall physical health emerges as of importance in overcoming postural and balance issues [72].

One of the highlighted aspects is the effect of exercises focused on increasing muscle strength on balance and postural control in the long term. Particularly, it has been demonstrated that exercises aimed at strengthening muscles around the back, hips, and both upper and lower extremities make significant contributions. Research indicating that strength training exercises yield better results in the long term underscores their importance in rehabilitation programs for improving static balance, functional dynamic balance, postural control, and walking efficiency in BCS [73]. Additionally, exercises such as Tai-Chi-Chuan or Qigong have been reported to enhance significantly the balance and postural control performance of BCS, thereby emphasizing the importance of sensory-based training in balance improvement [74]. Furthermore, yoga exercises have been found to promote relaxation in patients and improve posture, thus demonstrating positive effects on both physical and mental health in BCS [75]. Moreover, complex decongestive therapy has been observed to improve balance, especially in the presence of upper extremity lymphedema [76]. Therefore, by considering all clinical conditions accompanying surgery with a multidimensional perspective, the effectiveness of treatments can be significantly enhanced.

Exercise training programs based on cardiovascular endurance have been recognized as highly effective methods for increasing cardiovascular endurance, functional capacity, and physical activity levels [77]. Particularly, aerobic-based exercises, which have significant effects on both physical and mental health, are known to improve overall body fitness and mood, thus enhancing quality of life. A study has shown that Nordic walking exercises promote improvement in thoracic and lumbar posture in BCS, while aquatic exercises also lead to significant postural improvement in the thoracic region [78]. Aerobic exercises, which involve symmetrical body movements at their core and thus contribute significantly to balance from a biomechanical standpoint, come in various forms, and it has been suggested that their implementation as aquatic exercises may improve postural alignment and trunk muscle endurance more effectively than traditional methods [79].

Furthermore, although not specific to breast cancer, various manual therapy techniques, ranging from myofascial tissue techniques aimed at increasing joint mobility, have been observed to be effective on posture. Research indicates that soft tissue techniques may be effective in the medium and long term, particularly in postural abnormalities associated with muscle tension/imbalance, especially in the head, neck, and upper thoracic region. Myofascial relaxation techniques applied to region-specific muscles, particularly in cases of anterior tilt of the head, lateral tilt of the neck, and protrusion of the shoulders, are considered to be significant options. On the other hand, it has been observed that joint-oriented applications such as scapular mobilization and cervical mobilization are not as effective in correcting posture as myofascial techniques. Moreover, while mobilizations may not have significant effects on scoliosis, joint and myofascial techniques applied particularly to thoracic kyphosis may have postural corrective effects. Similarly, corrective effects are also observed around the pelvic girdle [80]. In BCS, considering the potential effects of various and multiple treatments such as surgery, chemotherapy, and hormone therapy on muscles, bones, soft tissues, and overall physical health, appropriate manipulative treatment methods can be included as complementary to the program. Especially, the consideration of soft tissue techniques is crucial during this process. In fact, it has been shown that myofascial relaxation techniques applied to muscles associated with the shoulder girdle and neck, particularly in breast cancer patients, can be an effective option for correcting postural abnormalities such as shoulder girdle, neck, head, spinal curvatures, and thoracic kyphosis. This emphasizes the clinical importance of using myofascial releasing techniques in this population [59].

Another approach emphasized for achieving postural alignment is Pilates-like posture correction exercises. A balanced muscle system is necessary to maintain and sustain balance and postural alignment. Therefore, it is necessary to include Pilates exercises aimed at increasing strength, endurance, and flexibility, as well as improving postural alignment and balance. Research conducted on BCS has shown that Pilates exercises, when applied appropriately, lead to improvements in patients' postural alignment and balance. By combining isometric and isotonic contractions of core muscles, especially those between the shoulders and pelvic floor and the abdominal region, strengthening and increasing endurance, Pilates exercises have been highlighted as an approach with significant effects on body alignment and spinal posture [81].

In summary, breast cancer treatment involves highly radical and impactful methods on posture and balance. Among these treatment methods, such as surgery, chemotherapy, and hormone therapy, have significant effects on the body, including various side effects like pain, lymphedema, neuropathy, and muscle weakness. Postural and balance disorders, particularly due to their functional effects on daily life, are significant issues. Managing these problems requires a comprehensive, long-term treatment program that takes a multidimensional treatment approach following medical and surgical interventions. Especially, surgical and complementary approaches for postural and balance disorders are highlighted. Surgical options, particularly results from autologous reconstructive surgeries, have corrective effects on posture, while implant breast reconstruction surgeries also impact posture positively. However, for both posture and balance improvement, appropriate physiotherapy approaches and exercise programs must be included in treatment programs to ensure their permanence and long-term sustainability. Early-stage interventions focusing on joint mobility and posture correction exercises, supported by strength training exercises in the long term, should be integrated as part of daily life. Moreover, postural correction exercises such as Pilates and yoga, along with balance-based exercise practices, should be considered as supportive approaches. It is recommended that combined, purposeful, appropriately intensive, and individualized approaches be implemented to reduce postural and balance disorders and improve overall health for patients with breast cancer.

References

1. Miaskowski C, Mastick J, Paul SM, Topp K, Smoot B, Abrams G, et al. Chemotherapy-induced neuropathy in cancer survivors. J Pain Symptom Manag. 2017;54(2):204–218.e2.
2. Hsieh KL, Wood TA, An R, Trinh L, Sosnoff JJ. Gait and balance impairments in breast cancer survivors: a systematic review and meta-analysis of observational studies. Arch Rehabil Res Clin Transl. 2019;1(1):100001.
3. Monfort SM, Pan X, Loprinzi CL, Lustberg MB, Chaudhari AMW. Impaired postural control and altered sensory organization during quiet stance following neurotoxic chemotherapy: a preliminary study. Integr Cancer Ther. 2019;18:1534735419828823.
4. Kolb NA, Smith AG, Singleton JR, Beck SL, Stoddard GJ, Brown S, et al. The association of chemotherapy-induced peripheral neuropathy symptoms and the risk of falling. JAMA Neurol. 2016;73(7):860–6.
5. Atanes Mendes Peres AC, de Oliveira D, Latorre MR, Yugo Maesaka J, Filassi JR, Chada Baracat E, Alves Gonçalves Ferreira E. Body posture after mastectomy: comparison between immediate breast reconstruction versus mastectomy alone. Physiother Res Int. 2017;22(1):e1642.
6. Birelliwar A, Dhankar S. Evaluation of posture and quality of life in females undergone modified radical mastectomy: a research protocol. Indian J Forensic Med Toxicol. 2021;15(1):963–5.
7. Wang AB, Housley SN, Flores AM, Kircher SM, Perreault EJ, Cope TC. A review of movement disorders in chemotherapy-induced neurotoxicity. J NeuroEng Rehabil. 2021;18(1):16.
8. Mangone M, Bernetti A, Agostini F, Paoloni M, De Cicco FA, Capobianco SV, et al. Changes in spine alignment and postural balance after breast cancer surgery: a rehabilitative point of view. Biores Open Access. 2019;8(1):121–8.
9. Monfort SM, Pan X, Patrick R, Singaravelu J, Loprinzi CL, Lustberg MB, et al. Natural history of postural instability in breast cancer patients treated with taxane-based chemotherapy: a pilot study. Gait Posture. 2016;48:237–42.
10. Serel S, Sefa Özden N, Aydınlı Y, Akkaya Z, Uzun Ç, Bayar S. Effects of delayed breast reconstruction on the thoracolumbar vertebrae in patients undergoing unilateral mastectomy: a retrospective cohort study. J Plast Reconstr Aesthet Surg. 2022;75(9):3022–9.
11. Serel S, Tuzlalı ZY, Akkaya Z, Uzun Ç, Kaya B, Bayar S. Physical effects of unilateral mastectomy on spine deformity. Clin Breast Cancer. 2017;17(1):29–33.
12. Ahn SY, Bok SK, Song Y, Lee HW, Jung JY, Kim JJ. Dynamic body posture after unilateral mastectomy: a pilot study. Gland Surg. 2020;9(5):1235–43.
13. Evans ES, Ketcham CJ, Hibberd JC, Cullen ME, Basiliere JG, Murphy DL. Examination of clinical and laboratory measures of static and dynamic balance in breast cancer survivors. Physiother Theory Pract. 2021;37(11):1199–209.
14. Głowacka I, Nowikiewicz T, Hagner W, Nowacka K, Sowa M, Zegarski W. Sagittal plane postural changes in female patients with breast cancer after different surgical techniques. Breast J. 2017;23(1):109–11.
15. Montezuma T, Guirro ECO, Vaz MMOLL, Vernal S. Changes in postural control in mastectomized women. J Cancer Ther. 2014;5(6):493–9.
16. Rangel J, Perez CS, Oliveira R, Guirro ECO. Effects of breast cancer treatment on posture: a current review. Int J Phys Ther Rehabil. 2019;2019(5):152–5.
17. Surmeli M, Ozdemir OC. Examination of the relationship between upper limb function, posture and quality of life in patients with and without lymphedema after breast cancer surgery. Konuralp Med J. 2019;11(3):432–9.
18. Tenda Y, Miyashita M, Yamada A, Shimizu C, Nakayama K, Honma N, et al. Older patients' experience of living with cognitive impairment related to hormone therapy for breast cancer. Eur J Oncol Nurs. 2022;57:102115.
19. Zou B, Li H, Liu J, Xu Z, Chen H, Li H, et al. Status and manifestations of sleep disorders and the status of drugs used to help fall sleep in Chinese breast cancer women at initial diagnosis and during chemotherapy. Res Sq. 2019.
20. Głowacka-Mrotek I, Sowa M, Nowikiewicz T, Siedlecki Z, Hagner W, Zegarski W. Foot posture in female patients 5 years after breast-conserving surgery: a case–control study. Breast Cancer. 2018;25(3):325–33.
21. Celenay ST, Ucurum SG, Kaya DO. Comparison of spinal alignment and mobility in women with and without post modified radical mastectomy unilateral lymphoedema. Clin Breast Cancer. 2020;20(3):e295–300.
22. Rasmussen GHF, Madeleine P, Arroyo-Morales M, Voigt M, Kristiansen M. Pain sensitivity and shoulder function among breast cancer survivors compared to matched controls: a case-control study. J Cancer Surviv. 2023;17(1):150–9.
23. Korucu TS, Ucurum SG, Tastaban E, Ozgun H, Kaya DO. Comparison of shoulder-arm complex pain, function, and scapular dyskinesia in women with and without unilateral lymphedema after breast cancer surgery. Clin Breast Cancer. 2021;21(3):e285–93.
24. Lang AE, Murphy M, Dickerson CR, Stavness I, Kim SY. Shoulder dysfunction in breast cancer survivors: can treatment type or musculoskeletal factors identify those at higher risk? Rehabil Oncol. 2021;39(3):143.
25. Lipps DB, Leonardis JM, Dess RT, McGinnis GJ, Marsh RB, Strauss JB, et al. Mechanical properties of the shoulder and pectoralis major in breast

cancer patients undergoing breast-conserving surgery with axillary surgery and radiotherapy. Sci Rep. 2019;9(1):17737.
26. Shital K, Kajol K, Sandeep S, Pise S. Correlation between postural impairment and lymphedema in breast cancer survivors. Asian Pac J Health Sci. 2022;9(2):125–9.
27. Surmeli M, Cinar Ozdemir O. The effect of upper limb lymphedema in posture of patients after breast cancer surgery. J Back Musculoskelet Rehabil. 2022;35(4):829–37.
28. Głowacka-Mrotek I, Tarkowska M, Nowikiewicz T, Hagner-Derengowska M, Goch A. Assessment of postural balance in women treated for breast cancer. Medicina (Mex). 2020;56(10):505.
29. Głowacka-Mrotek I, Tarkowska M, Leksowski L, Nowikiewicz T, Zegarski W. Evaluation of late postural complications in breast cancer patients undergoing breast-conserving therapy in relation to the type of axillary intervention-cross-sectional study. J Clin Med. 2021;10(7):1432.
30. Basar S, Bakar Y, Keser I, Kaba H, Güzel NA, Özdemir ÖÇ, et al. Does lymphedema affect the postural stability in women after breast cancer? Top Geriatr Rehabil. 2012;28(4):287.
31. Liu R, Xie H, Wang Y, Wang Q, Xie X, Zhang X. Impact of unilateral mastectomy on body posture: a prospective longitudinal observational study. Asia-Pac J Oncol Nurs. 2024;11(2):100336.
32. Haddad CAS, Saad M, Perez MDCJ, Miranda Júnior F. Assessment of posture and joint movements of the upper limbs of patients after mastectomy and lymphadenectomy. Einstein (Sao Paulo). 2013;11:426–34.
33. Głowacka I, Nowikiewicz T, Siedlecki Z, Hagner W, Nowacka K, Zegarski W. The assessment of the magnitude of frontal plane postural changes in breast cancer patients after breast-conserving therapy or mastectomy—follow-up results 1 year after the surgical procedure. Pathol Oncol Res. 2016;22(1):203–8.
34. Lee JS, Park E, Lee JH, Lee J, Park HY, Yang JD, et al. Alteration in skeletal posture between breast reconstruction with latissimus dorsi flap and mastectomy: a prospective comparison study. Gland Surg. 2021;10(5):1587–97.
35. Malicka I, Hanuszkiewicz J, Stefanska M, Barczyk K, Wozniewski M. Relation between trunk muscle activity and posture type in women following treatment for breast cancer. J Back Musculoskelet Rehabil. 2010;23:11–9.
36. Gutkin PM, Kapp DS, von Eyben R, Dirbas FM, Horst KC. Impact of mastectomy for breast cancer on spinal curvature: considerations when treating patients with scoliosis. Breast J. 2020;26(10):1973–9.
37. Koralewska A, Domagalska-Szopa M, Szopa A. Influence of the external breast prosthesis on the postural control of women who underwent mastectomy: cross-sectional study. Front Oncol. 2022;12:920211.
38. Burkhart SS, Morgan CD, Ben Kibler W. The disabled throwing shoulder: spectrum of pathology part III: the SICK scapula, scapular dyskinesis, the kinetic chain, and rehabilitation. Arthroscopy. 2003;19(6):641–61.
39. Pollock AS, Durward BR, Rowe PJ, Paul JP. What is balance? Clin Rehabil. 2000;14(4):402–6.
40. Bowden MG, Embry AE, Gregory CM. Physical therapy adjuvants to promote optimization of walking recovery after stroke. Stroke Res Treat. 2011;2011:e601416.
41. French HP, Hager CK, Venience A, Fagan R, Meldrum D. Psychometric properties and domains of postural control tests for individuals with knee osteoarthritis: a systematic review. Int J Rehabil Res. 2020;43(2):102.
42. Ivanenko Y, Gurfinkel VS. Human postural control. Front Neurosci. 2018;12:171.
43. Marchesi G, De Luca A, Squeri V, De Michieli L, Casadio M, Canessa A. A lifespan approach to balance in static and dynamic conditions: the effect of age on balance abilities. Front Neurol. 2022;13:801142.
44. Streckmann F, Kneis S, Leifert JA, Baumann FT, Kleber M, Ihorst G, et al. Exercise program improves therapy-related side-effects and quality of life in lymphoma patients undergoing therapy. Ann Oncol. 2014;25(2):493–9.
45. Tofthagen C, Overcash J, Kip K. Falls in persons with chemotherapy-induced peripheral neuropathy. Support Care Cancer. 2012;20(3):583–9.
46. Vallabhajosula S, Deaterly CD, Madzima TA. Comparison of forward and backward gait characteristics between those with and without a history of breast cancer. Gait Posture. 2019;74:162–8.
47. Winters-Stone K, Torgrimson B, Horak F, Eisner A, Nail L, Leo M, et al. Identifying factors associated with falls in postmenopausal breast cancer survivors: a multi-disciplinary approach. Arch Phys Med Rehabil. 2011;92(4):646–52.
48. Zeltzer AA, Anzarut A, Hamdi M. A review of lymphedema for the hand and upper-extremity surgeon. J Hand Surg. 2018;43(11):1016–25.
49. Smoot B, Wong J, Cooper B, Wanek L, Topp K, Byl N, et al. Upper extremity impairments in women with or without lymphedema following breast cancer treatment. J Cancer Surviv. 2010;4(2):167–78.
50. Marchica P, D'arpa S, Magno S, Rossi C, Forcina L, Capizzi V, et al. Integrated treatment of breast cancer-related lymphedema: a descriptive review of the state of the art. Anticancer Res. 2021;41(7):3233–46.
51. Doro E, Azzollini V, Ghilli M, Roncella M, Chisari C. Postural alterations in breast cancer survivors: proposal of the PABS evaluation protocol based on a systematic review. Eur J Phys Rehabil Med. 2023;59(3):406–13.
52. Jare SN, Malawade M. Effect of graded theraband exercise on myofascial dysfunctions in breast cancer survivors. Indian J Forensic Med Toxicol. 2021;15(1):634–9.
53. Vikmoen O, Wiestad TH, Thormodsen I, Nordin K, Berntsen S, Demmelmaier I, et al. Effects of high and low-to-moderate intensity exercise during (neo-)adjuvant chemotherapy on muscle cells, cardiorespiratory fitness, and muscle function in women with breast

cancer: protocol for a randomized controlled trial. JMIR Res Protoc. 2022;11(11):e40811.
54. Bertoli J, de Souza Bezerra E, Dias Reis A, Amice da Costa Barros Ê, Gobbo LA, Forte Freitas Júnior I. Long-term side effects of breast cancer on force production parameters. J Strength Cond Res. 2022;36(5):1450.
55. Yuan RZ, Li KP, Wei XL, Zheng W, Ye Y, Wang MY, et al. Effects of free range-of-motion upper limb exercise based on mirror therapy on shoulder function in patients after breast cancer surgery: study protocol for a randomized controlled trial. Trials. 2021;22(1):815.
56. Clark PG, Cortese-Jimenez G, Cohen E. Effects of reiki, yoga, or meditation on the physical and psychological symptoms of chemotherapy-induced peripheral neuropathy: a randomized pilot study. J Evid-Based Complement Altern Med. 2012;17(3):161–71.
57. Monfort SM, Pan X, Patrick R, Ramaswamy B, Wesolowski R, Naughton MJ, et al. Gait, balance, and patient-reported outcomes during taxane-based chemotherapy in early-stage breast cancer patients. Breast Cancer Res Treat. 2017;164(1):69–77.
58. Yildiz F, Alaguney ME. Factors associated with the employment status of breast cancer survivors: a single center cross-sectional study. Int J Community Med Public Health. 2020;7(8):2874–9.
59. Rao MS, Pattanshetty RB. Effect of myofascial release, stretching, and strengthening on upper torso posture, spinal curvatures, range of motion, strength, shoulder pain and disability, and quality of life in breast cancer survivors. Physiother Res Int. 2022;27(2):e1939.
60. Stubblefield MD, Keole N. Upper body pain and functional disorders in patients with breast cancer. PM R. 2014;6(2):170–83.
61. Bovbjerg DH, Keefe FJ, Soo MS, Manculich J, Van Denburg A, Zuley ML, et al. Persistent breast pain in post-surgery breast cancer survivors and women with no history of breast surgery or cancer: associations with pain catastrophizing, perceived breast cancer risk, breast cancer worry, and emotional distress. Acta Oncol. 2019;58(5):763–8.
62. Pang L, Li W, Yao S, Jing Y, Yin X, Cheng H. Psychological distress is involved in CRCI in breast cancer survivors via mediating cytokine levels. Cancer Med. 2023;12(10):11806–15.
63. Mallard J, Hucteau E, Schott R, Trensz P, Pflumio C, Kalish-Weindling M, et al. Early skeletal muscle deconditioning and reduced exercise capacity during (neo)adjuvant chemotherapy in patients with breast cancer. Cancer. 2023;129(2):215–25.
64. Sbitany H. Breast reconstruction. Surg Clin N Am. 2018;98(4):845–57.
65. Zhang H, Gao Y, Ying J, Yu H, Guo R, Xiong J, et al. Bibliometric analysis of global research on breast reconstruction after mastectomy for breast cancer from 2011 to 2021. J Cosmet Dermatol. 2023;22(7):2071–82.
66. Wu W, Cheng S, Deng H, Wu J, Mao K, Cao M. Impact of breast cancer subtype defined by immunohistochemistry hormone receptor and HER2 status on the incidence of immediate postmastectomy reconstruction. Medicine (Baltimore). 2016;95(3):e2547.
67. Heng SSL, Gan YH, Yahya MM, Haron J, Wan Sulaiman WA. Changes in spinal alignment of women who underwent unilateral mastectomy with immediate autologous breast reconstruction compared to mastectomy without breast reconstruction. Clin Breast Cancer. 2022;22(8):e863–73.
68. Jeong JH, Choi B, Chang SY, Kim EK, Kang E, Heo CY, et al. The effect of immediate breast reconstruction on thoracic spine alignment after unilateral mastectomy. Clin Breast Cancer. 2018;18(3):214–9.
69. Hojan K, Manikowska F, Chen BP, Lin CC. The influence of an external breast prosthesis on the posture of women after mastectomy. J Back Musculoskelet Rehabil. 2016;29(2):337–42.
70. Bula A, Tatar K, Wysocka R, Chyrek K, Piejko L, Nawrat-Szołtysik A, et al. Effect of physical activity on static and dynamic postural balance in women treated for breast cancer: a systematic review. Int J Environ Res Public Health. 2023;20(4):3722.
71. Mazuquin B, Sunemi MMO, Silva MPPE, Sarian LOZ, Williamson E, Bruce J. Current physical therapy care of patients undergoing breast reconstruction for breast cancer: a survey of practice in the United Kingdom and Brazil. Braz J Phys Ther. 2021;25(2):175–85.
72. Foley MP, Hasson SM. Effects of a community-based multimodal exercise program on health-related physical fitness and physical function in breast cancer survivors: a pilot study. Integr Cancer Ther. 2016;15(4):446–54.
73. Vollmers PL, Mundhenke C, Maass N, Bauerschlag D, Kratzenstein S, Röcken C, et al. Evaluation of the effects of sensorimotor exercise on physical and psychological parameters in breast cancer patients undergoing neurotoxic chemotherapy. J Cancer Res Clin Oncol. 2018;144(9):1785–92.
74. Fong S, Choi A, Luk W, Yam T, Leung J, Chung J. Bone mineral density, balance performance, balance self-efficacy, and falls in breast cancer survivors with and without qigong training: an observational study. Integr Cancer Ther. 2018;17(1):124–30.
75. O'Neill M, Samaroo D, Lopez C, Tomlinson G, Santa Mina D, Sabiston C, et al. The effect of yoga interventions on cancer-related fatigue and quality of life for women with breast cancer: a systematic review and meta-analysis of randomized controlled trials. Integr Cancer Ther. 2020;19:1534735420959882.
76. Bilek F, Deniz G, Gulkesen A. The effect of complex decongestive therapy on spatio-temporal parameters and balance in women with breast cancer-related upper extremity unilateral lymphedema. Clin Biomech. 2023;102:105890.
77. Ramos PGF, Júdice PB, Nobre I, Carraça EV. Home-based exercise interventions' impact on breast cancer survivors' functional performance: a systematic review. J Cancer Surviv. 2024. https://doi.org/10.1007/s11764-024-01545-y.

78. Hanuszkiewicz J, Malicka I, Barczyk-Pawelec K, Woźniewski M. Effects of selected forms of physical activity on body posture in the sagittal plane in women post breast cancer treatment. J Back Musculoskelet Rehabil. 2015;28(1):35–41.
79. Hanuszkiewicz JM, Woźniewski M, Malicka I. The relationship between sagittal spinal curvatures and isokinetic trunk muscle endurance after aquatic exercise training in survivors of breast cancer. Acta Bioeng Biomech. 2020;22(1):21–30.
80. Santos TS, Oliveira KKB, Martins LV, Vidal APC. Effects of manual therapy on body posture: systematic review and meta-analysis. Gait Posture. 2022;96:280–94.
81. Fretta TB, Boing L, Baffa AP, Borgatto AF, Coutinho de Azevedo Guimarães A. Mat pilates method improve postural alignment women undergoing hormone therapy adjunct to breast cancer treatment. Clinical trial. Complement Ther Clin Pract. 2021;44:101424.

Shoulder Function

12

Emine Baran and İrem Düzgün

12.1 Introduction

The emergence of new and effective methods for the diagnosis and treatment of breast cancer has led to an increase in cancer survival. At the same time, cancer and cancer-related treatments are often associated with side effects that threaten the physical, psychological, and social well-being of patients in the short and long term [1].

A variety of treatment approaches, such as breast surgery (mastectomy, breast-conserving surgery), axillary surgery (axillary lymph node dissection—ALND, sentinel lymph node biopsy—SLNB), radiotherapy (RT), chemotherapy (CT), hormone therapy, and immunotherapy, are individually planned and implemented specifically for patients with breast cancer. Since the type of breast cancer, stage, metastatic status, physiological, anatomical, and biomechanical characteristics of the patients, and the treatment approaches applied to the patients may vary, a wide range of treatment-related morbidities can be seen in patients in the breast, shoulder region, and/or the entire upper extremity [2].

Problems such as scarring, fibrosis, decreased elasticity and tension of the pectoral muscles and soft tissues in the surgical site, lymphedema, nerve damage, pain, sensory problems, axillary web syndrome, shoulder kinematics and range of motion (ROM) deficits, and loss of strength can commonly occur after breast cancer treatment [1, 3]. Myofascial and nerve dysfunction, adhesive capsulitis, and pain often affect shoulder strength and ROM. Protraction of the shoulder due to the shortening of the pectoral muscles and narrowing of the subacromial space can affect the biomechanics of rotator cuff muscles on the surgical side. All these impairments can lead to disability in various areas of a patient's functioning. Women experience limitations in activities of daily living, functionality, work, and leisure time activities, thereby their quality of life decreases after breast cancer treatment [2–5]. Upper extremity pain, shoulder ROM, hand grip strength, and the number of comorbidities after breast cancer treatment are also associated with a functional level, as defined by the International Classification of Functioning Disability and Health (ICF) [2].

Difficulty performing activities of daily living with the upper extremities is very common after breast cancer treatment, with a prevalence rate of 60% 1 year after surgery [3, 6]. Therefore, restoring optimal upper extremity function is one of the primary goals of postoperative physical therapy. According to the current literature, morbidity rates, severity, time of onset, and risk factors associated with medical treatments can vary widely in the affected upper extremities of patients with breast cancer. However, the lack of timely referral of patients to physical therapy for

E. Baran (✉) · İ. Düzgün
Faculty of Physical Therapy and Rehabilitation, Hacettepe University, Ankara, Turkey

Y. Bakar, A. Tuğral (eds.), *Managing Side Effects of Breast Cancer Treatment*, https://doi.org/10.1007/978-3-031-75480-7_12

the management of potential cancer treatment-related problems, the misconception that their problems would resolve on their own, and/or the lack of awareness of the potential benefits of physical therapy interventions may increase the morbidity of upper extremity and shoulder as well as treatment costs [7, 8]. In this context, this chapter discusses shoulder problems seen in women after breast cancer treatment, risk factors associated with medical treatments, assessment methods, functional limitations caused by morbidities, and evidence-based physical therapy approaches.

12.2 Evaluation of Shoulder Problems Associated with Breast Cancer Treatment

The shoulder region consists of the glenohumeral, scapulothoracic, acromioclavicular, and sternoclavicular joints. In addition to the joints of the shoulder girdle, shoulder problems can also be originated from damage to structures such as connective tissue, muscle tissue, ligaments, cervical spine, rib cage, or nerve tissue [9]. Therefore, a thorough evaluation of the shoulder complex is required.

Postural changes in the upper trunk, upper extremities, shoulder girdle, and neck; limited shoulder girdle ROM; biomechanical changes; and loss of strength, pain, and shoulder dysfunction are common following breast cancer treatment. These problems should be evaluated and treated preoperatively if possible, otherwise as early as possible postoperatively [2].

12.2.1 Medical History

The medical history of patients who develop or are likely to develop shoulder problems after breast cancer treatment should include demographic, physical, and medical information. Treatments for breast cancer, type of breast surgery (mastectomy, lumpectomy, etc.), type of axillary surgery (ALND, SLNB), CT agents, RT fields, dose, regular medications, and existing comorbidities should be elicited. The number of removed or sampled positive lymph nodes, the presence of metastasis, and planned future treatment approaches should be recorded [10–12].

The patient's discomfort in daily life, factors that increase or decrease symptoms, treatments received in the past, and the extent to which the patient has benefited from prior treatments should be recorded. In addition, whether the patient had any shoulder problems during the preoperative period should be questioned.

12.2.2 Inspection and Palpation

During the inspection, findings such as scars and incision marks, open wounds, skin color changes (brown, purple, etc.), swelling, and atrophy of the extremities and trunk should be evaluated within the scope of the examination of shoulder and upper body posture. During palpation, the elasticity of connective tissue, skin temperature, edema, scar tissue, and muscle tone should be evaluated [10–12].

12.2.3 Posture

Following breast cancer treatment, shoulder protraction, scapular misalignment, breast asymmetry, and thoracic asymmetry as a result of more aggressive surgery, increased thoracic kyphosis and differences in arm swing may occur. Since the pectoral muscles are excised in more aggressive surgeries, such as radical mastectomy, and the entire breast is removed in modified radical mastectomy, a marked inward collapse of the thorax may be observed. In cases where the radiation dose is higher in RT, muscle, and connective tissue may lose elasticity in both the pectoral and axillary regions, causing the skin to appear tighter [13].

Methods such as photogrammetry, radiography, raster stereography, plumb line assessment, tape measurement, and observational assessments have been used to evaluate posture after breast cancer treatment [13–15]. Postural changes are reported in 82.3% of women undergoing breast cancer treatment [13]. In a study of postmastectomy women, shoulder girdle and trunk asymmetry and an increase in thoracic kyphosis were observed. Elevation of the scapula on the surgical side has also been reported. This may be due to impaired activation and coordination of the stabilizing muscles of the scapula and weakening of the shoulder girdle muscles [16]. The scapular region is the area where of greatest changes occur in terms of both posture and functional problems [17]. Evaluation of scapular position and motion is thought to guide the rehabilitation of shoulder pain following surgery and in case of lymphedema. While scapular dyskinesia can practically be evaluated via observation in the clinic, scapular motion at different angles can be assessed via 3D analysis. Observational evaluation should focus on the prominence of the inferomedial edge of the scapula in terms of its symmetry with respect to the contralateral side during elevation of the arm.

Pain associated with breast cancer itself and related treatments can also cause patients to adopt an antalgic posture. Maintaining this posture for prolonged periods can lead to an increase in tightness and tension of the connective tissues and muscles, which can lead to further postural deformities. It is important to provide proper posture training before these compensatory habits develop. Fibrosis that may develop in tissues as a result of RT may also aggravate this condition. The change in mass distribution in the trunk after unilateral mastectomy may cause a change in the center of gravity can also affect posture [13–15]. Changes in posture may occur due to any of these reasons may be a risk factor for musculoskeletal problems in the future.

12.2.4 Range of Motion (ROM)

Reduced shoulder ROM is one of the most commonly reported problems following breast cancer treatment. A range of motion of 160–180° is considered normal for shoulder flexion/abduction. A decrease of 10% compared to that of the unaffected arm indicates a limitation of normal ROM [18].

The studies generally use methods such as manual goniometers, digital inclinometers, computerized goniometers, and photogoniometers to assess shoulder ROM. Some studies used subjective ROM limitation data defined by the physician or patient [19–21]. The potential effects of ALND, SLNB, RT, type of surgery, and CT application on shoulder ROM may vary. A systematic review of the effect of ALND on shoulder ROM reported that shoulder abduction/flexion ROM was limited in 1–67% of patients [3]. Patients who underwent ALND had higher rates of limitation in shoulder ROM after surgery compared to those who underwent SLNB in both the short and long term [5, 22]. When the effect of the type of surgery on shoulder ROM was analyzed, it was found that mastectomy increased the limitation of shoulder ROM more than breast-conserving surgery did [23]. These results may be due to the greater extent of tissue trauma associated with mastectomy and ALND.

Shoulder ROM was analyzed in those who received axillary RT and those who did not, and axillary RT was found to be more risky in terms of limitation of the shoulder ROM [24, 25]. However, both axillary and thoracic RT are responsible for greater shoulder ROM limitations than thoracic RT alone [5]. Although it has been reported that 90% of the expected damage from RT can be seen in an average of 3.7–4.2 years later [26], patients who have brachial plexopathy symptoms in the affected extremity are diagnosed 8–20 years after RT [27]. RT damages the pectoral muscles, causing them to reduce their size and shortening them. During recovery, these muscles may undergo fibrotic changes. Due to fibrosis, problems such as impingement syndrome and rotator cuff damage may also occur with limited shoulder ROM [26, 28, 29]. During humeral elevation, the scapulothoracic joint contributes 60° to shoulder flexion and abduction. Humerothoracic limitations can also be caused by alterations in scapular kinematics [28]. Moreover, an analysis of the effect of CT on shoulder ROM revealed that CT was a risk factor for shoulder limitation in the context of breast cancer treatment. Shoulder abduction morbidity is commonly associated with ALND, followed by systemic CT and axillary RT [18].

Women with severe lymphedema had lower shoulder abduction scores than women without lymphedema. However, the affected shoulder ROM of those with moderate and severe lymphedema was lower than the unaffected shoulder ROM [11, 30]. The reasons for decreased ROM in patients with lymphedema have been reported as prevented shoulder movement due to the probable increase in periarticular adipose tissue as a result of increased body mass index [31], the tension in the connective tissue caused by the increase in the subcutaneous layer because of lymphedema [30], and the possibility that prolonged exposure to lymphedema may lead to an increase in shoulder pathology [32]. Women who receive more aggressive treatment for breast cancer and develop lymphedema require more careful musculoskeletal evaluation to maintain maximum shoulder ROM after treatment.

The scapulothoracic joint has been evaluated by using observational assessments, the lateral scapular shift test, radiographic assessment, and electromagnetic assessment methods in the literature [11, 15, 33, 34]. During upper limb movements, the humerus moves in synchronization and harmony with the scapula. This synchronized movement is also referred to as the scapulohumeral rhythm [35]. Recent studies have shown that postmastectomy women have an impaired scapulohumeral rhythm with decreased scapular upward rotation, increased internal rotation, and decreased posterior tilt in the scapular plane during humerothoracic elevation [36, 37]. Moreover, scapular movements may be affected by complications related to breast cancer treatment (scar tissue, fibrosis, decreased muscle activity, etc.) [38]. The ability to achieve pain-free shoulder ROM may also be associated with the optimal posterior tilt, upward rotation, and external rotation of the scapula. Considering that humeral abduction is correlated with scapular upward rotation, deviations in scapular motion may be another factor limiting pain-free shoulder ROM [39]. Lymphedema may also exacerbate these findings [11, 40]. The weight of the limb due to chronic lymphedema can strain the shoulder girdle and scapular muscles. Prolonged weight bearing may result in the limitation of upward scapular rotation. In addition, subcutaneous fluid accumulation due to lymphedema can limit humerothoracic and scapulothoracic movements [11, 41].

12.2.5 Strength

Strength assessment of the upper extremity and shoulder girdle muscles of patients after breast cancer treatment has been performed by hand dynamometer or manual isometric muscle strength measurement, dynamic weight lifting, evaluation of isokinetic movements, biomechanical measurements, and subjective complaints of loss of strength. In some studies, radiographic methods were used for specific evaluation of muscles, and electromyographic measurements were also used to evaluate muscle activation [10, 12, 29, 42, 43].

Systematic reviews have reported that 9–28% of women experience a subjective loss of upper extremity strength [5, 25]. Axillary RT has been shown to be a risk factor in terms of causing loss of shoulder flexor, adductor, and internal rotator strength. In addition, ALND increases the likelihood of pectoral muscle injury, which may result in a decrease in shoulder strength. When managing physical therapy after breast cancer treatment, special attention should be given to shoulder dysfunction in patients who underwent ALND, especially in those who received axillary RT. It is recommended that physical therapy should be started at the time of RT implementation [42].

Strength values were reported to be lower in the scapular abduction and upward rotation, scapular depression and adduction, internal rotation, external rotation, scaption, and horizontal adduction in breast cancer survivors than in healthy controls [12]. In addition, a decrease in the upper trapezius, rhomboid, and serratus anterior muscle activity on the surgical side was demonstrated, and EMG activity showed that this decrease in muscle activity was not directly limited in the treatment area [29]. It has also been reported that the dynamic concentric strength of the shoulder protractors, retractors, and extensors of the affected arm was lower than that of the unaffected arm at an average of 28 months after surgery [44].

Compared with those who underwent SLNB, women who underwent ALND had lower shoulder internal rotation strength 5 years after surgery. However, the loss of shoulder external rotation strength persisted for 5 years in both the SLNB and ALND groups [45]. The major internal rotator muscles of the shoulder are the subscapularis, pectoralis major, teres major, and latissimus dorsi, and these muscles are part of the anatomy of the axillary fossa [45]. Both ALND and RT affect the axillary fossa and pectoral region and may damage the aforementioned underlying structures. Shoulder abduction and scaption depend primarily on the deltoid and supraspinatus muscles, which are not part of the axillary fossa. Although abduction is affected most in terms of shoulder ROM, the situation may be different regarding loss of strength. Therefore, shoulder abduction ROM may not be indicative of all shoulder pathologies.

12.2.6 Pain

Visual analog scales or questionnaires such as the McGill Pain Questionnaire and the Shoulder Pain and Disability Index have generally been used to assess pain in breast cancer patients. Several studies have used pressure pain algometry to assess pain thresholds and tolerance [20, 46, 47]. The prevalence of shoulder and/or arm pain and breast and/or scar tissue pain was reported to be in the range of 9–68% and 15–72% within 6–56 months after surgery, respectively. However, several studies have reported that arm and breast pain can persist in more than 20% of patients 30 months after surgery [25].

Patients undergoing ALND have been reported to have a worse pain prognosis than those undergoing SLNB, and ALND has also been reported to increase the risk of pain during movement. A larger surgical field affected in the axillary region during ALND is not only associated with prolonged tissue healing but also a greater risk of damage to the brachial plexus. This may be one of the prominent reasons for increased pain as a result of ALND [5, 25]. There are studies reporting brachial plexopathy as a result of the concurrent use of RT and CT (taxanes) [48]. In a cohort study comparing those who received CT and those who did not, CT was reported to be a risk factor for increased pain [49]. Risk factors for persistent pain include younger age (<55 years), ALND, RT, tamoxifen use, and shorter duration after surgery [46, 50]. Zoledronic acid, a type of chemotherapeutic agent, was also reported to be a risk factor for arthralgia and bone pain [51].

In a study investigating the relationship between arm-shoulder problems and insomnia symptoms in breast cancer survivors, 37% of patients reported arm-shoulder pain, and insomnia was significantly more common in those with arm-shoulder pain than those without. In this context, management of arm-shoulder pain is also essential for the prevention of insomnia [52]. Pain following breast cancer treatment has been found to be associated with a decrease in muscle strength, range of motion, participation in work, use of the affected arm for leisure time activities, and frequency of lifting objects or doing housework [22]. The motor function of upper extremity muscles may be inhibited by pain and can affect a person's behavior; moreover, pain-related anxiety may further lead to the avoidance of certain activities. In some patients, pain catastrophizing scenarios may also be observed [2]. In a study examining pain intensity, fatigue, central sensitization, illness beliefs, pain catastrophizing, and kinesiophobia in postmastectomy women, kinesiophobia was found to be the most important factor in pain-related disability [53].

12.2.7 Shoulder Function

Restricted upper extremity ROM, pain, loss of strength, and postural dysfunction after breast cancer treatment lead to limitations in women's activities of daily living, functionality, work, and leisure time activities, and thus a decrease in quality of life may occur. These impairments have been associated with the level of functioning as defined by the ICF [2, 3, 5]. Previous studies have used the Disabilities of the Arm, Shoulder and Hand Questionnaire, Penn Shoulder Scale, Shoulder Pain and Disability Index, and Constant-Murley Scale to assess functional impairment that may result from upper extremity and shoulder problems in women with breast cancer [2, 20, 54, 55].

Different modalities in breast cancer treatment may have unique effects on functional status. Health-related quality of life, including physical functioning, psychological functioning, level of independence, social relationships, and environmental factors, was assessed by using specifically developed questionnaires in women undergoing ALND. A total of 25–35% of patients reported problems in activities of daily living (housework, lifting heavy objects, etc.), 21% reported that they have to rest their affected arm frequently, 24% had to perform specific exercises for the affected arm, and 22% had to learn to do things with the unaffected arm. In addition, 37% of women reported having to give up a hobby or sport because of ALND [56]. In a cohort study, both ALND and SLNB patients reported a decrease in arm and shoulder function and social and work-related activities in the short and long term after surgery; however, ALND patients were found to have an avoidance pattern in arm use more than SLNB patients have [5, 57]. In the first year after surgery, 39–44% of those who underwent ALND, 18–19% of those who underwent SLNB, 42–31% of those who underwent mastectomy, and 12–18% of those who underwent breast conserving surgery exhibited a remarkable decrease in activities of daily living. Postoperative upper extremity dysfunction may be mainly related to pectoral muscle tension at 3 and 6 months and lymphedema at 12 months [58].

It has been reported that 90% of the effects of RT in arm/shoulder tissues occur within the first 3.9 years after RT, with the maximum effects of arm/shoulder problems occurring approximately 4 years after RT [26]. Axillary RT has been associated with greater functional impairment in work and/or activities of daily living than thoracic RT, and thoracic RT was associated with greater functional impairment than no RT [5]. It has been reported that 34% of those who received CT (cyclophosphamide, epirubicin, and fluorouracil vs. cyclophosphamide, epirubicin, and docetaxel) were unable to perform daily activities due to treatment related side effects [46].

In general, 31% of patients show a decrease in upper limb activity after breast cancer treatment. Within 1 year of surgery, activity levels do not reach presurgery levels. It has been reported that 83% of patients return to work 10 months after surgery, but use of the affected arm for leisure activities was reduced and associated with pain and numbness when lifting objects or doing household chores. ALND and axillary RT are important risk factors for reduced activities of daily living [3]. In a study that assessed occupational, sports, home, and total physical activity levels before and 12 months after surgery, activity levels were found to be decreased significantly after surgery and did not recover in the first year [59]. Upper extremity pain, limited shoulder ROM, decreased hand grip strength, and a high number of comorbidities were found to be associated with decreased upper extremity function [2].

12.3 Physiotherapy and Rehabilitation Approaches for Breast Cancer-Related Shoulder Problems

Breast cancer treatments cause problems in the upper extremities, most commonly in the shoulder girdle. Analysis of potential upper extremity problems and approaches to prevention/reduction/improvement should be planned and implemented from the preoperative period. To reduce the risk of the development/progression of lymphedema following breast cancer treatment, it is important that compression garments should be worn during upper extremity exercises which should be performed in compatible with patients' functional level and their intensity and type should be characterized by free of causing any fatigue. More aggressive treatments for breast cancer can cause more functional impairment in the shoulder girdle. Further attention should be given to the evaluation and physiotherapy of patients undergoing treatments such as mastectomy, ALND, axillary RT, and systemic CT. However, limitations in ROM, pain, loss of strength, and postural abnormalities associated with shoulder dysfunction are modifiable risk factors. Early diagnosis and treatment of these problems will prevent the onset/progression of functional disability [2, 4, 60].

In the literature, ROM (passive, active-assisted, active) exercises, stretching exercises, myofascial modalities, mobilization techniques, strengthening exercises, scapular-oriented exercises, aerobic, Pilates, yoga exercises, aquatic exercises, and mirror therapy have been used to treat the shoulder girdle after breast cancer treatment. These treatments can be used individually or in combination depending on the status of a patient's shoulder dysfunction [4, 55, 61, 62].

12.3.1 Range of Motion Exercises

Axillary surgery and RT increase the risk of ROM limitations, especially shoulder flexion, abduction, and external rotation. Depending on the patient's functional status, passive, active-assisted, and active ROM exercises are used to prevent shoulder ROM limitations in the early postoperative period. These exercises activate physiological mechanisms as a result of muscle contraction and may also increase the blood flow to surrounding tissues [62]. In one study, patients with breast cancer performed active shoulder ROM exercises, postural exercises, progressive resistance exercises, and proprioceptive neuromuscular facilitation pattern exercises for 30 min twice daily during hospitalization, and then they participated in an 8-week home program after discharge. The control group received no treatment. The patients in the study group had better shoulder ROM scores at postoperative day 5 and the following months [4].

Several studies have been conducted on the timing of exercise after breast cancer treatment and concluded that the beginning of exercise on postoperative days 1–3 and day 5 can be defined as early exercise and delayed exercise, respectively. Postoperative slinging of the shoulder, which has been practiced in the past, is no longer indicated, and more active approaches are recommended [61]. The shoulder flexion ROM was greater in those who started the exercise on the first postoperative day than in those who started the exercise on the seventh postoperative day according to the 2-week treatment results; however, no difference was found between the groups in 1 month In another study, the shoulder ROM values of patients who began exercise on the first postoperative day and those who began exercise on the 14th postoperative day were compared. Shoulder flexion and abduction ROM values were better in the early ROM group up to 2 years postoperatively. There was no difference in pain between the groups [4]. In a study that evaluated the effects of starting pendulum, finger ladder, and pulley exercises at three different times after surgery, the first group started on day 3 after surgery, the second group started on day 6, and the third group started after catheter removal. No difference in ROM was found between the groups at 6 months after surgery. When the amount of drainage was compared between those groups in that study, the amount of wound drainage fluid was found to be lower in those who started exercising later [63]. Lauridsen et al. [21] applied strengthening exercises, active stretching, venous pump exercises, and stretching relaxation exercises under the supervision of a physiotherapist for a total of 12 sessions, 2 sessions per week, 60 min per session. Postoperative exercises started at 6 weeks in the first group and at 26 weeks in the second group. At postoperative weeks 7 and 26, the first group had better Constant-Shoulder Scores. However, no difference was found between the groups at 56 weeks [62]. It was observed that ROM exercises limited to 90° shoulder elevation during the first week after ALND did not increase the risk of potential complications in patients compared to those who started exercising 1 week after surgery [62].

Early shoulder exercises, which are carefully performed under the guidance of a physiotherapist after breast cancer treatment, can have beneficial effects on shoulder ROM, strength, pain, and shoulder function in patients.

In postmastectomy patients, passive ROM exercises should be started in the first phase for the shoulder girdle. Exercises should be gentle and controlled, and patients should not be forced. Active and forceful shoulder movements should be avoided in the early postoperative period. At this stage, active hand and forearm exercises can be performed while the shoulder is positioned in a resting position (shoulder elevated 15–20° supported by pillows). In later stages, active-assisted and active shoulder ROM exercises can be performed in a controlled manner. For those with shoulder ROM less than 90°, ROM exercises can be performed on the edge of the treatment table, and as ROM increases, exercises can be performed with a ball (Fig. 12.1). Starting ROM exercises in the scapular plane and progressing to the sagittal and frontal planes may be preferred due to pain tolerance and biomechanical principles. It is well known that the scapular plane is a plane in which the soft tissues of the shoulder girdle are in an optimal position and are therefore more tolerable at initial stages. It is important to remember that most activities of daily living are performed in this position. Exercises such as pendulum exercises and finger ladders, which are relatively well tolerated, can be included in the treatment plan to increase shoulder mobility [64, 65] (Fig. 12.2).

12.3.2 Stretching Exercises

Shoulder ROM limitations may occur as a result of axillary surgery, RT applied to supraclavicular and infraclavicular lymph nodes, tissue infection and damage, and pectoral muscle tightness and atrophy. Stretching exercises may contribute to the remodeling of damaged connective tissue and prevent muscle fiber shortening and negative physiological adaptations [62]. Although studies evaluating the isolated efficacy of stretching exercise after breast cancer treatment are quite limited, the available evidence has shown conflicting results regarding improvements in ROM [4]. However, a minimum of 90° shoulder abduction and lateral rotation is required for the positioning of a patient in RT after breast cancer surgery. Due to the attachment of the pectoralis major to the humerus, shortening of the pectoralis muscle will make it difficult to arm positioning for RT. Therefore, studies suggest that stretching exercises are necessary to maintain shoulder ROM. After wound healing is fully completed, tolerable and pain free mild stretching exercises are recommended to improve shoulder ROM. The primary goal is to return patients to optimal shoulder ROM prior to RT. Patients undergoing RT should be very cautious with stretching exercises. Because RT decreases the flexibility of muscle, connective tissue, and nerve tissue, stretching exercises that are not performed at an appropriate dose may cause damage to muscle, connective tissue, and/or nerve tissue in patients [62] (Figs. 12.3 and 12.4).

In addition to shoulder girdle biomechanics, the cervical and thoracic regions are also affected after breast cancer treatment. In particular, specific exercises with the aim of increasing the flexibility of the upper trapezius, levator scapula, and rhomboid muscles should be included in the treatment plan. Stretching these muscles has been shown to be effective in reducing shoulder girdle pain.

12.3.3 Myofascial Treatment

The musculoskeletal system is a complex network of interconnected tissues that must work together in harmony to provide proper movement. When muscles and fascia are injured after breast cancer treatments, shoulder girdle function may also be affected. Myofascial therapy involves manual, noninvasive approaches used in the treatment of problems such as tension and pain in muscles and fascia [20, 66]. In the literature, upper extremity trigger point treatment, myofascial massage, and myofascial release techniques specific to the pectoralis major, cervical spine, diaphragm, scar adhesions, chest, thorax, and

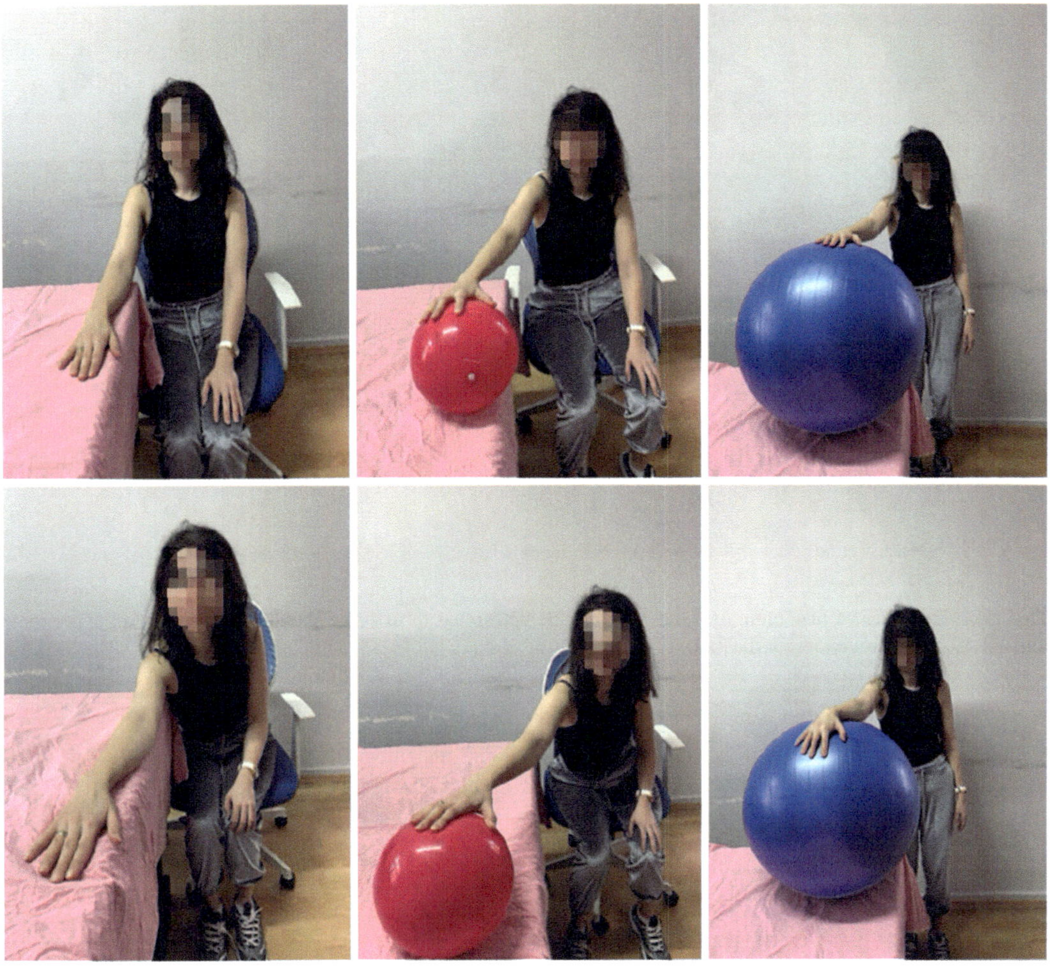

Fig. 12.1 Examples of ROM exercises on the edge of the treatment table. As the ROM increases, ball exercises may be preferred. Progression of exercises should be based on the level of ROM

shoulder have been used in patients following breast cancer treatment. Myofascial treatments appear to have a positive effect on pain intensity, functionality, and ROM, but no additional benefit beyond shoulder abduction has been statistically demonstrated. Beneficial effects on quality of life and mood are generally expected. Painful muscle trigger points (especially around the cervical and pectoral muscles) may occur in 45% of breast cancer patients in the long term. It is recommended that myofascial release techniques and trigger point compression may be beneficial in patients following breast cancer treatment and should therefore be added to treatment as needed [20, 67]. Based on our clinical experience, we can say that myofascial release, especially when applied to the thoracic and cervical spine, has a positive effect on the patient's pain and can be safely applied.

12.3.4 Mobilization

In a study of 257 patients included after breast cancer treatment, the effect of passive mobilization was investigated. The patients were divided into four groups: The control group, shoulder mobilization group, arm massage group, and shoulder mobilization and arm massage group. The applications started on the first postoperative

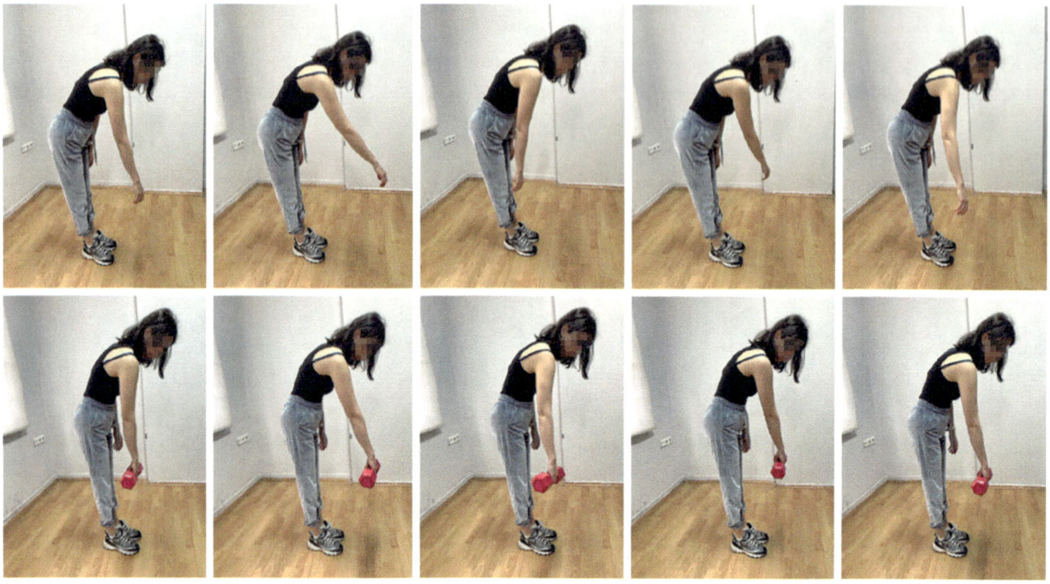

Fig. 12.2 Examples of pendulum exercises that can be performed to increase shoulder ROM with an appropriate amount of weight or without for the patient

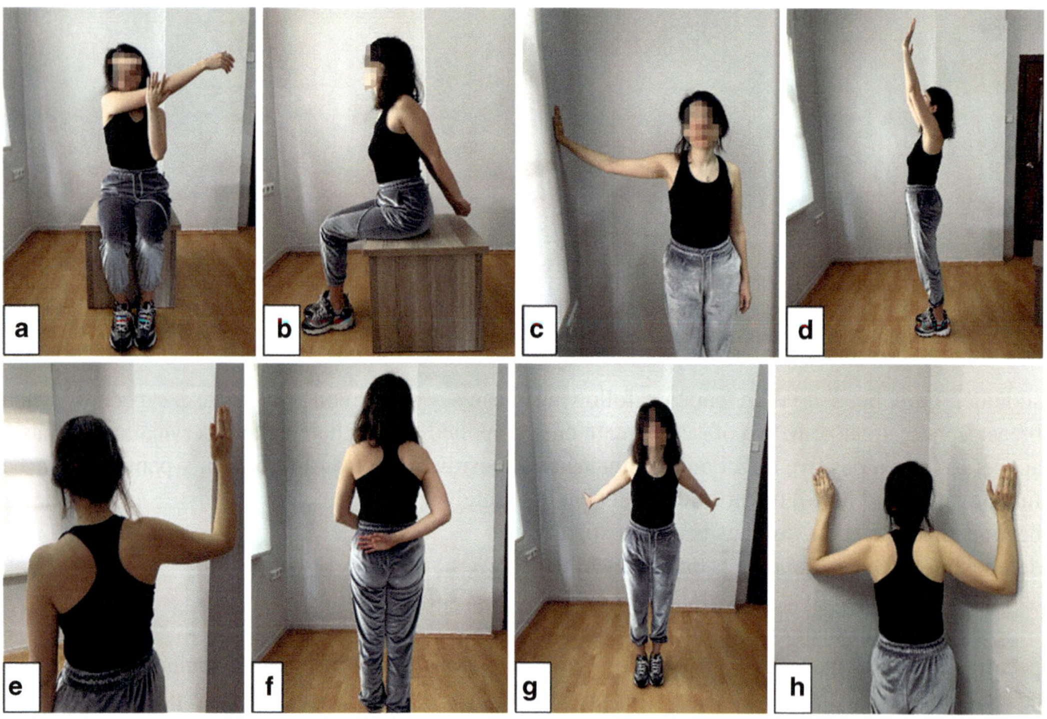

Fig. 12.3 Examples of stretching exercises: (**a**) posterior capsule stretching, (**b**, **c**) anterior capsule stretching, (**d**) raising and stretching the arms overhead, (**e**) unilateral corner stretch, (**f**) external rotator stretch, (**g**, **h**) pectoral stretching

day, and the treatments were applied for 7 days. After 1 week of treatment, the shoulder ROM values were greater in the mobilization and massage groups. After the treatment, the patients

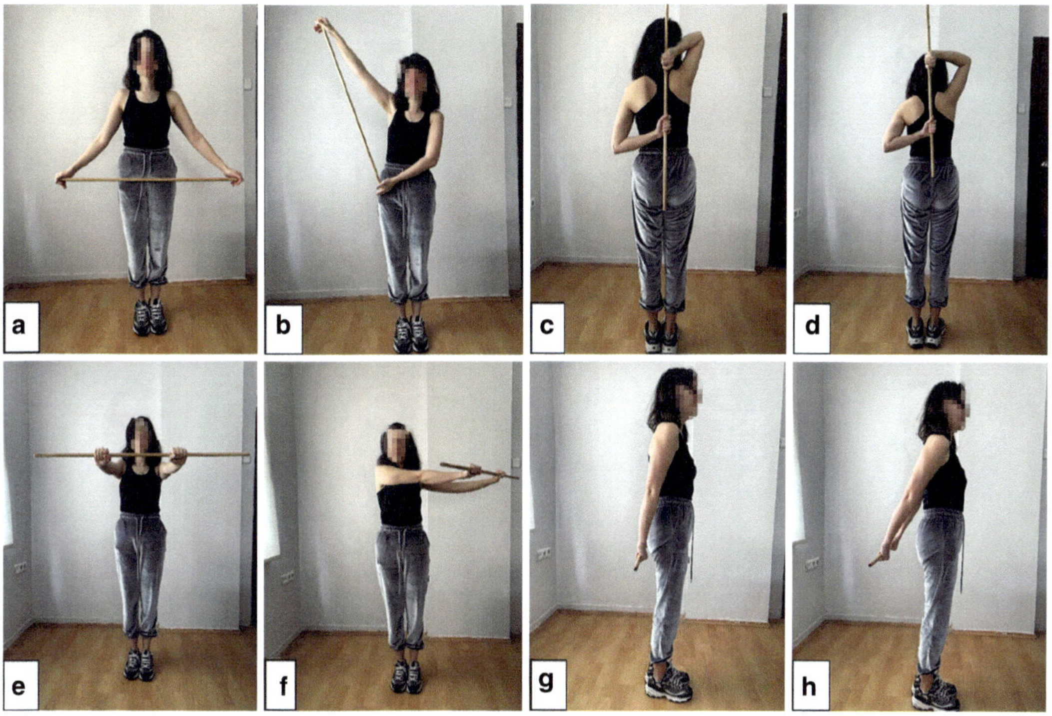

Fig. 12.4 ROM and stretching exercises with the exercise bar: (**a**, **b**) shoulder abduction, (**c**, **d**) shoulder internal-external rotation, (**e**, **f**) horizontal shoulder abduction and adduction, (**g**, **h**) shoulder hyperextension

continued the physiotherapy program, and no difference was observed between the groups in terms of shoulder ROM at 3 months. At 8–24 months postoperatively, pain intensity was lower in the mobilization groups than in the other groups [4].

The mobilization methods used in the clinic were found to be effective. In a randomized controlled trial, passive mobilization of the scapulothoracic joint was reported to be effective in reducing pain and improving functional recovery of the upper extremity after breast cancer treatment and was recommended as a part of physical therapy in the first year after surgery [68]. It is particularly appropriate to perform passive scapular mobilization prior to performing stabilization exercises.

12.3.5 Strengthening Exercises

There is an increased risk of loss of muscle mass and strength as a result of pathophysiological changes associated with breast cancer treatment. Breast cancer is more common in women over the age of 50, at which age 10% of muscle mass is already lost. Aging is a risk factor for loss of muscle mass and strength. Strengthening exercises can help to prevent loss of muscle mass and strength. The most affected muscles due to breast cancer treatment are the muscles around the shoulder, and impairment of these muscles is associated with a decrease in activities of daily living. Strengthening the muscles around the shoulder and scapula is important for preventing postural problems, reducing associated pain, and restoring function [4, 62] (Fig. 12.5). When performing strengthening exercises, the exercises should be individualized to the risk of lymphedema development/progression, should be free of causing fatigue during performing, and the exercises should be performed with compression garments. Strengthening exercises can be done by using dumbbells, elastic bands, and various positions against gravity. Isometric, isotonic, and eccentric exercises are beneficial for restoring

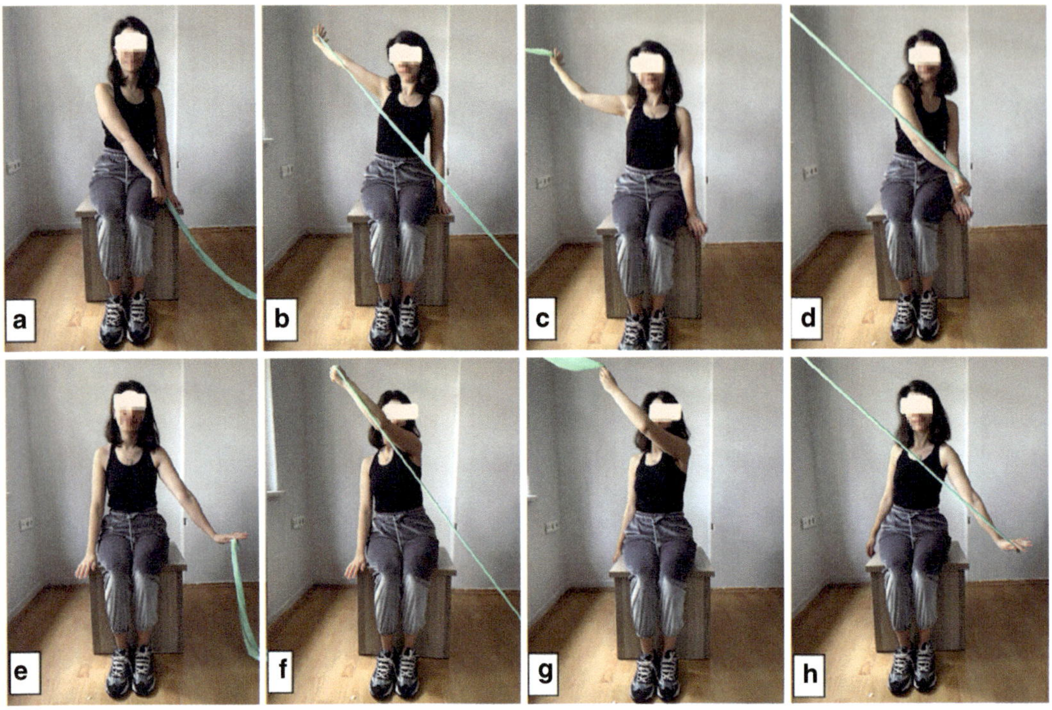

Fig. 12.5 Examples of strengthening exercises in the proprioceptive neuromuscular facilitation pattern with an elastic band: (**a**, **b**) flexion with elastic resistance, (**c**, **d**) extension with elastic resistance, (**e**, **f**) flexion with elastic resistance, (**g**, **h**) extension with elastic resistance

muscle function [47, 69]. A systematic review reported that resistance training improved the quality of life more than routine care or alternative exercise modalities in cancer patients [70]. A meta-analysis revealed that resistance training improved upper extremity muscle strength up to 1 year after cancer treatment [71].

12.3.6 Scapula-Oriented Exercises

Considering the kinematics of shoulder movement, breast cancer treatments have been reported to affect glenohumeral translation and scapulohumeral rhythm and may lead to scapular dyskinesia. As a complication of these treatments, particularly shortening of the pectoralis major and minor muscles may cause limitations in shoulder movement. It has been reported that scapula-oriented ROM, stretching, strengthening, and stabilization exercises performed after breast cancer treatment significantly improve upper extremity pain, strength, physical function, social function, and quality of life [72].

Lymphedema may increase scapular dyskinesia and upper extremity dysfunction [11]. In a randomized controlled trial of patients with breast cancer-related lymphedema, the study group received complex decongestive physiotherapy and scapulothoracic stabilization exercises, while the control group received complex decongestive physiotherapy only. According to the study results, scapulothoracic stabilization exercises were found to be effective in improving scapulothoracic muscle function and posture [73].

The importance of scapula-focused rehabilitation for shoulder problems has been recognized by many researchers, and scapular stabilization exercises have been incorporated into rehabilitation protocols. It is thought that increasing scapular stabilization after breast cancer treatment may prevent secondary shoulder problems. Strengthening exercises that specifically target the lower trapezius, middle trapezius, and serratus anterior may help to increase scapular stabilization. In the exercises to be performed, it is believed that the principle of low weight, high repetition, focusing on endurance, rather than high weight, focusing on increasing strength, is more appropriate. After increasing activation of scapular stabilizer muscles, focusing on the rotator cuff and finally the deltoid muscles might be an appropriate strengthening protocol [64] (Figs. 12.6 and 12.7).

12.3.7 Aerobic Exercises

Aerobic exercise can improve upper limb function, cardiopulmonary function, and quality of life after breast cancer surgery. Rehabilitation guidelines for breast cancer recommend active participation in aerobic exercise to improve patients' health-related physical fitness and prevent cancer recurrence [74].

A randomized controlled trial evaluated the effects of 16 weeks of aerobic and strengthening exercise on shoulder function in women who were overweight or obese after breast cancer treatment. The study group performed aerobic exercise at 65–80% of the maximum heart rate (150 min of aerobic exercise and 2 or 3 days of resistance exercise per week) intensity and resistance exercises for upper- and lower-extremity based on the recommendations of the American College of Sports Medicine. Patients were asked to choose one of the following for aerobic exercise: treadmill (walking/running), rowing machine, or stationary bicycle. Aerobic exercise

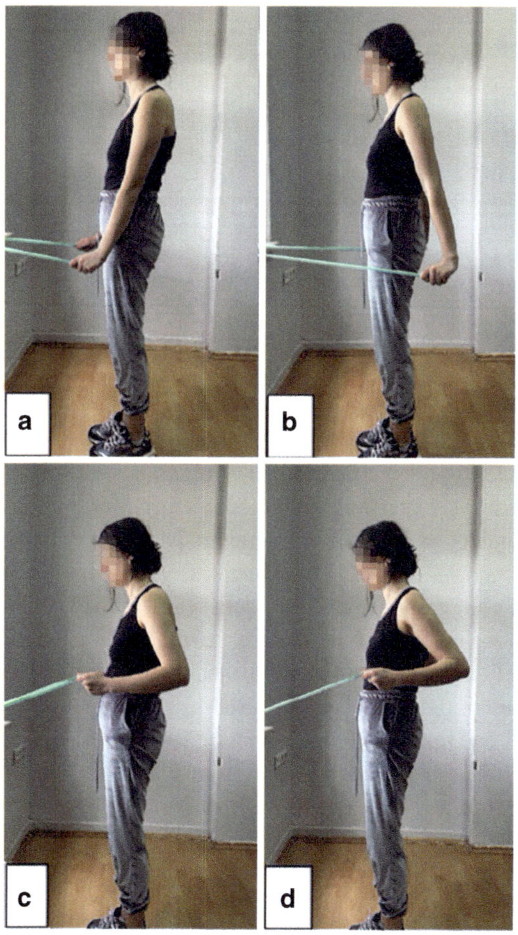

Fig. 12.6 Examples of scapular retraction exercises with elastic bands: (**a**-**b**) with elbows extended, (**c**-**d**) with elbows flexed

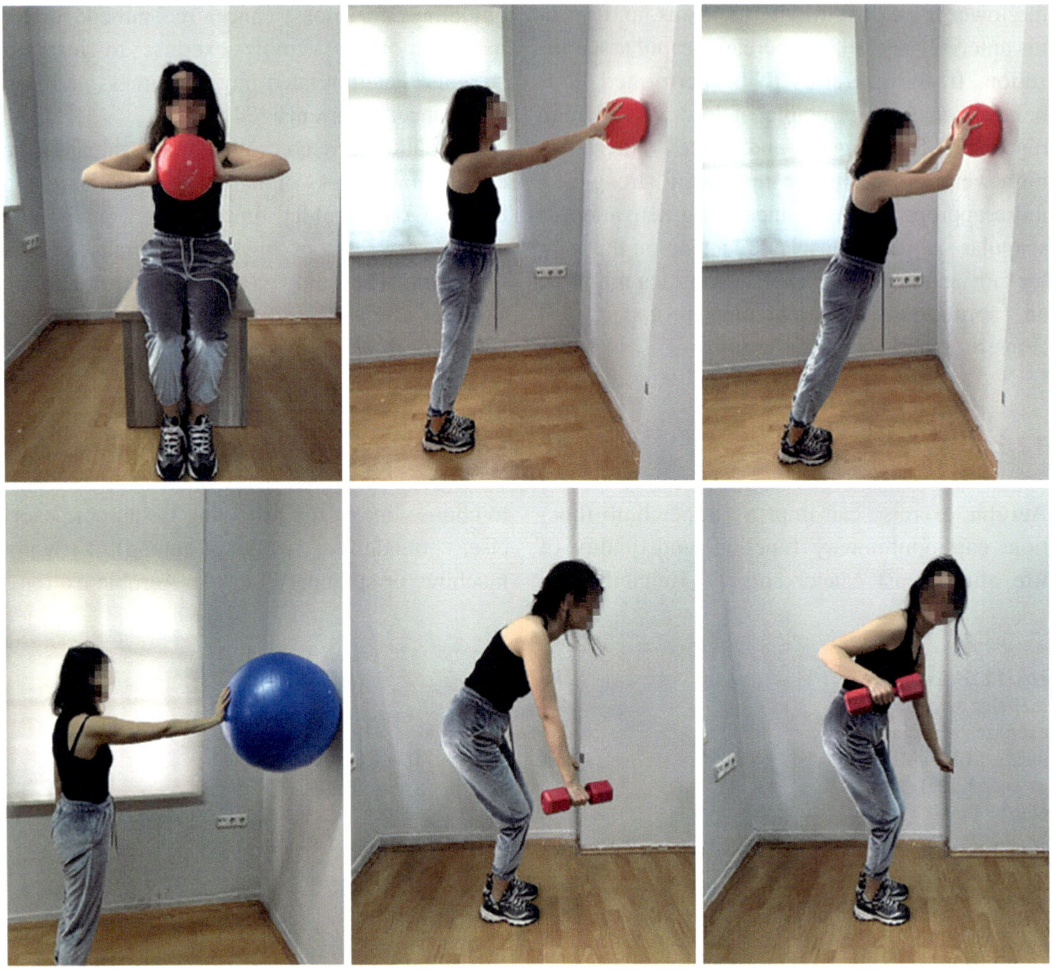

Fig. 12.7 Examples of scapular stabilization exercises

was performed 3 days per week. For resistance exercises, 10 repetitions of leg press, lunges, knee extension, knee flexion, chest press, seated rows, triceps extension, and biceps curls were used, and 3 sets of these exercises were performed 2 days a week. The exercises were performed with compression garments. The control group received only routine care. At the end of the study, 16 weeks of aerobic and resistance exercise improved shoulder ROM, strength, activity, and upper extremity function [54].

In a randomized controlled trial investigating the effect of aerobic exercise with walking poles on shoulder function, the study group performed walking exercises with walking poles for 20 min twice a week for 8 weeks. The control group performed 20 min of aerobic exercise without using walking poles. Both groups performed similar resistance exercises. At the end of the study, upper extremity muscle endurance was found to be better in the walking poles group, and it was reported that walking exercises with walking poles may be effective in improving shoulder function [75].

Aerobic exercise not only increases health-related physical fitness in both healthy people and patients but is also an effective approach for preventing cancer recurrence in cancer survivors. Therefore, specifically planned aerobic exercises for the patient (frequency, intensity, duration, type of exercise, exercise that the patient enjoys, progression) should be included in the physiotherapy and rehabilitation approaches of patients after breast cancer treatment.

12.3.8 Pilates Exercises

Pilates is an exercise approach that integrates the mind and body. It combines light- to moderate-intensity physical exercise with mindfulness. In this way, Pilates can improve both the physical and psychological outcomes of patients with breast cancer. Pilates exercise may also be effective in treating biomechanical dysfunction resulting from cancer treatment by increasing the awareness of the body and kinesthetic sense compared to traditional exercises. Pilates-based exercises after breast cancer treatment focus on core stabilization, spinal flexibility, and shoulder girdle ROM. Improvements in endurance and stability are achieved through the progression of exercise [76, 77].

Systematic reviews have reported the beneficial effects of Pilates exercise on shoulder ROM, pain, muscular strength and endurance, cardiorespiratory fitness, upper extremity function, mood, and quality of life in breast cancer survivors and have emphasized that exercise can reduce the impact of treatment-related symptoms. Patient compliance and adherence rates in Pilates exercises have been found to be quite high. Pilates is recommended as a safe exercise regimen for women with breast cancer [76, 77].

12.3.9 Yoga

Yoga is an integrated system of breathing (pranayama), postures (asana), meditation, and relaxation that improves the biopsychosocial functioning of an individual [78]. Yoga exercises such as diaphragmatic breathing, systematic relaxation, alternate nostril breathing, and shoulder and neck movements have been shown to improve general health, physical function, role functioning, emotional status, and quality of life and these exercises are also able to reduce symptoms such as pain, fatigue, insomnia, and loss of appetite in women with breast cancer undergoing CT [79]. A randomized controlled trial examined the effect of 8 weeks of yoga on shoulder and spinal movements. The study group focused on ROM, posture, and kinematic movement patterns of the shoulder and spine, and core and shoulder stabilization during yoga sessions. The control group received routine care. At the end of the study, improvements in lumbopelvic posture, shoulder ROM, and shoulder abduction strength were noted [78]. In a study investigating the effect of hatha yoga on breast cancer patients, restorative yoga, a gentle therapeutic yoga that uses self-massage techniques to relieve pain and techniques to rest and support the body in seated positions, was used. At the end of the study, improvements were observed in shoulder abduction, shoulder flexion, pain, depression and anxiety symptoms, and quality of life [80].

12.3.10 Aquatic Exercises

Water has the potential to provide a comfortable environment, reduce joint stress with additional beneficial effects such as hydrostatic pressure and buoyancy, increase neck–shoulder mobility, and reduce pain. In various clinical populations, aquatic exercise has been shown to improve muscle strength, balance, flexibility, and functional exercise capacity, and patients can adapt better to aquatic exercise [81, 82].

A systematic review examining the efficacy of aquatic exercise in breast cancer survivors reported that compared with land-based exercise interventions, aquatic exercise was better tolerated with higher rates of exercise adherence and showed greater improvements in pain, shoulder ROM, trigger points, lymphedema, cardiorespiratory fitness, muscle strength, body composition, respiratory function, cancer-related fatigue, psychological problems, and health-related quality of life [83].

12.3.11 Mirror Therapy

Mirror therapy is a classic and effective method for improving motor and sensory function of the extremities. Benefits of mirror therapy have been demonstrated in patients with shoulder pain, limited range of motion, and adhesive capsulitis [84, 85]. In a randomized controlled trial investigating the effect of mirror therapy-based upper extremity ROM exercises on shoulder function following breast cancer treatment, the control group received free ROM exercises, while the mirror therapy group received free ROM exercises as part of mirror therapy. The interventions were performed from the first postoperative day and lasted for 8 weeks. At the end of the study, mirror therapy was found to increase shoulder flexion and abduction ROM in patients without nerve injury, improve arm and shoulder function in daily life, and reduce pain and kinesiophobia [86]. Although there are not enough studies, it is emphasized that mirror therapy has the potential to improve shoulder function in breast cancer patients and should be supported by further research.

12.4 Conclusion

Given the wide range of breast cancer treatment options and the side effects of multimodal treatment, complex shoulder dysfunction can occur. Reduced shoulder function, or difficulty performing activities of daily living, is very common after breast cancer treatment. Reduced function has a negative impact on the quality of life, ability to participate in the community, well-being, and life satisfaction of breast cancer survivors. Patients who undergo mastectomy, ALND, axillary RT procedures, or intensive systemic CT may be at greater risk for shoulder dysfunction. It is recommended that patients undergoing treatment for breast cancer should be evaluated for shoulder function, preferably prior to surgery, in order to determine treatment strategies. Restoring optimal shoulder function should be one of the first goals of postoperative physical therapy. Specific exercises and techniques (i.e., mobilization approaches, myofascial techniques, aerobic exercises, Pilates, yoga exercises, etc.) should be used individually or in combination, depending on the patient's needs aiming to treat identified dysfunctions in the baseline evaluation.

References

1. Macdonald ER, Amorim NML, Hagstrom AD, Markovic K, Simar D, Ward RE, et al. Evaluating the effect of upper-body morbidity on quality of life following primary breast cancer treatment: a systematic review and meta-analysis. J Cancer Surviv. 2023;18:1517.
2. De Groef A, Van der Gucht E, Dams L, Evenepoel M, Teppers L, Toppet-Hoegars J, et al. The association between upper limb function and variables at the different domains of the international classification of functioning, disability and health in women after breast cancer surgery: a systematic review. Disabil Rehabil. 2022;44(8):1176–89.
3. Hidding JT, Beurskens CH, van der Wees PJ, van Laarhoven HW, Nijhuis-van der Sanden MW. Treatment related impairments in arm and shoulder in patients with breast cancer: a systematic review. PLoS One. 2014;9(5):e96748.
4. De Groef A, Van Kampen M, Dieltjens E, Christiaens MR, Neven P, Geraerts I, et al. Effectiveness of postoperative physical therapy for upper-limb impairments after breast cancer treatment: a systematic review. Arch Phys Med Rehabil. 2015;96(6):1140–53.
5. Levangie PK, Drouin J. Magnitude of late effects of breast cancer treatments on shoulder function: a systematic review. Breast Cancer Res Treat. 2009;116:1–15.
6. De Groef A, Meeus M, De Vrieze T, Vos L, Van Kampen M, Christiaens M-R, et al. Pain characteristics as important contributing factors to upper limb dysfunctions in breast cancer survivors at long term. Musculoskelet Sci Pract. 2017;29:52–9.
7. Stout NL, Pfalzer LA, Springer B, Levy E, McGarvey CL, Danoff JV, et al. Breast cancer-related lymphedema: comparing direct costs of a prospective surveillance model and a traditional model of care. Phys Ther. 2012;92(1):152–63.
8. Cheville AL, Tchou J. Barriers to rehabilitation following surgery for primary breast cancer. J Surg Oncol. 2007;95(5):409–18.
9. Chang L-R, Anand P, Varacallo M. Anatomy, shoulder and upper limb, glenohumeral joint. In: StatPearls. Treasure Island, FL: StatPearls Publishing; 2023.
10. Lang AE, Kim SY, Dickerson CR, Milosavljevic S. Measurement of objective shoulder function following breast cancer surgery: a scoping review. Phys Ther Rev. 2020;25(4):253–68.

11. Baran E, Yildiz Tİ, Gursen C, Üzelpasaci E, Özgül S, Düzgün İ, et al. The association of breast cancer-related lymphedema after unilateral mastectomy with shoulder girdle kinematics and upper extremity function. J Biomech. 2021;121:110432.
12. Harrington S, Padua D, Battaglini C, Michener LA, Giuliani C, Myers J, et al. Comparison of shoulder flexibility, strength, and function between breast cancer survivors and healthy participants. J Cancer Surviv. 2011;5:167–74.
13. Rangel J, Perez C, Oliveira R, Guirro E. Effects of breast cancer treatment on posture: a current review. Int J Phys Ther Rehabil. 2019;5:152.
14. Mangone M, Bernetti A, Agostini F, Paoloni M, De Cicco FA, Capobianco SV, et al. Changes in spine alignment and postural balance after breast cancer surgery: a rehabilitative point of view. Biores Open Access. 2019;8(1):121–8.
15. Korucu TS, Ucurum SG, Tastaban E, Ozgun H, Kaya DO. Comparison of shoulder-arm complex pain, function, and scapular dyskinesia in women with and without unilateral lymphedema after breast cancer surgery. Clin Breast Cancer. 2021;21(3):e285–93.
16. Rostkowska E, Bak M, Samborski W. Body posture in women after mastectomy and its changes as a result of rehabilitation. Adv Med Sci. 2006;51:287–97.
17. Crosbie J, Kilbreath SL, Dylke E, Refshauge KM, Nicholson LL, Beith JM, et al. Effects of mastectomy on shoulder and spinal kinematics during bilateral upper-limb movement. Phys Ther. 2010;90(5):679–92.
18. Ashikaga T, Krag DN, Land SR, Julian TB, Anderson SJ, Brown AM, et al. Morbidity results from the NSABP B-32 trial comparing sentinel lymph node dissection versus axillary dissection. J Surg Oncol. 2010;102(2):111–8.
19. Siqueira RBA, Freitas-Junior R, Lopes PS, Lagares MS, Viana FP, Mesquita TMJC, et al. Hydrotherapy following breast cancer surgery Phase II trial on hydrotherapy in women following breast cancer surgery. Breast J. 2020;26(5):1107–10.
20. Lara-Palomo IC, Castro-Sánchez AM, Córdoba-Peláez MM, Albornoz-Cabello M, Ortiz-Comino L. Effect of myofascial therapy on pain and functionality of the upper extremities in breast cancer survivors: a systematic review and meta-analysis. Int J Environ Res Public Health. 2021;18(9):4420.
21. Lauridsen MC, Christiansen P, Hessov I. The effect of physiotherapy on shoulder function in patients surgically treated for breast cancer: a randomized study. Acta Oncol. 2005;44(5):449–57.
22. Levy EW, Pfalzer LA, Danoff J, Springer BA, McGarvey C, Shieh C-y, et al. Predictors of functional shoulder recovery at 1 and 12 months after breast cancer surgery. Breast Cancer Res Treat. 2012;134:315–24.
23. Sugden E, Rezvani M, Harrison J, Hughes L. Shoulder movement after the treatment of early stage breast cancer. Clin Oncol. 1998;10(3):173–81.
24. Tsai RJ, Dennis LK, Lynch CF, Snetselaar LG, Zamba GK, Scott-Conner C. The risk of developing arm lymphedema among breast cancer survivors: a meta-analysis of treatment factors. Ann Surg Oncol. 2009;16:1959–72.
25. Lee TS, Kilbreath SL, Refshauge KM, Herbert RD, Beith JM. Prognosis of the upper limb following surgery and radiation for breast cancer. Breast Cancer Res Treat. 2008;110:19–37.
26. Bentzen SM, Overgaard M, Thames HD. Fractionation sensitivity of a functional endpoint: impaired shoulder movement after post-mastectomy radiotherapy. Int J Radiat Oncol Biol Phys. 1989;17(3):531–7.
27. Fathers E, Thrush D, Huson SM, Norman A. Radiation-induced brachial plexopathy in women treated for carcinoma of the breast. Clin Rehabil. 2002;16(2):160–5.
28. Ludewig PM, Borstad JD. The shoulder complex. In: Joint structure and function: a comprehensive analysis, vol. 4. New York: McGraw Hill; 2005. p. 233–71.
29. Shamley DR, Srinanaganathan R, Weatherall R, Oskrochi R, Watson M, Ostlere S, et al. Changes in shoulder muscle size and activity following treatment for breast cancer. Breast Cancer Res Treat. 2007;106:19–27.
30. Smoot B, Wong J, Cooper B, Wanek L, Topp K, Byl N, et al. Upper extremity impairments in women with or without lymphedema following breast cancer treatment. J Cancer Surviv. 2010;4(2):167–78.
31. Gilleard W, Smith T. Effect of obesity on posture and hip joint moments during a standing task, and trunk forward flexion motion. Int J Obes. 2007;31(2):267–71.
32. Jang D-H, Kim M-W, Oh S-J, Kim JM. The influence of arm swelling duration on shoulder pathology in breast cancer patients with lymphedema. PLoS One. 2015;10(11):e0142950.
33. Fisher MI, Levangie PK. Oncology section task force on breast cancer outcomes: scapular assessment. Rehabil Oncol. 2013;31(1):11–8.
34. Kara D, Harput G, Duzgun I. Shoulder-abduction angle and trapezius muscle activity during scapular-retraction exercise. J Athl Train. 2021;56(12):1327–33.
35. Shamley D, Srinaganathan R, Oskrochi R, Lascurain-Aguirrebeña I, Sugden E. Three-dimensional scapulothoracic motion following treatment for breast cancer. Breast Cancer Res Treat. 2009;118:315–22.
36. Shamley D, Lascurain-Aguirrebeña I, Oskrochi R, Srinaganathan R. Shoulder morbidity after treatment for breast cancer is bilateral and greater after mastectomy. Acta Oncol. 2012;51(8):1045–53.
37. Ribeiro IL, Camargo PR, Alburquerque-Sendin F, Ferrari AV, Arrais CL, Salvini TF. Three-dimensional scapular kinematics, shoulder outcome measures and quality of life following treatment for breast cancer—a case control study. Musculoskelet Sci Pract. 2019;40:72–9.
38. Shamley D, Lascurain-Aguirrebeña I, Oskrochi R. Clinical anatomy of the shoulder after treatment for breast cancer. Clin Anat. 2014;27(3):467–77.
39. Forte FC, de Castro MP, de Toledo JM, Ribeiro DC, Loss JF. Scapular kinematics and scapulohumeral rhythm during resisted shoulder abduction—impli-

cations for clinical practice. Phys Ther Sport. 2009;10(3):105–11.
40. Herrera JE, Stubblefield MD. Rotator cuff tendonitis in lymphedema: a retrospective case series. Arch Phys Med Rehabil. 2004;85(12):1939–42.
41. Haddad CAS, Saad M, Perez MCJ, Miranda JF. Assessment of posture and joint movements of the upper limbs of patients after mastectomy and lymphadenectomy. Einstein (Sao Paulo). 2013;11:426–34.
42. Johansson K, Ingvar C, Albertsson M, Ekdahl C. Arm lymphoedema, shoulder mobility and muscle strength after breast cancer treatment? A prospective 2-year study. Adv Physiother. 2001;3(2):55–66.
43. Patel DI, Gonzalez A, Moon C, Serra M, Bridges PB, Hughes D, et al. Exercise and creatine supplementation to augment the adaptation of exercise training among breast cancer survivors completing chemotherapy: protocol for an open-label randomized controlled trial (the THRIVE study). JMIR Res Protoc. 2022;11(4):e26827.
44. Merchant C, Chapman T, Kilbreath S, Refshauge K, Krupa K. Decreased muscle strength following management of breast cancer. Disabil Rehabil. 2008;30(15):1098–105.
45. Belmonte R, Messaggi-Sartor M, Ferrer M, Pont A, Escalada F. Prospective study of shoulder strength, shoulder range of motion, and lymphedema in breast cancer patients from pre-surgery to 5 years after ALND or SLNB. Support Care Cancer. 2018;26(9):3277–87.
46. Andersen KG, Jensen M-B, Kehlet H, Gärtner R, Eckhoff L, Kroman N. Persistent pain, sensory disturbances and functional impairment after adjuvant chemotherapy for breast cancer: cyclophosphamide, epirubicin and fluorouracil compared with docetaxel + epirubicin and cyclophosphamide. Acta Oncol. 2012;51(8):1036–44.
47. Tuğral A, Bakar Y, Akyol M. The characteristics of pain tolerance in patients who underwent unilateral breast cancer surgery: the effect of handedness and surgical site to assess the potential musculoskeletal symptoms and function. Clin Breast Cancer. 2022;22(7):e729–35.
48. Hickey BE, Francis DP, Lehman M. Sequencing of chemotherapy and radiotherapy for early breast cancer. Cochrane Database Syst Rev. 2013;(4):CD005212.
49. Sheridan D, Foo I, O'Shea H, Gillanders D, Williams L, Fallon M, et al. Long-term follow-up of pain and emotional characteristics of women after surgery for breast cancer. J Pain Symptom Manag. 2012;44(4):608–14.
50. Kanematsu M, Morimoto M, Honda J, Nagao T, Nakagawa M, Takahashi M, et al. The time since last menstrual period is important as a clinical predictor for non-steroidal aromatase inhibitor-related arthralgia. BMC Cancer. 2011;11:1–6.
51. Zhou W-B, Zhang P-L, Liu X-A, Yang T, He W. Innegligible musculoskeletal disorders caused by zoledronic acid in adjuvant breast cancer treatment: a meta-analysis. J Exp Clin Cancer Res. 2011;30:1–7.
52. Dahl AA, Nesvold I-L, Reinertsen KV, Fosså SD. Arm/shoulder problems and insomnia symptoms in breast cancer survivors: cross-sectional, controlled and longitudinal observations. Sleep Med. 2011;12(6):584–90.
53. Van der Gucht E, Dams L, Meeus M, Devoogdt N, Beintema A, Penen F, et al. Kinesiophobia contributes to pain-related disability in breast cancer survivors: a cross-sectional study. Support Care Cancer. 2020;28(9):4501–8.
54. Sweeney FC, Demark-Wahnefried W, Courneya KS, Sami N, Lee K, Tripathy D, et al. Aerobic and resistance exercise improves shoulder function in women who are overweight or obese and have breast cancer: a randomized controlled trial. Phys Ther. 2019;99(10):1334–45.
55. Beurskens CH, van Uden CJ, Strobbe LJ, Oostendorp RA, Wobbes T. The efficacy of physiotherapy upon shoulder function following axillary dissection in breast cancer, a randomized controlled study. BMC Cancer. 2007;7:166.
56. Ververs JMMA, Roumen RMH, Vingerhoets AJJM, Vreugdenhil G, Coebergh JWW, Crommelin MA, et al. Risk, severity and predictors of physical and psychological morbidity after axillary lymph node dissection for breast cancer. Eur J Cancer. 2001;37(8):991–9.
57. Land SR, Kopec JA, Julian TB, Brown AM, Anderson SJ, Krag DN, et al. Patient-reported outcomes in sentinel node-negative adjuvant breast cancer patients receiving sentinel-node biopsy or axillary dissection: National Surgical Adjuvant Breast and Bowel Project Phase III Protocol B-32. J Clin Oncol. 2010;28(25):3929.
58. Yang EJ, Park WB, Seo KS, Kim SW, Heo CY, Lim JY. Longitudinal change of treatment-related upper limb dysfunction and its impact on late dysfunction in breast cancer survivors: a prospective cohort study. J Surg Oncol. 2010;101(1):84–91.
59. Devoogdt N, Van Kampen M, Geraerts I, Coremans T, Fieuws S, Lefevre J, et al. Physical activity levels after treatment for breast cancer: one-year follow-up. Breast Cancer Res Treat. 2010;123(2):417–25.
60. Baran E, Özçakar L, Özgül S, Aksoy S, Akbayrak T. Upper limb sensory evaluations and ultrasonographic skin measurements in breast cancer-related lymphedema receiving complex decongestive physiotherapy. Support Care Cancer. 2021;29:6545–53.
61. McNeely ML, Campbell K, Ospina M, Rowe BH, Dabbs K, Klassen TP, et al. Exercise interventions for upper-limb dysfunction due to breast cancer treatment. Cochrane Database Syst Rev. 2010;(6):CD005211.
62. Bruce J, Mazuquin B, Mistry P, Rees S, Canaway A, Hossain A, et al. Exercise to prevent shoulder problems after breast cancer surgery: the PROSPER RCT. Health Technol Assess. 2022;26(15):1.
63. Bendz I, Olsen MF. Evaluation of immediate versus delayed shoulder exercises after breast cancer surgery including lymph node dissection—a randomised controlled trial. Breast. 2002;11(3):241–8.

64. Duzgun I, Eraslan LS, Yildiz TI, Demirci S. Shoulder rehabilitation. In: The shoulder. Cham: Springer; 2017. p. 215–55.
65. Singh C, De Vera M, Campbell KL. The effect of prospective monitoring and early physiotherapy intervention on arm morbidity following surgery for breast cancer: a pilot study. Physiother Can. 2013;65(2):183–91.
66. Mauntel TC, Clark MA, Padua DA. Effectiveness of myofascial release therapies on physical performance measurements: a systematic review. Athl Train Sports Health Care. 2014;6(4):189–96.
67. De Groef A, Van Kampen M, Dieltjens E, De Geyter S, Vos L, De Vrieze T, et al. Identification of myofascial trigger points in breast cancer survivors with upper limb pain: interrater reliability. Pain Med. 2017;19(8):1650–6.
68. Paolucci T, Bernetti A, Bai AV, Capobianco SV, Bonifacino A, Maggi G, et al. The recovery of reaching movement in breast cancer survivors: two different rehabilitative protocols in comparison. Eur J Phys Rehabil Med. 2021;57(1):137–47.
69. Luz RPC, Simao Haddad CA, Rizzi S, Elias S, Nazario ACP, Facina G. Complex therapy physical alone or associated with strengthening exercises in patients with lymphedema after breast cancer treatment: a controlled clinical trial. Asian Pac J Cancer Prev. 2018;19(5):1405–10.
70. Cramp F, James A, Lambert J. The effects of resistance training on quality of life in cancer: a systematic literature review and meta-analysis. Support Care Cancer. 2010;18(11):1367–76.
71. Strasser B, Steindorf K, Wiskemann J, Ulrich CM. Impact of resistance training in cancer survivors: a meta-analysis. Med Sci Sports Exerc. 2013;45(11):2080.
72. Lee SA, Kang J-Y, Kim YD, An AR, Kim S-W, Kim Y-S, et al. Effects of a scapula-oriented shoulder exercise programme on upper limb dysfunction in breast cancer survivors: a randomized controlled pilot trial. Clin Rehabil. 2010;24(7):600–13.
73. Pirincci CS, Dalyan M, Delialioglu SU, Celenay ST. Effects of scapulothoracic stabilization exercises on scapular function, posture, and balance in lymphedema after mastectomy: a randomized controlled trial. Women Health. 2023;63(4):251–65.
74. Yang Y, Gu D, Qian Y, Wang H, Chai X. Effectiveness of aerobic exercise on upper limb function following breast cancer treatment: a systematic review and meta-analysis. Ann Palliat Med. 2021;10(3):3396–403.
75. Sprod LK, Drum SN, Bentz AT, Carter SD, Schneider CM. The effects of walking poles on shoulder function in breast cancer survivors. Integr Cancer Ther. 2005;4(4):287–93.
76. Pinto-Carral A, Molina AJ, de Pedro Á, Ayán C. Pilates for women with breast cancer: a systematic review and meta-analysis. Complement Ther Med. 2018;41:130–40.
77. Espíndula RC, Nadas GB, Rosa MI, Foster C, Araújo FC, Grande AJ. Pilates for breast cancer: a systematic review and meta-analysis. Rev Assoc Med Bras. 2017;63:1006–12.
78. Loudon A, Barnett T, Piller N, Immink MA, Visentin D, Williams AD. The effects of yoga on shoulder and spinal actions for women with breast cancer-related lymphoedema of the arm: a randomised controlled pilot study. BMC Complement Altern Med. 2016;16(1):343.
79. Prakash K, Saini SK, Pugazhendi S. Effectiveness of yoga on quality of life of breast cancer patients undergoing chemotherapy: a randomized clinical controlled study. Indian J Palliat Care. 2020;26(3):323–31.
80. Sudarshan M, Petrucci A, Dumitra S, Duplisea J, Wexler S, Meterissian S. Yoga therapy for breast cancer patients: a prospective cohort study. Complement Ther Clin Pract. 2013;19(4):227–9.
81. Torres-Ronda L, Alcázar XSID. The properties of water and their applications for training. J Hum Kinet. 2014;44(1):237–48.
82. Dionne A, Goulet S, Leone M, Comtois A-S. Aquatic exercise training outcomes on functional capacity, quality of life, and lower limb lymphedema: pilot study. J Altern Complement Med. 2018;24(9–10):1007–9.
83. Mur-Gimeno E, Postigo-Martin P, Cantarero-Villanueva I, Sebio-Garcia R. Systematic review of the effect of aquatic therapeutic exercise in breast cancer survivors. Eur J Cancer Care. 2022;31(1):e13535.
84. Louw A, Puentedura EJ, Reese D, Parker P, Miller T, Mintken PE. Immediate effects of mirror therapy in patients with shoulder pain and decreased range of motion. Arch Phys Med Rehabil. 2017;98(10):1941–7.
85. Başkaya MÇ, Erçalık C, Karataş Kır Ö, Erçalık T, Tuncer T. The efficacy of mirror therapy in patients with adhesive capsulitis: a randomized, prospective, controlled study. J Back Musculoskelet Rehabil. 2018;31(6):1177–82.
86. Yuan R, Wei X, Ye Y, Wang M, Jiang J, Li K, et al. The effects of the mirror therapy on shoulder function in patients with breast cancer following surgery: a randomized controlled trial. J Cancer Surviv. 2024;18(5):1574–89.

13 Axillary Web Syndrome: Management and Implications for Function

Ege Nur Atabey Gerlegiz and Serap Özgül

13.1 Introduction

Breast cancer is the most common cancer in women, and it is the second leading cause of mortality after lung cancer [1]. Technological improvements in the diagnosis and treatment of breast cancer have led to a significant increase in breast cancer survival. Surgical techniques, particularly sentinel lymph node biopsy (SLNB) and axillary lymph node dissection (ALND), play an important role in breast cancer management for early detection, prognosis prediction, treatment planning, and prevention of possible recurrence [2]. As the survival rate of breast cancer increases, rapid recovery after surgery and improvement in quality of life becomes increasingly important. However, various short- and long-term complications may occur as a result of axillary surgery [3, 4]. These complications include pain, paresthesias, lymphedema, decreased range of motion of the shoulder joint, and axillary web syndrome (AWS) [5].

Patients may develop AWS after surgical intervention on axillary lymph nodes. This syndrome is characterized by the formation of fibrous bands or lymphatic cords in the axillary region that restrict shoulder motion, causing pain, and dysfunction [3].

E. N. Atabey Gerlegiz (✉) · S. Özgül
Faculty of Physical Therapy and Rehabilitation, Department of Fundamental Physiotherapy and Rehabilitation, Hacettepe University, Ankara, Turkey

Physical therapy is the first line of treatment for AWS, which helps to increase range of motion, reduce pain, and improve function [6, 7]. In addition, medications and surgical interventions can be tried in some patients. In this section, after reviewing the epidemiology, etiology, prevalence, and pathogenesis of AWS, symptoms associated with AWS, risk factors, and diagnosis, we will discuss the evidence-based practices preferred for managing AWS and improving function.

13.2 Epidemiology

Although AWS is a common complication after breast cancer surgery, it causes significant morbidity in the early and late postoperative periods it it is being neglected. Ferrandez and Serin [8] first defined AWS as superficial lymphatic thrombosis in 1996. Moskovitz et al. [3], conducted a retrospective analysis of 750 patients who underwent ALND surgery between 1980 and 1996. They reported that 44 patients developed axillary nodules, which limited shoulder abduction between 1 and 8 weeks following surgery. Moskovitz et al. termed this syndrome AWS in 2001, with a reported incidence of 6% after breast cancer surgery [3]. However, later research has revealed that AWS is a prevalent postoperative consequence of breast cancer, with an incidence that can reach up to 91%. The incidence rate var-

Y. Bakar, A. Tuğral (eds.), *Managing Side Effects of Breast Cancer Treatment*, https://doi.org/10.1007/978-3-031-75480-7_13

ies depending on the type of axillary surgery, the frequency of follow-up after surgery, and the diagnostic criteria for AWS [9].

In the past, AWS was regarded to be a benign condition that occurred in the early postoperative period and caused only minor limitations. However, Koehler et al. [10] indicate that AWS may occur in the early postoperative period and become a chronic condition, lasting for years, and may recur after the fibrotic bands are resolved.

13.3 Etiology and Pathophysiology

The etiology of AWS is not completely understood. AWS is known by a variety of names in the literature, such as cording, axillary cord, axillary string, vascular string, lymphatic cord, fibrotic band, Mondor disease, and violin string phenomenon [11].

According to reports, the etiology of AWS is related to the lymphovenous damage and fibrotic origin, but hypercoagulability caused by superficial and venous stasis, as well as tissue damage after axillary surgery, can also contribute to this process. As a result, thrombosis develops in the upper extremity lymphatic vessels, axillary lymphatic vessels, and large superficial vessels, which can cause AWS [3, 8].

After ALND, the incidence of AWS is much higher compared to SLNB. As the extent of surgery and the number of lymph nodes sampled or removed increase, so does the risk of developing AWS [3, 12, 13]. In addition, AWS may occur when individuals have extended axillary lymphadenopathy [12, 14, 15].

13.4 Symptoms

AWS is a condition characterized by the presence of palpable or visible cords or fibrotic bands in the affected axillary region, upper extremity, chest, or trunk following breast cancer surgery [5]. These fibrotic bands are sensitive to palpation and shoulder movement and can cause pain, limited range of motion, numbness, loss of function, and psychosocial symptoms [11]. In AWS, 1–3 fibrotic bands like palpable violin strings usually appear under the skin (Figs. 13.1 and 13.2). During shoulder flexion and abduction, fibrotic bands become more visible, stiff, and painful. Hyperemia, local temperature increase, or systemic symptoms associated with AWS are not observed. In some cases, fibrotic bands or cords may appear as subcutaneous nodules similar to cases of metastasis in breast cancer [16, 17].

In 20% of patients, AWS extends beyond the axillary region, continues to the anterior and middle part of the arm, extending to the antecubital fossa, and reaching the base of the thumb and the

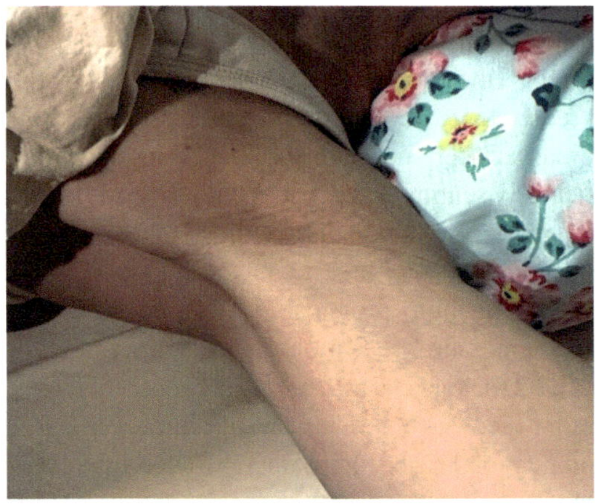

Fig. 13.1 Axillary web syndrome with the appearance of a single fibrotic band following breast cancer surgery

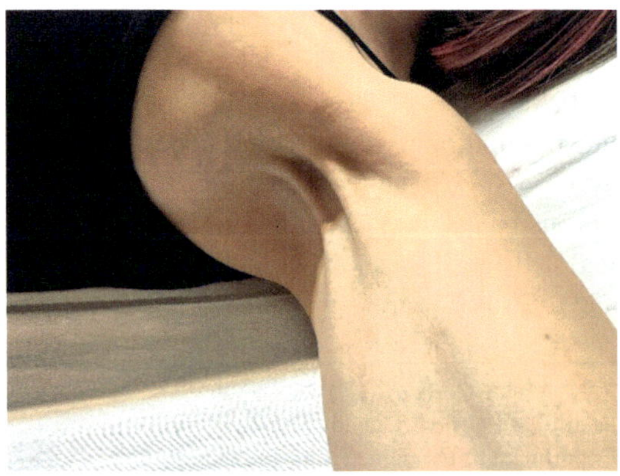

Fig. 13.2 Axillary web syndrome with the appearance of a double fibrotic band following breast cancer surgery

radial part of the wrist [9, 18]. AWS can cause shoulder limitation and pain, potentially delaying the use of adjuvant applications after breast cancer surgery. This can make it difficult to achieve the arm-shoulder position required for radiation therapy [5, 19].

13.5 Risk Factors

AWS is associated with several risk factors, including the type and extent of surgery, presence of postoperative seroma, breast reconstruction, complications, intercostal nerve injury during surgery, younger age, low body mass index, ethnicity, and presence of hypertension [13, 14, 17, 20, 21].

13.6 Axillary Web Syndrome and Lymphedema

AWS and lymphedema have similar pathophysiology. For this reason, AWS is also thought to be a risk factor for lymphedema. However, the literature is conflicting on this issue. Ryans et al. [22] found that patients with AWS have a higher risk of developing lymphedema in the first year after surgery. Furthermore, patients with AWS are three times more likely to develop lymphedema during the first month after breast cancer surgery than women without AWS. Wariss et al. [23] discovered that the incidence rates of AWS (35.9%) and lymphedema (31.4%) following surgery were similar in a 10-year prospective research.However, this study opposed previous findings by not including AWS as a risk factor for lymphedema.

13.7 Evaluation and Diagnosis

AWS is diagnosed with a physical examination [17, 20]. Following surgery, a cord-like nodule develops in the axilla, and cords resembling violin strings appear that extend to the chest wall, abdominal wall, axilla, arm, antecubital fossa, and hand on the ipsilateral side. Diagnosis of AWS is based on cord appearance, extremity pain, limited shoulder abduction and flexion, and numbness in the affected extremity [17, 24]. The evaluation should include the recording of the cord's location, number, length, depth, and palpability well as ultrasonographic (US) assessment of subcutaneous tissue thickness, subcutaneous reflex testing, skin echo density, joint range of motion, and pain [10, 16, 20, 25]. Furthermore, imaging techniques such as magnetic resonance imaging (MRI) have been used to diagnose AWS. However, research reports that MRI cannot accurately identify AWS. For this reason, the US is the most reliable method as it allows movement to the patient's arm while the diagnostic test is being carried out [25, 26].

13.8 Treatment Approaches

After breast cancer surgery, pain in the affected extremity, limitation of movement, and skin and subcutaneous tissue symptoms can cause anxiety in patients. In addition, prolonged pain leads to muscle atrophy, shoulder joint inflammation, and myofascial syndrome [17, 25]. All these impacts reduce the quality of life.

There are limited well-designed, evidence-based intervention studies for AWS management. The majority of studies on AWS consist of retrospective and case studies [7, 11, 17].

AWS treatment options include physical therapy, medical therapy, fat grafting, percutaneous injection, mesotherapy, and surgery [27]. Physical therapy and rehabilitation for AWS are first-line practices that include safe methods. However, no study in the literature has demonstrated that one physiotherapeutic application is superior to another. There is no clear information on application protocols and strategies. More research is needed to understand the prevention and treatment of AWS [6, 17, 28].

Table 13.1 Physiotherapy and rehabilitation interventions for AWS in breast cancer

Manual therapy interventions	Exercises interventions	Other approaches
Myofascial release techniques	Stretching exercises	Moist heat
Scar tissue manipulation	Mobilization exercises	Aqua lymphatic therapy
Manual lymph drainage	Resistance training	Kinesio-taping
Cord manipulation	Endurance training	Compression therapy
Soft tissue manipulation		

13.9 Physical Therapy Approaches

Physical therapy can help prevent AWS, manage pain, reduce symptoms including numbness and tingling, improve function, and decrease the progression of AWS [6].

Physical therapy modalities include patient education, exercise, manual therapy, and other approaches. Physical therapy begins with patient education. After patient education, other physical therapy approaches can be used including active resistive shoulder exercises, abduction cord manipulation, stretching exercises, fascial mobilization techniques, therapeutic massage applications with passive shoulder movements, myofascial release techniques, scar tissue mobilization, manual lymphatic drainage (MLD), kinesio-taping, compression, axillary and arm moist heat applications [6, 11, 17] (Table 13.1).

13.10 Patient Education

Patient awareness of AWS should be improved before and after breast cancer surgery, and patient education is very important in this regard. Patient education begins in the preoperative period and continues in the postoperative period. Individuals should be assessed for the risk of developing AWS, and education should include a discussion of the potential risk factors for AWS. In addition, patients should be informed that AWS is not associated with metastasis, which will alleviate their anxiety and increase their cooperation in treatment [17, 29].

13.11 Exercise Interventions

Exercise programs for AWS aim to reduce arm pain, improve shoulder function, and resolve the axillary cord. Exercise approaches for AWS range from gravity-assisted programs to resistance exercises.

According to studies, a qualified physical therapist should stretch the muscles pectoralis major and minor, biceps brachii, triceps brachii, rotator cuff, latissimus dorsi, intercostal muscles, and muscles in the cervical region passively before moving on to active stretching [16, 30–32]. It is recommended that the range of motion achieved from stretching should be maintained by using the elastic band and the bicycle ergometer exercises [30, 33]. Postural exercises for the trunk and shoulders, as well as diaphragmatic breathing exercises, should be included in a holistic treatment approach [6, 30].

Wyrick et al. [33], in 31 individuals who had AWS after breast cancer surgery, developed a combined exercise program that included active mobilization, soft tissue stretching, progressive resistance exercises, Airdyne cycling training, and a home exercise program. If the patients had lymphedema, MLD, compression bandaging, and intermittent pneumatic compression were also used. After 10 weeks of treatment, the cord resolved and the shoulder range of motion in abduction and flexion improved ($52 \pm 21°$ and $39 \pm 20°$, respectively).

Torres et al. [24] conducted a randomized controlled experiment in which the intervention group received active shoulder exercises and MLD, whereas the control group received standard PNF-based shoulder exercises and care. The treatment continued for 3 weeks, 3 days a week. According to the findings, pain intensity, shoulder range of motion, and quality of life measures improved much more than the control group after the treatment program in the intervention group.

According to Koeheler et al. [34], the physiotherapist plays an important role in the management of AWS. Exercises are first introduced under the supervision of a physiotherapist, a home program should be created in subsequent sessions, and the exercises should be continued independently at home in the context of AWS. Patients who learn and implement the exercises correctly can continue and achieve their treatment by implementing a home program.

13.12 Manipulative Treatment Interventions

Manual therapy modalities are often recommended along with exercise interventions to reduce pain and achieve functional recovery in the management of AWS. In the literature, manual therapy modalities for AWS include myofascial release techniques, scar tissue massage, and MLD techniques [11, 31, 34].

13.13 Myofascial Release Techniques

Myofascial release techniques include axillary cord massage at the painless border, cord manipulation, cord mobilization, passive skin traction, and myofascial traction [10, 16, 19, 30–32].

In the majority of the existing research, details of the application or protocols of myofascial release techniques were not reported. In contrast, Kepics et al. [30] included intervention details in their study. In practice, after initial superficial palpation, progressive fascial mobilization of deeper tissues is needed. During fascial manipulation, the elbow is extended as much as possible, and the extremity is placed in slight abduction with the forearm in supination. Once the patient is in the appropriate position, the patient is asked to perform flexion and extension of the wrist. Active mobilization is performed at various degrees of shoulder abduction depending on the length of the cord. While in the same position, myofascial release techniques and transverse tissue massage are applied to the areas where the cord is attached and to the surgical scar. During treatment, avoid focusing on a single point, and in the final stage, the cord should be mobilized and the extremity placed in a stretched position [30].

Lattanzi et al. [19] performed soft tissue mobilization, skin traction technique, and myofascial release techniques in the first week of individuals who developed AWS 10 days after surgery. In the second week, the elongation technique, skin traction, and scar tissue massage were performed, as well as home stretching exercises were implemented. After treatment, an increase in shoulder range of motion, resolving the cord, and an increase in muscle strength and functionality were reported.

In their case report, De Sire et al. [28] performed MLD, myofascial release techniques with soft tissue mobilization, scar tissue massage, active shoulder exercises, and stretching in individuals who developed AWS 1 month following the breast cancer surgery. The rehabilitation program is scheduled for 3 weeks, 3 sessions per week, and each session lasted for 45 min. After treatment, significant improvement in shoulder range of motion (increase in flexion to 170° vs. 80° and increase in abduction to 100° vs. 170°) and improvement in quality of life and functionality were reported.

Josenhans et al. [31] found that myofascial release techniques increased shoulder flexion and abduction ranges of motion by 20–40° at each treatment session.

According to Agostini et al. [6], manual therapy is strictly contraindicated if the patient is receiving radiotherapy or has axillary metastases, and treatment should be scheduled at least 2 weeks after the completion of radiotherapy and the area diagnosed with secondary neoplasia should be avoided.

13.14 Scar Tissue Massage

Scar tissue massage is used to dissolve adhesions in deeper layers. Scar tissue massage can be performed with perpendicular, parallel, or circular movements on the scar tissue [19, 30, 31].

13.15 Manual Lymphatic Drainage

Manual lymphatic drainage (MLD) is one of the possible treatment options for AWS. MLD has been found to reduce lymphatic vessel inflammation and increase joint range of motion by facilitating the reabsorption of lymphatic fluid [24, 30]. Cho et al. [35] performed MLD on 41 patients with AWS, 3–5 sessions per week for 4 weeks. The research reported that MLD significantly reduced pain, increased range of motion and muscle strength, and reduced the risk of postoperative lymphedema in the affected extremity. It was also found that MLD combined with exercise therapy was more effective than exercise alone.

13.16 Initiation, Duration, and Frequency of Physical Therapy for Axillary Web Syndrome

There is no consensus on the optimal time to begin rehabilitation following surgery in AWS. According to Josenhans [31], only 50% of patients are included in rehabilitation within the first 4 weeks after surgery, with the remaining 50% being able to participate in rehabilitation programs months or years later.

According to existing systematic reviews reported that the characteristics of rehabilitation in AWS are 2–3 sessions per week, with each session lasting an average of 30–45 min, and continuing for 4–5 weeks. However, for patients who have severe upper extremity functional limitations and require radiation therapy, an intense rehabilitation program of 5 sessions per week with a duration of 3–10 weeks is recommended [6, 11, 19, 25, 30–32]. As a result, the beginning time of the therapy, duration, frequency, and follow-up periods of treatment were quite heterogeneous in studies focusing on AWS.

13.17 Pharmacological Agents

The literature reports the use of various pharmacological agents to improve compliance and tolerance to physical therapy interventions as well as to manage pain in the treatment of AWS. In this context, the use of nonsteroidal anti-inflammatory drugs, opioids, and salicylates is recommended in patients with AWS [36–38]. However, to the best of our knowledge, there are no studies that have evaluated the efficacy of these medications alone when recommended in combination with physical therapy interventions.

13.18 Surgical Techniques

Spinal cord resection surgery has been attempted in the past in individuals whose functionality and quality of life were severely impaired by AWS [39]. However, it has been found that surgery does not provide effective results on functionality and increases the risk of lymphedema and recurrence of AWS. Furthermore, considering the high success rate of noninvasive treatments, surgical methods are rarely used in AWS nowadays.

13.19 Conclusion

Axillary web syndrome (AWS) is an important complication that causes physical, social, and psychological effects in individuals undergoing breast cancer surgery and consequently reduces their quality of life. Physical therapy should be considered the first-line option for AWS. However, the existing literature is limited to case reports, retrospective studies, and randomized controlled trials with small sample sizes. A better understanding of the etiology, pathophysiology, and risk factors of AWS will help to develop strategies for prevention, early diagnosis, and treatment. Clinical practice, especially in primary care management of AWS, should be expanded and the level of evidence increased.

References

1. Siegel RL, Miller KD, Wagle NS, Jemal A. Cancer statistics, 2023. CA Cancer J Clin. 2023;73(1):17–48.
2. Fan Y-J, Li J-C, Zhu D-M, Zhu H-L, Zhao Y, Zhu X-B, et al. Efficacy and safety comparison between axillary lymph node dissection with no axillary surgery in patients with sentinel node-positive breast cancer: a systematic review and meta-analysis. BMC Surg. 2023;23(1):209.
3. Moskovitz AH, Anderson BO, Yeung RS, Byrd DR, Lawton TJ, Moe RE. Axillary web syndrome after axillary dissection. Am J Surg. 2001;181(5):434–9.
4. Kootstra JJ, Dijkstra PU, Rietman H, de Vries J, Baas P, Geertzen JH, et al. A longitudinal study of shoulder and arm morbidity in breast cancer survivors 7 years after sentinel lymph node biopsy or axillary lymph node dissection. Breast cancer Res Treat. 2013;139:125–34.
5. Marco E, Trépanier G, Chang E, Mauti E, Jones JM, Zhong T. Postmas-tectomy functional impairments. Curr Oncol Rep. 2023;25(12):1445–53.
6. Agostini F, Attanasi C, Bernetti A, Mangone M, Paoloni M, Del Monte E, et al. Web axillary pain syndrome—literature evidence and novel rehabilitative suggestions: a narrative review. Int J Environ Res Public Health. 2021;18(19):10383.
7. Lippi L, de Sire A, Losco L, Mezian K, Folli A, Ivanova M, et al. Axillary web syndrome in breast cancer women: what is the optimal rehabilitation strategy after surgery? A systematic review. J Clin Med. 2022;11(13):3839.
8. Ferrandez J-C, Serin D. Rééducation et cancer du sein. Amsterdam: Elsevier Masson; 2006.
9. Figueira PV, Haddad CA, de Almeida Rizzi SK, Facina G, Nazario AC. Diagnosis of axillary web syndrome in patients after breast cancer surgery: epidemiology, risk factors, and clinical aspects: a prospective study. Am J Clin Oncol. 2018;41(10):992–6.
10. Koehler L, Day A, Hunter D, Blaes A, Haddad T, Shanley R. Five-year cumulative incidence of axillary web syndrome and comparison in upper extremity movement, function, pain, and lymphedema in survivors of breast cancer with and without axillary web syndrome. Arch Phys Med Rehabil. 2022;103(9):1798–806.
11. Yeung W, McPhail SM, Kuys SS. A systematic review of axillary web syndrome (AWS). J Cancer Surviv Res Pract. 2015;9:576–98.
12. Verbelen H, Gebruers N, Eeckhout F-M, Verlinden K, Tjalma W. Shoulder and arm morbidity in sentinel node-negative breast cancer patients: a systematic review. Breast Cancer Res Treat. 2014;144:21–31.
13. Torres Lacomba M, Mayoral del Moral O, Coperias Zazo JL, Yuste Sánchez MJ, Ferrandez J-C, Zapico Goñi Á. Axillary web syndrome after axillary dissection in breast cancer: a prospective study. Breast Cancer Res Treat. 2009;117:625–30.
14. Schuitevoerder D, White I, Fortino J, Vetto J. Axillary web syndrome: an underappreciated complication of sentinel node biopsy in melanoma. Am J Surg. 2016;211(5):846–9.
15. Clarke SA, Mortimer P, Powell BW. Axillary web syndrome following sentinel node biopsy for melanoma. J Plast Reconstr Aesthet Surg. 2013;66(12):1810–1.
16. Wei P, Zhu L, Chen K, Jia W, Hu Y, Su F. Axillary web syndrome following secondary breast-conserving surgery: a case report. World J Surg Oncol. 2013;11:1–4.
17. Elan Y, Xiongwei L, Xiao L. Diagnosis and treatment of axillary web syndrome: an overview. CJPRS. 2020;2(2):128–36.
18. Dinas K, Kalder M, Zepiridis L, Mavromatidis G, Pratilas G. Axillary web syndrome: incidence, pathogenesis, and management. Curr Prob Cancer. 2019;43(6):100470.
19. Lattanzi JB, Giuliano S, Meehan C, Sander B, Wootten R, Zimmerman A. Recommendations for physical and occupational therapy practice from the perspective of clients undergoing therapy for breast cancer-related impairments. J Allied Health. 2010;39(4):257–64.
20. Bergmann A, Mendes VV, de Almeida Dias R, do Amaral E Silva B, da Costa Leite Ferreira MG, Fabro EAN. Incidence and risk factors for axillary web syndrome after breast cancer surgery. Breast Cancer Res Treat. 2012;131:987–92.
21. Akezaki Y, Nakata E, Kikuuchi M, Tominaga R, Kurokawa H, Hamada M, et al. Influence of and risk factors for axillary web syndrome following surgery for breast cancer. Acta Med Okayama. 2021;75(1):39–44.
22. Ryans K, Davies CC, Gaw G, Lambe C, Henninge M, VanHoose L. Incidence and predictors of axillary web syndrome and its association with lymphedema in women following breast cancer treatment: a retrospective study. Support Care Cancer. 2020;28:5881–8.
23. Wariss BR, Costa RM, Pereira ACPR, Koifman RJ, Bergmann A. Axillary web syndrome is not a risk factor for lymphoedema after 10 years of follow-up. Support Care Cancer. 2017;25:465–70.
24. Torres-Lacomba M, Prieto-Gómez V, Arranz-Martín B, Ferrandez JC, Yuste-Sánchez MJ, Navarro-Brazález B, et al. Manual lymph drainage with progressive arm exercises for axillary web syndrome after breast cancer surgery: a randomized controlled trial. Phys Ther. 2022;102(3):pzab314.
25. Leduc O, Sichere M, Moreau A, Rigolet J, Tinlot A, Dare S, et al. Axillary web syndrome: nature and localization. Lymphology. 2009;42(4):176–81.
26. Koehler L, Hunter D, Haddad TC, Blaes A, Hirsch A, Ludewig P. Characterizing axillary web syndrome: ultrasonographic efficacy. Lymphology. 2014;47(4):156.
27. Evans HEL, Forbes CC, Galvao DA, Vandelanotte C, Newton RU, Wit-tert G, et al. Evaluating a web- and telephone-based personalised exercise intervention for individuals living with metastatic prostate cancer

(ExerciseGuide): protocol for a pilot randomised controlled trial. Pilot Feasibility Stud. 2021;7(1):16.
28. De Sire A, Losco L, Cisari C, Gennari A, Boldorini R, Fusco N, et al. Axillary web syndrome in women after breast cancer surgery referred to an Oncological Rehabilitation Unit: which are the main risk factors? A retrospective case-control study. Eur Rev Med Pharmacol Sci. 2020;24(15):8028–35.
29. Testa A, Iannace C, Di Libero L, Caracciolo F. Strengths of early physical rehabilitation programs in surgical breast cancer patients: results of a randomized control study. BMC Proc. 2013;7(Suppl 1):O5.
30. Kepics JM. Physical therapy treatment of axillary web syndrome. Rehabil Oncol. 2004;22(1):21.
31. Josenhans E. Physiotherapeutic treatment for axillary cord formation following breast cancer surgery. Pt_ Zeitschrift für Physiotherapeuten. 2007;59(9):868–78.
32. Fourie W, Robb K. Physiotherapy management of axillary web syndrome following breast cancer treatment: discussing the use of soft tissue techniques. J Physiother. 2009;95(4):314–20.
33. Wyrick SL, Waltke LJ, Ng AV. Physical therapy may promote resolution of lymphatic coding in breast cancer survivors. Rehabil Oncol. 2006;24(1):29–34.
34. Koehler L, Haddad T, Hunter D, Tuttle T. Axillary web syndrome following breast cancer surgery: symptoms, complications, and management strategies. Breast Cancer (Dove Med Press). 2018;11:13–9.
35. Cho Y, Do J, Jung S, Kwon O, Jeon JY. Effects of a physical therapy program combined with manual lymphatic drainage on shoulder function, quality of life, lymphedema incidence, and pain in breast cancer patients with axillary web syndrome following axillary dissection. Support Care Cancer. 2016;24:2047–57.
36. Aydogan F, Belli AK, Baghaki S, Karabulut K, Tahan G, Uras C. Axillary web syndrome after sentinel node biopsy. Breast Care. 2008;3(4):277–8.
37. Cheville AL, Tchou J. Barriers to rehabilitation following surgery for primary breast cancer. J Surg Oncol. 2007;95(5):409–18.
38. Craythorne E, Benton E, Macfarlane S. Axillary web syndrome or cording, a variant of mondor disease, following axillary surgery. Arch Dermatol. 2009;145(10):1199–200.
39. Marcus R, Pawade J, Vella E. Painful lymphatic occlusion following axillary lymph node surgery. Br J Surg. 1990;77(6):683.

14 Upper Back and Neck Problems and Management in Breast Cancer Survivorship

Özlem Ülger, Müzeyyen Öz, and Yasemin Özel Aslıyüce

14.1 Introduction

Advances in modern medicine have dramatically improved the cure rates of many diseases, but cancer continues to threaten human lives. Around the world, people are diagnosed with cancer every day [1].

Breast cancer is the second most common cancer. In 2023, it is estimated that there will be nearly 2 million new cancer cases and 609,820 cancer-related deaths in the United States, while this rate is anticipated to reach 22 million with new cases in the trajectory of the next 20 years [2, 3]. Breast cancer alone accounts for 31% of female cancers and is the leading cause of cancer-related disability-adjusted life years (DALYs), deaths, and years of life lost (YLL) globally [4].

Currently, the elective treatment of breast cancer is surgery with complete or partial mastectomy, often with sentinel lymph node biopsy and subsequent complete axillary lymph node dissection, if necessary. Depending on the stage and histology of the malignancy, surgery may be combined with neoadjuvant and adjuvant systemic treatment, including locoregional radiotherapy, chemotherapy, and hormone therapy [5]. As a result of constantly updated methods and pharmacological agents against cancer, treatment modalities have become increasingly effective and increased the survival rates of patients. However, these multimodal treatments are associated with side effects that can negatively affect the patient's functionality and quality of life [6]. Therefore, a new goal, which aims to help breast cancer survivors (BCS) cope with the short-, medium-, and long-term effects and treatment of the disease as they return to daily life, has been set [7].

Upper body problems and dysfunction associated with the side effects of multimodal interventions are common in BCS [8]. This chapter focuses on upper body and neck problems and provides a framework for the management of these consequences among BCS.

14.2 Upper Back and Neck Problems in Breast Cancer Survivorship

14.2.1 Postural Problems

Posture is the optimal positioning of each part of the body in relation to the whole body. Postural changes can occur in the body due to internal factors (i.e. disease) and external conditions (i.e. injury). The adverse effects of breast cancer treatment can negatively affect the functioning of the postural regulatory system due to potential consequences of breast cancer treatment related to

Ö. Ülger (✉) · M. Öz · Y. Ö. Aslıyüce
Faculty of Physical Therapy and Rehabilitation, Hacettepe University, Ankara, Turkey

Y. Bakar, A. Tuğral (eds.), *Managing Side Effects of Breast Cancer Treatment*,
https://doi.org/10.1007/978-3-031-75480-7_14

both the musculoskeletal and nervous systems [9]. There are various causes of unfavorable changes in posture and trunk balance in women undergoing breast cancer treatment (Fig. 14.1). These changes affect the ability of the spine to transfer normal loads and function properly.

Resection of the pectoralis minor muscle during radical mastectomy results in atrophy and fibrosis of the pectoralis major muscle [10]. This leads to depression of the rib cage due to the impaired motor function of this muscle. The long thoracic and thoracodorsal nerves may also be injured during axillary lymph node resection. Injury to the long thoracic nerve results in paralysis of the serratus anterior muscle and causes a condition called winged scapula (WS). Injury to the thoracodorsal nerve causes paralysis of the latissimus dorsi muscle, resulting in reduced glenohumeral joint mobility and a prominent protrusion of the scapular angle [9]. Radiotherapy can cause tissue fibrosis in the irradiated area, mainly affecting the anterolateral chest wall [11]. Chemotherapy, on the other hand, can affect the muscular system, causing metabolic changes and leading to muscle fiber loss, dysfunction, and atrophy [12].

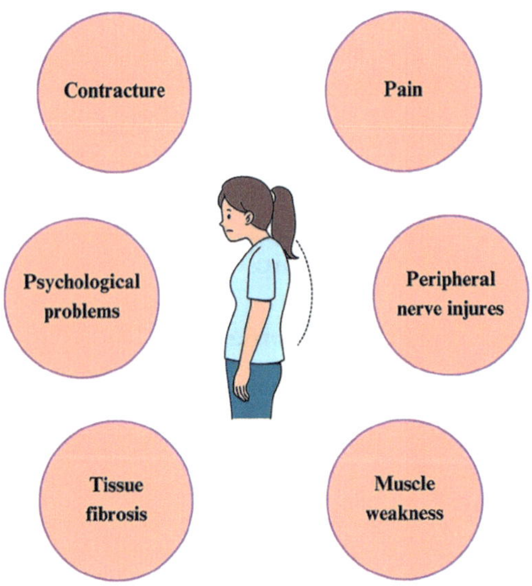

Fig. 14.1 Causes affecting the posture in breast cancer survivors

Although the upper extremities are affected mostly in the case of post-mastectomy lymphedema, the chest and upper back areas can also be affected. Both unilateral lymphedema and post-mastectomy breast abscesses are not confined to the upper limb on the operated side, as they are part of a kinematic chain with neighboring elements. The overload caused by increased volume due to lymphedema might affect spinal alignment and mobility [9]. In addition to the biomechanical effects on posture, there may also be a significant psychosocial problem in patients with unilateral modified radical mastectomy. Women define themselves as incomplete in relation to the loss of a feminine part of the body following mastectomy [13]. Studies have reported a "half-woman complex" and a deterioration in body image and quality of life [14]. Additional stress, particularly on the spine, may occur owing to the changes in body integrity and unilateral lymphedema, as well as perceptions, awareness, and emotions related to posture.

Studies of posture in women with breast cancer have reported abnormalities in the sagittal plane (i.e., thoracic hyperkyphosis) and frontal plane (i.e., shoulder descent or elevation, asymmetric scapular position, and scoliosis) [9, 15, 16]. Serel et al. [17] used radiographic examination to detect spinal deformity in patients with unilateral mastectomy and showed that women with unilateral mastectomy can develop long-term spinal deformity, especially scoliosis. Toprak Çelenay et al. [18] compared spinal alignment and mobility in women with and without unilateral lymphedema after modified radical mastectomy. They found that sagittal thoracic curvature and frontal tilt angle towards the unaffected side increased in women with unilateral lymphedema. The authors also noted that these changes can cause scoliosis, balance problems, chest mobility, and respiratory problems. As a result of aforementioned studies, these changes in postural alignment in people with breast cancer should be taken into account in the assessment, follow-up, and rehabilitation program when planning the management of the disease.

14.2.2 Pain and Myofascial Dysfunction

Upper body pain is a common problem among BCS. Pain limits physical functioning, reduces quality of life, and has adverse psychosocial effects [19]. About 25–60% of BCS report the presence of pain [20]. Modern breast cancer treatment includes surgery of the breast (lumpectomy and mastectomy), axillary interventions (sentinel lymph node biopsy and axillary lymph node dissection), and adjuvant therapies such as radiotherapy, chemotherapy, and endocrine therapy. These may contribute to the development of pain with different characteristics [21–23]. Treatment-related central sensitization of perceive pain has been reported in people with breast cancer [24, 25] (Fig. 14.2). A decrease in the pressure pain threshold and increased pain sensitivity in the upper trunk have been reported as signs of this condition. Caro-Morán et al. [26] conducted a study to determine the sensitivity of the anterior and dorsal parts of the shoulder region to tenderness in BCS. They found lower pressure pain thresholds in the upper part of the upper trapezius muscle (at the site of musculotendinous insertion), the anterior part of the deltoid muscle and the pectoralis tendon compared to healthy controls.

Approximately 44.8% of BCS experience myofascial pain, which can be defined as intense, deep pain originating in one or more muscles or fasciae [27]. The fascial system is a structural component, support unit, and framework for posture and mobility with its rich sympathetic innervation. Functions of fascial system are to support, stabilize and cushion the musculoskeletal system. After surgery, as a defensive response to trauma, the fascia tightens, loses flexibility, and becomes constricted, thereby causing pain [28].

14.2.3 Decreased Range of Motion

Breast cancer treatment modalities affect the entire neuromuscular, musculoskeletal, and lymphovascular systems through complex interrelated processes, especially around the shoulder girdle, resulting in a reduced range of motion of the arm, shoulder, and neck [26] (Fig. 14.3). BCS may experience postoperative scarring, nerve dysfunction, protective posture, and shortening of the soft tissues of the anterior chest wall, including the pectoralis major and minor muscles [8]. In addition, radiotherapy (i.e. supraclavicular site) can cause skin changes, fibrosis, and stiffness, which all can affect the extensibility of the neck muscles. Shortening of the pectoral muscles

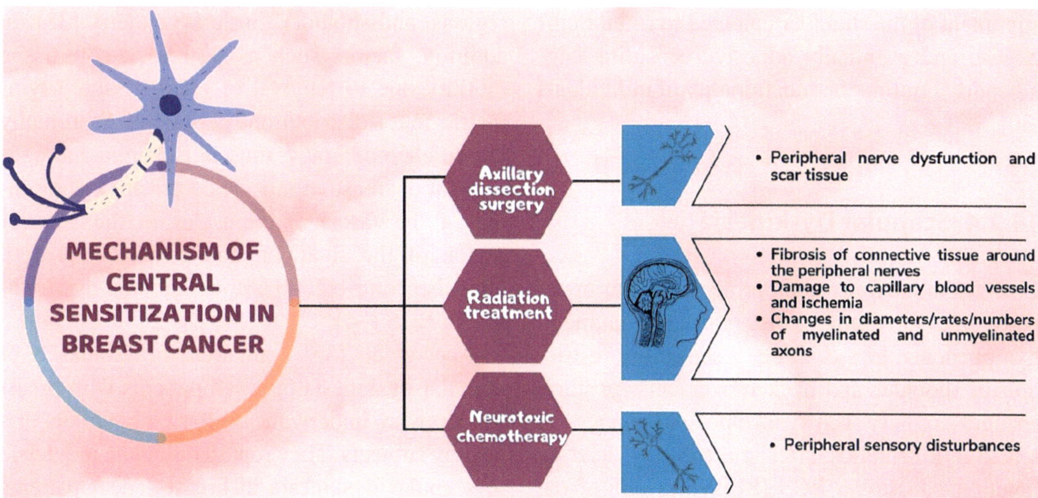

Fig. 14.2 Possible mechanisms of treatment related central sensitization in breast cancer

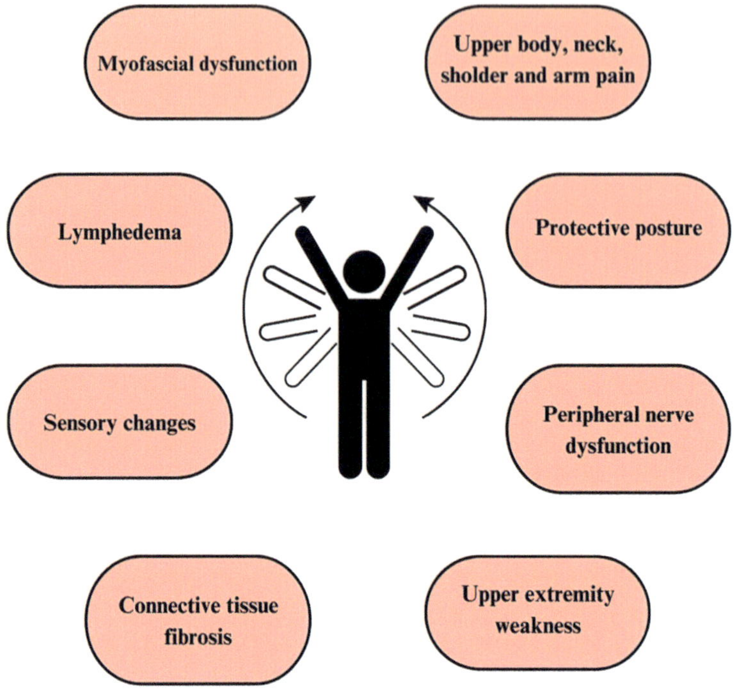

Fig. 14.3 Factors affecting range of motion in relation to breast cancer treatment

and associated soft tissues can cause the shoulder girdle to be positioned forward, and soft tissue fibrosis from radiotherapy can aggravate this misalignment [21, 29]. These changes are thought to affect the size of the subacromial space, increasing stress on the structures crossing this space and altering the biomechanics of the shoulder and neck, causing pain, reduced joint mobility, and dysfunction. In particular, misalignment of the shoulder can lead to rotator cuff disease and eventually adhesive capsulitis, significantly limiting the functionality of individuals [30].

14.2.4 Scapular Dyskinesia

Changes in anatomy and biomechanics of upper body are common after cancer treatment. Lymphedema, loss of axillary sensation, restriction in shoulder and neck movements, postural changes, axillary web syndrome, and changes in scapular kinematics after mastectomy lead to functional losses in BCS [8]. WS is one of the most common physical problems after radical mastectomies, especially after removing axillary lymph nodes and damage to the thoracic nerve innervating the serratus anterior muscle [31]. In a systematic review, the global incidence of WS was reported as 16.79% in BCS [32].

Scapular dyskinesia, characterized by scapular winging and/or abnormal scapular rhythm during function, can cause loss of function in the upper extremities and neck, pain in associated regions, and shoulder girdle asymmetry [33]. In addition, factors such as decreased soft tissue motility due to removal of breast tissue, asymmetric mass distribution, peripheral neuropathy due to chemotherapy, muscle ischemia and consequent decrease in muscle contraction, shortening of the fascia and muscles in the anterior region of the shoulder, and protective posture may also contribute to scapulohumeral dysrhythmia in BCS [34].

Acet et al. [35] compared the incidence of scapular dyskinesia between patients with breast cancer who underwent axillary dissection and healthy subjects. They reported that the incidence of scapular dyskinesia in breast cancer patients was 53.06% which was significantly higher compared to the control group Zabit et al. [36] compared healthy controls with mastectomized breast cancer patients and found that the incidence of scapular dyskinesia were 63.64% and 3.03% in breast cancer patients and healthy controls, respectively. Considering these higher rates, it can be said that it would be beneficial to include scapular dyskinesia in clinical evaluations and to study it in detail.

14.2.5 Cervical Radiculopathy

Cervical radiculopathy is an important cause of neck pain, upper limb pain, and muscle weakness in BCS [29]. Although cervical radiculopathy in these individuals is not directly related to the cancer and its treatments, it may mimic or aggravate other conditions (i.e. perceived pain, compensated posture, rotator cuff weakness). Pain associated with radiculopathy may be neuropathic in origin, following a dermatomal distribution of the affected nerve root(s). Alternatively, it may be caused by muscle spasms within the myotome of the affected nerve root(s). Both neuropathic and myofascial pain can often coexist in people with radiculopathy. People with breast cancer may have radiculopathy due to neurotoxic chemotherapy. It can cause pain and weakness in the upper extremities if the cervical nerve root is involved [37]. In particular, when the upper (C5-6) cervical nerve root is involved, pain may be radiated to the upper lateral aspect of the arm, thereafter the rotator cuff muscles may weaken, leading to shoulder dysfunction, rotator cuff impingement and adhesive capsulitis [8].

14.2.6 Muscle Weakness

Diminished upper extremity and periscapular muscle strength are one of the significant problems associated with mastectomy, axillary lymphadenectomy, and adjuvant therapies. Some chemotherapeutic agents (i.e., taxanes) cause oxidative stress in skeletal muscles, resulting in muscle weakness and increased fatigue [38]. The trapezius, rhomboid major and minor, pectoralis major and minor, serratus anterior, and latissimus dorsi muscles are often affected in strength in patients receiving chemotherapy [39, 40]. Studies have reported that scapula alata develops as a result of potential damage to the long thoracic nerve and/or serratus anterior muscle during axillary lymphadenectomy [41]. While the potential effects of surgery on the muscles are more commonly emphasized in the existing studies in the literature, it is thought that scapular dyskinesia may also occur as a result of radiotherapy to the trapezius, rhomboid, and serratus anterior muscles, which may lead to a decrease in muscle strength. One study [36] compared the physical characteristics, upper extremity function, and quality of life of BCS and healthy individuals. The results showed that the prevalence of scapular dyskinesia was higher in BCS. Upper extremity muscle strength, upper extremity function, and varied quality of life subscales were reduced in BCS compared to healthy women. The authors also suggested that the higher prevalence of scapular dyskinesia may be due to reduced scapular muscle strength.

14.2.7 Lymphedema

Lymphoedema is caused by a disruption of the lymphatic system, initially leading to the accumulation of protein-rich fluid in the interstitial space and eventually manifesting itself clinically as chronic swelling of the arm, breast, shoulder, neck, and/or trunk [42]. The estimated incidence of lymphedema is between 6% and 30%, and in most cases, it occurs within the first 6 months after surgery [43]. In addition to limb swelling, lymphedema can cause heaviness, skin changes, joint immobility, susceptibility to infection, and various other sequelae. Lymphedema is not usually painful but may predispose the patient to other painful conditions such as rotator cuff disease and adhesive capsulitis [29].

In summary, BCS have varied upper body and neck problems that affect their functionality and quality of life due to the side effects of multimodal treatment. Complex processes in the skin, lymphovascular, neuromuscular, and musculoskeletal systems can cause these problems. Therefore, it would be beneficial to plan and determine individualized treatment programs for the management of upper body and neck problems with a comprehensive clinical assessment of these contributing systems.

14.3 Physiotherapy and Rehabilitation in Upper Back and Neck Problems

Today, despite major advances in pharmaceutical and surgical technologies, pain and reduced quality of life in cancer patients are still recognized as major problems that need to be addressed. Many cancer patients develop opioid intolerance due to pain. The World Health Organization (WHO) defines opioid-tolerant patients as "patients taking at least 60 mg of oral morphine per day, 25 μg of transdermal fentanyl per hour, 30 mg of oral oxycodone per day, 8 mg of oral hydromorphone per day, 25 mg of oral oxymorphone per day, or an equianalgesic dose of another opioid for 1 week or more" [44]. Sometimes patients may have a condition or intolerance to opioid use.

In conclusion, physiotherapy and rehabilitation modalities have an important role to play in relieving pain and other symptoms in cancer patients. In cancer rehabilitation, it is important to understand whether pain or other symptoms are caused by an oncological condition [45]. In particular, any tumor-related fracture or metastasis should be excluded. Patients diagnosed with breast cancer may need physiotherapy and rehabilitation during chemotherapy, radiotherapy, other pharmacological treatments, or after surgery for upper back and neck problems [46]. The physiotherapeutic approaches used in this group of patients are summarized in this section.

14.3.1 Exercise Approaches

Exercise is the most commonly used physiotherapy modality for cervical and upper thoracic problems related to breast cancer and can be given for a variety of purposes. These goals may vary according to the patient's clinical condition and the stage of diagnosis or treatment. Depending on the purpose and the muscles involved, range of motion, stretching, strengthening, relaxation, stabilization, and aerobic exercise may be preferred. Alternative approaches such as Nordic walking, aquatic exercise, yoga, Pilates, Tai chi, and dance therapy may also be used. During breast cancer treatment, especially after surgery, the biomechanical alignment of the body can adversely be affected. This can lead to postural problems, myofascial dysfunction, decreased range of motion, and upper back and cervical pain which were discussed previously [47]. The primary aims of the exercise program in this case are to prevent the adverse effects of the disease or its treatment, to correct the impaired biomechanical alignment, to increase the range of motion of the joint that is restricted for various reasons, to reduce pain, and to improve the level of function.

In addition to anatomical and biomechanical problems, cancer patients may also experience cardiopulmonary problems, fatigue, and psychosocial issues. As a result, the clinical presentation of cancer patients is complex and multifaceted. Therefore, exercise programs typically serve multiple purposes. There is low-level evidence that exercise reduces mortality and recurrence specifically for breast cancer [48–50]. There is moderate- to high-level evidence for the beneficial effects of exercise on pain, fatigue, functional status, and quality of life in patients with breast cancer [49, 51, 52]. In addition, these interventions have been shown to have positive effects as well as reducing the risk of complications related to the disease, surgery, or other treatments [52–54]. According to the practice guidelines, participating in an exercise program is generally not recommended in case of severe fatigue, anemia, or ataxia [48].

14.3.2 General Principles of Exercise Practices

It is important to understand the disease management process and potential complications that may arise in breast cancer patients, as their clinical presentation and treatment complications differ from those of people experiencing pain for other reasons. In addition, when prescribing exercise, it is important to carefully determine the frequency, intensity, time, and type (FITT) parameters [55]. Aerobic exercise is generally preferred at an intensity between 50% and 75% of the heart rate reserve or between 11 and 14 according to the rating of perceived exertion. Aerobic exercise can be safely used during or after chemotherapy in people with cancer [55, 56]. It is important to note that for patients using beta-blockers, it is recommended to adjust the intensity to 40–45% of maximum heart rate or rating of perceived exertion to 13 [55]. The appropriate timing of postoperative exercise in breast cancer patients may vary depending on the type and purpose of the exercise since there is a need for early mobilization with the importance of allowing sufficient time for healing and recovery. In this manner, it is recommended that stretching exercises can be initiated as early as the first week after surgery, while progressive strengthening exercises should be postponed until the fourth to sixth week after surgery [57]. It is important to carefully determine the parameters of strengthening exercises to avoid side effects or excessive fatigue due to the "loading principle" feature of these exercises. According to the literature, these exercises are usually recommended for 2–3 times a week.

Resistance is usually determined using the 1 repetition maximum (1RM) method. The program is usually designed as one set of 10–12 repetitions at 50% of 1RM for the first few weeks. During the second week, it is recommended to increase the number of sets to 2. In the fourth week, it is recommended to gradually increase the weight to 75% of 1RM [58, 59]. Given the highly variable clinical status of cancer patients during and after treatment, it is crucial to monitor patients closely and to adjust exercise prescription accordingly. This dynamic process must be considered to ensure the best possible therapeutic outcomes [60]. As with many other medical issues, it is important to prioritize the principle of doing no harm when rehabilitating people with cancer. By following aforementioned guidelines, we can ensure the safety and well-being of people undergoing cancer rehabilitation. To achieve this, it is important to understand and follow the principles outlined in the current guidelines. These guidelines provide important information about 'things to look out for' during exercise program (Table 14.1).

14.3.3 Exercise Applications for Upper Back and Neck Regions

Studies have shown that a personalized exercise program can reduce pain severity and improve spinal alignment and posture in the upper back and neck. In a study conducted by Rao et al., 22 BCS participated in a 3-week exercise program and completed 12 sessions of myofascial release following. The study aimed to increase the strength of several muscles, including the trapezius, rhomboid, supraspinatus, and serratus anterior, while also stretching the upper trapezius and levator scapula muscles. The strengthening program was designed to be of low to moderate intensity, with each exercise consisting of two sets of ten repetitions. The stretching exercises required participants to hold the stretching position for 45 s and perform 3 repetitions with 15 s of rest in between. The program resulted in observed improvements in posture and spinal curvature, improvements in neck and shoulder pain and increases in range of motion, strength, and quality of life [28]. According to a study published in 2020, upper body and joint stabilization exercises were performed in the pool and on land in breast cancer survivors. Aquatic exercises were found to be more tolerable and more effective for postural correction [62]. Another study of 66 BCS showed that 8 weeks (24 sessions) of supervised low-intensity aquatic exercise provided more improvement in neck pain and trigger points in the upper trapezius, sternocleidomastoid and levator scapula muscles than traditional exercise. The content of the exercises in this study were reported to be as follows: an hour-long session consisted of a 10-min warm up at a slow pace, stretching exercises, 35 min of low-level endurance and core stabilization exercises,

Table 14.1 Factors to consider when designing an exercise program for breast cancer patients

• The exercise program is a versatile treatment option that can be used at any stage of breast cancer treatment, including during chemotherapy, radiotherapy, other pharmacological treatments as well as after surgery
• When a patient is undergoing hormone therapy, it is important to thoroughly review his/her assessment and rehabilitation program to identify any potential risk of fractures
• It is important to ensure that there is no metastasis to any part of the body. If so, the assessment and rehabilitation process may need to be reviewed
• It is advisable to have an examination of the upper extremities, shoulders, upper back, and neck to identify any underlying conditions before beginning an exercise
• It may take up to 8 weeks before you can start exercising after surgery, and you should consult your physiotherapist and doctor
• It should be noted that people with cancer may have an increased risk of cardiovascular events during exercise compared to healthy people
• It is recommended that medical treatment should be given prior to any exercise program or physiotherapy approach in case of a secondary complication of cancer arising in the upper extremity or shoulder
• If there is any visible swelling or increase in symptoms in the upper extremity or shoulder, it is recommended that the upper body exercise program stopped and the patient is referred to a doctor
• It is recommended that patients with lymphedema should wear compression garments during exercise
• It is recommended that the Borg rating of perceived exertion scale is used to assess fatigue during exercise
• It is important to recognize that patients' exercise tolerance may vary from session to session. Therefore it is important to monitor their progress closely
• It is recommended that a one repetition maximum (1-RM) test is done before performing strengthening exercises. It is important to note that the 1-RM test is safe for patients with breast cancer and those at risk of lymphedema
• If strengthening exercises are interrupted for any reason, it is recommended that the intensity of the exercise for each interrupted week should be the same as that of the previous 2 weeks. This will help to maintain progress and prevent setbacks
• Yoga is safe, provided that upper limb complications are taken into account
• There is insufficient evidence for Pilates or other specialized sports [61]

Table 14.2 The most common exercise barriers in patients with breast cancer [59]

Treatment-related illness
Conflicting appointment
Non-treatment-related illness
Surgery
Hospitalization
Work
Difficult prescription
Staff error in providing prescription

and then relaxation exercises focused on the neck and shoulder region for the last 15 min. The exercises were gradually increased in intensity and duration over 8 weeks [63]. A study investigated the effects of Nordic walking, aquatic exercise, and general exercise on sagittal posture in 60 BCS. All three-exercise program were scheduled in a similar way for 8 weeks. For the aquatic exercise content, balance coordination exercises were used after strengthening the abdominal, back and extremity muscles. Resistance in the water was increased by walking forward and backward. Nordic walking was found to be the most effective method of reducing thoracic kyphosis. In the aquatic exercise group, it was found that kyphotic posture decreased but lumbar lordosis increased. General exercises had no significant effect on kyphotic posture [64].

In conclusion, the literature on exercise interventions for upper back and neck problems is limited but provides valuable information. Exercise programs were generally adjusted to low or low-moderate intensity. Exercise can be used both during and after breast cancer treatment. According to the researchers, there is a need for studies to determine the optimal dose of the neck and upper back exercises, especially in patients with breast cancer. In addition, many studies indicate that there are serious barriers to exercise participation and adherence in this patient population (Table 14.2). The most common of these barriers are treatment-related problems (fatigue, nausea, dizziness, etc.) (33%) [59]. Clearly, future research is needed to better define these barriers and the steps to these barriers overcome.

14.3.4 Manual Therapy

Some manual therapy techniques may relatively be contraindicated in cancer patients according to several studies [65, 66]. However, there are also studies reporting that manual therapy increases the range of motion in breast, neck, and head cancer survivors [66, 67]. Myofascial tension in breast cancer patients can lead to neck and upper back problems. Manual therapy techniques have been shown to have a positive effect on pain and quality of life [68]. Myofascial release techniques, ischemic compression, and Maitland's mobilization techniques (grades 1–2) are the most commonly used muscle energy techniques in the context of manual therapy [68]. In a study of 21 BCS receiving adjuvant therapy, one session of myofascial induction therapy to optimize the fascial system was associated with a reduction in neck pain and an increase in range of motion. In another study of 44 BCS, multimodal therapy consisting of manual therapy (massage) and exercise was shown to reduce pain and general hyperalgesia in the shoulder and neck region [69]. Many important parameters, such as the level of pressure applied during manual therapy, hand position, and how to monitor tissue response, remain to be investigated in the literature. However, experts in the field agree that contact during manual therapy for BCS should be prolonged (120–300 s), gentle, and painless [70].

14.3.5 Electrotherapy

Many electrical and electrotherapeutic agents are avoided in cancer patients to prevent potential recurrence and side effects. Laser therapy, electrical stimulation, microwave, and thermal therapy are not recommended due to insufficient evidence to support their use and considered to be contraindicated in patients with neoplasms [57]. Therapeutic ultrasound is strictly contraindicated even in patients who are not at risk of metastasis, as it increases cellular activity [57]. However, transcutaneous electrical nerve stimulation (TENS) can be used safely for regional pain associated with cancer. The National Comprehensive Cancer Network has reached a consensus that TENS is particularly useful for people who cannot take analgesics because of contraception or for whom medication is ineffective [57]. Peripheral neuropathy is a serious problem that significantly reduces the quality of life of cancer patients. TENS has been shown to be an effective method for the management of cancer-related neuropathic pain. Yong et al. investigated the effect of low frequency electrical stimulation on peripheral neuropathy in breast cancer patients following chemotherapy. The application was performed for at least 120 min per day for more than 14 days. According to the results, the pain caused by peripheral neuropathy decreased. It was reported that no serious adverse effects were observed during the study and only 19 out of 36 people experienced mild to moderate side effects (diarrhea, lymphedema, limb edema, flu-like symptoms, febrile neutropenia, back pain, gastritis, pain in the extremities, adhesive capsulitis of the shoulder and dermatitis) [71]. A protocol study published in 2022 examines the effect of TENS on proinflammatory cytokines applied to the upper back and neck. The hypothesis of this study, the results of which have not yet been published, is that a single 30-min session of TENS applied to the upper back and neck will reduce pain and the level of serum proinflammatory cytokines [72]. Scrambler therapy, which has become popular in recent years, is also used for cancer-related pain and results are showing that it is able to reduce pain [73, 74].

14.3.6 Complementary Therapies

In recent years, holistic approaches have been favored for cancer patients due to the nature and course of the disease. A review of the literature shows that complementary therapies are frequently used in cancer survivors [75–77]. Pilates exercises are recommended as a complementary therapy for cancer patients. The main purpose of using this approach in breast cancer patients is to strengthen the mind–body relationship, increase body awareness, maintain and correct spinal alignment and flexibility. It also provides relaxation, stress control and pain relief because it is performed in conjunction with breathing [78]. A study published in 2021 examined the effect of Pilates exercises, performed 3 days a week for 16 weeks, on the posture of breast cancer patients receiving hormone therapy. Each exercise session was planned to have 10 min of warm-up, 40 min of exercise and 10 min of relaxation, as recommended in the guidelines for breast cancer patients. The results of the study showed that this program had positive effects on postural alignment [79]. Another complementary approach used in breast cancer patients is yoga. In a study of 28 patients with breast cancer-related lymphedema, patients attended a 90-min weekly yoga session with a yoga instructor and practiced yoga on video for 45 min at home daily. The exercises in the yoga session were chosen according to the principles of engaging the spinal stabilizing muscles while focusing on gentle joint movements of the shoulder and spine, posture, and kinematic movement patterns. According to the results of this research, there was an improvement in postural alignment and an increase in upper extremity muscle strength after an 8-week yoga program [80]. In a study of 10 postmenopausal women with stage 1–3 breast cancer, a yoga program was practiced of 2 days a week for 8 weeks. Results showed that back flexibility and postural stability increased and pain decreased [81]. In addition, yoga has many general positive effects, such as reducing regional pain, stress, anxiety, sleep problems, and fatigue as well as increasing muscle strength and postural control in people with breast cancer [82]. Tai chi is another complementary approach often favored by breast cancer patients. In a study of 12 BCS included, Tai Chi was shown to have beneficial effects on strength and mobility of shoulder [83]. However, no study investigated the effects of Tai Chi on the spine in breast cancer. Nevertheless, there is still a need for studies in high level evidence, particularly on complementary approaches based on mind-body integrity.

14.3.7 Preventive Rehabilitation and Physical Activity

It is well known that the upper back and neck, spinal alignment, and posture of breast cancer patients are negatively affected during treatment. Patients have to cope with many problems, including spinal problems caused by the cancer and its treatment. Treatment of additional problems is therefore difficult in the long term. In this respect, approaches to prevent possible problems are very important for cancer patients [84]. In recent years, several physiotherapeutic approaches have been developed in the literature to prevent spinal misalignment and a range of related problems. A study of 94 BCS included, it was reported that these approaches have the capability to reduce the risk of developing side effects in related structures [84, 85]. Although there is a paucity of literature on preventive rehabilitation, the most commonly used modality is exercise training. Regular physical activity has been shown to have a positive effect on maintaining body alignment and trunk symmetry, as well as stabilizing effect on the scapula and shoulder girdle in post-mastectomy women [15]. Studies emphasize that the preventive use of scapular and spinal stabilization, strengthening and stretching exercises should also be assessed for safety [84, 86]. Guidelines in this area state that the risk of spinal problems caused by cancer and its treatment can be reduced by performing 150 min of moderate-intensity or 75 min of vigorous aerobic exercise and large muscle strengthening exercises at least twice a week [55, 61, 87]. Another published guideline for cancer survivors reported that 20 min of moderate-intensity walking 3 days a week reduced the risk of both spine-related and generalized clinical outcomes [88]. Future studies are expected to focus more on preventive approaches, given the difficulty and cost of the management of cancer-related consequences [89].

14.4 Conclusion

The role of physiotherapy is utmost importance in increasing range of motion, reducing pain, maintaining and preserving physical performance, and improving condition, health and well-being in patients with breast cancer. Restoring postural stability, which is well known to be compromised after breast cancer, is one of the most important solutions for normal functioning. Physiotherapy can prevent further deterioration of the spine and general posture. It will also help prevent neck and surrounding problems. Physiotherapy will help to increase support, mobility, strength and knowledge, reduce pain, prevent and manage component changes due to lymphedema.

A multi-component exercise program is necessary to address multiple spinal conditions. In conclusion, considering that significant spinal dysfunction persists in breast cancer survivors, significant changes in spinal motion, decreased spinal stability, and disability in activities of daily living can be treated with exercise and various physiotherapy approaches.

References

1. Akram M, Iqbal M, Daniyal M, Khan AU. Awareness and current knowledge of breast cancer. Biol Res. 2017;50:1–23.
2. Ferlay J, Soerjomataram I, Dikshit R, Eser S, Mathers C, Rebelo M, et al. Cancer incidence and mortality worldwide: sources, methods and major patterns in GLOBOCAN 2012. Int J Cancer. 2015;136(5):E359–86.
3. Siegel RL, Miller KD, Wagle NS, Jemal A. Cancer statistics, 2023. CA Cancer J Clin. 2023;73(1):17–48.
4. Kocarnik JM, Compton K, Dean FE, Fu W, Gaw BL, Harvey JD, et al. Cancer incidence, mortality, years of life lost, years lived with disability, and disability-adjusted life years for 29 cancer groups from 2010 to 2019: a systematic analysis for the global burden of disease study 2019. JAMA Oncol. 2022;8(3):420–44.
5. Youlden DR, Cramb SM, Dunn NA, Muller JM, Pyke CM, Baade PD. The descriptive epidemiology of female breast cancer: an international comparison of screening, incidence, survival and mortality. Cancer Epidemiol. 2012;36(3):237–48.
6. Lovelace DL, McDaniel LR, Golden D. Long-term effects of breast cancer surgery, treatment, and survivor care. J Midwifery Womens Health. 2019;64(6):713–24.
7. Bodai BI, Tuso P. Breast cancer survivorship: a comprehensive review of long-term medical issues and lifestyle recommendations. Perm J. 2015;19(2):48.
8. Stubblefield S, Keole N. Upper body pain and functional disorders in patients with breast cancer. PM R. 2014;6(2):170–83.
9. Malicka I, Barczyk K, Hanuszkiewicz J, Skolimowska B, Woźniewski M. Body posture of women after breast cancer treatment. Ortop Traumatol Rehabil. 2010;12(4):353–61.
10. Merson M, Pirovano C, Balzarini A, Luini A, Biasi S, Galimberti V, et al. The preservation of minor pectoralis muscle in axillary dissection for breast cancer: functional and cosmetic evaluation. Eur J Surg Oncol. 1992;18(3):215–8.
11. Brooks C. Radiation therapy: guidelines for physiotherapists. Physiotherapy. 1998;84(8):387–95.
12. Visovsky C. Muscle strength, body composition, and physical activity in women receiving chemotherapy for breast cancer. Integr Cancer Ther. 2006;5(3):183–91.
13. Koçan S, Gürsoy A. Body image of women with breast cancer after mastectomy: a qualitative research. J Breast Health. 2016;12(4):145.
14. Chwałczyńska A, Woźniewski M, Rozek-Mróz K, Malicka I. Quality of life in women after mastectomy. Wiad Lek. 2004;57(5–6):212–6.
15. Rostkowska E, Bak M, Samborski W. Body posture in women after mastectomy and its changes as a result of rehabilitation. Adv Med Sci. 2006;51(2):287–97.
16. Ciesla S, Bak M. The effect of breast reconstruction on maintaining a proper body posture in patients after mastectomy. In: Breast reconstruction—current techniques. London: IntechOpen; 2012. p. 83–102.
17. Serel S, Tuzlalı ZY, Akkaya Z, Uzun Ç, Kaya B, Bayar S. Physical effects of unilateral mastectomy on spine deformity. Clin Breast Cancer. 2017;17(1):29–33.
18. Celenay ST, Ucurum SG, Kaya DO. Comparison of spinal alignment and mobility in women with and without post modified radical mastectomy unilateral lymphoedema. Clin Breast Cancer. 2020;20(3):e295–300.
19. Moloney N, Sung JMW, Kilbreath S, Dylke E. Prevalence and risk factors associated with pain 21 months following surgery for breast cancer. Support Care Cancer. 2016;24:4533–9.
20. Gärtner R, Jensen M-B, Nielsen J, Ewertz M, Kroman N, Kehlet H. Prevalence of and factors associated with persistent pain following breast cancer surgery. JAMA. 2009;302(18):1985–92.
21. Cheville AL, Tchou J. Barriers to rehabilitation following surgery for primary breast cancer. J Surg Oncol. 2007;95(5):409–18.

22. Johansson S, Svensson H, Larsson L-G, Denekamp J. Brachial plexopathy after postoperative radiotherapy of breast cancer patients: a long-term follow-up. Acta Oncol. 2000;39(3):373–82.
23. Andersen KG, Jensen M-B, Kehlet H, Gärtner R, Eckhoff L, Kroman N. Persistent pain, sensory disturbances and functional impairment after adjuvant chemotherapy for breast cancer: cyclophosphamide, epirubicin and fluorouracil compared with docetaxel + epirubicin and cyclophosphamide. Acta Oncol. 2012;51(8):1036–44.
24. Fernandez-Lao C, Cantarero-Villanueva I, Fernández-de-Las-Peñas C, Del-Moral-Avila R, Arendt-Nielsen L, Arroyo-Morales M. Myofascial trigger points in neck and shoulder muscles and widespread pressure pain hypersensitivtiy in patients with postmastectomy pain: evidence of peripheral and central sensitization. Clin J Pain. 2010;26(9):798–806.
25. Caro-Morán E, Díaz-Rodríguez L, Cantarero-Villanueva I, Galiano-Castillo N, Arroyo-Morales M, Fernández-Lao C. Nerve pressure pain hypersensitivity and upper limb mechanosensitivity in breast cancer survivors: a case–control study. Pain Med. 2014;15(10):1715–23.
26. Caro-Morán E, Fernández-Lao C, Diaz-Rodriguez L, Cantarero-Villanueva I, Madeleine P, Arroyo-Morales M. Pressure pain sensitivity maps of the neck-shoulder region in breast cancer survivors. Pain Med. 2016;17(10):1942–52.
27. Lacomba MT, Del Moral OM, Zazo JLC, Gerwin RD, Goñí AZ. Incidence of myofascial pain syndrome in breast cancer surgery: a prospective study. Clin J Pain. 2010;26(4):320–5.
28. Rao MS, Pattanshetty RB. Effect of myofascial release, stretching, and strengthening on upper torso posture, spinal curvatures, range of motion, strength, shoulder pain and disability, and quality of life in breast cancer survivors. Physiother Res Int. 2022;27(2):e1939.
29. Stubblefield MD, Custodio CM. Upper-extremity pain disorders in breast cancer. Arch Phys Med Rehabil. 2006;87(3):96–9.
30. Ebaugh D, Spinelli B, Schmitz KH. Shoulder impairments and their association with symptomatic rotator cuff disease in breast cancer survivors. Med Hypotheses. 2011;77(4):481–7.
31. Rizzi SK, Haddad CAS, Giron PS, Pinheiro TL, Nazário ACP, Facina G. Winged scapula incidence and upper limb morbidity after surgery for breast cancer with axillary dissection. Support Care Cancer. 2016;24:2707–15.
32. Plaza Meza MP, Marín Fermín T, Maffulli N. Diagnosis and epidemiology of winged scapula in breast cancer patients: a systematic review and meta-analysis. Br Med Bull. 2021;140(1):23–35.
33. Lin J, Lim HK, Yang JL. Effect of shoulder tightness on glenohumeral translation, scapular kinematics, and scapulohumeral rhythm in subjects with stiff shoulders. J Orthop Res. 2006;24(5):1044–51.
34. Lee CH, Chung SY, Kim WY, Yang SN. Effect of breast cancer surgery on chest tightness and upper limb dysfunction. Medicine. 2019;98(19):e15524.
35. Acet N, Guzel NA, Keser I, Kurukahvecioglu O. Scapular dyskinesis in patients with breast cancer. Ann Med Res. 2020;27:2311.
36. Zabit F, Iyigun G. A comparison of physical characteristics, functions and quality of life between breast cancer survivor women who had a mastectomy and healthy women. J Back Musculoskelet Rehabil. 2019;32(6):937–45.
37. Caridi JM, Pumberger M, Hughes AP. Cervical radiculopathy: a review. HSS J. 2011;7(3):265–72.
38. Gilliam LA, St. Clair DK. Chemotherapy-induced weakness and fatigue in skeletal muscle: the role of oxidative stress. Antioxid Redox Signal. 2011;15(9):2543–63.
39. Gerber L, Lampert M, Wood C, Duncan M, D'Angelo T, Schain W, et al. Comparison of pain, motion, and edema after modified radical mastectomy vs. local excision with axillary dissection and radiation. Breast Cancer Res Treat. 1992;21:139–45.
40. Shamley DR, Srinanaganathan R, Weatherall R, Oskrochi R, Watson M, Ostlere S, et al. Changes in shoulder muscle size and activity following treatment for breast cancer. Breast Cancer Res Treat. 2007;106:19–27.
41. Duncan MA, Lotze MT, Gerber LH, Rosenberg SA. Incidence, recovery, and management of serratus anterior muscle palsy after axillary node dissection. Phys Ther. 1983;63(8):1243–7.
42. Hayes SC, Johansson K, Stout NL, Prosnitz R, Armer JM, Gabram S, et al. Upper-body morbidity after breast cancer: incidence and evidence for evaluation, prevention, and management within a prospective surveillance model of care. Cancer. 2012;118(S8):2237–49.
43. McNeely ML, Binkley JM, Pusic AL, Campbell KL, Gabram S, Soballe PW. A prospective model of care for breast cancer rehabilitation: postoperative and postreconstructive issues. Cancer. 2012;118(S8):2226–36.
44. Cherny NI, Fallon MT. Opioid therapy. In: Oxford textbook of palliative medicine. Oxford: Oxford University Press; 2021. p. 372.
45. Swarm RA, Paice JA, Anghelescu DL, Are M, Bruce JY, Buga S, et al. Adult cancer pain, version 3.2019, NCCN clinical practice guidelines in oncology. J Natl Compr Cancer Netw. 2019;17(8):977–1007.
46. Ficarra S, Thomas E, Bianco A, Gentile A, Thaller P, Grassadonio F, et al. Impact of exercise interventions on physical fitness in breast cancer patients and survivors: a systematic review. Breast Cancer. 2022;29(3):402–18.
47. Ucurum SG, Felekoglu E, Naz I, Kaya DO, Bayram KB, Alacacioglu A. Investigation of the relationship between spinal posture and mobility to respiratory muscle strength and pulmonary functions in unilateral breast cancer surgery survivors: a cross-sectional study. Support Care Cancer. 2023;31(12):714.

48. del-Rosal-Jurado A, Romero-Galisteo R, Trinidad-Fernández M, González-Sánchez M, Cuesta-Vargas A, Ruiz-Muñoz M. Therapeutic physical exercise post-treatment in breast cancer: a systematic review of clinical practice guidelines. J Clin Med. 2020;9(4):1239.
49. Santos WD, Gentil P, de Moraes RF, Ferreira Junior JB, Campos MH, de Lira CA, et al. Chronic effects of resistance training in breast cancer survivors. Biomed Res Int. 2017;2017:8367803.
50. Gradishar WJ, Anderson BO, Balassanian R, Blair SL, Burstein HJ, Cyr A, et al. Breast cancer, version 4.2017, NCCN clinical practice guidelines in oncology. J Natl Compr Cancer Netw. 2018;16(3):310–20.
51. Yeo S, An S, Cheong I, Park W, Hwang J. Changes in muscle tone and stiffness around shoulder associated with radiotherapy in breast cancer patients. Ann Phys Rehabil Med. 2018;61:e142.
52. Runowicz C, Leach C, Henry N, Henry K, Mackey H, Cowens-Alvarado R, et al. American Cancer Society/American Society of Clinical Oncology breast cancer survivorship care guideline. J Clin Oncol. 2016;34:611–35.
53. Meneses-Echávez JF, Correa-Bautista JE, González-Jiménez E, Schmidt Rio-Valle J, Elkins MR, Lobelo F, et al. The effect of exercise training on mediators of inflammation in breast cancer survivors: a systematic review with meta-analysis. Cancer Epidemiol Biomarkers Prev. 2016;25(7):1009–17.
54. Kyu HH, Bachman VF, Alexander LT, Mumford JE, Afshin A, Estep K, et al. Physical activity and risk of breast cancer, colon cancer, diabetes, ischemic heart disease, and ischemic stroke events: systematic review and dose-response meta-analysis for the global burden of disease study 2013. BMJ. 2016;354:i3857.
55. Kirkham AA, Bonsignore A, Bland KA, McKenzie DC, Gelmon KA, Van Patten CL, et al. Exercise prescription and adherence for breast cancer: one size does not FITT all. Med Sci Sports Exerc. 2018;50(2):177–86.
56. Courneya KS, Mackey JR, Jones LW. Coping with cancer: can exercise help? Phys Sportsmed. 2000;28(5):49–73.
57. Harris SR, Schmitz KH, Campbell KL, McNeely ML. Clinical practice guidelines for breast cancer rehabilitation: syntheses of guideline recommendations and qualitative appraisals. Cancer. 2012;118(S8):2312–24.
58. Courneya KS, McKenzie DC, Mackey JR, Gelmon K, Friedenreich CM, Yasui Y, et al. Effects of exercise dose and type during breast cancer chemotherapy: multicenter randomized trial. J Natl Cancer Inst. 2013;105(23):1821–32.
59. Gerland L, Baumann FT, Niels T. Resistance exercise for breast cancer patients? Evidence from the last decade. Breast Care. 2021;16(6):657–63.
60. Medeiros Torres D, Jorge Koifman R, da Silva SS. Impact on fatigue of different types of physical exercise during adjuvant chemotherapy and radiotherapy in breast cancer: systematic review and meta-analysis. Support Care Cancer. 2022;30(6):4651–62.
61. Schmitz KH, Courneya KS, Matthews C, Demark-Wahnefried W, Galvão DA, Pinto BM, et al. American College of Sports Medicine roundtable on exercise guidelines for cancer survivors. Med Sci Sports Exerc. 2010;42(7):1409–26.
62. Hanuszkiewicz JM, Woźniewski M, Malicka I. The relationship between sagittal spinal curvatures and isokinetic trunk muscle endurance after aquatic exercise training in survivors of breast cancer. Acta Bioeng Biomech. 2020;22(1):21–30.
63. Cantarero-Villanueva I, Fernández-Lao C, Fernández-de-Las-Peñas C, Lopez-Barajas IB, Del-Moral-Ávila R, de la-Llave-Rincón AI, et al. Effectiveness of water physical therapy on pain, pressure pain sensitivity, and myofascial trigger points in breast cancer survivors: a randomized, controlled clinical trial. Pain Med. 2012;13(11):1509–19.
64. Hanuszkiewicz J, Malicka I, Barczyk-Pawelec K, Woźniewski M. Effects of selected forms of physical activity on body posture in the sagittal plane in women post breast cancer treatment. J Back Musculoskelet Rehabil. 2015;28(1):35–41.
65. Maltser S, Cristian A, Silver JK, Morris GS, Stout NL. A focused review of safety considerations in cancer rehabilitation. PM R. 2017;9(9):S415–28.
66. Yao C, Cheng Y, Zhu Q, Lv Z, Kong L, Fang M. Clinical evidence for the effects of manual therapy on cancer pain: a systematic review and meta-analysis. Evid Based Complement Alternat Med. 2021;2021:6678184.
67. Thomas A, D'Silva C, Mohandas L, Pais SM, Samuel SR. Effect of muscle energy techniques V/S active range of motion exercises on shoulder function post modified radical neck dissection in patients with head and neck cancer—a randomized clinical trial. Asian Pac J Cancer Prev. 2020;21(8):2389.
68. Pattanshetty RB, Patil SN. Role of manual therapy for neck pain and quality of life in head and neck cancer survivors: a systematic review. Indian J Palliat Care. 2022;28(1):99–112.
69. Fernández-Lao C, Cantarero-Villanueva I, Fernández-de-las-Peñas C, del Moral-Ávila R, Castro-Sánchez AM, Arroyo-Morales M. Effectiveness of a multidimensional physical therapy program on pain, pressure hypersensitivity, and trigger points in breast cancer survivors: a randomized controlled clinical trial. Clin J Pain. 2012;28(2):113–21.
70. Ajimsha M, Al-Mudahka NR, Al-Madzhar J. Effectiveness of myofascial release: systematic review of randomized controlled trials. J Bodyw Mov Ther. 2015;19(1):102–12.
71. Song SY, Park JH, Lee JS, Kim JR, Sohn EH, Jung MS, et al. A randomized, placebo-controlled trial evaluating changes in peripheral neuropathy and quality of life by using low-frequency electrostimulation on breast cancer patients treated with chemotherapy. Integr Cancer Ther. 2020;19:1534735420925519.

72. do Carmo Almeida TC, Zatta SM, da Silva Paiva L, de Carvalho LEW, Schoueri J, de Abreu LC, et al. Reduction on proinflammatory cytokines after application of transcutaneous electrical nerve stimulation (TENS) in patients with a breast cancer: a nonrandomized, open, and single-arm study protocol with paired analysis. Mediat Inflamm. 2022;2022:1350813.
73. Lee SC, Park KS, Moon JY, Kim EJ, Kim Y-C, Seo H, et al. An exploratory study on the effectiveness of "Calmare therapy" in patients with cancer-related neuropathic pain: a pilot study. Eur J Oncol Nurs. 2016;21:1–7.
74. Notaro P, Dell'Agnola CA, Dell'Agnola AJ, Amatu A, Bencardino KB, Siena S. Pilot evaluation of scrambler therapy for pain induced by bone and visceral metastases and refractory to standard therapies. Support Care Cancer. 2016;24:1649–54.
75. Stan DL, Collins NM, Olsen MM, Croghan I, Pruthi S. The evolution of mindfulness-based physical interventions in breast cancer survivors. Evid Based Complement Alternat Med. 2012;2012:758641.
76. Cheung MN, Loo TY. Tai Chi Chuan improves cytokine expression levels and quality of life in post chemotherapy breast cancer survivors. World J Adv Res Rev. 2021;10(3):322–33.
77. Saraswathi V, Latha S, Niraimathi K, Vidhubala E. Managing lymphedema, increasing range of motion, and quality of life through yoga therapy among breast cancer survivors: a systematic review. Int J Yoga. 2021;14(1):3.
78. Espíndula RC, Nadas GB, Rosa MID, Foster C, Araújo FC, Grande AJ. Pilates for breast cancer: a systematic review and meta-analysis. Rev Assoc Med Bras (1992). 2017;63(11):1006–12.
79. de Bem FT, Boing L, do Prado Baffa A, Borgatto AF, de Azevedo Guimarães AC. Mat Pilates method improve postural alignment women undergoing hormone therapy adjunct to breast cancer treatment. Clinical trial. Complement Ther Clin Pract. 2021;44:101424.
80. Loudon A, Barnett T, Piller N, Immink MA, Visentin D, Williams AD. The effects of yoga on shoulder and spinal actions for women with breast cancer-related lymphoedema of the arm: a randomised controlled pilot study. BMC Complement Altern Med. 2016;16(1):1–15.
81. Galantino ML, Desai K, Greene L, DeMichele A, Stricker CT, Mao JJ. Impact of yoga on functional outcomes in breast cancer survivors with aromatase inhibitor-associated arthralgias. Integr Cancer Ther. 2012;11(4):313–20.
82. Hsueh E-J, Loh E-W, Lin JJ-A, Tam K-W. Effects of yoga on improving quality of life in patients with breast cancer: a meta-analysis of randomized controlled trials. Breast Cancer. 2021;28:264–76.
83. Fong SS, Ng SS, Luk W, Chung JW, Chung LM, Tsang WW, et al. Shoulder mobility, muscular strength, and quality of life in breast cancer survivors with and without Tai Chi Qigong training. Evid Based Complement Alternat Med. 2013;2013:787169.
84. Rangel J, Perez C, Oliveira R, Guirro E. Effects of breast cancer treatment on posture: a current review. Int J Phys Ther Rehabil. 2019;5:152.
85. Rangel J, Tomás MT, Fernandes B. Physical activity and physiotherapy: perception of women breast cancer survivors. Breast Cancer. 2019;26(3):333–8.
86. Peres ACAM, de Oliveira Latorre MdRD, Maesaka JY, Filassi JR, Baracat EC, Ferreira EAG. Body posture after mastectomy: comparison between immediate breast reconstruction versus mastectomy alone. Physiother Res Int. 2017;22(1).
87. Piercy KL, Troiano RP, Ballard RM, Carlson SA, Fulton JE, Galuska DA, et al. The physical activity guidelines for Americans. JAMA. 2018;320(19):2020–8.
88. Campbell KL, Neil SE, Winters-Stone KM. Review of exercise studies in breast cancer survivors: attention to principles of exercise training. Br J Sports Med. 2012;46(13):909–16.
89. Kraschnewski JL, Schmitz KH. Exercise in the prevention and treatment of breast cancer: what clinicians need to tell their patients. Transl J Am Coll Sports Med. 2017;2(15):92–6.

Respiratory Problems and Management in Breast Cancer Survivors: What Should We Focus On?

15

Melda Saglam and Hamide Sahin Yildiz

15.1 Respiratory Challenges in Breast Cancer Survivors

As breast cancer treatment has advanced, survivors often face long-term health challenges, including respiratory issues. These respiratory challenges can arise from various factors, such as cancer itself, treatment-related complications, and other comorbidities.

Respiratory problems in breast cancer survivors (BCS) can manifest as dyspnea, reduced respiratory muscle strength, exercise intolerance, and impaired lung function. These issues can significantly impact survivors' quality of life, limiting their ability to perform daily activities and participate in physical exercise. Understanding and managing these respiratory challenges are essential to improving the overall health and well-being of BCS.

This chapter explores the respiratory challenges faced by BCS, focusing on the underlying causes, clinical manifestations, and impact on quality of life. Additionally, we discuss current approaches to managing these respiratory issues, including pulmonary rehabilitation and physical activity interventions. By highlighting these challenges and potential management strategies, we aim to provide valuable insights for healthcare providers and researchers working to improve the lives of BCS.

15.1.1 The Effects of Metastasis on Lungs

Metastatic breast cancer can have significant effects on the lungs, as breast cancer cells can spread to the lungs through the bloodstream or lymphatic system. Lung metastases have been found in 57–77% of individuals in autopsy research on breast cancer metastatic patterns [1, 2]. According to the reports, the median overall survival for patients with breast cancer who had only lung metastasis following systemic treatment was 22.5 months [3].

The process of metastasis involves the creation of a "pre-metastatic niche" in the secondary organ, a critical step for successful cancer cell colonization. This process unfolds in distinct phases: priming, licensing, initiation, and progression. During priming, tumor-derived factors target the bone marrow, triggering the remodeling of the secondary organ to create a more hospitable environment. Immune suppression and

M. Saglam (✉)
Faculty of Physical Therapy and Rehabilitation, Department of Cardiorespiratory Physiotherapy and Rehabilitation, Hacettepe University, Ankara, Turkey
e-mail: msaglam@hacettepe.edu.tr

H. Sahin Yildiz
Kizilcahamam Vocational School of Health Services, Department of Physical Therapy and Rehabilitation, Ankara University, Ankara, Turkey
e-mail: hmdsahin@ankara.edu.tr

Y. Bakar, A. Tuğral (eds.), *Managing Side Effects of Breast Cancer Treatment*,
https://doi.org/10.1007/978-3-031-75480-7_15

changes in the extracellular matrix further facilitate cancer cell colonization. Primary tumors of breast cancer influence lung metastasis by secreting factors that recruit bone marrow-derived cells to the lung, creating a conducive environment for metastasis. Further research is needed to identify biomarkers for predicting organ-specific metastasis, including the use of exosomes [4].

Metastasis in specific organs is influenced by the microenvironment of those organs. According to the hypothesis of Stephen Paget (1889), cancer cells (the "seed") preferentially grow in selected organs (the "soil") if conditions are favorable for growth. James Ewing proposed a competing theory in the early 1900s, suggesting that physiological blood flow patterns regulate organ-specific metastasis. For breast cancer, the lung's physical characteristics support Ewing's theory, as tumor cells encounter the lung's capillary bed first after entering the bloodstream. Although tumor cells can easily extravagate into the lung tissue, the transition to micro metastases, and macro metastases are rare and requires optimal collaboration between tumor cells and the lung microenvironment. Therefore, Paget's and Ewing's theories are likely complementary in understanding metastasis of breast cancer to the lung [5, 6].

Breast cancer subtypes show different propensities to spread to specific organs. Lymph node involvement and tumor size can influence how metastasis progresses and a patient's survival chances. Clinical determination of metastasis risk to specific organs often relies on the tumor's molecular or histopathological subtype. Metastasis is a multistep process involving local invasion, entry into blood or lymph vessels, circulation as circulating tumor cells, exit from the bloodstream, adaptation in the target organ, and eventually formation of macro metastases. Specific mutations, such as in TP53, CDKN2A, PTEN, PIK3CA, and RB1, can contribute to invasion and metastasis. Genomic studies, including those by The Cancer Genome Atlas and the International Cancer Genome Consortium, have identified genes frequently mutated in metastatic breast cancer, such as TP53, ESR1, GATA3, KMT2C, NCOR1, AKT1, NF1, RIC8A, and RB1 [7, 8].

Perou et al. classified breast cancer into four main clinical subtypes based on gene expression profiles and receptor status (estrogen receptor [ER], progesterone receptor [PR], human epidermal growth factor receptor 2 [HER2]) as well as proliferation status as assessed by Ki67: luminal A (ER+/PR+), luminal B (ER+/PR+/HER2−/+/Ki67+), HER2 overexpressing (ER−/PR−/HER2+), and basal-like/triple-negative (TN) (ER−/PR−/HER2−) [9]. While bone tissue is the most common site for metastasis across all subtypes, TN breast cancer has a higher tendency to metastasize to the lung, occurring in approximately 32% of patients compared to 21% of luminal A/B and 25% of HER2+ patients [10]. However, the mechanisms by which breast cancer molecular subtype influences metastasis to the lung are not yet fully understood.

Metastatic breast cancer subtypes exhibit distinct metastasis patterns. HR-positive/HER2-positive and triple-negative tumors are more likely to recur in the lungs compared to HR-positive/HER2-negative tumors. HER2-enriched and triple-negative subtypes have a particularly high prevalence of lung metastases. A retrospective analysis at M.D. Anderson Cancer Center found that patients with lung-only metastases who underwent surgical removal (pulmonary metastasectomy) had a significantly longer median overall survival (35–75.6 months) and a 5-year survival rate of 38–54% [2].

The effects of breast cancer metastasis on the lungs can vary depending on the size and location of the metastatic tumors. Small tumors may not cause any symptoms initially, but as the tumors grow, they can lead to symptoms such as cough, shortness of breath, chest pain, and wheezing. In some cases, lung metastases can cause complications such as pneumonia, pneumothorax, or pulmonary hemorrhage. The impact of metastasis on the respiratory system in general is described below.

Impact on lung function: Metastasis of breast cancer in the lungs can lead to the development of metastatic tumors in the lung tissue. These tumors can grow and interfere with normal lung function, leading to symptoms such as cough, shortness of breath, and decreased exercise tolerance. In severe cases, lung metastases can cause respiratory failure and significantly impact quality of life [2, 11].

Effect on lung structure: Metastatic tumors in the lungs can disrupt the normal structure and function of the lung tissue. This can lead to inflammation, fibrosis, and impaired gas exchange, which can further contribute to respiratory symptoms and decrease lung function [12].

Treatment considerations: The management of lung metastasis from breast cancer is complex and often involves a combination of systemic therapies (chemotherapy, hormonal therapy, and targeted therapy) and local treatments (surgery, radiation therapy) aimed at controlling the growth of metastatic tumors and improving related symptoms. Palliative care may also be provided to improve quality of life and manage respiratory symptoms.

Despite advances in treatment, lung metastasis from breast cancer is associated with a poor prognosis, with a median survival typically ranging from months to a few years [12].

15.1.2 Treatment-Related Respiratory Complications

Most short-term adverse effects involved the musculoskeletal system, skin, and the general/unspecified category across all age groups. However, a study found BCS reported experiencing back and abdominal pain, common infections (respiratory and urinary), and psychological problems (depression and sleeplessness) more frequently requiring them to be examined more often by their medical professionals [13].

The transition from cancer treatment to survivorship is often challenging and may leave some unmet needs. While information exists about potential late effects for each treatment modality, several studies found that follow-up care could be improved. Patients often report feeling unprepared for posttreatment because they lack information about potential late effects and their duration. Additionally, patients have indicated that they have significant unmet needs for support, information, or education regarding physical limitations or impairments [14].

de Ligt et al. found that cough, shortness of breath, and fatigue were the most frequently reported treatment-related respiratory symptoms in BCS [14]. Cough and nasal complaints became more common symptoms within five years of diagnosis, but interestingly, cough seemed to become less frequent over time. Cancer treatment, including surgery, chemotherapy, hormone therapy, and radiation, can all have negative side effects on the respiratory system (Fig. 15.1).

15.1.2.1 Surgical Treatment

Surgical site infections account for 2–19% of complications following breast surgery [15]. According to a study by de Blacam and colleagues, the most frequent complication following all treatments was superficial and deep surgical site infections, accounting for 5.6% of the 26,988 patients' morbidity rate following lumpectomy and mastectomy [16] The rate of surgical site infections can be influenced and varied by several factors, including the type of surgery, the accuracy of reporting, and characteristics of patients such as obesity, diabetes mellitus, smoking, kidney problems, prior radiation therapy, and skin conditions [15]. Despite appearing mild, these infections were more commonly reported by BCS of all ages up to 14 years after diagnosis [17]. This suggests potential long-term effects on the immune system. Current breast cancer survivorship guidelines do not address these infections. Perhaps because no prior research has specifically addressed this problem, or because BCS does not clearly link these infections to breast cancer, it has not been documented [17]. This kind of problem can lead to extended hospital stays, low patient satisfaction, longer treatment times for adjuvant therapy, and higher treatment costs [15].

Surgery can have several negative effects on the respiratory system, including immobilization and postoperative pain, reduced cough reflex, circulatory problems, and postural abnormalities [5–7]. These factors can all contribute to a decrease in both the range of motion of the dia-

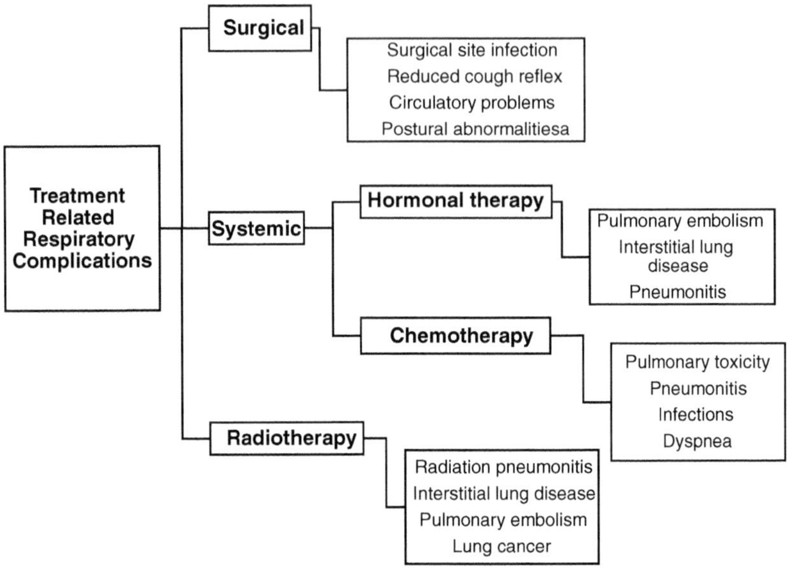

Fig. 15.1 Treatment-related respiratory complications

phragm and overall thoracic mobility, ultimately reducing respiratory muscle efficiency and leading to fatigue [18].

15.1.2.2 Radiotherapy

Radiotherapy-induced respiratory side effects are uncommon in breast cancer survivors but can develop, especially if treatment involves radiating the chest wall or lymph nodes near the lungs. Studies suggest that women with breast cancer who receive chest radiation may have a lower maximum oxygen uptake compared to healthy individuals, potentially affecting their cardiorespiratory capacity. Additionally, it can also lead to decreased respiratory and exercise capacity, likely due to limitations in chest wall mobility [18].

Some potential respiratory side effects of radiotherapy in BCS include:

Radiation pneumonitis: This refers to the initial cellular damage in the alveolar space that evolves into an acute inflammatory process, typically manifesting within 4–12 weeks following the conclusion of radiotherapy [19]. Symptoms may include cough, shortness of breath, fever, and chest discomfort. Most cases are mild and resolved with supportive care, but severe cases may require medical intervention.

Interstitial lung disease: Radiation therapy, in rare cases, can cause lung tissue fibrosis, leading to interstitial lung disease. This can further increase the risk of lung parenchymal injury, loss of type II pneumocytes, surfactant loss, and basement membrane edema, all of which can impair respiratory performance and limit physical activity participation [20]. It may worsen into lung fibrosis, causing a restrictive lung pattern. Symptoms of restrictive lung problems may include progressive shortness of breath, cough, and fatigue.

Pulmonary embolism: Radiation therapy can increase the risk of thrombosis, causing a pulmonary embolism. Symptoms of a pulmonary embolism can develop suddenly and include shortness of breath, chest pain, and coughing up blood. Prompt medical attention is essential for this potentially life-threatening condition [21].

Lung cancer: While rare, radiation therapy for breast cancer can slightly increase the long-term risk of developing lung cancer, particularly in patients with a history of smoking or other risk factors [22].

Furthermore, there is a decrease in respiratory muscle strength, along with notable alterations in pulmonary function tests, following locoregional radiotherapy [23].

15.1.2.3 Chemotherapy

Chemotherapy can have various respiratory side effects in BCS, although they are less common compared to radiation therapy [24].

Some potential respiratory side effects of chemotherapy in BCS include:

Pulmonary toxicity: Certain chemotherapy drugs, like bleomycin, methotrexate, and gemcitabine, can cause damage the lungs, leading to symptoms such as cough, shortness of breath, and difficulty with exercising. This condition, known as chemotherapy-induced pulmonary toxicity, can be acute or chronic and may require treatment with corticosteroids or other medications [24, 25].

Pneumonitis: Chemotherapy-induced pneumonitis is an inflammatory reaction in the lungs that can occur as a side effect of certain chemotherapy drugs. Symptoms may include cough, fever, and shortness of breath [26].

Increased susceptibility to infections: Chemotherapy can weaken the immune system, increasing the risk of respiratory infections such as pneumonia. BCS undergoing chemotherapy should be vigilant for signs of infection and seek prompt medical attention if symptoms develop [27].

Exacerbation of preexisting respiratory conditions: Chemotherapy can worsen preexisting respiratory conditions, such as asthma or chronic obstructive pulmonary disease (COPD), leading to increased symptoms and exacerbations. Close monitoring and management of these conditions are essential during chemotherapy treatment [28].

Hematologic side effects: Some chemotherapy drugs can affect the bone marrow, leading to anemia, leukopenia, and thrombocytopenia. Severe anemia or thrombocytopenia can result in symptoms such as shortness of breath or increased risk of bleeding, respectively [29].

Dyspnea, a common respiratory symptom experienced by BCS undergoing systemic chemotherapy, is believed to be primarily caused by paclitaxel, a frequently used chemotherapeutic agent. Paclitaxel has been linked to various respiratory symptoms, including non-productive cough, wheezing, and shortness of breath [23]. In the study by de Ligt et al., treatment with chemotherapy, particularly when combined with trastuzumab, was found to be significantly associated with an increased risk of fatigue, respiratory (cough, shortness of breath, and complaints nose), and gastrointestinal problems (nausea, diarrhea, and dry mouth), central nervous system (hypersensitivity for light or sound, headache, dizziness, and neuralgia) and skin health problems (hair loss and skin problem) [14].

Briasoulis et al. [30] documented a 9% incidence of interstitial pneumonia or pulmonary fibrosis linked to lung injury from chemotherapy. Similarly, Krengli et al. [31] reported a 4.9% incidence of grade I pneumonitis, which resolved with medical intervention.

15.1.2.4 Hormone Therapy

Hormone therapy for breast cancer, particularly with drugs like tamoxifen or aromatase inhibitors, is generally well-tolerated. However, there have been some reports of respiratory side effects associated with these medications, though they are rare. Tamoxifen and certain chemotherapy drugs can lead to pulmonary toxicity, impacting lung function tests and causing respiratory muscle weakness [32]. This highlights the importance of monitoring respiratory function, especially for BCS experiencing exertional dyspnea. Antihormonal therapy was associated with increased fatigue and reproductive system health problems, but completed therapy showed a reduction in central nervous system issues such as hypersensitivity to light or sound, headache, and dizziness. Decreased menopausal symptoms may be due to non-compliance with antihormonal treatment, emphasizing the need for longitudinal studies to understand ongoing cancer-related late effects and their impact on the quality of life of BCS. Some potential respiratory side effects of hormone therapy in *BCS* may include interstitial lung disease, pneumonitis, and pulmonary embolism [33]. There is a small increased risk of pulmonary embolism with hormone therapy. Especially using tamoxifen is linked to a 1.95 times higher likelihood of developing deep vein thrombosis or pulmonary embolism in BCS [34].

Hormone therapy can exacerbate preexisting respiratory conditions such as asthma or chronic obstructive pulmonary disease, leading to increased symptoms and exacerbations.

Palliative Care: In breast cancer survivors, palliative care plays a crucial role in managing respiratory side effects, especially in advanced or metastatic cases. Palliative care focuses on improving the quality of life by addressing symptoms and providing support.

15.2 Identifying Respiratory Problems

15.2.1 Common Respiratory Symptoms

Patients describe symptoms as subjective experiences that disrupt their usual activities, sensations, or emotions, often caused by an illness. The cumulative impact of all symptoms related to a disease and/or treatment on an individual's ability to function as they did before to the onset of the disease and/or therapy is known as the "symptom burden." Qualitative research has confirmed that this burden can significantly limit patients' ability to walk, work, interact socially, and maintain their mental well-being. In spite of the fact that breast cancer patients may live longer than those with other cancers, they may feel uncertain due to side effects from therapy, worry of recurrence or advancement, and the weight of their remaining symptoms [35].

Accurate symptom assessment and communication between patients and health professionals are crucial for optimal symptom management in cancer care. While improved communication is known to lead to better outcomes, identifying the most effective methods for symptom monitoring remains a challenge. However, healthcare professionals can significantly enhance their ability to monitor cancer-related symptoms, especially those specific to certain populations or treatments (e.g., breast cancer), by utilizing valid and reliable patient-reported outcome measures (PROMs) [35].

Cancer-associated symptoms often occur together and can have a common or related cause. This means that one symptom can influence the occurrence and severity of others. Some of the most common respiratory symptom clusters identified in BCS as shortness of breath (dyspnea), cough, chest pain, and wheezing.

A key finding is the frequent occurrence of fatigue-sleep disturbance and psychological symptom clusters among patients at all stages of cancer treatment, even before treatment begins. Studies showed that fatigue-sleep disturbance can persist even after treatment completion [36]. Similarly, psychological symptoms, especially anxiety and depression, can be present before, during, and/or after treatment, often co-occurring with the pain-fatigue-sleep disturbance cluster. The co-occurrence of symptom clusters like pain-fatigue-sleep disturbance and the psychological cluster could be due to changes in molecular pathways associated with these clusters, such as dysregulation of the hypothalamic–pituitary–adrenal axis, altered serotonin neurotransmission, or increased production of pro-inflammatory cytokines [37].

Another important finding is that the composition of symptom clusters among BCS seems to change over time. Studies on people who have survived breast cancer are mostly cross-sectional and concentrate on the initial two years following diagnosis. On the other hand, longer-term research projects that monitor survivors for over five years following diagnosis are required. This is significant because it can take up to 10 years following diagnosis for certain health repercussions, such as heart failure. As a result, longitudinal research can offer important new perspectives on the requirements and long-term health consequences of BCS [17].

15.2.2 Screening and Monitoring

Screening and monitoring for respiratory symptoms in BCS are crucial for early detection and management.

15.2.2.1 Screening

Clinical assessment and patient history: During routine clinical visits, healthcare providers should actively inquire about respiratory symptoms such as shortness of breath, cough, chest pain, or wheezing. Any new or worsening symptoms should be thoroughly evaluated, including their onset, duration, and severity. It is also important to assess smoking history and other risk factors for lung disease.

In addition to this information, a comprehensive history should include:

Current medications: This includes prescription drugs, over-the-counter medications, and herbal supplements.

Recent infections: A history of recent illnesses like cold, flu, or pneumonia can be helpful.

Patient-reported symptoms: Several patient-reported symptom scales can assess respiratory symptoms in breast cancer patients. The MD Anderson Symptom Inventory and the European Organization for Research and Treatment of Cancer Quality of Life Questionnaire include items on shortness of breath and cough severity [38–41]. The functional assessment of cancer therapy-breast measures physical well-being, which may capture respiratory symptoms. The National Comprehensive Cancer Network Distress Thermometer assesses difficulty breathing. These scales help understand symptom severity and guide interventions for improved symptom management and quality of life.

Dyspnea assessment: Dyspnea is a complex symptom influenced by various factors, including physiological, psychological, social, and environmental factors. To effectively address dyspnea, understanding the individual's experience is crucial. Various assessment tools such as questionnaires, scales, and physiological tests like spirometry, respiratory muscle strength, and cardiopulmonary exercise tests can help to diagnose and manage dyspnea comprehensively.

The most commonly used instruments include the Borg Scale, Visual Analog Scale, Modified Medical Research Council Dyspnea Scale, and Cancer Dyspnea Scale [42].

Cough assessment: In assessing cough in BCS, a thorough history is essential, including questions about the onset, duration, and progression of the cough. Clinicians should inquire about any associated symptoms, such as sputum production, hemoptysis (coughing up blood), chest pain, or shortness of breath, which can provide clues to the underlying cause. They should also ask about any exacerbating or alleviating factors, such as specific activities, positions, or environmental exposures. Objective measures can help quantify the severity and impact of cough on a patient's quality of life [43].

Fatigue-sleep disturbance assessment: Clinicians can use standardized tools like the Brief Fatigue Inventory or the Functional Assessment of Cancer Therapy-Fatigue to quantify the severity and impact of fatigue. For sleep disturbances, tools like the Pittsburgh Sleep Quality Index or the Insomnia Severity Index can be used to assess sleep quality, latency, duration, and disturbances. Assessing how fatigue and sleep disturbances affect a patient's daily activities, work, social interactions, and overall quality of life is crucial. Patients may also report cognitive difficulties (e.g., "chemo brain") related to fatigue and sleep disturbances [37, 44].

15.2.2.2 Monitoring

For patients undergoing a set of/multifaceted treatments, close monitoring of respiratory symptoms is essential. This can involve regular assessments by healthcare providers and keeping track of symptoms at home. Monitoring tools like spirometry or pulse oximetry may be used to assess lung function and oxygen levels. Reduced muscle oxygenation can contribute to exercise intolerance, which is commonly observed in individuals with respiratory symptoms [45]. This can manifest as fatigue, weakness, and reduced endurance during physical activity. Monitoring muscle oxygenation can help assess the potential side effects of treatment on muscle health and function. Adequate muscle oxygenation is essential for the function of respiratory muscles, including the diaphragm and intercostal muscles. These muscles play a crucial role in breathing, and any impairment in their oxygenation can lead to respiratory symptoms such as dyspnea. Noninvasive methods, like near-infrared spectroscopy and cardiopulmonary exercise testing, can be used to monitor muscle oxygenation in breast cancer patients. These methods provide valuable insights into muscle health and function, guiding tailored interventions to improve overall physical function in this population.

Pulmonary function tests: Pulmonary function testing (PFT) is widely utilized in clinical settings due to its safe and cost-effective nature, as well as its ability to objectively indicate early respiratory system changes. They include spirometry, lung volume tests, and diffusion capacity tests (DLCO). PFT is important for evaluating respiratory symptoms in breast cancer patients. PFT assesses lung function, detects respiratory abnormalities, and evaluates the impact of cancer treatment on the lungs. They help to identify preexisting lung conditions and guide treatment decisions. Its utility extends beyond clinical use, as parameters like forced vital capacity (FVC) and forced expiratory volume in 1 s (FEV_1) provide valuable insights into lung elasticity, airway size, and resistance to airflow. Given the potential challenges related to systemic chemotherapy and radiotherapy, which can impact airway elasticity and resistance, PFT emerges as an optimal choice for detecting early respiratory issues [23].

There was a notable decline in pulmonary function tests, both FVC and FEV_1 among patients, not only before and after chemotherapy but also following the completion of radiotherapy, displaying a significant linear trend. Many studies suggest that these declines are reversible within approximately a year after systemic treatment [31]. Although these declines may not have significant clinical implications, they could be interpreted/viewed as early indicators of potential respiratory function decline.

Spyropoulou et al. suggest that the decrease in DLCO may signify interstitial damage from inflammatory infiltrates, resulting in restricted lung function among women undergoing chemotherapy [19]. DLCO is highly sensitive to drug-related lung damage. Additionally, the reduction in FVC and FEV_1, without a change in their ratio, suggests a restrictive lung injury, possibly due to an acute inflammatory process in the alveolar space. While the deterioration in maximum expiratory flow between 25% and 75% of FVC could suggest evolving bronchiolar damage, its lack of significant change supports the likelihood of restrictive lung injury [19].

Additionally, patients of advanced age and/or those who have undergone mastectomy should be closely monitored, as they may be more susceptible to respiratory complications related to systemic treatment.

Posture Assessment: Women's posture and upper body are greatly influenced by their breasts. Because of its anatomical location, thoracic curvature changes may be the main outcome of breast-related procedures. But, in terms of possible compensatory mechanisms, it is also crucial to take into account other spinal curvatures [46]. Postural changes, especially in the sagittal plane of the spine, are commonly seen after breast cancer surgery and can progress over time [47]. These changes in spine biomechanics can lead to adaptive changes in the thorax, potentially affecting respiratory muscles and chest wall motion, which can impact breathing patterns and respiratory volume.

Research on this issue has shown that postural changes following breast cancer surgery can negatively affect respiratory volume and muscle strength, even in healthy women [47]. Additionally, these changes in posture may increase the risk of respiratory complications, particularly in relation to pulmonary functions and the possibility of radiotherapy and chemotherapy-induced pulmonary toxicity.

In a different study, women who had unilateral breast cancer surgery showed a correlation between their pulmonary functioning, spinal posture, and spinal mobility [47]. It was shown that thoracic frontal mobility was linked to a decrease in peak expiratory flow (PEF), while thoracic curvature angle was linked to a decrease in FEV_1 and subcostal mobility. Greater overall spinal inclination movement was associated with decreased maximal inspiratory pressure (MIP), while greater lumbar mobility was linked to enhanced FVC. These results emphasize how critical to evaluate and treat postural abnormalities in breast cancer patients in order to maintain respiratory health and general quality of life. Diaphragmatic mobility and thoracic kyphosis were negatively correlated; respiratory functions were impacted by decreased diaphragmatic mobility along with increased thoracic kyphosis, which resulted in a decrease in FEV_1 [47].

Research on the specific link between posture and respiration in breast cancer is ongoing, and the potential for improvement is promising. Pulmonary rehabilitation programs focusing on posture correction and breathing exercises can be a valuable tool for breast cancer patients to manage these complications and improve their overall well-being.

Respiratory muscle strength assessment: Respiratory muscle strength can be affected in breast cancer patients due to systemic treatments and surgery, as well as reduced physical activity levels and changes in breathing patterns [48]. While assessing respiratory symptoms and function is crucial in breast cancer patients, formal respiratory muscle strength assessment is not routinely included in the standard evaluation process. However, in the following certain situations, respiratory muscle strength assessment might be considered:

Severe or persistent respiratory symptoms: If symptoms are particularly severe or unresponsive to initial treatment, muscle strength testing could provide additional insights.

Pre-existing lung condition: For patients with preexisting lung conditions such as COPD, muscle strength assessment might be helpful to draw a conclusion on overall respiratory function.

Prehabilitation before surgery: In some cases, prehabilitation programs that incorporate respiratory muscle training exercises may be implemented before surgery to improve strength and endurance.

There is limited research on respiratory muscle strength in breast cancer patients. Santos et al. observed a 33% decrease in MIP and a 25% decrease in expiratory muscle strength (MEP) after 5–6 weeks of radiotherapy. In contrast, Vardar-Yağlı et al. found that, five years after diagnosis and treatment, respiratory muscle strength, as measured by MIP and MEP, was similar between breast cancer patients and healthy individuals. These findings imply that, unlike the acute decrease seen with radiotherapy, respiratory muscle strength remains stable in the long term for breast cancer patients [48]. O'Donnell et al. identified that a reduction in inspiratory capacity and static inspiratory muscle strength, as well as a faster and shallower breathing pattern, and higher ratings of breathlessness intensity during exercise, were indicative of significant dynamic inspiratory muscle weakness. The study suggests that simple tests can be used to identify potentially reversible factors such as inspiratory muscle weakness in patients with breast cancer [49].

Assessments of the respiratory muscles can be performed using both invasive and noninvasive techniques. The most commonly used method is mouth pressure measurement of respiratory muscles that assessed MIP and/or MEP.

Exercise capacity assessment: The issue of exercise capacity in BCS is increasingly problematic, with recent research emphasizing the significance of physical activity and overall survival rates in this population [50]. Numerous treatments can burden survivors with various long-term side effects, which can diminish their quality of life and make them more vulnerable to future illnesses and premature death. To address these adverse effects, researchers have introduced a range of exercise interventions during, immediately after, and years after, following primary treatment, respectively.

In BCS who are stable and not receiving any treatment, several factors may contribute to dyspnea and exercise intolerance. These include the effects of the cancer itself, adverse effects of chemotherapy and/or radiotherapy, and deconditioning due to lack of physical activity. The underlying mechanisms are likely complex and may involve increased ventilatory demand due to ventilation-perfusion abnormalities, reduced ventilatory capacity from inspiratory muscle weakness, compromised dynamic respiratory mechanics from peripheral airway dysfunction or lung restriction, decreased lung diffusion capacity from microvascular injury, cardiocirculatory impairment, or a combination of these factors. O'Donnell et al. identified a correlation between dyspnea and exercise intolerance in breast cancer survivors, which is related not only to increased ventilatory demand but also to a decrease in inspiratory capacity, likely attributable to inspiratory muscle weakness [49]. There are several ways to objectively demonstrate this exercise intolerance in patients with breast cancer such as field and laboratory tests. The most commonly used field test that indirectly measures aerobic capacity is the 6-minute walk test (6 MWT). The 6 MWT is valuable for designing exercise programs and evaluating, and monitoring breast cancer survivors, as it is linked to their psychological and physiological well-being, quality of life, cancer-related symptoms, and body composition. The 6 MWT protocol can guide exercise prescriptions for breast cancer survivors and serve as a useful tool for immediate assessments of aerobic capacity in clinical settings [51].

Cardiopulmonary exercise testing (CPET) is a comprehensive assessment that evaluates the responses of cardiovascular, pulmonary, and muscular systems to exercise. During CPET, the individual typically performs incremental exercise on a treadmill or stationary bike while wearing a mask to measure their breathing and gas exchange. When evaluating a breast cancer patients' cardiopulmonary fitness, CPET is regarded as the gold standard method [52]. Peak oxygen uptake (VO_{2peak}), which represents the maximal respiratory and cardiovascular performance during exercise, is measured by using this technique.

Physical activity assessment: Assessing physical activity in breast cancer patients is crucial for understanding their overall health and well-being. There are several methods to assess physical activity levels, including questionnaires or objective measures such as accelerometers or pedometers.

Activities of daily living and quality of life: Respiratory complications in patients with breast cancer can have a significant impact on functional limitations and quality of life. Assessing the impact of respiratory symptoms on activities of daily life in breast cancer patients is important for understanding the full scope of their functional limitations and for developing appropriate interventions to improve their quality of life. This assessment may involve using standardized tools to measure activities of daily life and evaluating how respiratory symptoms affect a patient's ability to perform specific tasks. By addressing respiratory symptoms and their impact on activities of daily life, healthcare providers can help improve the overall well-being and functional status of breast cancer patients. Understanding how symptoms like dyspnea or difficulty walking and climbing stairs impact daily activities provides valuable insight.

Functional Assessment of Cancer Therapy-Breast and European Organization for Research and Treatment of Cancer Quality of Life Questionnaire are widely used questionnaires that assess the quality of life in breast cancer patients [39, 40].

15.2.2.3 Imaging

Imaging plays a crucial role in evaluating respiratory symptoms in breast cancer patients. Chest X-rays offer a quick and initial assessment, while computed tomography (CT) scans provide detailed images of the lungs and surrounding structures. Positron emission tomography (PET) scans, often combined with CT scans (PET/CT), can help determine metabolic activity in suspicious areas, potentially indicating cancer spread. Magnetic resonance imaging (MRI) and bone scans may be used in specific situations to gather additional information. Ultrasound can also be a valuable tool for certain purposes. These imaging tests work together to diagnose conditions like lung metastases, guiding treatment decisions and ensuring optimal patient care [53].

15.3 Comprehensive Respiratory Management Strategies

Effective management of respiratory problems in BCS requires a multidisciplinary approach aimed at addressing underlying causes and optimizing respiratory function. Collaboration between oncologists, pulmonologists, and physiotherapists is very important in the treatment of respiratory problems in breast cancer patients. Following breast cancer treatment, individuals may experience various respiratory impairments, including reduced lung capacity and respiratory muscle strength. These impairments can result from treatments such as chemotherapy and radiation therapy, as well as from physical inactivity during treatment and recovery periods. A recognized way to preserve and enhance respiratory capacity, quality of life, and posttreatment side effects of breast cancer is respiratory physiotherapy, which combines a variety of techniques targeted at preventing, treating, and stabilizing cardiorespiratory diseases [18]. Individualized treatment plans tailored to the respiratory problems of patients with breast cancer should be made.

15.3.1 Role of Physical Activity and Pulmonary Rehabilitation in Improving Respiratory Function

Important factors in enhancing respiratory function among breast cancer patients are physical activity and pulmonary rehabilitation. Breast cancer treatment like surgery, chemotherapy, and radiation therapy can decrease lung capacity, reduce respiratory muscle strength, and impair overall lung function.

Physical activity, encompassing aerobic and strength exercise training, and flexibility exercises, has been shown to improve lung function, increase respiratory muscle strength, and enhance overall cardiorespiratory fitness. Engaging in regular physical activity also promotes better oxygen utilization and delivery throughout the body, which is vital for eliminating the perception of dyspnea and fatigue often experienced during cancer treatment [54].

Additionally, personalized pulmonary rehabilitation programs combine aerobic and resistance exercise training with patient education, self-management, and psychological support to improve lung function, exercise tolerance, and overall quality of life in patients with various lung conditions [55, 56]. Few studies are investigating the effectiveness of these programs specifically for breast cancer survivors with respiratory issues that are designed to address the respiratory limitations caused by breast cancer and its treatment [57–60]. Patient education incorporates proper breathing mechanics and management of respiratory symptoms. Breathing exercises and relaxation techniques help to improve lung function and manage shortness of breath. Supervised exercise training tailored to individual needs and gradually increased intensity, promoting improved lung capacity and exercise tolerance. Psychological support addresses the emotional and psychological impact of respiratory issues and can significantly enhance overall well-being.

Studies have demonstrated that pulmonary rehabilitation programs effectively improve lung function, increase exercise capacity, and reduce symptoms like shortness of breath and fatigue in BCS [57]. For example, a randomized controlled trial assigned 50 women with post-mastectomy syndrome to either conditional swimming and Pilates exercises or a combination of aqua aerobics, swimming, and recreational aerobics. Both groups followed their workout regimens three times a week for 48 weeks. The study showed that all respiratory function parameters except maximal voluntary ventilation rose significantly in both groups during a year-long exercise training. These findings suggest that individualized physical rehabilitation programs may be useful in helping patients with post-mastectomy syndrome to restore their ability to breathe [58].

Additionally, pulmonary rehabilitation has been shown to improve the quality of life, reduce healthcare utilization, and even enhance psychological well-being. For cancer patients, particularly those with breast cancer, exercise may be an effective treatment for breathlessness. A meta-analysis of 11 intervention groups from 10 randomized controlled trials, including 3 studies on breast cancer, found that dyspnea perception was considerably lower in the exercise group compared to the control group [59]. Vardar Yagli et al suggested that both aerobic exercise and yoga are beneficial for BCS for improving muscle strength and functional exercise may provide additional relief from fatigue [60].

By incorporating endurance and resistance exercise training and complementary therapies into survivorship care plans, healthcare providers can support BCS in achieving optimal respiratory function and enhancing their quality of life posttreatment.

15.3.1.1 Breathing Exercises

Breathing exercises are important for patients with breast cancer. Incorporating breathing exercises into the care plan of BCS can significantly enhance their respiratory function and overall well-being. These exercises, often part of pulmonary rehabilitation programs, aim to increase lung capacity and pulmonary ventilation, correct breathing errors, re-establish a proper breathing pattern, reduce and control dyspnea, enhance relaxation, improve thorax mobility, and improve quality of life of breast cancer patients [61]. For BCS who may experience compromised lung function due to treatments such as chemotherapy or radiation therapy, breathing exercises offer a non-invasive and empowering approach to manage respiratory symptoms.

There are many breathing exercise techniques such as diaphragmatic breathing, pursed-lip breathing, segmental breathing, and controlled breathing patterns not only promote relaxation but also aid in clearing airway secretions and improving oxygenation. These exercises can be easily integrated into daily routines, empowering BCS to take an active role in their recovery and fostering a sense of control over their respiratory health. Breathing exercises are beneficial throughout cancer treatment, from the preoperative period to palliative care, helping to manage symptoms at each stage.

Diaphragmatic breathing, also known as deep breathing, is particularly effective for increasing lung capacity. Pursed-lip breathing can also be used—with diaphragmatic breathing. This technique involves inhaling slowly through the nose and exhaling with pursed lips, altering breathing mechanics. It helps regulate breathing during activities that may cause shortness of breath.

Diaphragmatic breathing has an impact on the brain and cardiovascular, respiratory, and gastrointestinal systems through the modulation of the autonomic nervous function. Shahirai et al. investigated the impact of diaphragmatic breathing, muscle relaxation, and body image on the quality of life of older patients with breast or prostate cancer. Fifty patients were divided into intervention and control groups [62]. The intervention group showed improvement in physical functioning and overall quality of life scores immediately and again at 6 weeks, while the control group did not experience significant changes. While few studies focus specifically on breast cancer patients, deep slow breathing exercises are recommended for 5 min/session, 3–5 times a day, for at least 4 weeks.

A case series study in 5 radiotherapy-treated breast cancer patients demonstrated improved pulmonary function and exercise capacity after using an incentive spirometer and positive expiratory pressure (PEP) mask as respiratory physiotherapy [63].

To reduce stress and anxiety, relaxation breathing techniques encourage using total lung capacity and slow, deep breaths. Many different relaxation breathing techniques are shown as effective. This can involve specific breathing patterns, such as inhaling slowly through the nose for a set count and exhaling slowly through the mouth. Relaxation breathing technique helps regulate the autonomic nervous system, which controls stress [64]. Relaxation breathing technique can be used immediately after surgery, as it allows the patient to focus all energy on healing. A study was administered in breathing exercises to breast cancer patients undergoing outpatient chemotherapy. These exercises, used alongside regular care, improved the patients' functional status by reducing chemotherapy-induced nausea, vomiting, and retching [65].

Breathing exercises, like pranayama, are a common element of comprehensive therapies like yoga for breast cancer treatment. Studies show that pranayama, a specific breathing technique used in yoga, offers similar benefits for breast cancer patients including a reduction in fatigue and an improvement in quality of life in patients receiving radiation therapy and/or chemotherapy [66, 67]. Pranayama breathing exercises involve stretching the lungs, which sends signals to the nervous system to promote relaxation. This leads to a calmer state of mind, reduced sensitivity to negative physical sensations, and lower anxiety—all of which improve the quality of life for patients undergoing radiation therapy or chemotherapy [64].

15.3.1.2 Adjunct Therapies with Breathing Exercises

Breathing exercises have been combined with other techniques such as soft tissue techniques, thoracic mobilization, and kinesiotaping for helping to restore proper thoracic mobility and enhance the function of the respiratory muscles in the operated area, thereby improving respiratory system functions [68, 69]. There was no evidence of additional benefit from these interventions. More studies are needed in this regard.

15.3.1.3 Respiratory Muscle Training

Respiratory muscle training (RMT) holds promise as a targeted intervention to address respiratory impairments in BCS [70]. Following breast cancer treatment, individuals may experience reduced respiratory muscle strength and endurance, leading to symptoms such as dyspnea and decreased exercise tolerance [48]. RMT involves specific exercises designed to strengthen the muscles involved in breathing, including the diaphragm, intercostal muscles, and accessory respiratory muscles. By engaging in RMT, BCS can improve their respiratory muscle function, enhance lung capacity, and alleviate symptoms of breathlessness. Research has shown that RMT can have numerous benefits for BCS. Not only does it improve respiratory muscle function and lung capacity, but it also reduces dyspnea and enhances overall physical performance [71]. Furthermore, RMT has been linked to improvements in quality of life, as survivors experience less breathlessness during daily activities and have increased confidence in their ability to engage in physical exercise. In a recent study, 98 breast cancer patients underwent inspiratory muscle training in addition to a rehabilitation program for 3 months. It was shown that there was a greater decrease in dyspnea perception and a greater increase in respiratory muscle endurance and cycling endurance time in the inspiratory muscle training group compared to the control group [71]. Integrating RMT into rehabilitation programs tailored to the needs of BCS can offer targeted support for improving respiratory health and enhancing overall well-being. Rehabilitation programs should include a combination of RMT exercises, aerobic training, and strength training to address the multifaceted nature of respiratory impairments in this population. Further research exploring the effectiveness of RMT in this population is warranted to optimize survivorship care strategies and promote long-term respiratory function and quality of life.

15.3.2 Lifestyle Management for Respiratory Health

15.3.2.1 Smoking Cessation and Environmental Modifications

While breast cancer itself does not directly impact the lungs, smoking is a significant risk factor for both breast cancer and respiratory problems. Quitting smoking is crucial for breast cancer patients. Smoking cessation programs provide support and strategies to help patients to end tobacco use. Alongside quitting, environmental modifications can further improve respiratory function [72]. This can involve reducing exposure to secondhand smoke and air pollutants, both indoors and outdoors. By combining smoking cessation with these environmental changes, breast cancer patients can potentially improve their lung function and overall well-being.

15.3.3 Pharmacological Management of Respiratory Symptoms

Pharmacological interventions for respiratory symptoms include opioids, inhaled bronchodilators and corticosteroids, benzodiazepines and antidepressants, and supplemental oxygen [73]. Treatment of respiratory symptoms is not specific to breast cancer. It is usually more commonly used at the end of the disease or in palliative care. Pharmacological management of respiratory symptoms in breast cancer is often targeted at the underlying cause. For instance, if a patient experiences a cough or shortness of breath due to drug-induced lung injury from chemotherapy, corticosteroids like prednisone may be used to reduce inflammation. In cases with pleural effusion, diuretics can help remove excess fluid and improve breathing. Opioids may be prescribed for severe, persistent breathlessness, although this approach is used cautiously due to potential side effects and the need for careful monitoring. It is important to note that some targeted therapies for breast cancer, like CDK 4/6 inhibitors, can also cause respiratory problems. In these cases, close monitoring and potentially interrupting treatment may be necessary. Ultimately, the specific medications used will depend on the cause of the respiratory symptoms and a patient's individual needs [74].

Breast cancer treatments can weaken the immune system, making individuals more susceptible to respiratory infections. Immunizations for influenza, pneumococcus (pneumonia), and other common respiratory viruses can provide important protection. Alongside vaccinations, frequent handwashing, maintaining distance from those who are sick, and wearing a mask in crowded places are all crucial infection prevention strategies. By staying up-to-date on immunizations and practicing good hygiene, women with breast cancer can significantly reduce their risk of developing respiratory complications [75].

15.4 Patient Education and Self-Management

Breast cancer patients often experience a whirlwind of emotions and information following diagnosis. Empowering them with knowledge about respiratory health concerning breast cancer can significantly improve their overall well-being. Understanding potential respiratory side effects from treatment, like drug-induced lung injury, shortness of breath, or cough, allows patients to recognize symptoms early and report them to their healthcare team. Knowledge about managing these side effects, such as breathing exercises or medication options, can foster a sense of control and reduce anxiety. Additionally, information on quitting smoking, maintaining a healthy weight, and dietary choices that support lung health empowers patients to make proactive decisions that benefit both their respiratory health and overall breast cancer management.

Learning self-management techniques, such as breathing exercises or positioning strategies for improved comfort, can equip patients with tools to alleviate symptoms. The activity pacing approach helps patients with cancer manage their energy levels. It teaches them to find a balance between rest and activity by staying moderately active and avoiding getting too tired or resting for too long. Think of it like a steady rhythm instead of bursts of activity followed by crashes. While research has not specifically looked at activity pacing for shortness of breath (dyspnea), the benefits seen in managing fatigue and pain from cancer likely apply here as well [76].

Support groups or online communities specifically for breast cancer patients can also provide a safe space to share experiences, ask questions, and gain valuable insights from others who experience similar challenges. By providing these resources, healthcare professionals can empower patients to become active participants in managing their respiratory health and overall well-being throughout their breast cancer journey.

15.5 Future Research

Despite strides in breast cancer treatment, there is still room for improvement regarding respiratory outcomes in breast cancer survivors. A key area for further research involves determining the long-term impact of specific treatment regimens on lung function. This knowledge can help tailor treatment plans to minimize respiratory side effects. Investigating the effectiveness of personalized pulmonary rehabilitation programs specifically designed for BCS with varying respiratory complications is crucial. By focusing on these areas, researchers can pave the way for improved respiratory health and overall well-being for BCS.

15.6 Conclusion

In conclusion, prioritizing proactive respiratory care within breast cancer survivorship programs is no longer an afterthought but a critical necessity. Early detection, education, and personalized interventions can significantly improve the quality of life for breast cancer survivors by mitigating the side effects of treatment, promoting self-management, and fostering a proactive approach to lung health. By prioritizing lung health alongside cancer recurrence and prevention, survivorship programs can empower BCS to breathe easier and live fuller lives after their cancer journey.

References

1. Lee Y-TNM. Breast carcinoma: pattern of metastasis at autopsy. J Surg Oncol. 1983;23:175–80.
2. Xiao W, Zheng S, Liu P, Zou Y, Xie X, Yu P, et al. Risk factors and survival outcomes in patients with breast cancer and lung metastasis: a population-based study. Cancer Med. 2018;7(3):922–30.
3. Yhim HY, Han SW, Oh DY, Han W, Im SA, Kim TY, et al. Prognostic factors for recurrent breast cancer patients with an isolated, limited number of lung metastases and implications for pulmonary metastasectomy. Cancer. 2010;116(12):2890–901.
4. Liu Y, Cao X. Characteristics and significance of the pre-metastatic niche. Cancer Cell. 2016;30(5):668–81.
5. Paget S. The distribution of secondary growths in cancer of the breast. Lancet. 1889;133:571–3.
6. Ewing J. Neoplastic diseases: a treatise on tumors. 3rd ed. Philadelphia: Saunders; 1928. p. 77–89.
7. Medeiros B, Allan AL. Molecular mechanisms of breast cancer metastasis to the lung: clinical and experimental perspectives. Int J Mol Sci. 2019;20(9):2272.
8. Brown D, Smeets D, Szekely B, Larsimont D, Szasz AM, Adnet PY, et al. Phylogenetic analysis of metastatic progression in breast cancer using somatic mutations and copy number aberrations. Nat Commun. 2017;8:14944.
9. Charles M, Perou TS, Eisen MB, van de Rijn M, Jeffreyk SS, Rees CA, Pollack JR, et al. Molecular portraits of human breast tumours. Nature. 2000;406:747–52.
10. Wu Q, Zhu S, Wu J, Chen C, Liu Q, Wei W, et al. Breast cancer subtypes predict the preferential site of distant metastases: a SEER based study. Oncotarget. 2017;8:27990–6.
11. Smith I. Goals of treatment for patients with metastatic breast cancer. Semin Oncol. 2006;33:2–5.
12. Lin S, Mo H, Li Y, Guan X, Chen Y, Wang Z, et al. Clinicopathological characteristics and survival outcomes in patients with synchronous lung metastases upon initial metastatic breast cancer diagnosis in han population. BMC Cancer. 2021;21(1):1330.
13. Heins MJ, Korevaar JC, Rijken PM, Schellevis FG. For which health problems do cancer survivors visit their general practitioner? Eur J Cancer. 2013;49(1):211–8.
14. de Ligt KM, Heins M, Verloop J, Smorenburg CH, Korevaar JC, Siesling S. Patient-reported health problems and healthcare use after treatment for early-stage breast cancer. Breast. 2019;46:4–11.
15. Al-Hilli Z, Wilkerson A. Breast surgery: management of postoperative complications following operations for breast cancer. Surg Clin North Am. 2021;101(5):845–63.
16. de Blacam C, Ogunleye AA, Momoh AO, Colakoglu S, Tobias AM, Sharma R, et al. High body mass index and smoking predict morbidity in breast cancer surgery: a multivariate analysis of 26,988 patients from the National Surgical Quality Improvement Program Database. Ann Surg. 2012;255(3):551–5.
17. Heins MJ, de Ligt KM, Verloop J, Siesling S, Korevaar JC. Adverse health effects after breast cancer up to 14 years after diagnosis. Breast. 2022;61:22–8.
18. Vinolo-Gil MJ, Martin-Valero R, Martin-Vega FJ, Rodriguez-Huguet M, Perez-Cabezas V, Gonzalez-Medina G. Respiratory physiotherapy intervention strategies in the sequelae of breast cancer treatment: a systematic review. Int J Environ Res Public Health. 2022;19(7):3800.
19. Despina Spyropoulou ML, Tsiamita M, Spiropoulos K, Kardamakis D. Pulmonary function testing in women with breast cancer treated with radiotherapy and chemotherapy. In Vivo. 2009;23:867–72.
20. Ciesla S, Polom K. The effect of immediate breast reconstruction with becker-25 prosthesis on the preservation of proper body posture in patients after mastectomy. Eur J Surg Oncol. 2010;36(7):625–31.
21. Guy JB, Bertoletti L, Magne N, Rancoule C, Mahe I, Font C, et al. Venous thromboembolism in radiation therapy cancer patients: findings from the RIETE registry. Crit Rev Oncol Hematol. 2017;113:83–9.
22. Brown LC, Mutter RW, Halyard MY. Benefits, risks, and safety of external beam radiation therapy for breast cancer. Int J Women's Health. 2015;7:449–58.
23. Tugral A, Aribas Z, Akyol M, Bakar Y. Understanding changes in pulmonary function and functional status in breast cancer patients after systemic chemotherapy

and radiotherapy: a prospective study. BMC Pulm Med. 2024;24(1):83.
24. Tao JJ, Visvanathan K, Wolff AC. Long term side effects of adjuvant chemotherapy in patients with early breast cancer. Breast. 2015;24:149–53.
25. Dorothy A, White MO, Godwin TA, Stover DE. Chemotherapy-associated pulmonary toxic reactions during treatment for breast cancer. Arch Intern Med. 1984;144:953–6.
26. Omarini C, Thanopoulou E, Johnston SR. Pneumonitis and pulmonary fibrosis associated with breast cancer treatments. Breast Cancer Res Treat. 2014;146(2):245–58.
27. Vento S, Cainelli F, Temesgen Z. Lung infections after cancer chemotherapy. Lancet Oncol. 2008;9(10):982–92.
28. Mo H, Jazieh KA, Brinzevich D, Abraham J. A review of treatment-induced pulmonary toxicity in breast cancer. Clin Breast Cancer. 2022;22(1):1–9.
29. Kassem L, Shohdy KS, Lasheen S, Abdel-Rahman O, Bachelot T. Hematological adverse effects in breast cancer patients treated with cyclin-dependent kinase 4 and 6 inhibitors: a systematic review and meta-analysis. Breast Cancer. 2018;25(1):17–27.
30. Evangelos Briasoulis NP. Noncardiogenic pulmonary edema: an unusual and serious complication of anticancer therapy. Oncologist. 2001;6:153–61.
31. Krengli M, Sacco M, Loi G, Masini L, Ferrante D, Gambaro G, et al. Pulmonary changes after radiotherapy for conservative treatment of breast cancer: a prospective study. Int J Radiat Oncol Biol Phys. 2008;70(5):1460–7.
32. Curigliano G, Mayer EL, Burstein HJ, Winer EP, Goldhirsch A. Cardiac toxicity from systemic cancer therapy: a comprehensive review. Prog Cardiovasc Dis. 2010;53(2):94–104.
33. Franzoi MA, Agostinetto E, Perachino M, Del Mastro L, de Azambuja E, Vaz-Luis I, et al. Evidence-based approaches for the management of side-effects of adjuvant endocrine therapy in patients with breast cancer. Lancet Oncol. 2021;22(7):e303–e13.
34. Lin HF, Liao KF, Chang CM, Lin CL, Lai SW, Hsu CY. Correlation of the tamoxifen use with the increased risk of deep vein thrombosis and pulmonary embolism in elderly women with breast cancer: a case-control study. Medicine. 2018;97(51):e12842.
35. Whisenant MS, Strunk FA, Tripathy D, Williams LA. What symptoms are important to patients? Developing a symptom burden measure for women with breast cancer. Support Care Cancer. 2019;27(12):4639–47.
36. So WK, Law BM, Ng MS, He X, Chan DN, Chan CW, et al. Symptom clusters experienced by breast cancer patients at various treatment stages: a systematic review. Cancer Med. 2021;10(8):2531–65.
37. Kwekkeboom KL, Tostrud L, Costanzo E, Coe CL, Serlin RC, Ward SE, et al. The role of inflammation in the pain, fatigue, and sleep disturbance symptom cluster in advanced cancer. J Pain Symptom Manag. 2018;55(5):1286–95.
38. Mendoza TR, Zhao F, Cleeland CS, Wagner LI, Patrick-Miller LJ, Fisch MJ. The validity and utility of the M. D. Anderson symptom inventory in patients with breast cancer: evidence from the symptom outcomes and practice patterns data from the Eastern Cooperative Oncology Group. Clin Breast Cancer. 2013;13(5):325–34.
39. Miriam AG, Sprangers MG, Arraras JI, Franklin J, te Velde A, Muller M, Franzini L, Williams A, de Haes HCJM, Hopwood P, Cull A, Aaronson NK. The European Organization for Research and treatment of cancer breast cancer-specific quality-of-life questionnaire module: first results from a three-country field study. J Clin Oncol. 1996;14:2756–68.
40. Marianne J, Brady DFC, Mo F, Bonomi AE, Tulsky DS, Lloyd SR, Deasy S, Cobleigh M, Shiomoto G. Reliability and validity of the functional assessment of cancer therapy-breast quality-of-life instrument. J Clin Oncol. 1997;15:974–86.
41. Michele Dabrowski AS, Boucher K, Bloch J, Norman L, Buys SS, Ward JH, Carlquist L, Lovell MM. Clinical experience with the NCCN distress thermometer in breast cancer patients. J Natl Compr Cancer Netw. 2007;5:104–11.
42. Mancini JJ. Assessment of dyspnea in advanced cancer patients. Support Care Cancer. 1999;7:229–32.
43. Morice AH, Fontana GA, Belvisi MG, Birring SS, Chung KF, Dicpinigaitis PV, et al. ERS guidelines on the assessment of cough. Eur Respir J. 2007;29(6):1256–76.
44. Kathleen Van Dyk PA. Cancer-related cognitive impairment in patients with a history of breast cancer. JAMA. 2021;326(17):1736–7.
45. Mouadh Hiraoui NG. Effects of multimodal training program on muscle deoxygenation in women with breast cancer: a randomized controlled trial. Physiol Int. 2022;109(2):246–60.
46. Ferrara PE, Gatto DM, Codazza S, Zordan P, Stefinlongo G, Ariani M, et al. An update on rehabilitative treatment of shoulder disease after breast cancer care. Musculoskelet Surg. 2024;108(1):31–45.
47. Ucurum SG, Felekoglu E, Naz I, Kaya DO, Bayram KB, Alacacioglu A. Investigation of the relationship between spinal posture and mobility to respiratory muscle strength and pulmonary functions in unilateral breast cancer surgery survivors: a cross-sectional study. Support Care Cancer. 2023;31(12):714.
48. Vardar-Yağli N, Şener G, Sağlam M, Inal Ince D, Çalik Kütükçü E, Arikan H, et al. Meme Kanseri Olan Kadinlarda Ve Sağlikli Kişilerde Pulmoner Fonksiyonlar Ve Solunum Kas Kuvvetinin Karşilaştirilmasi. Turk J Physiother Rehabil. 2015;25(3):19.
49. O'Donnell DE, Webb KA, Langer D, Elbehairy AF, Neder JA, Dudgeon DJ. Respiratory factors contributing to exercise intolerance in breast cancer survivors: a case-control study. J Pain Symptom Manag. 2016;52(1):54–63.
50. Dolan LB, Lane K, McKenzie DC. Optimal mode for maximal aerobic exercise testing in breast cancer survivors. Integr Cancer Ther. 2012;11(4):321–6.

51. Galiano-Castillo N, Arroyo-Morales M, Ariza-Garcia A, Sanchez-Salado C, Fernandez-Lao C, Cantarero-Villanueva I, et al. The six-minute walk test as a measure of health in breast cancer patients. J Aging Phys Act. 2016;24(4):508–15.
52. Jones LW, Eves ND, Haykowsky M, Joy AA, Douglas PS. Cardiorespiratory exercise testing in clinical oncology research: systematic review and practice recommendations. Lancet Oncol. 2008;9(8):757–65.
53. Brennan ME, Houssami N. Evaluation of the evidence on staging imaging for detection of asymptomatic distant metastases in newly diagnosed breast cancer. Breast. 2012;21(2):112–23.
54. Foulkes SJ, Edith P, Thompson Richard B, André LG, Haykowsky Mark J. A review on the role of exercise training to prevent a decline in cardiorespiratory fitness and cardiac function in breast cancer survivors. J Cardiopulm Rehabil Prev. 2024;44(1):5–14.
55. Peddle-McIntyre CJ, Singh F, Thomas R, Newton RU, Galvao DA, Cavalheri V. Exercise training for advanced lung cancer. Cochrane Database Syst Rev. 2019;2(2):CD012685.
56. McCarthy B, Casey D, Devane D, Murphy K, Murphy E, Lacasse Y. Pulmonary rehabilitation for chronic obstructive pulmonary disease. Cochrane Database Syst Rev. 2015;2:CD003793.
57. Perez-Dominguez B, Garcia-Cerdan P, Perpiña-Martinez S, Garcia-Isidoro S, Rodriguez-Rodriguez AM, Blanco-Diaz M. Effects of exercise on respiratory muscle function and functional capacity in patients with cancer. Systematic review. Clin Cancer Invest J. 2023;12(3):19–26.
58. Odinets T, Briskin Y, Pityn M. Effect of individualized physical rehabilitation programs on respiratory function in women with post-mastectomy syndrome. Physiother Theory Pract. 2019;35(5):419–26.
59. Nakano J, Hashizume K, Fukushima T, Ueno K, Matsuura E, Ikio Y, et al. Effects of aerobic and resistance exercises on physical symptoms in cancer patients: a meta-analysis. Integr Cancer Ther. 2018;17(4):1048–58.
60. Vardar Yagli N, Sener G, Arikan H, Saglam M, Inal Ince D, Savci S, et al. Do yoga and aerobic exercise training have impact on functional capacity, fatigue, peripheral muscle strength, and quality of life in breast cancer survivors? Integr Cancer Ther. 2015;14(2):125–32.
61. Liu X, Wang YQ, Xie J. Effects of breathing exercises on patients with lung cancer. Oncol Nurs Forum. 2019;46(3):303–17.
62. Shahriari M, Dehghan M, Pahlavanzadeh S, Hazini A. Effects of progressive muscle relaxation, guided imagery and deep diaphragmatic breathing on quality of life in elderly with breast or prostate cancer. J Educ Health Promot. 2017;6:1.
63. Pedrero Leal C, Yuste Sánchez MJ, Arranz MB. Efecto De La Espirometría Incentiva Y Máscara PEP En La Funci6n Pulmonar De Mujeres Tratadas De Cáncer De Mama Con Radioterapia: Estudio De Caso. Fisioterapia. 2019;41(6):337–41.
64. Qing-Hua Song R, Zhang Q-H, Ma M, Zhao X-P. Relaxation training during chemotherapy for breast cancer improves mental health and lessens adverse events. Int. J Clin Exp Med. 2013;6(10):979–84.
65. Aybar DO, Kilic SP, Cinkir HY. The effect of breathing exercise on nausea, vomiting and functional status in breast cancer patients undergoing chemotherapy. Complement Ther Clin Pract. 2020;40:101213.
66. Gündogdu F. The effects of pranayama or deep breathing exercises on fatigue and sleep quality in women receiving radiation therapy for breast cancer. Oncol Nurs Forum. 2023;50(4):509–20.
67. Dhruva A, Miaskowski C, Abrams D, Acree M, Cooper B, Goodman S, et al. Yoga breathing for cancer chemotherapy-associated symptoms and quality of life: results of a pilot randomized controlled trial. J Altern Complement Med. 2012;18(5):473–9.
68. Domaszewska K, Pienkowski T, Janiak A, Bukowska D, Laurentowska M. The influence of soft tissue therapy on respiratory efficiency and chest mobility of women suffering from breast cancer. Int J Environ Res Public Health. 2019;16:24.
69. Banerjee G, Rose A, Briggs M, Johnson MI. Could kinesiology taping help mitigate pain, breathlessness and abdominal-related symptoms in cancer? BMJ Case Rep. 2017;2017:216695.
70. Ray AD, Williams BT, Mahoney MC. Respiratory muscle training improves exercise performance and quality of life in cancer survivors: a pilot study. Rehabil Oncol. 2017;35(2):81–9.
71. Dahhak A, Devoogdt N, Langer D. Adjunctive inspiratory muscle training during a rehabilitation program in patients with breast cancer: an exploratory double-blind, randomized, controlled pilot study. Arch Rehabil Res Clin Transl. 2022;4(2):100196.
72. Parker BA, Pierce JP. Importance of smoking cessation to reduce breast cancer mortality. J Clin Oncol. 2016;34(12):1295–6.
73. Yamaguchi T, Goya S, Kohara H, Watanabe H, Mori M, Matsuda Y, et al. Treatment recommendations for respiratory symptoms in cancer patients: clinical guidelines from the Japanese Society for Palliative Medicine. J Palliat Med. 2016;19(9):925–35.
74. Hui D, Maddocks M, Johnson MJ, Ekstrom M, Simon ST, Ogliari AC, et al. Management of breathlessness in patients with cancer: ESMO clinical practice guidelines. ESMO Open. 2020;5(6):e001038.
75. Pardoll D. Cancer and the immune system: basic concepts and targets for intervention. Semin Oncol. 2015;42(4):523–38.
76. Getu MAWP, Addissie A, Seife E, Chen C, Kantelhardt EJ. The effect of cognitive behavioural therapy integrated with activity pacing on cancer-related fatigue, depression and quality of life among patients with breast cancer undergoing chemotherapy in ethiopia: a randomised clinical trial. Int J Cancer. 2023;152(12):2541–53.

Fine Motor Function in Breast Cancer: Special Focus on Sensation

16

Burcu Semin Akel, Halenur Evrendilek, and Zeynep Hoşbay

Breast cancer in women ranks as the most prevalent form of cancer globally, with 2.26 million newly diagnosed cases [1]. Patients with breast cancer generally receive multimodal treatments like chemotherapy, hormone therapy, radiotherapy, and/or surgery. Though these treatments are necessary, however, they might cause functional limitations, cognitive impairment, emotional challenges, and chemotherapy-induced peripheral neuropathy (CIPN) with other various adverse effects [2–4]. One of the most challenging symptoms is sensory disturbances and extended limitations during the execution of fine motor skills. Being aware of the risk of diminished fine motor function is necessary for women undergoing combined cancer treatment to support the patient multidisciplinary and to improve overall patient experiences and quality of life [5].

Fine motor skills are defined as small muscle movements requiring control, coordination, and accuracy during specific tasks. The hand is a complex organ for performing manual tasks such as grasping, drawing, using scissors, writing, carrying, and manipulating objects. This definition is also known as visual-motor integration, perceptual-motor skills, manual dexterity, hand–eye coordination, manual control, visuomotor skill, and graphomotor in literature [6, 7]. Hand use is influenced by aging, gender, and as well as previous injury, disease, or applied treatment [8]. Decreased unimanual and bimanual hand dexterity is determined both in dominant and non-dominant hands of women with breast cancer after a multi-modal treatment with surgery and chemotherapy or surgery, chemotherapy, and radiotherapy [5].

16.1 Neural and Sensory Mechanism of Manual Dexterity

Right before grasping an object, the hand preshapes into different postures depending on the size and shape of the object. This involves coordinated flexion, extension and spreading of the fingers, with a tendency for independent thumb motion [9, 10]. Sophisticated functions and dexterity of the hand are enabled by neural control of the musculoskeletal structures. The primary motor cortex (M1) has a critical role in the dexterity of manual behavior, control of the manual application of forces, and effectiveness of selectivity on muscle recruitment. As a dynamic process, the corticospinal input is strongest for the forearm muscles during the reach toward an object; and shifts to the intrinsic hand muscles as the hand closes over an object [11]. M1 also has

B. S. Akel (✉) · H. Evrendilek
Physiotherapy and Rehabilitation, T.C. Istanbul Kultur University, Istanbul, Turkey

Z. Hoşbay
Physiotherapy and Rehabilitation, T.C. Istanbul Kultur University, Istanbul, Turkey

Physiotherapy and Rehabilitation, Biruni University, İstanbul, Turkey

Y. Bakar, A. Tuğral (eds.), *Managing Side Effects of Breast Cancer Treatment*,
https://doi.org/10.1007/978-3-031-75480-7_16

a modulating role on spinal reflexes and gating sensory inputs that ensure stabilization on the hand and wrist. One of the important parts of the brain is the posterior parietal cortex for visuomotor transformation that helps successful motor planning interaction by assuring visual guidance from objects' location and shape [12].

Beyond these sophisticated neural mechanisms, two exquisite sensory systems for manual dexterity are critical: tactile and proprioceptive sensitivity. While proprioception tracks the hand motion, touch gives information about the object. Patients who lose their senses due to peripheral neuropathies, immune diseases, cancer, or deficiencies might develop movement disorders.

The palmar surface of the hand is conferred around 17,000 nerve fibers that carry one of the four types of mechanoreceptors [13]. While rapidly adapting fibers innervate Meissner and Pacinian corpuscles, slowly adapting type 1 fiber innervates Merkel receptors, and slowly adapting type 2 fiber innervates Ruffini-like endings. While Meissner and Pacinian corpuscles have sensitivity to skin vibrations, Merkel receptors are sensitive to light pressure which is important for static discrimination of the shapes, rough textures, and edges. Ruffini-like endings respond to cutaneous stretch produced by digit or limb movements. Proprioceptive signals are conveyed from mechanoreceptors in the muscle and tendons and cutaneous mechanoreceptors. Muscle spindles and Golgi tendon organs are sensitive to limb conformation and applied forces [14].

16.2 Fine Motor Skills in Breast Cancer Patients

Chemotherapy (CT), which is a common effective, standard, and proven care for patients, has detrimental neurotoxic effects on nerves and related structures [15, 16]. As a consequence of chemotherapeutic treatments, CIPN is the most common neurological side effect ranging from 30% to 60%, and has a critical impact on quality of life, and physiological and psychological health [17, 18]. Dose intensity, cumulative dose exposure, therapy duration, and other medications may affect the incidence of CIPN. As an accepted side effect of CT drugs, CIPN manifests sensory disturbances and results in a decrease in quality of life and functional capacity for cancer survivors. It occurs due to the disruption of the neuronal electrical activity caused by CT which leads to damage to peripheral nerve fibers. CIPN can cause a variety of sensory, motor, and autonomic symptoms [16, 19]. Cancer survivors experiencing CIPN with hypersensitivity and loss of sensation can report symmetrical numbness, tingling, discomfort, reduced handgrip strength, skin sensation, and pain, particularly in the distal part of both the upper and lower body as stock and glove-like distribution. These symptoms can increase the risk of falls and injuries and negatively impact both fine motor skills (such as dressing, writing, and buttoning) and gross motor abilities [20–22]. CT agents such as anthracyclines have inhibiting effects on the mitochondrial function which results in a decrease in muscle strength and activity tolerance [23]. Inducing muscle depletion in intrinsic muscles might affect fine motor function. Different treatment modalities might also cause different fine motor changes. It is found that neoadjuvant chemotherapy showed better Minnesota Manual Dexterity Test results compared to adjuvant chemotherapy [19].

One of the most troublesome long-term complications of surgery in breast cancer is secondary lymphedema, which is caused by interruption or damage of lymphatic circulation and leads to accumulation of lymph fluid regionally or generally in the interstitial space [24]. The incidence of secondary lymphedema is ranging from 12.5% to 56% within two years after completion of treatment [25–27].

Lymphedema has a negative impact on arm morbidity due to symptomatic arm or shoulder problems around the prevalence between 30% to 70% and has a critical impact on the quality of life in breast cancer survivors [26]. Lymphedema results in patient discomfort and functional impairment due to a reduction in the range of motion (ROM), muscle weakness, paresthesia, cervical radiculopathy, peripheral neuropathy, pain, musculoskeletal problems such as rotator cuff tendonitis, adhesive capsulitis, and neural compression. All possible pathologies can limit upper limb function and performance. Also, patients with lymphedema might experience disfigurement, emotional stress, and depression that causes activity limitations and reduced social participation by decreasing quality of life [28–30]. Early detection and management of lymphedema is important for better clinical outcomes and decreases the rate of breast cancer-related lymphedema (BCRL) by 50% [31].

The main symptoms of lymphedema are swelling, tightness, and heaviness. However, trophic changes, pain, and sensory symptoms such as paresthesia, numbness, or tenderness can also accompany the main symptoms [32]. Sensory changes after breast cancer treatment might be related to secondary damage of the intercostal brachial and thoracodorsal nerves. Symptoms such as pain and heaviness due to lymphedema can affect shoulder function [33, 34]. It is found that patients with BCRL have significantly decreased hand grip strength while fine motor test (Nine-Hole Peg and Box and Block) results were similar compared to ones without BCRL [35]. In lymphedema, changes in extracellular fluid volume may activate mechanoreceptors and cause self-reported perceived larger arm size and swelling [36]. Decreased sensitivity for mechanical stimuli and sensory perception at the affected side and negative self-reported body perception have been extensively described in BCRL [37, 38]. Although not fully understood, altered or diminished sensory input after treatment may negatively impact the bodily representation within the somatosensory cortex among lymphedema patients [39]. Also, peripheral sensitization can cause sensory abnormalities, pain, and increased excitability of nociceptors which might lead to nociplastic pain [38, 40, 41].

Cancer-related fatigue limits the physical functioning of breast cancer survivors which has a significant impact on the ability to live independently. Even though, caregiver support is important for the patient's quality of life, independence, psychosocial health, and treatment process management, the over-attention of caregivers might contribute to decreased physical activity demands of the patient which makes patients more vulnerable to the negative effects of physical inactivity. Caregiver burden is known to be associated with increased arm disability in breast cancer survivors; however, the disability may worsen with excessive care. Uncontrolled care and fatigue can impair fine motor dexterity [42, 43].

16.3 Assessment of Sensory and Fine Motor Skills

Women with breast cancer who are treated with surgery might have disturbed somatosensory functioning with a high prevalence of sensory loss and/or pain. Assessment of somatosensory and fine motor skills during the early stages of breast cancer treatment plays a key role in early intervention approaches [44, 45]. Physiotherapists possess the capability to conduct proactive evaluations and screenings encompassing both sensory and motor functionalities, inclusive of fine motor proficiency, leveraging appropriate tools and expertise. The principal outcome metrics, delineated henceforth, pertain primarily to fine motor capabilities. These encompass pain assessment metrics, sensory examinations such as tactile and pressure sensitivity evaluations, appraisal of manual grip strength, and evaluations of functional dexterity [19, 46].

16.4 Sensory Testing

Quantitative sensory testing (QST) can be used as a noninvasive technique to examine the function of the somatosensory nervous system. This test includes 7 tests to assess the functioning of myelinated A-alpha, A-beta, A-delta fibers, small unmyelinated C fibers, and corresponding central pathways by interpreting standardized stimuli tests and the self-reported sensory experience. It involves the systematic measurement of various sensory modalities such as touch, pressure, temperature, and pain perception. Table 16.1 shows the testing methods valid for women with breast cancer [47, 48]. Additionally 2 point discrimination, and vibration detection with a tuning fork can be evaluated. It takes 60–90 min to complete and cannot give the exact source of somatosen-

Table 16.1 Overview of the quantitative sensory testing protocol [47]

QST method	Device	Outcome	Test location
Mechanical detection threshold	Von Frey monofilaments	Geometric mean of first and last detected stimulus (mN)	Inner upper arm Lateral trunk Quadriceps
Mechanical pain threshold	Von Frey monofilaments	Geometric mean of first and last painful stimulus (mN)	Inner upper arm Lateral trunk Quadriceps
Pressure pain threshold	Digital algometer	Method of limits: arithmetic mean of two trials (kgf)	Upper trapezius Pectoral region Lateral trunk Quadriceps
Thermal detection threshold – Warmth detection threshold – Cold detection threshold	Thermode system (TSA II)	Method of limits: arithmetic mean of three trials (C°)	Inner upper arm Lateral trunk Quadriceps
Thermal pain threshold – Heat pain threshold – Cold pain threshold	Thermode system (TSA II)	Method of limits: arithmetic mean of three trials (C°)	Inner upper arm Lateral trunk Quadriceps
Temporal summation	Von Frey monofilament 256 mN	Difference in pain intensity between immediately after 30-s stimulation and after single stimulation (NRS)	Pectoral region
Conditional pain modulation	Two-thermode system (Q-sense)	Difference in pain intensity between conditioned test stimulus and test stimulus without conditioning (NRS)	Volar side lower arm – Conditioning stimulus: non-affected side – Test stimulus: affected side

kgf kilogram-force, *mN* millinewtons, *NRS* numerical rating scale, *s* seconds

sory dysfunction but it can be useful to identify underlying contributing pain mechanisms and pathophysiology, which can assist with targeted intervention strategies [38, 44, 47]. While testing, the patient is briefed about the procedure. This may involve removing restrictive clothing or ensuring the patient is in a comfortable position. Different sensory modalities are tested using specific stimuli. For example, tactile sensitivity may be assessed using a monofilament, pressure sensitivity with an algometer, temperature perception with thermodes, and pain perception with calibrated mechanical or thermal devices. The selected stimuli are applied to predetermined areas of the patient's body. These areas may include both affected and unaffected regions, depending on the condition being assessed. The patient's response to each stimulus is measured quantitatively [47, 48] (Table 16.1).

Therapists may prefer to conduct necessary assessments individually. Pain assessment can be done to understand the severity and threshold of sensory pain. *The Visual Analog Scale (VAS)* is a scale where 0 represents no pain and 10 represents the worst imaginable pain, and patients are asked to report a number corresponding to the severity of pain they are experiencing. This scale is the most preferred one for determining the level of pain. *A pressure algometer* is a tool used to examine the pressure pain threshold for both regional and widespread musculoskeletal pain (Fig. 16.1). It includes a system and an indicator that applies pressure to a surface area of 1 cm^2, converting the force to Newtons (N/cm^2) or kilograms (kgf/cm^2). These units can be converted to kilopascals (kPa), which is an internationally recognized unit of pressure measurement in pain tolerance [19, 49, 50]. It can be used as a part of

QST but also separately. Figure 16.1 shows the frequently used measurement points.

Light touch/pressure assessment can be conducted for mechanical detection or allodynia detection. The examination entails the use of a cotton tip, with its tip bent to a point, a Frey brush, or a fingertip. During the procedure, the patient's eyes remain closed. Patients are instructed to signal whenever they perceive the stimulus. This stimulus is systematically applied to various regions like the ulnar side of the hand, radial side of the hand, and volar side of the forearm to ascertain the boundaries of any sensory deficits. Augmented touch sensitivity is termed hyperesthesia, diminished sensation is termed hypoesthesia, and complete absence of sensation is termed anesthesia.

Semmes–Weinstein monofilament test can be used to evaluate sensory perception and tactile sensitivity and detect peripheral neuropathy. This test is one of the most commonly used tests in sensory assessment as a reliable, standardized, affordable, and easily administered method of obtaining quantitative sensory data. It involves applying nylon monofilaments of varying thicknesses (measured in grams of force) to the skin of the hand (Fig. 16.2). Typically, it is preferred to apply them distally on the palmar surface of the first, second, and fifth fingers, as well as the web area of the dorsal surface of the hand. The monofilament is held perpendicular to the skin and pressed until it bends slightly for 1.5 s, ensuring a consistent force, before being removed from the area prior to repeating the process. During testing, the patient is asked to verbally acknowledge perception by saying "yes" or "I felt," while their eyes remain closed. The examination begins with the smallest diameter monofilament (1.65 or 2.83) and progresses to larger diameters until the patient perceives the touch sensation. If there is no response to the last filament (6.65), it indicates an absent tactile sense.

Vibration perception threshold measurement can provide valuable information about the integrity of the sensory nervous system and help identify sensory deficits. In tracking vibration sensation, a tuning fork with a frequency of 30 cycles/s for Meissner corpuscles and 256 cycles/s

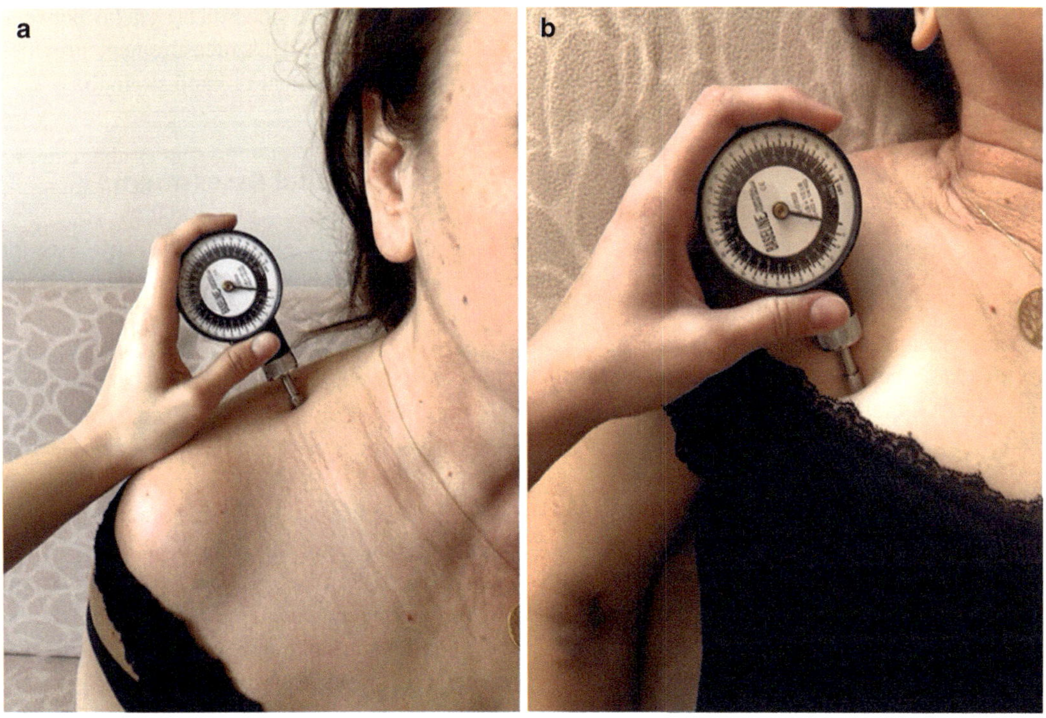

Fig. 16.1 Pressure pain threshold measurement with digital algometer (**a** upper trapezius muscle, **b** pectoral muscle)

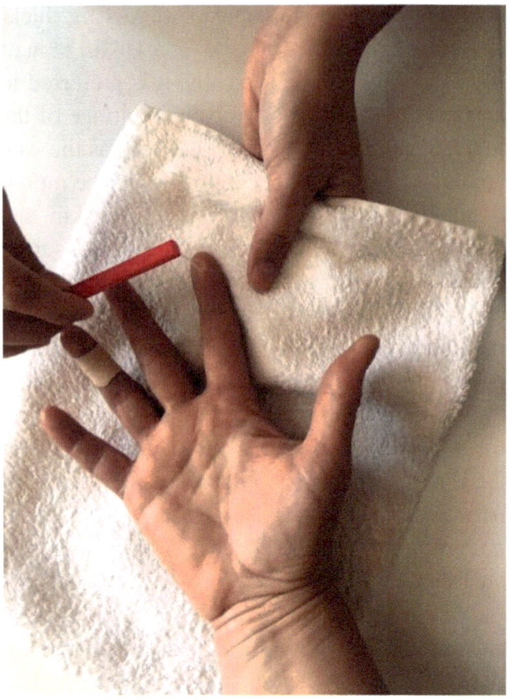

Fig. 16.2 Semmes weinstein monofilament testing

for Pacinian corpuscles is used. Utilizing a low-frequency tuning fork enables the evaluation of both initial nerve impairment and the subsequent restoration and reinnervation of previously affected nerves. The tuning fork is struck against the edge of the examination table and then applied to the skin to be tested. With eyes closed, the patient is asked if they perceive the vibration when it is placed firmly and vertically on a bony prominence at the extremities (radial and ulnar styloid processes, humerus epicondyles, olecranon, etc.). If perceived, then they are asked to indicate when the vibration stops. Thus, the duration of vibration perception is determined.

16.4.1 Grip Strength Measurement

A decrease in muscular functioning due to cancer itself or sensory changes has an impact on fine motor skills. Grip strength is measured in breast cancer patients as it serves as an indicator of physical function and overall health. It allows healthcare providers to assess the muscular function and to monitor changes over time. Additionally, grip strength is associated with activities of daily living and quality of life, so monitoring it can provide valuable insights into a patient's functional status and help guide rehabilitation interventions to improve fine motor strength and function.

Grip strength measurement involves using a handheld device called a hand dynamometer to assess grip strength. The hand dynamometer is designed to measure the maximum force generated by the muscles of the hand and forearm when squeezing the device. The measurement is done according to the recommendation of the American Society for Surgery of the Hand and the American Society of Hand Therapists. During testing, the patient sits with shoulder adduction and neutral rotation, elbow at 90°flexion, forearm in a neutral position, and wrist at 0 to 30° of dorsiflexion. The therapist gently supports the base of the dynamometer while placing it in the patient's hand and instructs the patient to grip it as tightly as possible. The patient is then asked to squeeze the handle as hard as possible without support. An average of three measurements are taken in kg/f for each side by a 60-s delay between each measurement. This measurement provides an objective assessment of hand strength.

16.5 Functional Assessments

The predominantly preferred dexterity tests for assessing fine motor function in patients with breast cancer are elaborated upon below.

Jebsen Taylor test: The Jebsen Hand Function Test, described by Jebson and colleagues in 1969, is a valid test for determining the functional capacity of the upper extremity. It is an objective test that evaluates hand and upper extremity functions in daily life activities. It is often considered the "gold standard" and norms for the Jebsen Taylor Hand Function Test are classified based on the maximum time required to complete the tests, dominant hand, age, and gender. This test consists of tasks involving common gripping types used in daily life and evaluates the speed of individuals in these tasks. It assesses both dominant and non-dominant hand skills and provides an objective assessment with 7 subtests. These 7 subtests include writing, turning cards, picking up small objects and placing them in a box, stacking checkers, simulating feeding, carrying large light objects, and carrying large heavy objects. The time taken to complete each subtest is measured with a stopwatch and recorded in seconds [5, 51].

Grooved pegboard test: The Grooved pegboard is a neuropsychological assessment tool used to assess fine motor coordination and dexterity. The test is a manipulative skill test consisting of a board with 25 holes and a set of pegs with a unique shape on one end. The pegs need to be rotated to the correct position to enter the holes. During the test, the individual is required to insert the pegs into the corresponding slots as quickly and accurately as possible, using one hand at a time. Performance on the test is evaluated based on the total time taken to complete it. The Grooved Pegboard Test demands a higher level of visual-motor coordination than conventional Pegboard assessments [52].

Purdue pegboard test (PPT): This test is a reliable, easily applicable, and time-efficient measure that assesses finger dexterity and hand coordination for both unilateral and bilateral fine motor skills. The test consists of nails, washers, and a pegboard apparatus. There are two parallel rows of 25 holes on both sides of the board. The nails and washers are placed in designated spaces on the board. The test comprises 5 sections, including 4 main subtests assessing the dominant hand, non-dominant hand, both hands, a combined evaluation of dominant + non-dominant + both hands, and an additional subtest where all activities are performed together.

It holds promise as a valuable assessment tool in the context of breast cancer. This standardized assessment evaluates fine motor dexterity and hand–eye coordination, offering insights into physical function and potential neurological effects. With its simplicity and ease of administration, the PPT can be effectively utilized in clinical settings without the need for specialized training. Its portability further enhances its utility, allowing for convenient use in various healthcare environments. In the realm of breast cancer survivorship care, the PPT shows potential for facilitating long-term monitoring, aiding in the early detection of motor impairments, and guiding interventions to optimize functional outcomes [5].

Archimedes spiral drawing test: This test is a neuropsychological assessment tool used to measure the speed and accuracy of fine motor skills, hand–eye coordination, and visuospatial abilities. During the test, the individual is asked to trace a spiral pattern starting from the center and gradually moving outward, using a pencil or pen and paper. The patients are not allowed to lean on their hands or arms. The goal is to maintain a consistent distance between each loop of the spiral while staying as close to the ideal spiral shape as possible with the dominant hand. Patients are asked to be as quick as possible. Performance on the test provides valuable information about motor control, precision, and spatial perception. The data can be collected in a computerized version by using an electronic drawing board and pen [53]. Movement time (s), length of drawing (cm), average speed, and speed variability (cm/s) can be recorded with this system and processed by software.

The Minnesota Manual Dexterity Test is a skill test applied to evaluate patients' ability to move small objects in different directions and assess hand–eye coordination and manual dexterity. It consists of a board in a 4 × 15 layout with a series of holes for a set of 60 circular pegs. The test has 5 parameters: placing, turning, displacing, one-hand turning and placing, and two-hand turning and placing. During the test, the individual is required to insert, turn, and remove the discs within a specific time frame, following a prescribed sequence of tasks. The individual is given at least one trial for each section, and the time spent for each section is recorded in seconds. Typically the test is done while standing however it can also be performed while sitting. As the test takes much more time than the other dexterity tests, it may give an insight into muscular endurance [19].

The Nine-Hole Peg test is used to determine the functional status of the hand. It consists of a square platform with 9 holes and 9 appropriate cylinders for these holes. The individual is asked to quickly pick up the 9 cylinders from a storage box, place them into the holes, and then return them to the storage box. Meanwhile, the time is measured in seconds using a stopwatch. The advantages of the test include its simplicity, portability, short duration, and low cost. However, its limitation lies in its inability to provide detailed information about the adequacy of daily life activities related to the upper extremity and its focus on factors such as endurance and speed rather than the nature of the activity, which may not adequately reflect the individual's functional capacity [54].

Moberg Pick-up Test: This test was initially developed by Moberg in 1958 and assesses sensory functioning, tactile gnosis, and fine motor proficiency. During the test, the patient is presented with a set of 12 small objects, such as coins or pins. The objects vary in size, shape, and texture, requiring the participant to utilize tactile sensation and manual dexterity to complete the task. The individual is asked to pick objects up one by one and place them in a small container. Participants use their free hand to stabilize the container. In this test, patients are instructed to close their eyes and verbally identify the objects as they place them. Time is recorded in seconds [55].

Patient-reported CIPN severity and upper-limb symptoms can be evaluated with outcome measures. The European Organization for Research and Treatment of Cancer Quality of Life Questionnaire-Core (EORTC-QLQ-CIPN20) is a valid, widely used patient-reported outcome measure that quantifies the quality of life. The test consists of 20 items that include upper limb functional activities like difficulty in writing (item 11) and manipulating small objects with the fingers (item 12). Fatigue, pain, and overall functioning are also covered within the questionnaire. The questionnaire is designed to be self-administered and higher scores indicate more severe CIPN. The sum score of these two items (S11 and S12; score range: 2–8) is used as a composite measure of patient-reported upper limb functional deficit severity [56].

16.6 Increasing Fine Motor Capacity by Sensory-Based Rehabilitation

Sensory-based reasons that can decrease fine motor skills were explained previously. The common problems that affect daily life and hand use of patients with BC are peripheral neuropathy and lymphedema [2]. Even though a treatment protocol is missing, there are some methods to cope with the problems. Education, self-management strategies, exercise, and skills training are commonly used for better functioning.

16.6.1 Educational Methods

Maladaptive cognitions exert a profound influence on sensory processing, perceived pain levels, disability, and the attitude towards rehabilitation among individuals dealing with side effects of cancer treatment [57]. In these cases, perceived symptoms can be consistently high despite the actual severity of the underlying pathology. The initial step toward addressing these challenges lies in enhancing patients' understanding of their condition [58]. Educational programs are offered for individuals dealing with breast cancer, however, they primarily focus on elucidating anatomical structures, medical interventions, and pharmaceutical options, and they often fall short of addressing the multidimensional nature of symptoms such as pain, neuropathy, and discomfort [59]. These symptoms not only impact physical health but also vitality, mood, social interactions, and various other dimensions of well-being. Therefore, comprehensive education should encompass the human components of biology, emotion, spirituality, and sociality [60].

To effectively manage the complexities associated with sensory symptoms, it is imperative to integrate psychosocial considerations into treatment strategies. Understanding the patient's individual circumstances and social environment is of paramount importance in tailoring interventions to their specific needs [5, 61]. A comprehensive assessment can help professionals understand patient experiences and develop a management plan. Open communication is needed among healthcare providers, cancer patients, and their families. Management is more effective when overall goals and limitations are understood, and both the patient and family are educated and involved in the decision-making process [62].

Education should delve into the physiology underlying sensory symptoms, including phenomena like numbness, pain, and hypersensitivity. Neuroscience-based educational interventions offer promising avenues for reconceptualizing pain perception [63, 64]. By elucidating that pain does not always reflect the actual state of tissue damage but rather represents the interpretation of potential injury threat to the nervous system, influenced by psychological factors such as anxiety, distress, cognitions, and beliefs, patients can gain valuable insights into their experiences and develop more effective coping mechanisms [65]. Patients and families are taught to replace anxious thoughts with helpful cognitions. During education, expected symptoms and their causes; biological knowledge like tissue health, inflammation, and neuroanatomy; factors contributing to the experience like self-efficacy, stress response, cognitive reconstructing for cancer, wrong beliefs related to symptom or exercise; activity-rest balance and useful coping strategies can be covered.

Sensory education programs aim to empower patients by providing them with knowledge and strategies to cope with the changes effectively. Through sensory education, patients learn about potential sensory alterations they may experience during treatment, understand the underlying causes, and discover techniques to mitigate discomfort and enhance their quality of life. Furthermore, sensory education fosters emotional resilience and empowers individuals to actively participate in their recovery journey. Coping with sensory changes and related challenges can emotionally be difficult for BC patients. By equipping them with knowledge and practical skills, sensory education not only enhances their ability to manage physical symptoms but also promotes psychological well-being. Through education and support, patients gain a sense of control over their bodies and develop confidence in navigating the complexities of life after breast cancer treatment. Overall, sensory education serves as a cornerstone in the comprehensive care approach for individuals affected by BC, empowering them to lead fulfilling lives beyond their diagnosis [66–69].

Self-management strategies play a pivotal role in empowering individuals to navigate the complexities of BC diagnosis, treatment, and survivorship. It is also helpful in managing sensory symptoms and participating in activities. These strategies encompass a broad range of practices aimed at enhancing patients' autonomy, resilience, and overall well-being throughout their journey. Education serves as a cornerstone, enabling patients to understand their condition, treatment options, and potential side effects. By equipping individuals with knowledge about healthy lifestyle choices, symptom management techniques, and available support resources, they can actively participate in decision-making processes and take control of their health. The process can be initiated by the person or the environment. Through a holistic approach encompassing education, self-awareness, and community engagement, self-management strategies empower individuals affected by BC to optimize their quality of life and cultivate a sense of agency in their healing journey. Coping with symptoms can be more successful with self-management strategies [66, 70].

16.7 Exercise

Regular and aerobic exercises, upper extremity mobility exercises, fine motor skills training, and sensorimotor training can be used in individuals with cancer to decrease sensory disturbances and increase fine motor functioning.

Regular exercise has been associated with numerous positive outcomes, including reductions in cancer-related fatigue, improvements in physical function, muscle strength, and cardiorespiratory fitness, as well as enhancements in psychological well-being, mood, and body image [71]. Exercise interventions tailored to the specific needs and preferences of BC patients with supervision have been shown to promote well-being, mitigate treatment-related side effects, and facilitate the management of side effects and symptoms [71–73]. According to the guidelines from the European Society of Medical Oncology, physical exercise stands out as the non-pharmacological approach backed by Level 1 quality evidence for effectively managing neuropathic pain [73, 74]. Sensory side effects and neuropathic pain that decrease fine motor skills are shown to be less with strength, endurance, and sensorimotor training programs in comparison to standard care. The severity of sensory adverse symptoms was less with strength and endurance training with or without sensorimotor training [75]. Moderate intensity is preferred for the exercise regimen and walking, and resistance training is advised. Exercise can be adapted according to illness-related symptoms [75].

Exercise for fine motor skills in BC rehabilitation is a critical component of comprehensive care aimed at restoring and maintaining upper extremity function. Numerous studies have highlighted the benefits of exercise interventions for fine motor skills in BC survivors. Exercise programs targeting fine motor skills typically encompass a variety of activities aimed at improving coordination, dexterity, strength, precision, and flexibility in the hands and fingers [5, 76–78]. These exercises may include gripping and releasing objects of varying sizes and textures, manipulating small objects, performing precision tasks, and engaging in activities that promote finger and hand movement. Research has shown that structured exercise programs can lead to significant improvements in hand function, grip strength, and overall upper extremity function. Moreover, exercise has been associated with reductions in pain, stiffness, and disability, ultimately enhancing movement quality for affected individuals [76, 77].

Upper extremity functioning exercises to increase fine motor skills should include the shoulder region. Resection of the pectoral fascia during mastectomies may restrict shoulder movement by causing adherence to subcutaneous tissue [79]. The limitations may limit circulatory functioning and cause edema and sensory disturbances. Shoulder mobilization, myofascial release, and active range of motion exercises are useful. However, rigorous harmful exercises should be avoided. Nerve mobilization exercises can have a positive effect on neural tension that may arise due to inflammation, nerve compression, or impaired blood supply to the area. Neural tissue mobilization is recognized as an intervention to treat sensory-motor impairments in BC survivors with lymphedema [80]. Intrinsic strengthening and stabilization exercises can be recommended for increasing fine motor skills.

Active exercises that simulate activities are more effective in the upper extremity rehabilitation of individuals with BC [81]. Mostly affected fine motor skills in cancer patients are stated as writing, cutting, opening a bottle/pack of chips or jar, squeezing toothpaste or cloth, and closing zip. Psycho-educational stimulation activities that are used for children with cancer showed a slight improvement in overall occupational performance in school which includes fine motor skills [82]. These activities should be enriched with sensory stimuli.

Exercise for fine motor skills in breast cancer rehabilitation can be integrated into multidisciplinary care approaches to optimize outcomes. Collaborative efforts involving healthcare professionals such as physical therapists, occupational therapists, and oncology specialists allow for comprehensive assessment and tailored interventions addressing individual needs [83]. Moreover, incorporating elements of patient education, behavioral counseling, and self-management strategies can enhance the effectiveness of exercise programs and empower patients to actively participate in their recovery process. Future research endeavors should focus on identifying the most effective exercise modalities, optimal timing and duration of interventions, and strategies to promote long-term adherence and sustainability, thereby maximizing functional outcomes and quality of life for breast cancer survivors can be achieved.

16.8 Sensorimotor Training

Sensory training in BC represents a targeted approach to addressing sensory impairments and challenges experienced by individuals undergoing treatment or in post-treatment phases [84]. BC treatments such as surgery, chemotherapy, and radiation therapy can lead to sensory alterations like numbness, tingling, and pain in the affected breast and surrounding areas. Sensory training programs aim to enhance sensory perception, promote rehabilitation, and improve the quality of life for BC survivors [85]. Among the goals of sensory re-education, is to retrain neural pathways and responses to stimuli to restore a patient's sensory perception [86, 87]. Through a combination of education, exercises, and sensory stimulation techniques, patients can regain sensory function, alleviate discomfort, and regain confidence in their bodies.

Education about sensory changes and their management strategies is a central part of sensory training in breast cancer. As mentioned before, patients are empowered with knowledge about the potential sensory alterations they may encounter during treatment, along with understanding the underlying mechanisms behind these changes [86, 87]. Furthermore, sensory training encompasses a variety of sensory stimulation exercises. These exercises may include tactile stimulation, proprioceptive training, and sensory integration activities designed to improve sensory perception and motor function. By engaging in targeted sensory training exercises, patients can enhance their sensory awareness, restore function, and improve their overall quality of life. Additionally, sensory training programs may incorporate mindfulness and relaxation techniques to help patients manage stress and enhance their emotional well-being amidst the challenges of BC treatment and recovery.

Desensitization may be needed which refers to a therapeutic approach aimed at reducing or managing the heightened sensitivity to stimuli experienced by individuals. Desensitization techniques seek to alleviate abnormal sensations such as pain, tingling, numbness, and hypersensitivity to touch, temperature, or pressure. Methods typically involve gradual exposure to stimuli that trigger discomfort or pain, with the goal of reducing the nervous system's response over time. This may include gentle touch, massage, temperature variations (such as warm and cold water baths), and texture exploration using different materials. By repeatedly exposing the affected areas to these stimuli in a controlled and gradual manner, the nervous system can adapt and become less reactive, leading to decreased sensitivity and improved tolerance to sensations [88, 89].

Exercises can involve manipulating different objects to stimulate the tactile sense and enhance fine motor skills. Examples of sensory exercises that can increase fine motor skills include:

Texture exploration: Encouraging individuals to touch and manipulate objects with varying textures, such as smooth, rough, soft, or bumpy surfaces, to enhance tactile discrimination and sensory processing.

Finger painting: Engaging in activities like finger painting with different textures of paint or materials, such as sand or pudding, to promote finger dexterity, hand–eye coordination, and sensory integration.

Bead threading: Using small beads or buttons to thread onto a string or wire, requiring precise finger movements and hand–eye coordination to manipulate the objects and string them together.

Playdough activities: Utilizing playdough or similar moldable materials to sculpt shapes, roll balls, or create intricate designs, which can improve hand strength, finger control, and fine motor coordination.

Pegboard games: Using peg boards and pegs of various sizes to practice inserting and removing pegs from the board, promoting hand–eye coordination, finger dexterity, and spatial awareness.

Sensory bins: Creating sensory bins filled with materials like rice, beans, or sand, along with hidden objects or small toys, encouraging individuals to search, scoop, pour, and manipulate the materials to develop fine motor skills and sensory exploration.

Sensory exercises that increase fine motor skills provide opportunities for individuals to engage in hands-on activities that stimulate their senses while promoting the development of precise hand movements, finger control, and overall coordination. Sensory education may also include techniques such as manual lymphatic drainage, exercises, and compression garments to reduce swelling and improve overall well-being.

16.9 Conclusion

In conclusion, the exploration of fine motor function in breast cancer patients, with a special emphasis on sensation, offers profound insights into the holistic impact of the disease and its treatments. Through a nuanced examination of sensory experiences and motor capabilities, this chapter underscores the importance of addressing the multifaceted challenges faced by individuals undergoing breast cancer treatment. By integrating knowledge from various disciplines, from oncology to neuroscience, we can develop more comprehensive strategies to support patients in preserving and enhancing their quality of life.

During rehabilitation, it is important to develop manual control, coordination, and accuracy for tasks like writing, using scissors, and manipulating objects. A motivational basis can help during the process. This motivation can be enhanced through patient education. Unfortunately, there is currently no structured educational program available that specifically focuses on sensory disturbances, even though there are promising programs that focus on pain. The exploration of sensory-based hand exercises in the context of breast cancer rehabilitation provides an excellent opportunity to enhance fine motor skills. By engaging in exercises tailored to promote sensory awareness and dexterity, individuals undergoing breast cancer treatment can regain confidence and independence in their daily activities. Exercises that focus on perceptual-motor skills, manual dexterity, and fine coordination are necessary to gain fine motor proficiency. Desensitization programs, nerve gliding exercises, mobility exercises, general physical activity exercises, and body awareness programs are recommended for overcoming sensory disturbances and increasing fine motor skills.

Moving forward, continued research and clinical interventions aimed at optimizing fine motor function and sensory perception hold promise for fostering resilience and well-being in breast cancer survivors.

References

1. Ferlay J, Colombet M, Soerjomataram I, Parkin DM, Piñeros M, Znaor A, et al. Cancer statistics for the year 2020: an overview. Int J Cancer. 2021. https://doi.org/10.1002/ijc.33588.
2. Bao T, Basal C, Seluzicki C, Li SQ, Seidman AD, Mao JJ. Long-term chemotherapy-induced peripheral neuropathy among breast cancer survivors: prevalence, risk factors, and fall risk. Breast Cancer Res Treat. 2016;159(2):327–33.
3. Kubo Y, Naito T, Mori K, Osawa G, Aruga E. Skeletal muscle loss and prognosis of breast cancer patients. Support Care Cancer. 2017;25(7):2221–7.
4. Ono M, Ogilvie JM, Wilson JS, Green HJ, Chambers SK, Ownsworth T, et al. A meta-analysis of cognitive impairment and decline associated with adjuvant chemotherapy in women with breast cancer. Front Oncol. 2015;5:59.
5. Grusdat NP, Stäuber A, Tolkmitt M, Schnabel J, Schubotz B, Schulz H. Routine cancer treatment regimens and its impact on fine motor dexterity in breast cancer. Oncol Res Treat. 2022;45(1-2):37–44.
6. Magill FN, editor. International encyclopedia of psychology. London: Fitzroy Dearborn; 1996.
7. Michel DE, Pinson J. Music therapy in principle and practice. 2nd ed. Springfield: Charles C Thomas; 2012. p. 223.
8. Kumar S. Muscle strength. Boca Raton: CRC Press; 2004. Available from: https://www.taylorfrancis.com/books/9781134202201.
9. Häger-Ross C, Schieber MH. Quantifying the independence of human finger movements: comparisons of digits, hands, and movement frequencies. J Neurosci. 2000;20(22):8542–50.
10. Ingram JN, Körding KP, Howard IS, Wolpert DM. The statistics of natural hand movements. Exp Brain Res. 2008;188(2):223–36.
11. Lemon RN, Johansson RS, Westling G. Corticospinal control during reach, grasp, and precision lift in man. J Neurosci. 1995;15(9):6145–56.
12. Sobinov AR, Bensmaia SJ. The neural mechanisms of manual dexterity. Nat Rev Neurosci. 2021;22(12):741–57.
13. Johansson RS, Vallbo AB. Tactile sensibility in the human hand: relative and absolute densities of four

types of mechanoreceptive units in glabrous skin. J Physiol. 1979;286(1):283–300.
14. Goodman JM, Bensmaia SJ. The neural mechanisms of touch and proprioception at the somatosensory periphery. In: The senses: a comprehensive reference. Amsterdam: Elsevier; 2020. p. 2–27. Available from: https://linkinghub.elsevier.com/retrieve/pii/B9780128054086000142.
15. Derksen TME, Bours MJL, Mols F, Weijenberg MP. Lifestyle-related factors in the self-management of chemotherapy-induced peripheral neuropathy in colorectal cancer: a systematic review. Evid Based Complement Alternat Med. 2017;2017:1–14.
16. Xu M, Wang F, Zhu X, Hao Z. Efficacy of cryotherapy on chemotherapy-induced peripheral neuropathy in patients with breast cancer: a propensity score-matched study. Ann Med Surg. 2023;85(6):2695–703.
17. Seretny M, Currie GL, Sena ES, Ramnarine S, Grant R, MacLeod MR, et al. Incidence, prevalence, and predictors of chemotherapy-induced peripheral neuropathy: a systematic review and meta-analysis. Pain. 2014;155(12):2461–70.
18. Streckmann F, Zopf EM, Lehmann HC, May K, Rizza J, Zimmer P, et al. Exercise intervention studies in patients with peripheral neuropathy: a systematic review. Sports Med Auckl N Z. 2014;44(9):1289–304.
19. Tuğral A, Arıbaş Z, Akyol M, Bakar Y. Assessment of sensorimotor and strength related function of breast cancer patients during systemic drug therapy: a prospective observational study. BMC Cancer. 2023;23(1):981.
20. Cox-Martin E, Trahan LH, Cox MG, Dougherty PM, Lai EA, Novy DM. Disease burden and pain in obese cancer patients with chemotherapy-induced peripheral neuropathy. Support Care Cancer. 2017;25(6):1873–9.
21. Holst-Wolf J, Tseng YT, Konczak J. The Minnesota haptic function test. Front Psychol. 2019;10:818.
22. McCrary JM, Goldstein D, Trinh T, Timmins HC, Li T, Menant J, et al. Balance deficits and functional disability in cancer survivors exposed to neurotoxic cancer treatments. J Natl Compr Cancer Netw. 2019;17(8):949–55.
23. Sorensen JC, Cheregi BD, Timpani CA, Nurgali K, Hayes A, Rybalka E. Mitochondria: inadvertent targets in chemotherapy-induced skeletal muscle toxicity and wasting? Cancer Chemother Pharmacol. 2016;78(4):673–83.
24. Mortimer PS. The pathophysiology of lymphedema. Cancer. 1998;83(12 Suppl):2798–802.
25. Engel J, Kerr J, Schlesinger-Raab A, Sauer H, Hölzel D. Axilla surgery severely affects quality of life: results of a 5-year prospective study in breast cancer patients. Breast Cancer Res Treat. 2003;79(1):47–57.
26. Kwan W, Jackson J, Weir LM, Dingee C, McGregor G, Olivotto IA. Chronic arm morbidity after curative breast cancer treatment: prevalence and impact on quality of life. J Clin Oncol. 2002;20(20):4242–8.
27. Petrek JA, Senie RT, Peters M, Rosen PP. Lymphedema in a cohort of breast carcinoma survivors 20 years after diagnosis. Cancer. 2001;92(6):1368–77.
28. Chachaj A, Małyszczak K, Pyszel K, Lukas J, Tarkowski R, Pudełko M, et al. Physical and psychological impairments of women with upper limb lymphedema following breast cancer treatment. Psychooncology. 2010;19(3):299–305.
29. Dawes DJ, Meterissian S, Goldberg M, Mayo NE. Impact of lymphoedema on arm function and health-related quality of life in women following breast cancer surgery. J Rehabil Med. 2008;40(8):651–8.
30. Nesvold IL, Dahl AA, Løkkevik E, Marit Mengshoel A, Fosså SD. Arm and shoulder morbidity in breast cancer patients after breast-conserving therapy versus mastectomy. Acta Oncol Stockh Swed. 2008;47(5):835–42.
31. Rafn BS, Christensen J, Larsen A, Bloomquist K. Prospective surveillance for breast cancer-related arm lymphedema: a systematic review and meta-analysis. J Clin Oncol. 2022;40(9):1009–26.
32. Gursen C, Dylke ES, Moloney N, Meeus M, De Vrieze T, Devoogdt N, et al. Self-reported signs and symptoms of secondary upper limb lymphoedema related to breast cancer treatment: systematic review. Eur J Cancer Care. 2021;30(5):e13440.
33. Crosbie J, Kilbreath SL, Dylke E, Refshauge KM, Nicholson LL, Beith JM, et al. Effects of mastectomy on shoulder and spinal kinematics during bilateral upper-limb movement. Phys Ther. 2010;90(5):679–92.
34. Stubblefield MD, Keole N. Upper body pain and functional disorders in patients with breast cancer. PM R. 2014;6(2):170–83.
35. Kim SJ. Impact of the type of compression materials on manual dexterity of patients with breast cancer-related lymphedema (BCRL). J Phys Ther Sci. 2012;24(10):969–73.
36. Brunelle CL, Roberts SA, Horick NK, Gillespie TC, Jacobs JM, Daniell KM, et al. Integrating symptoms into the diagnostic criteria for breast cancer-related lymphedema: applying results from a prospective surveillance program. Phys Ther. 2020;100(12):2186–97.
37. Baran E, Özçakar L, Özgül S, Aksoy S, Akbayrak T. Upper limb sensory evaluations and ultrasonographic skin measurements in breast cancer-related lymphedema receiving complex decongestive physiotherapy. Support Care Cancer. 2021;29(11):6545–53.
38. Dams L, Van der Gucht E, Meeus M, Devoogdt N, Smeets A, Penen F, et al. Quantitative sensory testing in women after surgery for breast cancer: a systematic review and narrative synthesis. Clin J Pain. 2021;37(7):538–64.
39. Harvie DS, Edmond-Hank G, Smith AD. Tactile acuity is reduced in people with chronic neck pain. Musculoskelet Sci Pract. 2018;33:61–6.
40. De Groef A, Devoogdt N, Gursen C, Moloney N, Warpy V, Daelemans J, et al. Sensory signs and symptoms in women with self-reported breast cancer-

related lymphedema: a case-control study close up. J Cancer Surviv Res Pract. 2022;16(5):1096–106.
41. Edwards RR, Mensing G, Cahalan C, Greenbaum S, Narang S, Belfer I, et al. Alteration in pain modulation in women with persistent pain after lumpectomy: influence of catastrophizing. J Pain Symptom Manag. 2013;46(1):30–42.
42. Giray E, Akyuz G. Assessment of family caregiver burden and its relationships between quality of life, arm disability, grip strength, and lymphedema symptoms in women with postmastectomy lymphedema: a prospective cross-sectional study. Eur J Breast Health. 2019;15(2):111–8.
43. Hayes SC, Battistutta D, Parker AW, Hirst C, Newman B. Assessing task 'burden' of daily activities requiring upper body function among women following breast cancer treatment. Support Care Cancer. 2005;13(4):255–65.
44. Mustonen L, Vollert J, Rice ASC, Kalso E, Harno H. Sensory profiles in women with neuropathic pain after breast cancer surgery. Breast Cancer Res Treat. 2020;182(2):305–15.
45. Dams L, Van der Gucht E, Haenen V, Devoogdt N, Smeets A, Morlion B, et al. Questionnaire-based somatosensory profiling in breast cancer survivors: are we there yet? Associations between questionnaires and quantitative sensory testing. Disabil Rehabil. 2023;45(11):1865–76.
46. Tofthagen C, Visovsky C, Dominic S, McMillan S. Neuropathic symptoms, physical and emotional well-being, and quality of life at the end of life. Support Care Cancer. 2019;27(9):3357–64.
47. Dams L, Haenen V, Van der Gucht E, Devoogdt N, Smeets A, Bernar K, et al. Absolute and relative reliability of a comprehensive quantitative sensory testing protocol in women treated for breast cancer. Pain Med Malden Mass. 2022;23(6):1162–75.
48. Rolke R, Baron R, Maier C, Tölle TR, Treede DR, Beyer A, et al. Quantitative sensory testing in the German Research Network on Neuropathic Pain (DFNS): standardized protocol and reference values. Pain. 2006;123(3):231–43.
49. Knoerl R, Gilchrist L, Kanzawa-Lee GA, Donohoe C, Bridges C, Lavoie Smith EM. Proactive rehabilitation for chemotherapy-induced peripheral neuropathy. Semin Oncol Nurs. 2020;36(1):150983.
50. Stoller S, Capozza S, Alberti P, Lustberg M, Kleckner IR. Framework to leverage physical therapists for the assessment and treatment of chemotherapy-induced peripheral neurotoxicity (CIPN). Support Care Cancer. 2023;31(5):293.
51. Smoot B, Wong J, Cooper B, Wanek L, Topp K, Byl N, et al. Upper extremity impairments in women with or without lymphedema following breast cancer treatment. J Cancer Surviv Res Pract. 2010;4(2):167–78.
52. Mortimer JE, Waliany S, Dieli-Conwright CM, Patel SK, Hurria A, Chao J, et al. Objective physical and mental markers of self-reported fatigue in women undergoing (neo)adjuvant chemotherapy for early-stage breast cancer. Cancer. 2017;123(10):1810–6.
53. Hoogendam YY, Schagen SB, Ikram MA, Boogerd W, Seynaeve C, Seidler RD, et al. Late effects of adjuvant chemotherapy for breast cancer on fine motor function. Psychooncology. 2015;24(12):1799–807.
54. Doubblestein D, Koehler L, Anderson E, Scheiman N, Stewart P, Schaverien M, et al. Development of a core outcome set for breast cancer-related lymphedema: a Delphi study. Breast Cancer Res Treat. 2024;205(2):359–70.
55. Cederlund R. The use of dexterity tests in hand rehabilitation. J Hand Surg. 1996;21(1):41.
56. Mahfouz FM, Li T, Joda M, Harrison M, Kumar S, Horvath LG, et al. Upper-limb dysfunction in cancer survivors with chemotherapy-induced peripheral neurotoxicity. J Neurol Sci. 2024;457:122862.
57. Rattanakrong N, Promma N, Saraboon C, Waongenngarm P. Physical impairments, sensory disturbance, and functional ability in a cancer patient with and without chemotherapy-induced peripheral neuropathy symptoms. Support Care Cancer. 2022;30(6):5055–62.
58. Yang EJ, Lee KS, Lim MC, Baek JY, Han JY, Yu ES, et al. Symptom perception and functioning in patients with advanced cancer. PLoS One. 2021;16(2):e0245987.
59. Noman S, Shahar HK, Abdul Rahman H, Ismail S, Abdulwahid Al-Jaberi M, Azzani M. The effectiveness of educational interventions on breast cancer screening uptake, knowledge, and beliefs among women: a systematic review. Int J Environ Res Public Health. 2020;18(1):263.
60. De Groef A, Meeus M, Heathcote LC, Wiles L, Catley M, Vogelzang A, et al. Treating persistent pain after breast cancer: practice gaps and future directions. J Cancer Surviv Res Pract. 2023;17(6):1698–707.
61. Sebri V, Pravettoni G. Tailored psychological interventions to manage body image: an opinion study on breast cancer survivors. Int J Environ Res Public Health. 2023;20(4):2991.
62. Dalal S, Tanco KC, Bruera E. State of art of managing pain in patients with cancer. Cancer J Sudbury Mass. 2013;19(5):379–89.
63. Adam R, Bond C, Murchie P. Educational interventions for cancer pain. A systematic review of systematic reviews with nested narrative review of randomized controlled trials. Patient Educ Couns. 2015;98(3):269–82.
64. Pas R, Leysen L, De Goeij W, Vossebeld L, Van Wilgen P, De Groef A, et al. Pain neuroscience education in cancer survivors with persistent pain: a pilot study. J Bodyw Mov Ther. 2020;24(4):239–44.
65. Dams L, Van Der Gucht E, Haenen V, Devoogdt N, Smeets A, Bernar K, et al. Effectiveness of pain neuroscience education on somatosensory functioning after surgery for breast cancer: a double-blinded randomized controlled trial. Anat Rec. 2024;307(2):248–72.
66. Ogle T, Alexander K, Miaskowski C, Yates P. Systematic review of the effectiveness of self-initiated interventions to decrease pain and sensory

disturbances associated with peripheral neuropathy. J Cancer Surviv. 2020;14(4):444–63.
67. Roszkowska M, Białczyk K. Coping styles and quality of life in breast cancer patients undergoing radiotherapy. Cancer. 2023;15(23):5515.
68. Tanay MAL, Armes J, Moss-Morris R, Rafferty AM, Robert G. A systematic review of behavioural and exercise interventions for the prevention and management of chemotherapy-induced peripheral neuropathy symptoms. J Cancer Surviv Res Pract. 2023;17(1):254–77.
69. Volcheck MM, Graham SM, Fleming KC, Mohabbat AB, Luedtke CA. Central sensitization, chronic pain, and other symptoms: better understanding, better management. Cleve Clin J Med. 2023;90(4):245–54.
70. van Dongen SI, de Nooijer K, Cramm JM, Francke AL, Oldenmenger WH, Korfage IJ, et al. Self-management of patients with advanced cancer: a systematic review of experiences and attitudes. Palliat Med. 2020;34(2):160–78.
71. Misiąg W, Piszczyk A, Szymańska-Chabowska A, Chabowski M. Physical activity and cancer care-a review. Cancer. 2022;14(17):4154.
72. Goldschmidt S, Schmidt ME, Steindorf K. Long-term effects of exercise interventions on physical activity in breast cancer patients: a systematic review and meta-analysis of randomized controlled trials. Support Care Cancer. 2023;31(2):130.
73. Hao J, Zhu X, Bensoussan A. Effects of nonpharmacological interventions in chemotherapy-induced peripheral neuropathy: an overview of systematic reviews and meta-analyses. Integr Cancer Ther. 2020;19:153473542094502.
74. Jordan B, Margulies A, Cardoso F, Cavaletti G, Haugnes HS, Jahn P, et al. Systemic anticancer therapy-induced peripheral and central neurotoxicity: ESMO-EONS-EANO clinical practice guidelines for diagnosis, prevention, treatment and follow-up. Ann Oncol. 2020;31(10):1306–19.
75. Crichton M, Yates PM, Agbejule OA, Spooner A, Chan RJ, Hart NH. Non-pharmacological self-management strategies for chemotherapy-induced peripheral neuropathy in people with advanced cancer: a systematic review and meta-analysis. Nutrients. 2022;14(12):2403.
76. Joaquim A, Leão I, Antunes P, Capela A, Viamonte S, Alves AJ, et al. Impact of physical exercise programs in breast cancer survivors on health-related quality of life, physical fitness, and body composition: evidence from systematic reviews and meta-analyses. Front Oncol. 2022;12:955505.
77. Mirandola D, Monaci M, Miccinesi G, Ventura L, Muraca M, Casini E, et al. Long-term benefits of adapted physical activity on upper limb performance and quality of life in breast cancer survivors. J Funct Morphol Kinesiol. 2017;2(4):38.
78. Wirtz P, Baumann FT. Physical activity, exercise and breast cancer - what is the evidence for rehabilitation, aftercare, and survival? A review. Breast Care. 2018;13(2):93–101.
79. Lauridsen MC, Christiansen P, Hessov I. The effect of physiotherapy on shoulder function in patients surgically treated for breast cancer: a randomized study. Acta Oncol. 2005;44(5):449–57.
80. Joshi D, Shah S, Shinde SB, Patil S. Effect of neural tissue mobilization on sensory-motor impairments in breast cancer survivors with lymphedema: an experimental study. Asian Pac J Cancer Prev. 2023;24(1):313–9.
81. De Groef A, Van Kampen M, Dieltjens E, Christiaens MR, Neven P, Geraerts I, et al. Effectiveness of postoperative physical therapy for upper-limb impairments after breast cancer treatment: a systematic review. Arch Phys Med Rehabil. 2015;96(6):1140–53.
82. Taverna L, Bellavere M, Tremolada M, Santinelli L, Rudelli N, Mainardi M, et al. Oncological children and well-being: occupational performance and HRQOL change after fine motor skills stimulation activities. Pediatr Rep. 2021;13(3):383–400.
83. Schmitz KH, Campbell AM, Stuiver MM, Pinto BM, Schwartz AL, Morris GS, et al. Exercise is medicine in oncology: engaging clinicians to help patients move through cancer. CA Cancer J Clin. 2019;69(6):468–84.
84. Melara RD, Root JC, Bibi R, Ahles TA. Sensory filtering and sensory memory in breast cancer survivors. Clin EEG Neurosci. 2021;52(4):246–53.
85. Lopez V, Klainin-Yobas P. Health promotion among cancer patients: innovative interventions. In: Haugan G, Eriksson M, editors. Health promotion in health care – vital theories and research. Cham: Springer; 2021.
86. Fagerlin A, Lakhani I, Lantz PM, Janz NK, Morrow M, Schwartz K, et al. An informed decision? Breast cancer patients and their knowledge about treatment. Patient Educ Couns. 2006;64(1-3):303–12.
87. Mohamed A, Attia A, Zakaria H, Wahman MM, Mahmoud NF, Mohammed AA, et al. Efficacy of a sensory re-education paradigm on postural stability in chemotherapy-induced peripheral neuropathy among breast cancer survivors: a randomized controlled trial (RCT). NeuroQuantology. 2022;20(9):3021.
88. Castells M. Rapid desensitization of hypersensitivity reactions to chemotherapy agents. Curr Drug Saf. 2006;1(3):243–51.
89. Cooper C, editor. Fundamentals of hand therapy: clinical reasoning and treatment guidelines for common diagnoses of the upper extremity. 2nd ed. Elsevier Mosby: St. Louis; 2014.

Exercise in Breast Cancer: A Key Factor for the Management of Side Effects of Breast Cancer

17

Gözde Kaya and Alper Tuğral

17.1 Exercise Prescription in Breast Cancer Survivors

A great body of evidence shows that exercise is the safest non-pharmacological intervention in terms of the cancer care continuum due to its numerous beneficial physiological effects. Guidelines for prescribing exercise in cancer patients generally follow the reports of the American College of Sports Medicine (ACSM) in which >150 min/week of moderate-intensity aerobic exercise or >75 min/week of vigorous-intensity aerobic exercise which are also in parallel for healthy individuals are suggested [1]. Although exercise is reported to be safe in each period of cancer treatment and survivorship, defining risk factors and thresholds are prerequisites for maintaining sustainable health benefits. In this regard, the prescription and individualizing of exercise in terms of its frequency, intensity, and duration, as well as considering the specific precautions are of utmost importance [2, 3]. However, since cancer has its unique features, the differentiation of living with cancer can considerably vary among cancer patients. Therefore, it is mandatory to individualize the prescription of physical activity and exercise for each cancer patient to optimize clinical outcomes [2].

Prescribing exercise is important especially in cancer patients when considering the frequency, type, intensity, and timing of exercise. Percentage of maximal oxygen uptake (VO_{2max}), heart rate reserve (HRR, range between resting heart rate and HR_{max}), and/or age-predicted heart rate (APHR, 220-age) are the options available to determine exercise intensity in case of the absence of cardiopulmonary exercise test (CPET). Moderate intensity refers to 40–60% of VO_{2max} [4], while vigorous intensity is between 60 and 85% of VO_{2max}. However, heart rate-based intensity calculation is common in which >70% HR_{max} is accepted as vigorous intensity [5]. CPET shows using the percentage of HRR overloads the intensity of exercise in breast cancer survivors due to increased resting heart rate while using the HR_{max} is more appropriate [5, 6]. Although these rates are usable in healthy individuals, a thorough adjustment of exercise intensity is needed for breast cancer patients. Studies reported that remarkably decreased VO_{2max} in patients with breast cancer compared to their healthy counterparts [7]. Nearly 20% (17–22%) decrease in VO_{2max} was reported in patients with breast cancer who completed their primary treatment [8, 9]. Systemic chemotherapy and locoregional radiotherapy were also reported to be responsible for various cardiopulmonary symptoms such as anthracycline-induced cardiomy-

G. Kaya · A. Tuğral (✉)
Faculty of Health Sciences, Department of Physical Therapy and Rehabilitation, Izmir Bakircay University, Izmir, Turkey
e-mail: gozde.kaya@bakircay.edu.tr; alper.tugral@bakircay.edu.tr

Y. Bakar, A. Tuğral (eds.), *Managing Side Effects of Breast Cancer Treatment*,
https://doi.org/10.1007/978-3-031-75480-7_17

opathy even many years later after the completion of systemic treatment [10]. Resting sinus tachycardia was also reported for nearly 50% of breast cancer survivors after an anthracycline-taxane combined regimen of chemotherapy and monoclonal antibodies such as trastuzumab [11]. The risk of death due to cardiovascular problems among breast cancer survivors was also reported to be 1.8 times higher [12]. Due to the increased resting heart rate, using HRR when determining exercise intensity is of utmost importance to be adjusted. Scharhag-Rosenberger et al. [6] also highlighted that exercise intensity would be too high or quite low when using HRR or VO_{2max}, respectively. On the other hand, ventilatory and blood lactate (bLa) thresholds are also available to determine exercise intensity due to their advantages in the ability to determine more accurately individual metabolic profiles and the absence of maximal exhaustion which would be an obstacle for many cancer survivors [13, 14]. Yet, determining these thresholds generally requires completing at least five stepwise incremental exercise protocols which are also not suitable for many ones due to diminished aerobic fitness [8, 15]. Studies suggested that using these submaximal thresholds such as bLa is as useful as VO_{2max} due to meeting the targeted intensity zone and more homogenous metabolic response [14]. It should be noted that these adjustments should thoroughly be implemented when adjusting exercise intensity to individualize exercise prescriptions in breast cancer survivors who already completed their primary treatment. Nonetheless, additional actions might also be required in breast cancer patients whose primary treatment is ongoing. In a nutshell, when following ACSM guidelines for exercise intensity to prescribe exercise for patients with breast cancer, HR_{max} shows itself as the most appropriate way to individualize exercise intensity by taking into account type, duration, and frequency of exercise as well as sociodemographic and clinical features of patients such as age.

According to the ACSM guideline, there is strong evidence level of the effect of aerobic exercise on cancer-related fatigue, quality of life, physical function, anxiety, and depression when the frequency of exercise is set at 2–3 times weekly for at least 30 min up to 60 [16]. Resistance exercise was also reported to have strong evidence levels to improve physical function, quality of life, and fatigue. In a meta-analysis, it was also highlighted that the duration and volume of the exercise were the most important parameters due to larger volumes and durations of exercise contributed to a larger increase in VO_{2max} in patients with cancer during their systemic treatment [17]. Huang et al. [18] also reported a significant dose–response relationship between duration and increase in VO_{2max} in healthy individuals, yet authors also underlined that the increase in VO_{2max} stopped after 45 min of exercise. Therefore, it is plausible to conclude that each set of exercises should ideally be no longer than that time frame. When it comes to resistance exercise, Physical Activity Guidelines for Americans (PAGA) suggests moderate or high-intensity training relatively for major muscle groups twice weekly [19]. Studies suggested that there is no need for specific exercise testing if cancer survivors would like to attend low-to-moderate activities such as walking as well as resistance training. Yet, exercise testing should be implemented as much as possible prior to participating in vigorous-intensity exercises by exercise specialists and/or physical therapists. Besides, exercise recommendations and prescriptions are usually suggested to rely on a symptom-based approach in oncology settings [3]. However, further evaluations might be necessary to implement an exercise protocol in patients with breast cancer specifically those who might suffer from neuropathy, balance loss, fatigue, bone metastasis, or preexisting or ongoing cardiac conditions some of which can also be counted for contraindication of exercise participation at some level [20]. In addition, specific evaluations should be applied in patients with breast cancer with a special focus on arm and shoulder morbidity, peripherally inserted central catheter (PICC) lines, and/or axillary web syndrome (which is separately discussed in another chapter).

American Society of Clinical Oncology (ASCO) guidelines also suggest evaluating the risk of bone fracture in patients with breast cancer who are under exposure to hormone treatment as well as for premenopausal women with treatment-induced ovarian failure [21]. Studies also stated that regular assessments of fracture risk by dual-energy X-ray absorptiometry (DEXA) should be included in routine clinical care; however, the National Cancer Comprehensive Network (NCCN) recommends the use of the FRAX algorithm (World Health Organization Fracture Risk Assessment Tool (FRAX)) to evaluate the potential bone fractures and losses [22, 23]. Nonetheless, there is no report that exercise is not safely applicable at each level of fracture risk. Loss of muscle mass can be another issue that might prevent and/or hinder participation a regular physical activity and exercise protocol in breast cancer patients. It is an undisputable problem when adjusting and prescribing exercise; however, weakness was reported to be an insufficient reason to not attend an exercise program. In contrast, it is reasonable to think that an indication [3].

Safety precautions when prescribing exercise carry great importance, especially for those who suffer from chemotherapy-induced peripheral neuropathy (CIPN) which is mostly characterized by an increased risk of falling due to decreased sensorial loss on plantar surfaces. ACSM guidelines also offer to perform a pre-exercise evaluation regarding neuropathy since patients with CIPN have difficulty with walking and/or dropping items which are potential risks, especially for patients with breast cancer. In these patient groups, setting a more stable environment for exercise such as implementing a stationary bike exercise or avoiding unstable exercises such as outdoor hiking might be more suitable for preventing potential injuries [3]. Upper body and arm morbidity should be carefully evaluated before beginning an exercise program in breast cancer survivors since potential problems associated with shoulder girdle might hinder participation or make exercise less safe in terms of limited range of motion, pain, and even clinical manifestation of lymphedema. Yet, studies also highlighted that light-intensity exercise for the upper body can be initiated even if there is a lack of thorough evaluation of the upper body in breast cancer survivors [3].

17.2 Contraindications

According to the NCCN guidelines, cancer patients should be encouraged to participate in a moderate level of physical activity during and after cancer treatment. However, in certain cases, a thorough pre-exercise evaluation should be implemented in patients such as those with higher fatigue, comorbidities, recent major surgery, cardiopulmonary complications, metastasis, and so forth. Some issues should be investigated in detail since fatigue may represent itself as a contraindication to exercise, yet NCCN suggests exercise as a treatment modality in fatigue with a higher evidence level [23]. Again, it is important to assess a patient with a symptom-based approach since there are limited suggestions in guidelines in some specific cases. For instance, in the case of anemia, there is insufficient data on whether patients with anemia can attend a low-to-moderate level of exercise. Nevertheless, data suggests that exercise has beneficial effects on hemoglobin in patients with breast cancer who suffer from treatment-related anemia [24]. On the other hand, cardiotoxicity, which is a common consequence after combined treatment regimens of breast cancer, should be further examined before participating in an exercise program. In summary, it should be noted that most of the contraindications are also prerequisites for exercise participation and an individualized symptom-based approach as well as increased awareness of symptom recognition are crucial for maintaining a sustainable exercise program among breast cancer survivors. Besides, exercise especially when it is initiated and supervised at a low to moderate level is safe, beneficial, and supportive for primary treatment.

17.3 Type of Exercises in Breast Cancer

Aerobic exercise, resistance exercise, combined aerobic and resistance exercise, Pilates, yoga, Tai Chi, Qigong, and aquatic exercises are among the exercise modalities suggested to be implemented for breast cancer patients according to the literature [25–27].

Research has indicated that aerobic and resistance exercises can effectively mitigate the treatment-related side effects in breast cancer patients [28]. Aerobic or anaerobic exercise training at moderate or high intensity has beneficial outcomes on fatigue, quality of life, sleep quality, and bone mineral density in breast cancer survivors [29]. Moreover, the combination of supervised aerobic and resistance exercises is particularly effective in improving physical function [30]. A variety of exercise modalities have been identified as having potential benefits for different symptoms. Furthermore, special attention should be given to ensuring that exercise programs are sustainable, individualized, and suitable for the needs of patients.

17.3.1 High-Intensity Interval Training in Breast Cancer

High-intensity interval training (HIIT) consists of brief bouts of exercise performed at an intensity above the anaerobic threshold that are interspersed with short bursts of low-intensity exercise or rest intervals [31]. Examining the effects of HIIT on cancer patients has come to prominence as an increasingly promising field of research [32]. Although there have been studies indicating positive outcomes of HIIT exercises for cancer patients, the findings addressing the safety and feasibility are relatively new [33, 34]. According to the systematic review and meta-analysis, HIIT is reported to be safe and feasible in cancer patients in the prehabilitation phase [33], and it has a positive effect on aerobic capacity, cancer-related fatigue, and pain [33, 35]. Although HIIT may be beneficial in cancer patients at all phases of treatment, it has been shown to be more effective in increasing cardiovascular fitness, particularly when initiated before treatment and continued for more than 8 weeks [36].

Regarding the impact of HIIT exercises on breast cancer patients, Chen et al. [32] determined that HIIT improved cardiorespiratory fitness (VO_2 peak) in breast cancer patients compared to patients with standard care. On the other hand, it was reported that moderate-intensity continuous exercise and HIIT produced similar results regarding cardiorespiratory fitness [32]. Additionally, HIIT may be beneficial for emotional symptoms, fatigue, and muscular strength [32]. Although further research is required to examine the effect of HIIT on various symptoms associated with breast cancer, it currently stands as a time-efficient alternative for moderate-intensity continuous exercise [32]. Despite the positive reports regarding the implementation of HIIT in cancer patients, further investigation is required to ascertain its safety, efficacy, and feasibility [37].

17.3.2 Mind-Body Exercises in Breast Cancer

A growing body of evidence shows that mind-body exercises (MBE) have promising effects on clinical outcomes in cancer patients. MBE can help to relieve symptoms of several forms of cancer. MBE may exhibit positive impacts on physical fitness, fatigue, sleep disturbances, and psychological problems for patients with various types and stages of cancer [38]. In their meta-analysis of 10 randomized controlled studies, Kuo et al. [39] determined that Baduanjin Qigong exercises may provide beneficial outcomes in terms of fatigue, sleep problems, and quality of life in cancer patients. Furthermore, it has been established that Qigong is helpful for improving CRF, Tai Chi Chuan for lowering anxiety, and yoga for improving quality of life and reducing depression, anxiety, and stress among cancer patients [40]. To specifically emphasize the effects of Baduanjin exercises on breast cancer patients, the results revealed that postoperative Baduanjin exercise improves patients' quality of life and psychological well-being [41]. Also, Tai Chi Chuan exercise has beneficial impacts on several aspects, including quality of life, pain, shoulder function, upper extremity muscle strength, and fatigue in breast cancer patients [42]. Moreover, Liuzijue and Tai Chi Chuan may effectively reduce symptoms of depression among breast cancer survivors [43]. It is worth mentioning that research has shown that Qigong and Tai Chi Chuan exercises exhibit a more significant therapeutic effect on fatigue and sleep disturbances among cancer patients in comparison to the active control groups [44]. More research is needed to establish conclusive findings, notwithstanding the promising positive effects of Qigong and Tai Chi Chuan exercises on cancer-related symptoms. Furthermore, investigation into their impact on mortality is also warranted [44].

According to the existing evidence from meta-analyses, yoga was found to be effective in enhancing the quality of life and reducing fatigue, anxiety, depression, stress, pain, and sleep problems among breast cancer patients [45–48]. However, it is necessary to conduct more well-designed, methodologically robust research with larger sample sizes to acquire more strong evidence for the efficacy of yoga in alleviating symptoms in breast cancer patients [47].

Pilates exercises are also effective in alleviating fatigue and improving the range of motion, mood, and quality of life in breast cancer patients [49, 50]. It is noteworthy that Pilates exercises have been claimed to be more beneficial than other exercise methods in enhancing upper extremity pain and function [50]. Nevertheless, the effect of Pilates exercises and other exercise programs on the range of motion in the shoulder joint and quality of life was found similar [50]. Further investigation into the impact of Pilates on symptoms associated with cancer, such as CRF [51], is warranted.

17.3.3 Aquatic Exercises in Breast Cancer

The aquatic therapeutic exercise, which incorporated stretching, breathing, endurance, strength, and mobility exercises, led to the alleviation of the side effects associated with breast cancer and its treatments [52]. There is evidence to suggest that aquatic exercises exhibit a high degree of adherence. This is crucial, as it will increase the benefits of exercise [52]. Aquatic exercises improve pain, shoulder joint range of motion, respiratory and muscular functions, cardiorespiratory fitness, and HRQOL in breast cancer patients [52]. Although breast cancer survivors benefit from aquatic therapeutic exercises for the alleviation of pain, and fatigue, and improved quality of life, the precise impact of these exercises on BCRL has yet to be determined [53]. In their meta-analysis involving five randomized controlled studies, Wang et al. [27] determined that aquatic exercises provided positive effects in terms of fatigue and quality of life. Further studies are needed to elucidate the effects of aquatic exercises on the symptoms of breast cancer patients [53]. Prior to implementing aqua therapies, it is necessary to rule out contraindicated conditions, including but not limited to open wounds, infections, and extremely low or high blood pressure [54]. Aside from these, aquatic therapeutic exercises for breast cancer patients are feasible and safe [52].

It is crucial to prioritize maintaining and improving the state of physical function due to its proven capability to predict both survival and mortality among cancer patients [55]. An improved survival function which is characterized by decreased rates of recurrence and mortality is one of the most significant effects of exercise for breast cancer patients [55, 56]. Research has established that exercise following a breast cancer diagnosis is associated with a 37% decrease in breast cancer-specific mortality. In addition, regular moderate exercise was associated with a 39% reduction in the all-cause mortality rate [55]. Growing evidence supports the benefits of exercise in breast cancer patients. Detailed exercise prescriptions are of utmost importance to promote the integration of research findings into clinical practice [57]. Furthermore, more knowledge is required to ascertain the most effective exercise regimens in terms of the frequency, intensity, duration, and type of exercise for the management of different cancer-related symptoms [28, 58, 59].

17.4 Resistance Exercise in Breast Cancer: Special Focus on Lymphedema

Breast cancer patients can face a wide variety of symptoms due to systemic treatment such as chemotherapy. Though these symptoms can vary in a wide range, mostly are attributable to diminished skeletal mass such as decreased force capacity, difficulty with daily life physical activities, climbing stairs, and so forth. Antineoplastic chemotherapy agents such as anthracyclines have been known to be responsible for deteriorated muscle metabolism via decreasing fiber cross-sectional area and motor neuron excitability [60, 61] which are also thereafter responsible for delayed treatment, dose reductions, and/or discontinuation of primary treatment. Besides, nearly 16% and 25% reductions were reported in muscle strength during the treatment for the upper and lower extremities, respectively [62]. It was also reported that a nearly 10% decrease in leg press strength after 12-week chemotherapy was evident which nearly equals the consequences of typical aging for over a decade [61]. Therefore, it is indisputable that there is a need for strengthening management options in patients with breast cancer.

Resistance exercise has been offered not only to increase muscle hypertrophy and strength but also to counteract the side effects of systemic treatment in breast cancer survivors. In addition, the mitigating of reliance on type-II muscle fibers which are less efficient compared to type-I can be achieved by the effect of the resistance exercise [63]. Yet, it has been suggested to avoid strenuous activity for breast cancer patients due to the increased risk of breast cancer-related lymphedema (BCRL) for a long time. Since BCRL is a relatively incurable chronic disease, suggestions were also gotten more rigid in patients with breast cancer who were free of clinical lymphedema. However, thanks to the efforts on this topic, it can be exactly said that resistance exercise is safe in patients with breast cancer in the context of increased risk of BCRL [64, 65]. On the contrary, studies suggested that resistance exercise is not only safe for patients with breast cancer but also has preventive features against BCRL [66]. Considering the intensity of resistance exercise, studies also reported that there was no significant change in acute response to the resistance exercise in extracellular fluid irrespective of load in patients with breast cancer [67, 68]. Hasenoehrl et al. [64] reported a significant reduction in BCRL due to resistance exercise. Rosenberg et al. [69] stated that only a small minority of breast cancer survivors prescribed a resistance exercise which is also disputable in terms of their ability to follow general guidelines. An exercise program without any resistance and mostly depending on aerobic training was also reported to be relatively harmful since it might cause to increase in the ratio of type I to type II muscle fibers which is also in line with aging. Although endurance activities are based on fibers type I, timely and rapid action of some muscle movements is necessary for some conditions such as preventing falling due to loss of balance especially for those who suffer from CIPN [70, 71].

Studies highlighted that even adding two sessions weekly of resistance exercise in breast cancer patients' home-based exercise program can yield a large increase in full-body muscular strength [72] without any increased risk for BCRL. An et al. [73] also reported a significantly superior effect of combined aerobic and resistance exercise programs to the higher dose aerobic exercise alone in a longer term. We also would like to state that patients with breast cancer can safely attend a progressive resistance exercise program starting with the low level with free loads and/or safely applicable stretch bands without any risk of increased or manifested BCRL according to our clinical experiences. Patients who have additional problems (i.e., pre-existing cardiac problems) can also attend a resistance exercise program after performing further evaluations and invidualizing of resistance exercise prescription in terms of intensity, frequency, and duration as we noted above. Resistance training has also varied effects on neuromuscular adaptations depending on its loading intensity which is greater in higher loads compared to lower [74]. In addition, it is also plausible to state that supervised resistance exercise is not only safe for preventing secondary injuries [69] but also for improving adherence to the program. Nevertheless, it was also noted that there is an increasing need for updating clinical exercise guidelines in terms of resistance training among breast cancer survivors [65].

17.5 The Effect of Exercise on Cancer-Related Symptoms

Breast cancer survivors may confront a multitude of disease or treatment-related physical, psychological, and psychosocial symptoms that reduce their quality of life [75]. These symptoms might manifest before treatment, worsen during treatment, and persist after treatment [76]. Acute or chronic symptoms such as fatigue, sleep disorders, neurocognitive impairment, pain, functional limitation, limited range of motion, muscle weakness, lymphedema, a decline in cardiopulmonary function, and peripheral neuropathy may occur due to side effects of multimodal treatment [75–77]. The experienced symptoms may vary based on the specific cancer treatment, including surgery, radiotherapy, hormonal therapy, biological therapy, and/or systemic chemotherapy [75, 77].

Exercise emerges as a prominent method for mitigating the side effects of cancer and related multimodal treatment and functional impairments [78]. Exercise provides many therapeutic benefits not only before and during, cancer treatment but also afterward [79]. There is high-level evidence that exercise improves survival rates in many types of cancer [55, 80]. It improves mental, physical, and social well-being, and overall quality of life and reduces the risk of cancer recurrence [79]. In addition to preventative and mitigating impacts of exercise on the side effects of treatment, it may also improve the tolerance and the completion of chemotherapy [81]. In this section, the effect of exercise on common cancer-related symptoms will be discussed.

17.5.1 Fatigue

Cancer-related fatigue (CRF) is one of the most prevalent and devastating symptoms in breast cancer patients [82]. CRF is described as persistent, physical, emotional, or cognitive exhaustion caused by cancer and its treatment, which is not proportionate to the activity performed and is responsible for impaired function [83]. Fatigue facilitates sedentary behavior in cancer patients, which leads to physical deconditioning. As a result, decreased muscle strength creates a vicious cycle by contributing to an increased perception of fatigue [58]. The vicious cycle of fatigue induces an increase in sleep problems, cognitive dysfunction, and physiological distress, as well as a decline in quality of life [58]. Frequently, anemia, pain, distress, and sleep disorders are present along with CRF [83]. Hence, a comprehensive approach in which comorbid symptoms should also be considered is necessary [83]. CRF, including mild, moderate, and severe forms, has been demonstrated to affect 70.7% of the population [84]. The prevalence of CRF is at its lowest point before treatment, with a moderate to severe fatigue rate of 30.8%. It reaches the highest level during treatment, with a moderate to severe fatigue rate of 46.1%. After treatment, the prevalence of CRF (moderate to severe fatigue rate 39.5%) gradually starts to diminish [84]. Nevertheless, disease-free survivals may continue to experience fatigue even in the long term after completion of treatment [85]. Therefore, actions should be taken to manage potential CRF as soon as possible after a diagnosis of cancer [83].

According to the existing research, exercise interventions are highly effective in alleviating CRF during and post-treatment [86]. Moreover, a meta-analysis of 113 randomized controlled trials showed that exercise approaches were significantly more effective than existing pharmaceutical treatments in the management of CRF [86]. The positive impacts of exercise on self-efficacy, muscle strength, aerobic capacity, autonomic nervous system balance, brain function, and anti-inflammatory effects may all contribute to alleviating CRF [87]. The efficacy of different exercise methods, including aerobic exercise, resistance exercise, combined exercise, and yoga, in managing CRF has been demonstrated in breast cancer patients [88]. A systematic review and meta-analysis involving 1793 participants concluded that exercise effectively reduces CRF in women with breast cancer who are undergoing adjuvant chemotherapy and/or radiotherapy [51]. Further, the studies reported that supervised resistance or combined exercises, which are reported to be more efficient than aerobic or resistance exercises alone, have remarkable effects on reducing CRF [51, 88]. On the other hand, the findings of a network meta-analysis indicated that yoga is the most effective exercise modality for managing CRF in breast cancer patients [88]. Possible explanations for this may include the therapeutic influence of yoga on sleep disturbances [89], inflammatory mechanisms, and dysfunction of the hypothalamic–pituitary–adrenal axis (i.e., serum cortisol levels) [90]. These factors are well-known factors associated with perceived fatigue in cancer patients [85, 89]. Tai Chi exercises have been suggested to be more effective in alleviating CRF in breast cancer patients when conducted in sessions lasting a minimum of 40 min for a duration of ≤6 weeks [91]. Consequently, for the management of CRF, it is recommended to provide supervised and structured exercise programs to breast cancer survivors [92]. While previous research has shown the effect of exercise approaches on CRF, further study is required to ascertain the optimal dosage that takes into account different exercise approaches.

17.5.2 Sleep Disorders

Sleep disorders are another prevalent and significant concern and it is experienced by over 50% of breast cancer survivors [93]. Breast cancer patients frequently face a variety of sleep disorders, the most prevalent of which are circadian rhythm disorders, sleep apnea, and chronic insomnia [94]. The prevalence and persistence of sleep disorders following the completion of treatment indicate that screening and management of sleep disorders should be prioritized [93, 94]. Anxiety, depression, fatigue, and intensity of pain have been identified as factors that are correlated with sleep disturbances among breast cancer patients [95–97]. Moreover, managing sleep disorders and associated complications is of the utmost importance to improve patients' quality of life, and mortality, and ensure healthy survival [98, 99]. A systematic review and meta-analysis of 13 randomized controlled trials revealed that supervised exercises increased subjective sleep quality and reduced sleep disturbances in breast cancer survivors [100]. Of the 13 studies considered, 10 used a combination of aerobic and resistance exercises, while 1 used mat Pilates or combined exercise and the others only employed aerobic exercise [100]. Various physical and mind–body exercise modalities, including yoga, Qigong, Thai Chi Chuan, resistance exercise, aerobic exercise, and a combination of aerobic and resistance exercise, have been used to manage sleep disorders in breast cancer patients [26]. Although evidence regarding the therapeutic effects of exercise on sleep disorders is growing, there is insufficient data regarding the potential effect of the prescription of exercise on sleep disorders in the context of its frequency, intensity, time, and type [101]. In addition, further research is needed to clarify the best exercise approach not only to reduce sleep problems but also to provide sustainable improved sleep quality [26].

17.5.3 Pain

Although there have been significant improvements in cancer treatment, the occurrence of chronic pain remains a significant side effect of these multimodal treatments [102]. The pain experienced by breast cancer patients can be categorized as nociceptive, neuropathic, central sensitization, or a combination of these [103]. Exercise interventions may effectively alleviate pain in breast cancer patients [104]. However, there is a scarcity of research examining the impact of exercise on pain associated with cancer and its treatment [59]. Rather than pain, the primary outcomes of the exercise interventions used in the studies are range of motion, strength, quality of life, fatigue, or lymphedema [105]. A recent systematic review and meta-analysis comprising 76 studies concluded that exercise may effectively manage pain in cancer patients [105]. However, it was noted that because of the heterogeneity of the studies, the level of evidence was poor [105]. Further methodologically robust studies are required to elucidate the potential role of exercise in the management of cancer-related pain [105]. Various exercise modalities, including Pilates, yoga, aerobic exercise, resistance exercise, combined aerobic, resistance, and flexibility exercises, high-intensity interval training, and dance movement therapy, have been demonstrated to be effective in reducing pain in breast cancer patients [105]. Nevertheless, further investigation is warranted due to the varied results of different types of exercise on pain were reported [105].

Determining the efficacy of exercise regimens could be a crucial step in the management of pain among breast cancer patients [59]. An increasing amount of evidence supports that exercise training may reduce the neuropathic pain associated with peripheral neuropathy [106]. Moreover, the systematic review and meta-analysis study showed that exercise performed before or during chemotherapy had a reducing effect on CIPN symptoms, which is a common side effect of (neo)adjuvant therapy in breast cancer patients [107]. Determining the optimal exercise intensity, frequency, duration, and type is crucial for the management of CIPN and neuropathic pain [106]. In addition, the potential impact of exercise in the presence of central sensitivity in cancer patients should be elucidated [104].

17.5.4 Upper Extremity Dysfunctions

Breast cancer patients may experience a wide variety of upper extremity impairments, such as reduced shoulder range of motion (ROM), reduced muscle strength, pain, and BCRL [108]. After completion of multimodal treatment (surgery, chemotherapy, or radiotherapy), breast cancer survivors who participate in aerobic exercise can see improvements in their ROM in shoulder flexion, abduction, internal rotation, and external rotation [109]. Studies also showed that aerobic exercise improves pain intensity, upper extremity functions, and muscle strength among patients who underwent breast cancer surgery [110]. Different surgical complications require specialized treatment protocols [110]; therefore, it is necessary to implement various exercise approaches alone or in combination. Upper extremity dysfunctions can be alleviated by using aerobic or resistance exercises [110]. To improve the shoulder ROM, shoulder and elbow exercises should specifically be incorporated into the treatment in addition to aerobic exercises [110]. Moreover, to prevent muscle dysfunction in breast cancer patients, it is recommended to include resistance training in rehabilitation programs as early as possible [62].

Timing is another crucial factor to consider when beginning ROM exercises following breast cancer surgery [111]. In light of existing research, low-quality data suggests that early ROM exercises may enhance shoulder flexion ROM [111]. Thus, the timing of postoperative exercises should be determined in a patient-centered manner [111]. Some studies show that various types of exercise have positive or neutral effects on reducing BCRL symptoms [112]. It has been stated that aerobic exercise, resistance exercise, Pilates, yoga, Qigong, stretching, and combined exercises may be used safely for BCRL management [112]. Even though research suggests that exercise interventions may decrease the incidence of BCRL more research is needed to elucidate this relationship [113]. Particular attention is paid to the effects of resistance exercise on BCRL. Therefore, we tried to discuss the effects of resistance exercises on BCRL in more detail.

17.5.5 Cognitive Impairment

Cancer and related treatments, such as chemotherapy, can negatively affect cognitive functions [114, 115]. Limited but promising evidence indicates that exercise has a beneficial effect on cognitive functions in breast cancer patients [114, 116]. For further knowledge, please see the relevant chapter.

17.5.6 Health-Related Quality of Life

Exercise interventions enhance breast cancer patients' health-related quality of life (HRQOL) and physical functioning, even during active systemic therapy [30, 117]. Hong et al. [117] determined in their meta-analysis that exercise interventions contributed to the improvement of HRQOL in breast cancer survivors. On the other hand, to observe the beneficial effects of exercise on symptoms and HRQOL, it is necessary to adjust the exercise dosage appropriately [117]. Specifically, the duration of exercise sessions is linearly correlated with improved HRQOL [117]. The optimal duration for exercise has been suggested to be a minimum of 45 min, and it has been established that sessions lasting less than 45 min do not produce any notable improvement in HRQOL [117].

17.6 Managing Exercise Barriers in Breast Cancer Survivors

Despite numerous benefits and higher-level evidence of the effect of exercise among breast cancer survivors, however, adherence to regular exercise and physical activity was reported to be dramatically low. Studies reported that patients with breast cancer tend to lower their physical activity levels from diagnosis to survivorship [118] and even some of them did not exercise at all [119]. Studies also highlighted the significant trend towards decreasing the level of physical activity over time [119]. Though it can be understandable various barriers to preventing a regular exercise program during and/or completion of the primary treatment among breast cancer patients such as fatigue, nausea, and weakness there are also a wide variety of issues that should be thoroughly addressed to eliminate potential barriers to implement a sustainable exercise habit. In this regard, lack of self-discipline, procrastination, inadequate social support, and/or lack of referral were reported to be some domains that should be critically documented to improve the level of participation in regular physical activity among cancer survivors. In contrast, it has been also reported that no significant change was observed even though some exercise barriers were improved among cancer survivors and therefore studies concluded that sociodemographic characteristics and exercise barriers are not associated with each other [119, 120]. Yet, the major barriers were reported as "being busy" or "lack of willpower" except for clinical and treatment-related issues [120]. Nonetheless, failing in patient education is also another problem that needs to be considered in detail. Not only patient and caregiver education but also timing is of utmost importance to build long-life regular exercise and physical activity habits among cancer patients. Studies also highlighted the importance of timing as early as possible [121]. Besides, it is also noteworthy to discuss that despite good levels of exercise beliefs among cancer survivors, the failure to adhere a regular exercise is a global problem among breast cancer survivors [118–121], and we think that this should be studied in an individualized manner.

To overcome and manage exercise barriers, technology-based mobile health applications were reported to be promising options for improving physical health and exercise adherence. When considering that we live in the era of smartphones, it is plausible to expect that smartphones can be useful for not only promoting physical activity and exercise but also for tracking potential changes that can be associated with secondary injuries. Pope et al. [122] reported that commercially available mobile applications and social media education had significant improvements in increased physical activity levels along with improved body composition. However, it should be noted that individualizing exercise prescriptions can also be accounted as a major contributor to improved physical activity. Studies also highlighted the significant impact of individualized prescription of exercise in terms of improving physical activity [123]. We think that not only individualizing exercise but also determining potential barriers to exercise among breast cancer patients are unique and indispensable parameters that should be addressed in detail and further especially for those who are not aware of the potential benefits of exercise. Therefore, it is logical to sum up these discussions that proper and timely patient education irrespective of experienced symptoms and perceived barriers to the exercise is of utmost importance, especially in patients with low levels of sociodemographic and socioeconomic background.

17.7 Conclusion

Exercise is the best non-pharmacological option that can be used safely for managing the side effects of multimodal breast cancer treatment due to its proven efficacy on symptom improvement. Yet, choosing the optimal dose, type, and frequency as well as customizing it individually may need further experience. In this manner, physical therapists may show themselves as the primary source of exercise counseling in oncology settings via their educational and experienced clinical background in musculoskeletal and nervous systems. In addition, patients who suffer from a fear of lymphedema can be supervised by a physical therapist in order to overcome their fears and improve their participation. However, it should be noted that management of these side effects can also bring the need for multidisciplinary team management in patients with breast cancer both during treatment and survivorship. Besides, digging into the potential barriers to participating in an exercise should improve the clinical outcomes through increased participation and adherence to the exercise.

References

1. Irwin ML. ACSM's guide to exercise and cancer survivorship. Indianapolis: ACSM; 2012.
2. Redondo M, Morales JS, Lucia A, Prieto I. Physical exercise in cancer: general recommendations might not be enough. Cancer Causes Control. 2020;31:83–4.
3. Wolin KY, Schwartz AL, Matthews CE, Courneya KS, Schmitz KH. Implementing the exercise guidelines for cancer survivors. J Support Oncol. 2012;10(5):171–7.
4. Thompson PD, Buchner D, Piña IL, Balady GJ, Williams MA, Marcus BH, et al. Exercise and physical activity in the prevention and treatment of atherosclerotic cardiovascular disease: a statement from the Council on Clinical Cardiology (Subcommittee on Exercise, Rehabilitation, and Prevention) and the Council on Nutrition, Physical Activity, and Metabolism (Subcommittee on Physical Activity). Circulation. 2003;107(24):3109–16.
5. Gil-Rey E, Quevedo-Jerez K, Maldonado-Martin S, Herrero-Román F. Exercise intensity guidelines for cancer survivors: a comparison with reference values. Int J Sports Med. 2014;35(14):e1–9.
6. Scharhag-Rosenberger F, Kuehl R, Klassen O, Schommer K, Schmidt ME, Ulrich CM, et al. Exercise training intensity prescription in breast cancer survivors: validity of current practice and specific recommendations. J Cancer Surviv. 2015;9:612–9.
7. Peel AB, Thomas SM, Dittus K, Jones LW, Lakoski SG. Cardiorespiratory fitness in breast cancer patients: a call for normative values. J Am Heart Assoc. 2014;3(1):e000432.
8. Jones LW, Courneya KS, Mackey JR, Muss HB, Pituskin EN, Scott JM, et al. Cardiopulmonary function and age-related decline across the breast cancer survivorship continuum. J Clin Oncol. 2012;30(20):2530–7.
9. Koch B, Schäper C, Ittermann T, Spielhagen T, Dörr M, Völzke H, et al. Reference values for cardiopulmonary exercise testing in healthy volunteers: The SHIP study. Eur Respir J. 2009;33(2):389–97.
10. Lipshultz SE, Adams MJ, Colan SD, Constine LS, Herman EH, Hsu DT, et al. Long-term cardiovascular toxicity in children, adolescents, and young adults who receive cancer therapy: pathophysiology, course, monitoring, management, prevention, and research directions: a scientific statement from the American Heart Association. Circulation. 2013;128(17):1927–95.
11. Jones L, Haykowsky M, Peddle C, Joy A, Pituskin E, Tkachuk L, et al. Cardiovascular risk profile of breast cancer patients treated with anthracycline-taxane containing adjuvant chemotherapy and/or trastuzumab. J Clin Oncol. 2006;24(18):666.
12. Bradshaw PT, Stevens J, Khankari N, Teitelbaum SL, Neugut AI, Gammon MD. Cardiovascular disease mortality among breast cancer survivors. Epidemiology. 2016;27(1):6–13.
13. Wolpern AE, Burgos DJ, Janot JM, Dalleck LC. Is a threshold-based model a superior method to the relative percent concept for establishing individual exercise intensity? A randomized controlled trial. BMC Sports Sci Med Rehabil. 2015;7:1–9.
14. Schneider J, Schlüter K, Sprave T, Wiskemann J, Rosenberger F. Exercise intensity prescription in

cancer survivors: ventilatory and lactate thresholds are useful submaximal alternatives to VO2 peak. Support Care Cancer. 2020;28:5521–8.
15. Dickhuth H-H, Yin L, Niess A, Roecker K, Mayer F, Heitkamp H-C, et al. Ventilatory, lactate-derived and catecholamine thresholds during incremental treadmill running: relationship and reproducibility. Int J Sports Med. 1999;20(2):122–7.
16. Chyu C, Halnon N. Exercise training in cancer survivors. Curr Oncol Rep. 2016;18(6):1–9.
17. Bjørke ACH, Sweegers MG, Buffart LM, Raastad T, Nygren P, Berntsen S. Which exercise prescriptions optimize VO_{2max} during cancer treatment?—a systematic review and meta-analysis. Scand J Med Sci Sports. 2019;29(9):1274–87.
18. Huang G, Wang R, Chen P, Huang SC, Donnelly JE, Mehlferber JP. Dose–response relationship of cardiorespiratory fitness adaptation to controlled endurance training in sedentary older adults. Eur J Prev Cardiol. 2016;23(5):518–29.
19. Xao-feng Y, Sheng-tao Y. Physical activity guidelines advisory committee report, 2008. Background & Process Review. 2011.
20. ACSM. ACSM's guidelines for exercise testing and prescription. Philadelphia: Lippincott Williams & Wilkins; 2013.
21. Hillner BE, Ingle JN, Chlebowski RT, Gralow J, Yee GC, Janjan NA, et al. American Society of Clinical Oncology 2003 update on the role of bisphosphonates and bone health issues in women with breast cancer. J Clin Oncol. 2003;21(21):4042–57.
22. Gralow JR, Biermann JS, Farooki A, Fornier MN, Gagel RF, Kumar RN, et al. NCCN task force report: bone health in cancer care. J Natl Compr Cancer Netw. 2009;7(Suppl_3):S1–S32.
23. Gradishar WJ, Moran MS, Abraham J, Aft R, Agnese D, Allison KH, et al. NCCN guidelines® insights: breast cancer, version 4.2021: featured updates to the NCCN guidelines. J Natl Compr Cancer Netw. 2021;19(5):484–93.
24. Ashem HN, Hamada HA, Abbas RL. Effect of aerobic exercise on immunoglobulins and anemia after chemotherapy in breast cancer patients. J Bodyw Mov Ther. 2020;24(3):137–40.
25. Ficarra S, Thomas E, Bianco A, Gentile A, Thaller P, Grassadonio F, et al. Impact of exercise interventions on physical fitness in breast cancer patients and survivors: a systematic review. Breast Cancer. 2022;29(3):402–18.
26. Kreutz C, Schmidt ME, Steindorf K. Effects of physical and mind-body exercise on sleep problems during and after breast cancer treatment: a systematic review and meta-analysis. Breast Cancer Res Treat. 2019;176(1):1–15.
27. Wang J, Chen X, Wang L, Zhang C, Ma J, Zhao Q. Does aquatic physical therapy affect the rehabilitation of breast cancer in women? A systematic review and meta-analysis of randomized controlled trials. PLoS One. 2022;17(8):e0272337.
28. Furmaniak AC, Menig M, Markes MH. Exercise for women receiving adjuvant therapy for breast cancer. Cochrane Database Syst Rev. 2016;9(9):Cd005001.
29. Schutz S, Aidar FJ, Souza RLM, Dos Santos JL, Voltarelli FA, Vieira Junior RC, et al. Different methods of physical training applied to women breast cancer survivors: a systematic review. Front Physiol. 2021;12:639406.
30. Andersen HH, Vinther A, Lund CM, Paludan C, Jørgensen CT, Nielsen D, et al. Effectiveness of different types, delivery modes and extensiveness of exercise in patients with breast cancer receiving systemic treatment - a systematic review and meta-analysis. Crit Rev Oncol Hematol. 2022;178:103802.
31. Laursen PB, Jenkins DG. The scientific basis for high-intensity interval training: optimising training programmes and maximising performance in highly trained endurance athletes. Sports Med. 2002;32(1):53–73.
32. Chen X, Shi X, Yu Z, Ma X. High-intensity interval training in breast cancer patients: a systematic review and meta-analysis. Cancer Med. 2023;12(17):17692–705.
33. Palma S, Hasenoehrl T, Jordakieva G, Ramazanova D, Crevenna R. High-intensity interval training in the prehabilitation of cancer patients-a systematic review and meta-analysis. Support Care Cancer. 2021;29(4):1781–94.
34. Wallen MP, Hennessy D, Brown S, Evans L, Rawstorn JC, Wong Shee A, et al. High-intensity interval training improves cardiorespiratory fitness in cancer patients and survivors: a meta-analysis. Eur J Cancer Care. 2020;29(4):e13267.
35. Wang L, Quan M, Nieman DC, Li F, Shi H, Bai X, et al. Effects of high-intensity interval training and combined high-intensity interval training programs on cancer-related fatigue and cancer pain: a systematic review and meta-analysis. Med Sci Sports Exerc. 2023;55(9):1620–31.
36. Lavín-Pérez AM, Collado-Mateo D, Mayo X, Humphreys L, Liguori G, James Copeland R, et al. High-intensity exercise to improve cardiorespiratory fitness in cancer patients and survivors: a systematic review and meta-analysis. Scand J Med Sci Sports. 2021;31(2):265–94.
37. Herranz-Gómez A, Cuenca-Martínez F, Suso-Martí L, Varangot-Reille C, Calatayud J, Blanco-Díaz M, et al. Effectiveness of HIIT in patients with cancer or cancer survivors: an umbrella and mapping review with meta-meta-analysis. Scand J Med Sci Sports. 2022;32(11):1522–49.
38. Duan L, Xu Y, Li M. Effects of mind-body exercise in cancer survivors: A systematic review and meta-analysis. Evid Based Complement Alternat Med. 2020;2020:7607161.
39. Kuo CC, Wang CC, Chang WL, Liao TC, Chen PE, Tung TH. Clinical effects of Baduanjin Qigong exercise on cancer patients: a systematic review and meta-analysis on randomized controlled trials. Evid Based Complement Alternat Med. 2021;2021:6651238.

40. Casuso-Holgado MJ, Heredia-Rizo AM, Gonzalez-Garcia P, Muñoz-Fernández MJ, Martinez-Calderon J. Mind-body practices for cancer-related symptoms management: an overview of systematic reviews including one hundred twenty-nine meta-analyses. Support Care Cancer. 2022;30(12):10335–57.
41. Ye XX, Ren ZY, Vafaei S, Zhang JM, Song Y, Wang YX, et al. Effectiveness of Baduanjin exercise on quality of life and psychological health in postoperative patients with breast cancer: a systematic review and meta-analysis. Integr Cancer Ther. 2022;21:15347354221104092.
42. Luo XC, Liu J, Fu J, Yin HY, Shen L, Liu ML, et al. Effect of Tai Chi Chuan in breast cancer patients: a systematic review and meta-analysis. Front Oncol. 2020;10:607.
43. Geng L, Duan Y, Li X, Yue S, Li R, Liu H, et al. Comparative efficacy of mind-body exercise for depression in breast cancer survivors: a systematic review and network meta-analysis. Worldviews Evid-Based Nurs. 2023;20(6):593–609.
44. Wayne PM, Lee MS, Novakowski J, Osypiuk K, Ligibel J, Carlson LE, et al. Tai Chi and Qigong for cancer-related symptoms and quality of life: a systematic review and meta-analysis. J Cancer Surviv. 2018;12(2):256–67.
45. Zhu J, Chen X, Zhen X, Zheng H, Chen H, Chen H, et al. Meta-analysis of effects of yoga exercise intervention on sleep quality in breast cancer patients. Front Oncol. 2023;13:1146433.
46. Hsueh EJ, Loh EW, Lin JJ, Tam KW. Effects of yoga on improving quality of life in patients with breast cancer: a meta-analysis of randomized controlled trials. Breast Cancer. 2021;28(2):264–76.
47. Hou L, Wang J, Mao M, Zhang Z, Liu D, Gao S, et al. Effect of yoga on cancer-related fatigue in patients with breast cancer: a systematic review and meta-analysis. Medicine. 2024;103(1):e36468.
48. Dong B, Xie C, Jing X, Lin L, Tian L. Yoga has a solid effect on cancer-related fatigue in patients with breast cancer: a meta-analysis. Breast Cancer Res Treat. 2019;177(1):5–16.
49. Espíndula RC, Nadas GB, Rosa MI, Foster C, Araújo FC, Grande AJ. Pilates for breast cancer: a systematic review and meta-analysis. Rev Assoc Med Bras. 2017;63(11):1006–12.
50. Pinto-Carral A, Molina AJ, de Pedro Á, Ayán C. Pilates for women with breast cancer: a systematic review and meta-analysis. Complement Ther Med. 2018;41:130–40.
51. Medeiros Torres D, Jorge Koifman R, da Silva SS. Impact on fatigue of different types of physical exercise during adjuvant chemotherapy and radiotherapy in breast cancer: systematic review and meta-analysis. Support Care Cancer. 2022;30(6):4651–62.
52. Mur-Gimeno E, Postigo-Martin P, Cantarero-Villanueva I, Sebio-Garcia R. Systematic review of the effect of aquatic therapeutic exercise in breast cancer survivors. Eur J Cancer Care. 2022;31(1):e13535.
53. Muñoz-Gómez E, Arnal-Gómez A, López Cascón A, Espí-López GV. Systematic review of aquatic therapeutic exercise efficacy in breast cancer survivors. Support Care Cancer. 2022;31(1):44.
54. Reger M, Kutschan S, Freuding M, Schmidt T, Josfeld L, Huebner J. Water therapies (hydrotherapy, balneotherapy or aqua therapy) for patients with cancer: a systematic review. J Cancer Res Clin Oncol. 2022;148(6):1277–97.
55. Salam A, Woodman A, Chu A, Al-Jamea LH, Islam M, Sagher M, et al. Effect of post-diagnosis exercise on depression symptoms, physical functioning and mortality in breast cancer survivors: a systematic review and meta-analysis of randomized control trials. Cancer Epidemiol. 2022;77:102111.
56. Akdeniz N, Kaplan MA, Küçüköner M, Urakçı Z, Laçin Ş, Ceylan EH, et al. The effect of exercise on disease-free survival and overall survival in patients with breast cancer. Ir J Med Sci. 2022;191(4):1587–97.
57. Neil-Sztramko SE, Winters-Stone KM, Bland KA, Campbell KL. Updated systematic review of exercise studies in breast cancer survivors: attention to the principles of exercise training. Br J Sports Med. 2019;53(8):504–12.
58. Piraux E, Caty G, Aboubakar Nana F, Reychler G. Effects of exercise therapy in cancer patients undergoing radiotherapy treatment: a narrative review. SAGE Open Med. 2020;8:2050312120922657.
59. De Groef A, Penen F, Dams L, Van der Gucht E, Nijs J, Meeus M. Best-evidence rehabilitation for chronic pain part 2: pain during and after cancer treatment. J Clin Med. 2019;8(7):979.
60. Mijwel S, Backman M, Bolam KA, Olofsson E, Norrbom J, Bergh J, et al. Highly favorable physiological responses to concurrent resistance and high-intensity interval training during chemotherapy: the OptiTrain breast cancer trial. Breast Cancer Res Treat. 2018;169:93–103.
61. Cešeiko R, Thomsen SN, Tomsone S, Eglītis J, Vētra A, Srebnijs A, et al. Heavy resistance training in breast cancer patients undergoing adjuvant therapy. Med Sci Sports Exerc. 2020;52(6):1239–47.
62. Klassen O, Schmidt ME, Ulrich CM, Schneeweiss A, Potthoff K, Steindorf K, et al. Muscle strength in breast cancer patients receiving different treatment regimes. J Cachexia Sarcopenia Muscle. 2017;8(2):305–16.
63. Wang E, Nyberg SK, Hoff J, Zhao J, Leivseth G, Tørhaug T, et al. Impact of maximal strength training on work efficiency and muscle fiber type in the elderly: implications for physical function and fall prevention. Exp Gerontol. 2017;91:64–71.
64. Hasenoehrl T, Palma S, Ramazanova D, Kölbl H, Dorner TE, Keilani M, et al. Resistance exercise and breast cancer–related lymphedema—a systematic review update and meta-analysis. Support Care Cancer. 2020;28:3593–603.
65. Wang L, Shi YX, Wang TT, Chen KX, Shang SM. Breast cancer-related lymphoedema and

resistance exercise: an evidence-based review of guidelines, consensus statements and systematic reviews. J Clin Nurs. 2023;32(9-10):2208–27.
66. Kilbreath SL, Refshauge KM, Beith JM, Ward LC, Lee M, Simpson JM, et al. Upper limb progressive resistance training and stretching exercises following surgery for early breast cancer: a randomized controlled trial. Breast Cancer Res Treat. 2012;133:667–76.
67. Cormie P, Singh B, Hayes S, Peake J, Galvão D, Taaffe D, et al. Acute inflammatory response to low-, moderate-, and high-load resistance exercise in women with breast cancer-related lymphedema. Integr Cancer Ther. 2016;15(3):308–17.
68. Bloomquist K, Oturai P, Steele ML, Adamsen L, Møller T, Christensen KB, et al. Heavy-load lifting: acute response in breast cancer survivors at risk for lymphedema. Med Sci Sports Exerc. 2018;50(2):187–95.
69. Rosenberg J, Hyde PN, Yancy WS Jr, Ford KM, Champ CE. Quantity of resistance exercise for breast cancer patients: does the dose match the objective? J Strength Cond Res. 2021;35(5):1467–76.
70. Korhonen MT, Cristea A, Alén M, Hakkinen K, Sipila S, Mero A, et al. Aging, muscle fiber type, and contractile function in sprint-trained athletes. J Appl Physiol. 2006;101(3):906–17.
71. Shaw CS, Swinton C, Morales-Scholz MG, McRae N, Erftemeyer T, Aldous A, et al. Impact of exercise training status on the fiber type-specific abundance of proteins regulating intramuscular lipid metabolism. J Appl Physiol. 2020;128(2):379–89.
72. Soriano-Maldonado A, Diez-Fernandez DM, Esteban-Simon A, Rodriguez-Perez MA, Artes-Rodriguez E, Casimiro-Artes MA, et al. Effects of a 12-week supervised resistance training program, combined with home-based physical activity, on physical fitness and quality of life in female breast cancer survivors: The EFICAN randomized controlled trial. J Cancer Surviv. 2023;17(5):1371–85.
73. An KY, Morielli AR, Kang DW, Friedenreich CM, McKenzie DC, Gelmon K, et al. Effects of exercise dose and type during breast cancer chemotherapy on longer-term patient-reported outcomes and health-related fitness: a randomized controlled trial. Int J Cancer. 2020;146(1):150–60.
74. Heggelund J, Fimland MS, Helgerud J, Hoff J. Maximal strength training improves work economy, rate of force development and maximal strength more than conventional strength training. Eur J Appl Physiol. 2013;113:1565–73.
75. Runowicz CD, Leach CR, Henry NL, Henry KS, Mackey HT, Cowens-Alvarado RL, et al. American Cancer Society/American Society of Clinical Oncology breast cancer survivorship care guideline. J Clin Oncol. 2016;34(6):611–35.
76. Palesh O, Scheiber C, Kesler S, Mustian K, Koopman C, Schapira L. Management of side effects during and post-treatment in breast cancer survivors. Breast J. 2018;24(2):167–75.
77. Casla S, Hojman P, Márquez-Rodas I, López-Tarruella S, Jerez Y, Barakat R, et al. Running away from side effects: physical exercise as a complementary intervention for breast cancer patients. Clin Transl Oncol. 2015;17(3):180–96.
78. Stout NL, Baima J, Swisher AK, Winters-Stone KM, Welsh J. A systematic review of exercise systematic reviews in the cancer literature (2005-2017). PM R. 2017;9(9):347–84.
79. Campos M, Feitosa RHF, Mizzaci CC, Flach M, Siqueira BJM, Mastrocola LE. The benefits of exercise in breast cancer. Arq Bras Cardiol. 2022;119(6):981–90.
80. McTiernan A, Friedenreich CM, Katzmarzyk PT, Powell KE, Macko R, Buchner D, et al. Physical activity in cancer prevention and survival: a systematic review. Med Sci Sports Exerc. 2019;51(6):1252–61.
81. Potiaumpai M, Schleicher EA, Wang M, Campbell KL, Sturgeon K, Schmitz KH. Exercise during chemotherapy: friend or foe? Cancer Med. 2023;12(9):10715–24.
82. Ruiz-Casado A, Álvarez-Bustos A, de Pedro CG, Méndez-Otero M, Romero-Elías M. Cancer-related fatigue in breast cancer survivors: a review. Clin Breast Cancer. 2021;21(1):10–25.
83. Berger AM, Mooney K, Alvarez-Perez A, Breitbart WS, Carpenter KM, Cella D, et al. Cancer-related fatigue, version 2.2015. J Natl Compr Cancer Netw. 2015;13(8):1012–39.
84. Kang YE, Yoon JH, Park NH, Ahn YC, Lee EJ, Son CG. Prevalence of cancer-related fatigue based on severity: a systematic review and meta-analysis. Sci Rep. 2023;13(1):12815.
85. Thong MS, van Noorden CJ, Steindorf K, Arndt V. Cancer-related fatigue: causes and current treatment options. Curr Treat Options in Oncol. 2020;21(2):17.
86. Mustian KM, Alfano CM, Heckler C, Kleckner AS, Kleckner IR, Leach CR, et al. Comparison of pharmaceutical, psychological, and exercise treatments for cancer-related fatigue: a meta-analysis. JAMA Oncol. 2017;3(7):961–8.
87. LaVoy EC, Fagundes CP, Dantzer R. Exercise, inflammation, and fatigue in cancer survivors. Exerc Immunol Rev. 2016;22:82–93.
88. Wu T, Yan F, Wei Y, Yuan C, Jiao Y, Pan Y, et al. Effect of exercise therapy on cancer-related fatigue in patients with breast cancer: a systematic review and network meta-analysis. Am J Phys Med Rehabil. 2023;102(12):1055–62.
89. Lin PJ, Kleckner IR, Loh KP, Inglis JE, Peppone LJ, Janelsins MC, et al. Influence of yoga on cancer-related fatigue and on mediational relationships between changes in sleep and cancer-related fatigue: a nationwide, multicenter randomized controlled trial of yoga in cancer survivors. Integr Cancer Ther. 2019;18:1534735419855134.
90. Oka T, Tanahashi T, Sudo N, Lkhagvasuren B, Yamada Y. Changes in fatigue, autonomic functions,

and blood biomarkers due to sitting isometric yoga in patients with chronic fatigue syndrome. Biopsychosoc Med. 2018;12:3.
91. Liu C, Qin M, Zheng X, Chen R, Zhu J. A meta-analysis: intervention effect of mind-body exercise on relieving cancer-related fatigue in breast cancer patients. Evid Based Complement Alternat Med. 2021;2021:9980940.
92. Meneses-Echávez JF, González-Jiménez E, Ramírez-Vélez R. Effects of supervised exercise on cancer-related fatigue in breast cancer survivors: a systematic review and meta-analysis. BMC Cancer. 2015;15:77.
93. Otte JL, Carpenter JS, Russell KM, Bigatti S, Champion VL. Prevalence, severity, and correlates of sleep-wake disturbances in long-term breast cancer survivors. J Pain Symptom Manag. 2010;39(3):535–47.
94. Otte JL, Davis L, Carpenter JS, Krier C, Skaar TC, Rand KL, et al. Sleep disorders in breast cancer survivors. Support Care Cancer. 2016;24(10):4197–205.
95. Weng YP, Hong RM, Chen VC, Tsai CJ, Yeh DC, Fang YH. Sleep quality and related factors in patients with breast cancer: a cross-sectional study in Taiwan. Cancer Manag Res. 2021;13:4725–33.
96. Hajj A, Hachem R, Khoury R, Nehme T, Hallit S, Nasr F, et al. Clinical and genetic factors associated with the breast cancer-related sleep disorders: The "CAGE-Sleep" study-a cross-sectional study. J Pain Symptom Manag. 2021;62(3):e46–55.
97. Fox RS, Ancoli-Israel S, Roesch SC, Merz EL, Mills SD, Wells KJ, et al. Sleep disturbance and cancer-related fatigue symptom cluster in breast cancer patients undergoing chemotherapy. Support Care Cancer. 2020;28(2):845–55.
98. Bach L, Kalder M, Kostev K. Depression and sleep disorders are associated with early mortality in women with breast cancer in the United Kingdom. J Psychiatr Res. 2021;143:481–4.
99. Aggeli P, Fasoi G, Zartaloudi A, Kontzoglou K, Kontos M, Konstantinidis T, et al. Posttreatment anxiety, depression, sleep disorders, and associated factors in women who survive breast cancer. Asia Pac J Oncol Nurs. 2021;8(2):147–55.
100. de Moura Ferraz Barbosa MP, de Jesus NT, Bergmann A, da Silva Alves Gomes VM, Sacomori C, Dantas D. Efficacy of supervised exercise on sleep of women who survived breast cancer: a systematic review with meta-analysis. J Cancer Surviv. 2024. https://doi.org/10.1007/s11764-024-01532-3.
101. Sturgeon KM, Kok DE, Kleckner IR, Guertin KA, McNeil J, Parry TL, et al. Updated systematic review of the effects of exercise on understudied health outcomes in cancer survivors. Cancer Med. 2023;12(24):22278–92.
102. Paice JA. Pain in cancer survivors: how to manage. Curr Treat Options in Oncol. 2019;20(6):48.
103. Leysen L, Adriaenssens N, Nijs J, Pas R, Bilterys T, Vermeir S, et al. Chronic pain in breast cancer survivors: nociceptive, neuropathic, or central sensitization pain? Pain Pract. 2019;19(2):183–95.
104. Nijs J, Leysen L, Pas R, Adriaenssens N, Meeus M, Hoelen W, et al. Treatment of pain following cancer: applying neuro-immunology in rehabilitation practice. Disabil Rehabil. 2018;40(6):714–21.
105. Cuthbert C, Twomey R, Bansal M, Rana B, Dhruva T, Livingston V, et al. The role of exercise for pain management in adults living with and beyond cancer: a systematic review and meta-analysis. Support Care Cancer. 2023;31(5):254.
106. Andersen Hammond E, Pitz M, Shay B. Neuropathic pain in taxane-induced peripheral neuropathy: evidence for exercise in treatment. Neurorehabil Neural Repair. 2019;33(10):792–9.
107. Brownson-Smith R, Orange ST, Cresti N, Hunt K, Saxton J, Temesi J. Effect of exercise before and/or during taxane-containing chemotherapy treatment on chemotherapy-induced peripheral neuropathy symptoms in women with breast cancer: systematic review and meta-analysis. J Cancer Surviv. 2023. https://doi.org/10.1007/s11764-023-01450-w.
108. Hidding JT, Beurskens CH, van der Wees PJ, van Laarhoven HW, Nijhuis-van der Sanden MW. Treatment related impairments in arm and shoulder in patients with breast cancer: a systematic review. PLoS One. 2014;9(5):e96748.
109. Yang Y, Gu D, Qian Y, Wang H, Chai X. Effectiveness of aerobic exercise on upper limb function following breast cancer treatment: a systematic review and meta-analysis. Ann Palliat Med. 2021;10(3):3396–403.
110. Lin Y, Chen Y, Liu R, Cao B. Effect of exercise on rehabilitation of breast cancer surgery patients: a systematic review and meta-analysis of randomized controlled trials. Nurs Open. 2023;10(4):2030–43.
111. Redemski T, Hamilton DG, Schuler S, Liang R, Michaleff ZA. Rehabilitation for women undergoing breast cancer surgery: a systematic review and meta-analysis of the effectiveness of early, unrestricted exercise programs on upper limb function. Clin Breast Cancer. 2022;22(7):650–65.
112. Panchik D, Masco S, Zinnikas P, Hillriegel B, Lauder T, Suttmann E, et al. Effect of exercise on breast cancer-related lymphedema: what the lymphatic surgeon needs to know. J Reconstr Microsurg. 2019;35(1):37–45.
113. Tendero-Ruiz L, Palomo-Carrión R, Megía-García-Carpintero Á, Pérez-Nombela S, López-Muñoz P, Bravo-Esteban E. The effect of therapeutic exercise in the prevention of lymphoedema secondary to breast cancer: a systematic review. Arch Med Sci. 2023;19(6):1684–92.
114. Jia M, Zhang X, Wei L, Gao J. Measurement, outcomes and interventions of cognitive function after breast cancer treatment: a narrative review. Asia Pac J Clin Oncol. 2021;17(4):321–9.
115. Oliveira MEC, Torres GSV, Franklin RG, Gomes KAL, Nóbrega WFS, Fernandes TP, et al. Cognitive impairments associated with chemotherapy in

women with breast cancer: a meta-analysis and meta-regression. Braz J Med Biol Res. 2023;56:e12947.
116. Jesús OJ, Luis CP, Matilde MF. Effects of exercise on cancer-related cognitive impairment in breast cancer survivors: a scoping review. Breast Cancer. 2023;30(6):885–909.
117. Hong F, Ye W, Kuo CH, Zhang Y, Qian Y, Korivi M. Exercise intervention improves clinical outcomes, but the "Time of Session" is crucial for better quality of life in breast cancer survivors: a systematic review and meta-analysis. Cancer. 2019;11(5):706.
118. Chan A, Ports K, Neo P, Ramalingam MB, Lim AT, Tan B, et al. Barriers and facilitators to exercise among adult cancer survivors in Singapore. Support Care Cancer. 2022;30(6):4867–78.
119. Hsu HT, Dodd MJ, Guo SE, Lee KA, Hwang SL, Lai YH. Predictors of exercise frequency in breast cancer survivors in Taiwan. J Clin Nurs. 2011;20(13-14):1923–35.
120. Ottenbacher AJ, Day RS, Taylor WC, Sharma SV, Sloane R, Snyder DC, et al. Exercise among breast and prostate cancer survivors—what are their barriers? J Cancer Surviv. 2011;5:413–9.
121. Clifford BK, Mizrahi D, Sandler CX, Barry BK, Simar D, Wakefield CE, et al. Barriers and facilitators of exercise experienced by cancer survivors: a mixed methods systematic review. Support Care Cancer. 2018;26:685–700.
122. Pope Z, Lee JE, Zeng N, Lee HY, Gao Z. Feasibility of smartphone application and social media intervention on breast cancer survivors' health outcomes. Transl Behav Med. 2019;9(1):11–22.
123. Gao Z, Ryu S, Zhou W, Adams K, Hassan M, Zhang R, et al. Effects of personalized exercise prescriptions and social media delivered through mobile health on cancer survivors' physical activity and quality of life. J Sport Health Sci. 2023;12(6):705–14.

18 Nutrition in Breast Cancer

Emine Merve Ekici

18.1 Nutritional Intervention in Cancer Treatment

Despite many advances in cancer treatment over the last hundred years, cancer remains a major cause of death and a public health problem. Cancer, which also has a significant impact on health expenditures in society, occurs in one out of every five people before the age of 75. Half of the people who develop the disease die due to cancer [1–4].

Breast cancer is the most common cancer and the leading cause of cancer death in women worldwide. Nonmodifiable risk factors for breast cancer include being female, older age, family history, genetic mutations, race, pregnancy, breastfeeding, menstruation, and menopause, which affect breast tissue density. Modifiable risk factors for breast cancer include hormonal replacement therapy, diethylstilbestrol, lack of physical activity, overweight/obesity, alcohol intake, smoking, inadequate vitamin supplements, processed food consumption, and exposure to chemicals. Nutritional status, which is one of the modifiable risk factors, is seen as an effective method in the prevention and treatment of cancer [5].

Physiological adaptations to nutrient intake have aspects that may influence cancer incidence, growth, and development. According to available data, it is estimated that one-third of the most common types of cancer can be prevented by dietary modification [1–4].

According to the results of preclinical models and early clinical trials conducted in recent years, some nutritional patterns have been shown to have a strong role in the prevention and treatment of cancer by preventing tumor formation, delaying tumor growth, and producing synergistic effects with various anticancer therapies [1, 6, 7]. Despite promising results, nutrition interventions have been overlooked in the clinic, especially in cancer treatment, due to a lack of robust evidence and large-scale clinical trials of nutrition interventions. The lack of well-controlled studies of cancer patients and unclear criteria for enrolling and grouping patients with both metabolic and different tumor profiles have made it difficult to identify nutritional therapeutics in these patients. However, scientific efforts to investigate the effects of nutritional therapeutics and nutritional interventions on cancer metabolism in oncology are ongoing [4].

E. M. Ekici (✉)
Gülhane Faculty of Health Sciences, Department of Nutrition and Dietetics, University of Health Sciences, Ankara, Turkey

Y. Bakar, A. Tuğral (eds.), *Managing Side Effects of Breast Cancer Treatment*,
https://doi.org/10.1007/978-3-031-75480-7_18

18.2 Current Evidence on the Relationship Between Nutrition and Cancer

The known widespread effects of nutrition on health and physiology suggest that nutritional interventions may also mediate antitumor effects. Diet may directly target cancer metabolism by eliminating nutrients preferred by tumors or may have a modulating effect on cancer-associated factors such as growth signaling, oxidative stress, and immunity [8].

There are some mechanisms mediating the nutrition-cancer interaction. First observed by Otto Warburg in the early twentieth century, "metabolic reprogramming" is considered to be one of the most important distinguishing features of cancer. The emergence of this feature revealed that energy and nutrients are used in tumor growth and migration [4, 9, 10]. The genetic heterogeneity of tumors and the different metabolic profiles of their tissues of origin cause cancer cells to prefer certain nutrients, making them vulnerable to changes in nutrient intake as a therapeutic intervention [8].

Under normal conditions, tissues utilize glucose to generate ATP by combining glycolysis and oxidative phosphorylation. Cancer cells typically metabolize glucose via aerobic glycolysis and ferment glucose to lactate independently of oxygen availability and mitochondrial function. This is an inefficient way to obtain ATP per unit of glucose compared to mitochondrial respiration; however, it allows for a much faster rate of glucose metabolism. Glycolysis also produces waste products such as lactate, which contributes to cancer growth and progression and can be incorporated into tricarboxylic acid cycle intermediates to feed tumors [11].

Fructose is another monosaccharide associated with cancer growth. Genes of the polyol pathway are known to be associated with epithelial mesenchymal transition (EMT) in human lung cancer samples and EMT-driven colon cancer models in mice [12]. Fructose has also been found to be a potent inducer of transketolase in pancreatic cancer cells and to induce cell proliferation through the phosphate pentose pathway [13]. Generally, it is known that there is a link between dietary intake of simple carbohydrates and tumor incidence and growth, both by directly feeding existing tumors and through metabolic reprogramming by facilitating uncontrolled cell growth. Cancer cells often prefer glucose as the primary nutrient for energy production, making glucose metabolism a fundamental element of cancer progression and a promising therapeutic target [8].

Amino acids are another nutrient associated with tumor formation. Cancer cells require protein synthesis to sustain growth and proliferation. In addition, some cancer types depend on exogenous sources of nonessential amino acids to sustain growth. For example, serine and glycine metabolism have been shown to be important in cancer proliferation, and dietary restrictions have been shown to inhibit tumor growth and increase survival in mouse models of intestinal cancer and lymphoma [14]. Furthermore, inhibition of the glutamate transporter ASCT2 has been shown to reduce the growth of gastric cancer, triple-negative breast cancer, and prostate cancer in various mouse models [15, 16]. These data suggest that some types of cancer require dietary sources of specific amino acids to sustain growth. There is also evidence that some metabolites derived from amino acid catabolism, such as polyamines and kynurenine derived from arginine and tryptophan, promote cancer growth and migration [8].

Lipids are the main component of biological membranes, serve as the body's main energy stores, and are involved in metabolism and hormone synthesis. Therefore, the alteration of lipid metabolism seen in cancer is expected [17]. Cancer cells are often associated with upregulation of lipid receptors and transporters. Increased expression of CD36, a fatty acid receptor, is strongly associated with poor prognosis in squamous cell lung carcinoma and in bladder and breast cancers. CD36 also appears to enhance cancer progression and metastatic potential in oral squamous epithelial cell carcinoma and ovarian cancer in response to lipids supplied via adipocytes, making it an attractive target for cancer therapy and prevention [18, 19].

18.3 Nutritional Therapy in Breast Cancer

The increasing trend in breast cancer incidence and mortality in underdeveloped and highly developed countries proves the urgency of measures, strategies, and calls for action that can be implemented to address cancer. Nutritional interventions and methods are one of these strategies. Many nutrients such as fatty acids, carbohydrates, vitamins B, and D, carotenoids, phytoestrogens, and dietary fiber have been identified to have a potential effect on tumor development in animal experiments and population studies, but there is little evidence from epidemiological studies [20, 21].

Issues such as measurement error in nutritional assessment, lack of adequate follow-up, and differences in the timing of exposure may contribute to differences between epidemiologic studies. Another source of variation not considered in epidemiological studies is genomic variation in tumor phenotypes. Disease outcomes, susceptibility to treatment, and risk factors may also vary between different types of breast cancer [21].

The role of some specific nutrients in the etiology of breast cancer has been suggested based on associations reported in epidemiologic studies, and attention has been drawn to the antioxidant properties of selected nutrients, their effect on epigenetic processes, DNA repair, DNA adducts, inflammation, regulation of gene expression, stimulation of growth factors or circulating levels of endogenous hormones. Energy balance, caloric intake, physical activity, body mass index (BMI), and metabolic rate are among other important factors that may influence breast cancer development [21].

18.4 Breast Cancer and Nutrients

18.4.1 Carbohydrate, Glycemic Load, and Glycemic Index and Fiber

Dietary carbohydrate intake is hypothesized to modulate cancer risk depending on the amount and type consumed. Carbohydrates belong to a broad category of biomolecules that function as preferred cellular energy substrates in their monosaccharide form. Besides their basic functions, carbohydrates exert a comprehensive range of cellular, physiological, and ecological effects. Noteworthy among these are microbial and epigenetic modulations, as well as endocrine and systemic changes resulting from their consumption, which could potentially influence cancer risk and progression [22].

The consumption of dietary carbohydrates has recently increased worldwide. Different types of carbohydrates, such as monosaccharides and disaccharides, now form one of the most important parts of the diet. It is often reported that the amount of simple sugar consumption is associated with the development of some types of cancer. In addition, large amounts of dietary fructose have also been reported to be associated with specific metabolic changes in the mammary glands that have been linked to the development of breast cancer [23].

The hypothesis that a carbohydrate-rich diet increases the risk of breast cancer dates back to the 1990s [24]. Although carbohydrates are recommended to constitute more than half of daily calories, some features in their metabolism have been found to be associated with breast cancer. Carbohydrates affect blood glucose and insulin levels. Although the relationship between breast cancer and dietary carbohydrates is not clear, it has been suggested that the effect of glucose on insulin levels may be associated with cancer risk. The intake of carbohydrates causes insulin secretion and affects the activity of insulin-like growth factor (IGF) and estrogen. Many studies have shown that high levels of IGF increase the risk of premenopausal breast cancer. Laboratory studies have shown that insulin increases the proliferation of breast cells [25].

In addition, it is thought that high-carbohydrate diets may also promote carcinogenesis through various mechanisms such as inducing oxidative stress and promoting body weight gain [23, 26].

In addition to total carbohydrate intake, carbohydrate quality can potentially influence breast cancer risk by affecting insulin resistance and plasma insulin and glucose levels [21]. Available data on the relationship between total carbohydrate intake or specific carbohydrate types, glycemic index (GI) glycemic load (GL), and breast cancer risk are conflicting. GI and GL are both measures of carbohydrate quality. Specifically, GI refers to the postprandial glucose response to a fixed amount of 50 g of carbohydrates from different foods. GL is the product of GI and the total available carbohydrate content in a given amount of food. Therefore, GL is a stronger predictor of postprandial glycemia and insulin response than GI [27].

A recent meta-analysis of prospective studies reported a significant positive association between the glycemic index, a measure of carbohydrate quality, and breast cancer risk [28]. In the EPIC study, high dietary carbohydrate and glycemic load were significantly associated with increased breast cancer in postmenopausal women [29].

These results, in agreement with those of the Women's Health Initiative, suggest that insulinogenic diets may influence breast cancer risk [30]. In support of this hypothesis, data from Mexico, where carbohydrates account for approximately 64% of caloric intake in the population, showed a strong positive association between carbohydrate intake as well as glycemic load and breast cancer among pre- and postmenopausal women [31]. High refined carbohydrate intake may have stronger associations with breast cancer risk in populations genetically predisposed to insulin resistance, such as in Mexico, especially when combined with obesity and physical inactivity [32].

The International World Cancer Research Fund (WCRF) review panel concluded that there is insufficient evidence of an association between dietary fiber and breast cancer risk [33]. The type of food consumed may be important in studies on dietary fiber. A recent prospective study showed that breast cancer risk was inversely associated with dietary fiber from vegetables but not with fiber from fruits, cereals, or other dietary sources. The specific biological mechanisms underlying the observed differences in the association of vegetable, fruit, and cereal fibers with breast cancer are still unclear. Other dietary factors may also be involved, as a combination of low fat and high fiber intake is associated with a significant reduction in breast cancer risk in premenopausal women [34]. In addition, dietary fiber has been hypothesized to reduce the risk of breast cancer by reducing circulating estrogen levels [35].

18.4.2 Lipids

Many studies have examined the relationship between dietary fatty acid intake and breast cancer risk [21, 36]. Western diets high in fat have been hypothesized to play a role in breast cancer pathophysiology [36]. Early ecologic studies showed that per capita dietary fat consumption was highly associated with breast cancer mortality. A study among Japanese immigrants showed increased breast cancer mortality rates in the USA compared to those observed in Japan, suggesting that environmental factors, including components of the Western diet, may play a role in reduced survival [37]. More recently, several studies in humans have investigated the relationship between dietary fat and breast cancer recurrence, mortality, and all-cause mortality [36, 38–40].

Dietary fats are hypothesized to play a key role in the etiology of breast cancer malignancy [41]. Accordingly, the roles of dietary fatty acid intake on membrane fluidity and function, inflammation, oxidative stress, regulation of gene expression, stimulation of growth factors, or effects on circulating levels of endogenous estrogens have been mostly mentioned [21, 36].

It seems that the effect of fatty acid types rather than total fat intake on breast cancer risk is important. However, there is still a need for larger and more comprehensive studies on this subject. In a meta-analysis, intake of N-3 fatty acids from seafood was associated with a 14% reduction in breast cancer risk [42]. In a case–control study conducted in Mexico, long-chain N-3 PUFA intake was associated with a reduced risk of breast cancer in obese women and the underlying mechanisms were reduced inflammation and improved adipokine and estrogen levels in adipose tissue induced by N-3 PUFA intake. In contrast, trans-fatty acids, whose main source worldwide is the industrial partial hydrogenation process of plant products, have been associated with an increased risk of breast cancer [41, 43]. The risk of natural trans-fatty acids produced by ruminants remains unclear [21].

In a randomized control study, the relationship between dietary fatty acid intake and breast cancer was examined. The study showed that high MUFA intake, especially in the premenopausal period, was associated with a decreased risk of breast cancer. Chronic inflammation is known to play a role in breast cancer development and progression by affecting tumor growth and metastasis and high insulin levels. MUFA has positive effects on inflammation and insulin sensitivity. In addition, diets high in MUFA are associated with reduced breast cancer risk through their effects on weight control and metabolism regulation. Furthermore, increasing MUFA intake in the diet may cause changes in the function and location of proteins important for tumor suppression [44].

18.4.3 Protein

Evidence on the association between dietary protein intake and breast cancer incidence and outcome is inconsistent. In 2016, a meta-analysis of 46 prospective cohort studies, nested case-control studies, and case–cohort studies showed that total red meat intake was associated with a 1.07-fold higher risk of breast cancer for each increase in red meat servings [45].

On the contrary, in the Nurses' Health Study (NHS), one of the most comprehensive studies in which 1982 women participated, higher dietary protein intake was found to be associated with higher survival in breast cancer. The reasons for this association are not yet fully known, and recent focus has been on the effects of protein quality on health In especially, the essential amino acids lysine, threonine, valine, isoleucine, leucine, methionine, phenylalanine, tryptophan and histidine are actively investigated for their roles in lean body mass maintenance, cell signaling, glucose metabolism, bone health and satiety. The branched-chain amino acids leucine, isoleucine, and valine modulate muscle protein synthesis through insulin signaling and are particularly abundant in dairy products. Besides its positive effects on weight loss, leucine inhibits skeletal muscle breakdown and stimulates muscle protein synthesis by increasing insulin sensitivity. Glutamine also increases insulin sensitivity in vivo [46].

In a study examining total daily protein, animal protein, and plant protein intake and breast cancer incidence and the causes of breast cancer, 100,024 women participated and were followed up for 3 years. At the end of the study, total protein intake was not associated with breast cancer incidence or risk of death after breast cancer development, whereas vegetable protein intake was associated with lower breast cancer incidence and decreased risk of death after breast cancer. In the same study, higher animal protein intake was associated with a higher incidence of breast cancer [47].

A systematic review and meta-analysis evaluated the association of certain foods and food groups (total meat, red meat, poultry, fish, processed meat, eggs, fruits, vegetables, dairy products, milk, yogurt, cheese, cereals, soybeans, nuts, and legumes) with breast cancer risk. At the end of the study, the findings of the present meta-analysis showed that high intakes of fruits, vegetables, soybeans, and cheese and low intakes of red meat and processed meat were associated with a reduced risk of breast cancer. This emphasizes the type and quality of protein intake rather than total protein intake [48].

Red meat consumption is high in North America and Western Europe, countries with the highest incidence of breast cancer. Although consumption of red meat, especially fried meat, has been shown to increase the risk, white meat and pork have not been associated and further studies are needed [25]. The relationship between dairy products and breast cancer is controversial, with some sources stating that dairy products reduce the risk, others that they increase it or that they are not associated. The effect of dairy products should be evaluated together with other nutrients.

Another point is the amount of fat contained in dairy products and further studies are needed [25].

Soy foods and soy products are rich in phytoestrogens, naturally occurring hormone-like compounds with weak estrogenic effects. Despite inconsistencies in the available data, there is a possibility of an inverse association between soy food consumption and breast cancer. Soy consumption appears to be higher in Asian societies than in Western societies, and this association is more pronounced in Asian societies [21]. Furthermore, soy consumption may be most important during childhood and adolescence, and this association has only been evaluated in Asian populations [49]. Thus, the effect of soy foods and soy products may vary depending on genetics, previous soy intake, time of exposure, and level of soy intake [21].

18.4.4 Vitamin D

Vitamin D is the precursor of 1,25-dihydroxyvitamin D in the organism and has a steroid hormone structure that plays a role in various processes in the body, including cancer-related pathways. The mechanisms by which 1,25-dihydroxyvitamin D may exert protective effects against cancer include induction of apoptosis, stimulation of cell differentiation, anti-inflammatory and antiproliferative effects, and inhibition of angiogenesis, invasion, and metastasis. Furthermore, a number of factors such as obesity, low physical activity, age, race, skin type, smoking, and living in high latitudes lead to low circulating levels of 25-hydroxyvitamin D [50].

It is possible that vitamin D plays a role in controlling normal breast cell growth and has the capacity to stop the growth of cancer cells in this region. This protective effect is believed to be largely supported by the chemopreventive effects of 1,25-hydroxyvitamin D (1,25OH2D or calcitriol), the bioactive form of vitamin D, a well-known calcium regulator [50].

In a meta-analysis including the results of 22 studies conducted between 2000 and 2018, 25(OH)D deficiency was directly associated with breast cancer, while total vitamin D and supplemental vitamin D intake showed an inverse relationship with this result and it was recommended that randomized controlled trials should be conducted at the end of the study [50].

The possible effects of vitamin D on breast cancer are summarized below:

- Decreased proliferation, increased cellular maturation, and apoptosis
- Inhibition of the renin-angiotensin system, restoration of the glomerular filtration barrier
- Reduction of inflammation, reduction of inflammatory cell accumulation
- It inhibits angiogenesis and regulates insulin secretion and activity [51]

18.5 General Nutrition Recommendations for Breast Cancer

- Consume a diet that provides at least 30 g/day of fiber from food.
- Include foods containing whole grains, non-starchy vegetables, fruit, and pulses (legumes) such as beans and lentils in most meals.
- Eat a diet high in all types of plant foods including at least five portions or servings (at least 400 g or 15 oz in total) of a variety of non-starchy vegetables and fruit every day.
- If you eat starchy roots and tubers as staple foods, eat non-starchy vegetables, fruit, and pulses (legumes) regularly too if possible.
- Limit consumption of processed foods high in fat, starches, or sugars—including "fast foods"; many pre-prepared dishes, snacks, bakery foods, and desserts; and confectionery (candy)
- If you eat red meat, limit consumption to no more than about three portions per week. Three portions are equivalent to about 350–500 g (about 12–18 oz) cooked weight. Consume very little, if any, processed meat.
- Do not consume sugar-sweetened drinks.
- One of our Cancer Prevention Recommendations is to limit alcohol con-

sumption. For cancer prevention, it's best not to drink alcohol.
- High-dose dietary supplements are not recommended for cancer prevention—aim to meet nutritional needs through diet alone [52].

18.6 Breast Cancer and Nutrition Models

A review examined the association between dietary patterns and/or major food groups and mortality and cancer recurrence in survivors of common cancer types, including breast cancer, before or after cancer diagnosis. It showed that reducing body fat after diagnosis reduced the risk of breast cancer recurrence and that adherence to a high-quality, low-fat diet after diagnosis was associated with a reduced risk of all-cause mortality in breast cancer survivors. Conversely, adherence to a Western diet before and after diagnosis was positively associated with overall mortality risk and breast cancer survival. Following a "prudent" diet was associated with a reduced risk of overall mortality and death from causes other than breast cancer while following a Western-type diet was considered an indicator of a worse prognosis after breast cancer diagnosis [53]. Accordingly, in the Women's Health Initiative (WHI) study, a large prospective cohort study of 2295 postmenopausal women followed for more than 12 years, diet quality was assessed using the Healthy Eating Index (HEI)-2010 score and it was shown that adherence to a lower quality diet after breast cancer diagnosis increased the risk of death from breast cancer [53, 54].

A report published in China collected 5 years of dietary information to assess breast cancer survival and found that high adherence to healthy eating patterns, namely the Chinese Food Pagoda (CHFP) and Dietary Approach to Stop Hypertension (DASH) diets, was associated with a 25–34% lower risk of overall mortality and a 36–40% lower risk of breast cancer-specific events [55]. A low-fat dietary pattern ($\leq$20% of total energy intake from fat) was implemented in a long-term follow-up of 16.1 years and was able to reduce the incidence of death after breast cancer in the intervention group compared to the usual diet [56].

Recently, the Mediterranean diet has been recognized worldwide as one of the healthiest dietary patterns, mainly due to its rich content of antioxidants and anti-inflammatory nutrients. The combination of dietary components has been suggested to play a common role in reducing inflammation and oxidative stress, thereby inhibiting the progression of various malignancies, including cardiovascular disease and cancer. Given its protective effects in reducing oxidative and inflammatory processes of cells and preventing deoxyribose nucleic acid damage, cell proliferation and survival, angiogenesis, inflammation, and metastasis, the Mediterranean diet may be an effective method for breast cancer prevention and treatment [57].

References

1. Taylor SR, Falcone JN, Cantley LC, Goncalves MD. Developing dietary interventions as therapy for cancer. Nat Rev Cancer. 2022;22(8):452–66.
2. Song M, Giovannucci E. Preventable incidence and mortality of carcinoma associated with lifestyle factors among white adults in the United States. JAMA Oncol. 2016;2(9):1154–61.
3. Parkin DM, Boyd L, Walker LC. The fraction of cancer attributable to lifestyle and environmental factors in the UK in 2010. Br J Cancer. 2011;105(2):S77–81.
4. Martínez-Garay C, Djouder N. Dietary interventions and precision nutrition in cancer therapy. Trends Mol Med. 2022;29(7):489–511.
5. Łukasiewicz S, Czeczelewski M, Forma A, Baj J, Sitarz R, Stanisławek A. Breast cancer—epidemiology, risk factors, classification, prognostic markers, and current treatment strategies—an updated review. Cancer. 2021;13(17):4287.
6. Kanarek N, Petrova B, Sabatini DM. Dietary modifications for enhanced cancer therapy. Nature. 2020;579(7800):507–17.
7. Tajan M, Vousden KH. Dietary approaches to cancer therapy. Cancer Cell. 2020;37(6):767–85.
8. Martínez-Garay C, Djouder N. Dietary interventions and precision nutrition in cancer therapy. Trends Mol Med. 2023;29(7):489–511.
9. Warburg O. On the origin of cancer cells. Science. 1956;123(3191):309–14.
10. Liberti MV, Locasale JW. The Warburg effect: how does it benefit cancer cells? Trends Biochem Sci. 2016;41(3):211–8.

11. Pérez-Tomás R, Pérez-Guillén I. Lactate in the tumor microenvironment: an essential molecule in cancer progression and treatment. Cancer. 2020;12(11):3244.
12. Schwab A, Siddiqui A, Vazakidou ME, Napoli F, Böttcher M, Menchicchi B, Ceppi P. Polyol pathway links glucose metabolism to the aggressiveness of cancer cells. Cancer Res. 2018;78(7):1604–18.
13. Ricciardelli C, Lokman NA, Cheruvu S, Tan IA, Ween MP, Pyragius CE, Oehler MK. Transketolase is upregulated in metastatic peritoneal implants and promotes ovarian cancer cell proliferation. Clin Exp Metastasis. 2015;32:441–55.
14. Maddocks OD, Athineos D, Cheung EC, Lee P, Zhang T, Van Den Broek NJ, Vousden KH. Modulating the therapeutic response of tumours to dietary serine and glycine starvation. Nature. 2017;544(7650):372–6.
15. Wang Q, Hardie RA, Hoy AJ, Van Geldermalsen M, Gao D, Fazli L, Holst J. Targeting ASCT2-mediated glutamine uptake blocks prostate cancer growth and tumour development. J Pathol. 2015;236(3):278–89.
16. Van Geldermalsen M, Wang Q, Nagarajah R, Marshall AD, Thoeng A, Gao D, Holst J. ASCT2/SLC1A5 controls glutamine uptake and tumour growth in triple-negative basal-like breast cancer. Oncogene. 2016;35(24):3201–8.
17. Santos CR, Schulze A. Lipid metabolism in cancer. FEBS J. 2012;279(15):2610–23.
18. Xu S, Chaudhary O, Rodríguez-Morales P, Sun X, Chen D, Zappasodi R, Kaech SM. Uptake of oxidized lipids by the scavenger receptor CD36 promotes lipid peroxidation and dysfunction in CD8+ T cells in tumors. Immunity. 2021;54(7):1561–77.
19. Pascual G, Avgustinova A, Mejetta S, Martín M, Castellanos A, Attolini CSO, Benitah SA. Targeting metastasis-initiating cells through the fatty acid receptor CD36. Nature. 2017;541(7635):41–5.
20. Michels KB, Mohllajee AP, Roset-Bahmanyar E, Beehler GP, Moysich KB. Diet and breast cancer: a review of the prospective observational studies. Cancer. 2007;109:2712–49.
21. Chajes V, Romieu I. Nutrition and breast cancer. Maturitas. 2014;77(1):7–11.
22. Maino Vieytes CA, Taha HM, Burton-Obanla AA, Douglas KG, Arthur AE. Carbohydrate nutrition and the risk of cancer. Curr Nutr Rep. 2019;8:230–9.
23. Pishdad S, Joola P, Bourbour F, Rastgoo S, Majidi N, Gholamalizadeh M, Doaei S. Association between different types of dietary carbohydrate and breast cancer. Clin Nutr ESPEN. 2021;46:259–63.
24. Sieri S, Pala V, Brighenti F, Agnoli C, Grioni S, Berrino F, Krogh V. High glycemic diet and breast cancer occurrence in the Italian EPIC cohort. Nutr Metab Cardiovasc Dis. 2013;23(7):628–34.
25. Yılmaz M, Atak N. Meme kanseri riskinin beslenme ile ilişkili faktörler açısından değerlendirilmesi. Turk J Public Health. 2014;12(1):51–60.
26. Quesada-Morúa MS, Hidalgo O, Morera J, Rojas G, Perez AM, Vaillant F, Fonseca L. Hypolipidaemic, hypoglycaemic and antioxidant effects of a tropical highland blackberry beverage consumption in healthy individuals on a high-fat, high-carbohydrate diet challenge. J Berry Res. 2020;10(3):459–74.
27. De Cicco P, Catani MV, Gasperi V, Sibilano M, Quaglietta M, Savini I. Nutrition and breast cancer: a literature review on prevention, treatment and recurrence. Nutrients. 2019;11(7):1514.
28. Choi Y, Giovannucci E, Lee JE. Glycaemic index and glycaemic load in relation to risk of diabetes-related cancers: a meta-analysis. Br J Nutr. 2012;108(11):1934–47.
29. Romieu I, Ferrari P, Rinaldi S, Slimani N, Jenab M, Olsen A, Clavel-Chapelon F. Dietary glycemic index and glycemic load and breast cancer risk in the European Prospective Investigation into Cancer and Nutrition (EPIC). Am J Clin Nutr. 2012;96(2):345–55.
30. Shikany JM, Redden DT, Neuhouser ML, Chlebowski RT, Rohan TE, Simon MS, Tinker L. Dietary glycemic load, glycemic index, and carbohydrate and risk of breast cancer in the Women's Health Initiative. Nutr Cancer. 2011;63(6):899–907.
31. Romieu I, Lazcano-Ponce E, Sanchez-Zamorano LM, Willett W, Hernandez-Avila M. Carbohydrates and the risk of breast cancer among Mexican women. Cancer Epidemiol Biomarkers Prev. 2004;13(8):1283–9.
32. Gómez LM, Hernández-Prado B, Morales MDC, Shamah-Levy T. Physical activity and overweight/obesity in adult Mexican population: the Mexican National Health and Nutrition Survey 2006. Salud Publica Mex. 2009;51:S621–9.
33. World Cancer Research Fund. Physical activity, and the prevention of cancer: a global perspective. Washington: AICR; 2007.
34. Ferrari P, Rinaldi S, Jenab M, Lukanova A, Olsen A, Tjønneland A, Romieu I. Dietary fiber intake and risk of hormonal receptor–defined breast cancer in the European Prospective Investigation into Cancer and Nutrition study. Am J Clin Nutr. 2013;97(2):344–53.
35. Wen W, Shu XO, Li H, Yang G, Ji BT, Cai H, Zheng W. Dietary carbohydrates, fiber, and breast cancer risk in Chinese women. Am J Clin Nutr. 2009;89(1):283–9.
36. Makarem N, Chandran U, Bandera EV, Parekh N. Dietary fat in breast cancer survival. Annu Rev Nutr. 2013;33:319–48.
37. Buell P. Changing incidence of breast cancer in Japanese-American women. J Natl Cancer Inst. 1973;51(5):1479–83.
38. Pierce JP, Natarajan L, Caan BJ, Parker BA, Greenberg ER, Flatt SW, Stefanick ML. Influence of a diet very high in vegetables, fruit, and fiber and low in fat on prognosis following treatment for breast cancer: the Women's Healthy Eating and Living (WHEL) randomized trial. JAMA. 2007;298(3):289–98.
39. Jaiswal McEligot A, Largent J, Ziogas A, Peel D, Anton-Culver H. Dietary fat, fiber, vegetable, and micronutrients are associated with overall survival in postmenopausal women diagnosed with breast cancer. Nutr Cancer. 2006;55(2):132–40.
40. Beasley JM, Newcomb PA, Trentham-Dietz A, Hampton JM, Bersch AJ, Passarelli MN, Willett WC. Post-diagnosis dietary factors and survival

after invasive breast cancer. Breast Cancer Res Treat. 2011;128:229–36.
41. Hu J, La Vecchia C, de Groh M, Negri E, Morrison H, Mery L, Canadian Cancer Registries Epidemiology Research Group. Dietary transfatty acids and cancer risk. Eur J Cancer Prev. 2011;20(6):530–8.
42. Zheng JS, Hu XJ, Zhao YM, Yang J, Li D. Intake of fish and marine n-3 polyunsaturated fatty acids and risk of breast cancer: meta-analysis of data from 21 independent prospective cohort studies. BMJ. 2013;346:f3706.
43. Chajès V, Thiébaut AC, Rotival M, Gauthier E, Maillard V, Boutron-Ruault MC, Clavel-Chapelon F. Association between serum trans-monounsaturated fatty acids and breast cancer risk in the E3N-EPIC Study. Am J Epidemiol. 2008;167(11):1312–20.
44. Guo F, Wang M, Guo X, Pu L, Sun M, Li S, Jin L. The association between fatty acid intake and breast cancer based on the NHANES and Mendelian randomization study. Cancer Epidemiol. 2021;73:101966.
45. Wu J, Zeng R, Huang J, Li X, Zhang J, Ho JCM, Zheng Y. Dietary protein sources and incidence of breast cancer: a dose-response meta-analysis of prospective studies. Nutrients. 2016;8(11):730.
46. Holmes MD, Wang J, Hankinson SE, Tamimi RM, Chen WY. Protein intake and breast cancer survival in the Nurses' Health Study. J Clin Oncol. 2017;35(3):325.
47. Pan K, Larson JC, Prentice RL, Mortimer JE, Neuhouser ML, Manson JE, Chlebowski RT. Protein intake by source and breast cancer incidence and mortality: The Women's Health Initiative. JNCI Cancer Spectr. 2020;4(6):pkaa101.
48. Kazemi A, Barati-Boldaji R, Soltani S, Mohammadipoor N, Esmaeilinezhad Z, Clark CC, Akbarzadeh M. Intake of various food groups and risk of breast cancer: a systematic review and dose-response meta-analysis of prospective studies. Adv Nutr. 2021;12(3):809–49.
49. Korde LA, Wu AH, Fears T, Nomura AM, West DW, Kolonel LN, Ziegler RG. Childhood soy intake and breast cancer risk in Asian American women. Cancer Epidemiol Biomarkers Prev. 2009;18(4):1050–9.
50. Hossain S, Beydoun MA, Beydoun HA, Chen X, Zonderman AB, Wood RJ. Vitamin D and breast cancer: a systematic review and meta-analysis of observational studies. Clin Nutr ESPEN. 2019;30:170–84.
51. de La Puente-Yagüe M, Cuadrado-Cenzual MA, Ciudad-Cabañas MJ, Hernández- Cabria M, Collado-Yurrita L. Vitamin D: and its role in breast cancer. Kaohsiung J Med Sci. 2018;34(8):423–7.
52. World Cancer Research Fund. Recommendations and public health and policy implications. Washington: American Institute for Cancer Research; 2018.
53. Cava E, Marzullo P, Farinelli D, Gennari A, Saggia C, Riso S, Prodam F. Breast cancer diet "BCD": a review of healthy dietary patterns to prevent breast cancer recurrence and reduce mortality. Nutrients. 2022;14(3):476.
54. Sun Y, Bao W, Liu B, Caan BJ, Lane DS, Millen AE, Snetselaar LG. Changes in overall diet quality in relation to survival in postmenopausal women with breast cancer: results from the Women's Health Initiative. J Acad Nutr Diet. 2018;118(10):1855–63.
55. Wang F, Cai H, Gu K, Shi L, Yu D, Zhang M, Shu XO. Adherence to dietary recommendations among long-term breast cancer survivors and cancer outcome associations. Cancer Epidemiol Biomarkers Prev. 2020;29(2):386–95.
56. Chlebowski RT, Aragaki AK, Anderson GL, Thomson CA, Manson JE, Simon MS, Prentice RL. Low-fat dietary pattern and breast cancer mortality in the Women's Health Initiative randomized controlled trial. J Clin Oncol. 2017;35(25):2919.
57. Güneş BD, Acar T, N. The effect of Mediterranean diet on prevention and treatment of breast cancer. J Adnan Menderes Univ Health Sci Fac. 2021;5(2):442–54.

Part III

Specific Problems in Breast Cancer Survivorship and Management

Management of Hematological Toxicity in Breast Cancer Patients

19

Fatoş Dilan Köseoğlu

19.1 Introduction

Breast cancer is among the most commonly diagnosed types of cancer worldwide, and managing breast cancer involves not only addressing the tumor itself but also the myriad of complications that can arise throughout the disease [1–3]. One significant aspect of breast cancer management is the monitoring and treatment of hematological complications. These complications can be present at diagnosis, during treatment, and throughout long-term follow-up, highlighting the complex interplay between the cancer, its treatment, and the patient's overall health.

In the sections that follow, it will be summarized the acute complications under the headings of paraneoplastic hematological syndromes, treatment-related toxicities, and ultimately thrombotic complications. These topics encompass a wide range of issues, from the direct effects of the tumor on the body's blood cells to the side effects of chemotherapy and other cancer therapies. Understanding these complications is crucial for providing comprehensive care to breast cancer patients, aiming to mitigate risks and manage symptoms effectively.

Additionally, it will also be explored the long-term hematological toxicities associated with breast cancer treatments, including the development of leukemia and other blood-related disorders. These late effects underscore the importance of vigilant monitoring and follow-up in breast cancer survivors, ensuring that any emerging issues are promptly addressed. Through this review, it was aimed to provide a concise yet comprehensive overview of the hematological challenges encountered in breast cancer management, emphasizing the need for a multidisciplinary approach to patient care.

19.2 Acute Hematological Complications

19.2.1 Hematological Paraneoplastic Syndromes

Paraneoplastic syndromes are a group of disorders that occur in patients with cancer, which are not directly related to the physical effects of the primary tumor or its metastases. These syndromes are caused by the immune system's response to the cancer or by substances produced by the tumor [4]. In the context of breast cancer, paraneoplastic syndromes can manifest through various hematological complications. Among these, hematologic paraneoplastic syndromes such as eosinophilia, granulocytosis, pure red cell aplasia, and thrombocytosis are noteworthy. These conditions are often asymptomatic and are

F. D. Köseoğlu (✉)
Department of Internal Medicine, Hematology Clinic, Cigli Training and Research Hospital, Izmir Bakırcay University, Izmir, Turkey

Y. Bakar, A. Tuğral (eds.), *Managing Side Effects of Breast Cancer Treatment*,
https://doi.org/10.1007/978-3-031-75480-7_19

usually detected after the diagnosis of cancer. They are more frequently associated with advanced stages of the disease [5, 6]. Their presence can provide valuable clues to the underlying malignancy and its progression. Interestingly, managing these paraneoplastic syndromes often does not require specific treatment. Instead, they generally improve with the treatment of the underlying cancer.

19.2.1.1 Eosinophilia

Eosinophilia in cancer patients represents a distinctive scenario from clonal eosinophilia, stemming from factors such as interleukin-3 (IL-3), interleukin-5 (IL-5), and granulocyte-macrophage colony-stimulating factor (GM-CSF) secreted by the tumor [5, 6]. This condition is commonly observed in hematological malignancies like lymphoma but can also appear in other types of cancer such as lung, gastrointestinal system, and gynecological malignancies [4]. Unlike primary eosinophilia, which may cause end-organ damage, cancer-related eosinophilia typically does not lead to such complications and is often asymptomatic. However, it can sometimes produce symptoms similar to asthma.

In the context of breast cancer, eosinophilia takes on additional significance due to the influence of sex hormones on immune responses [7]. The interaction between estrogen and progesterone and their receptors in breast tissue can contribute to tumor-associated tissue eosinophilia, which is not uncommon in breast cancer. While the presence of eosinophilia does not show a clear correlation with survival outcomes in breast cancer contrary to tumor-infiltrating lymphocytes, nevertheless, it provides insight into the complex interplay between the tumor microenvironment and the immune system [8]. The prognostic significance of blood eosinophil count has been highlighted in some studies, suggesting its potential value as a biomarker at diagnosis and relapse [9, 10]. The management of eosinophilia in cancer patients usually does not require specific treatment for the eosinophilia itself, as it often returns to normal with antineoplastic therapy targeting the underlying cancer [4]. This underscores the reactive nature of eosinophilia to the tumor environment rather than an independent disease process.

19.2.1.2 Granulocytosis

Granulocytosis is a condition that can occur in association with various types of tumors, including solid tumors, where it is present in about 15% of cases [4]. It has been frequently reported in cancers of the lung, gastrointestinal tract, brain, breast, and kidney. In breast cancer, granulocytosis is among the commonly noted hematological abnormalities. The underlying cause of this condition is often attributed to colony-stimulating factors synthesized by the tumor, which promote the proliferation of granulocytes [11–13].

Recent studies have shed light on the role of tumor-infiltrating neutrophils in creating a conducive microenvironment for tumor development [14, 15]. These neutrophils can release extracellular traps that not only support tumor growth but also facilitate the establishment of metastatic sites. Moreover, circulating neutrophils have been found to bind circulating tumor cells, assisting them in adhering to the vascular wall—a process that potentially enhances metastasis [16, 17]. This interaction underscores the importance of carefully examining granulocytosis in cancer patients, as it may not only reflect the presence of cancer but also contribute to its progression.

When diagnosing granulocytosis, it is crucial to consider differential diagnoses, including leukemias, to ensure accurate patient management. However, in the context of cancer, specific treatment for granulocytosis is often not administered. Instead, the focus is on the antineoplastic treatment of the underlying cancer, which can subsequently reduce granulocyte levels. It is noteworthy that, unless mature neutrophil counts rise significantly, leukostasis is unlikely to occur, negating the need for leukapheresis [4].

19.2.1.3 Pure Red Cell Aplasia

Pure red cell aplasia (PRCA) is a rare hematologic disorder characterized by a selective decrease in red blood cell production, with normal white cell and platelet counts. Among malignancies, thymoma is the most commonly associated with PRCA due to the presence of autoreactive T-cell clones that inhibit red blood cell formation [18, 19]. However, PRCA has also been reported in association with other malignancies such as leukemia, lymphoma, and myeloma, indicating a broader relevance across different types of cancer [20, 21].

In the context of breast cancer, there are documented cases where PRCA has been observed. For instance, a study by Slater et al. described a situation where a patient required frequent transfusions in the early stages of breast cancer but showed normalization of hematologic parameters following antineoplastic therapy [22]. Similarly, Harris and colleagues reported a case where short-term corticosteroid treatment combined with antineoplastic therapy led to remission. These instances highlight PRCA as a paraneoplastic syndrome that, while rare in breast cancer, can significantly impact patient management [23].

The treatment of PRCA in the setting of breast cancer, as these cases suggest, often involves addressing the primary malignancy along with early management of complications following international guidelines [24–26]. The efficacy of antineoplastic therapy in resolving PRCA indicates that the hematologic disorder is closely linked to the activity of the underlying cancer. Therefore, comprehensive management that includes both the specific treatment of PRCA (when necessary, such as corticosteroids) and primary cancer therapy is crucial for optimal clinical outcomes.

19.2.1.4 Thrombocytosis

Thrombocytosis is a common finding in various cancers and is often induced by the production of cytokines, notably interleukin-6 (IL-6), by the tumor or the tumor microenvironment. This condition is a part of the systemic response to inflammation and can be seen as a reflection of the inflammatory processes associated with cancer.

While the general frequency of thrombocytosis in breast cancer is not reported as particularly high, it has been shown to occur more frequently in specific types of cancer, such as inflammatory breast cancer [27, 28]. This subtype of breast cancer is characterized by rapid progression, greater local symptoms, and a higher propensity for metastasis, which may contribute to the observed increase in platelet counts.

Several studies have indicated that thrombocytosis can serve as a poor prognostic indicator in breast cancer [29–31]. Elevated platelet counts may contribute to a prothrombotic state, enhancing the potential for cancer cell dissemination and metastasis. Platelets can protect circulating tumor cells from immune surveillance and facilitate their adhesion to the endothelium, promoting metastatic spread. Additionally, the growth factors and cytokines released by platelets can support tumor growth and angiogenesis.

Given its association with poorer outcomes, thrombocytosis in breast cancer patients necessitates careful evaluation and management. It may also prompt more aggressive monitoring for metastasis and consideration of therapeutic strategies that address both the primary tumor and the associated inflammatory and thrombotic processes.

19.2.2 Treatment-Related Hematological Toxicities

19.2.2.1 Selective Estrogen Receptor Modulators (SERMs) (Tamoxifen)

Tamoxifen is a commonly used endocrine therapy for women with hormone receptor-positive metastatic breast cancer and is also recommended as an adjuvant therapy for the early stages of the disease. This medication works by blocking estrogen receptors in breast cancer cells, effectively slowing or halting tumor growth. Tamoxifen has been shown to decrease the risk of breast cancer recurrence and improve survival rates. It is widely considered one of the most important treatments for breast cancer and is used extensively worldwide [32].

While tamoxifen is generally safe, there have been rare reports of tamoxifen-related hematological toxicity that can have negative effects on blood and blood-forming tissues, potentially leading to venous thromboembolism and pulmonary embolism. According to one analysis, the incidence of venous thromboembolism due to tamoxifen use in breast cancer patients was 3.5%. Studies like ATLAS and aTTom have shown that the risk of pulmonary embolism increases with a longer duration of tamoxifen use. If a hematological complication develops, it is recommended to interrupt tamoxifen treatment and initiate antithrombotic therapies in accordance with appropriate venous thromboembolism or pulmonary embolism guidelines [33].

19.2.2.2 Aromatase Inhibitors (AIs) (Anastrazole, Letrozole, Examestane)

AIs are medications that target and inhibit aromatase, a key factor in estrogen biosynthesis. These inhibitors come in two types: nonsteroidal (such as anastrozole and letrozole) and steroidal (like exemestane). AIs are used to treat estrogen and/or progesterone-positive breast cancer in the adjuvant, neoadjuvant, and metastatic settings and are considered the gold standard for postmenopausal women [34].

While thromboembolic events are a rare side effect of AIs, they can still occur. A meta-analysis of 30,023 patients with postmenopausal breast cancer found that the incidence of venous thrombosis associated with AIs use was 1.6%. However, this was significantly lower than the incidence of thrombosis associated with tamoxifen use. In cases of thrombosis due to AIs use, it is recommended to interrupt treatment and start appropriate antithrombotic treatment regimens, as venous thrombosis may lead to acute thromboembolic events that could be life-threatening [35].

19.2.2.3 Selective Estrogen Receptor Downregulators (SERDs) (Fulvestrant)

Fulvestrant is a highly effective estrogen receptor downregulator that acts as a pure anti-estrogen without any partial agonist effects. It effectively blocks the trophic actions of estrogens while being well tolerated with minimal systemic side effects. Research has shown that the risk of drug-related thromboembolic events and anemia are similar to that of anastrozole (3.5% vs. 4%, $p = 0.68$; 4% vs. 9%, $p > 0.05$, respectively) [36, 37]. However, caution should be taken when administering the drug to patients with bleeding diatheses or on anticoagulants, as it is given by intramuscular injection [38]. To date, no other hematological side effects have been reported from the use of fulvestrant.

19.2.2.4 Monoclonal Antibodies (mAb) (Trastuzumab/Pertuzumab/Pembrolizumab/Sacituzumab)

Trastuzumab was a groundbreaking humanized mAb that targeted HER2 and achieved incredible success in treating breast cancer. By binding to the extracellular domain of HER2, it was able to inhibit intracellular HER2 signaling pathways, prevent cell cycle arrest, and facilitate antibody-dependent cell-mediated cytotoxicity. As a result, trastuzumab quickly became the go-to treatment for patients with HER2+ breast cancer, revolutionizing the way we approach this disease. Despite its efficacy, however, many patients eventually develop therapeutic resistance and experience relapse. To address this issue, a second humanized anti-HER2 mAb called pertuzumab was developed. Unlike trastuzumab, pertuzumab targets extracellular domain-II of HER2, preventing its heterodimerization with HER1, HER3, and HER4, which in turn blocks downstream tumor signaling [39].

The Phase II studies of trastuzumab revealed thrombocytopenia as the most commonly reported grade 3 or 4 laboratory abnormality and associated with dose-limited hematological toxicity. This condition can be observed as early as 1 day after treatment, with platelet counts reaching their lowest point by day eight and recovering by day 18 for most patients. Thrombocytopenia persisted and could sometimes worsen with repeated dosing, but it was not typically linked to significant bleeding events [40]. Studies have shown that trastuzumab treatment can cause transient thrombocytopenia, with up to 10.7% of patients experiencing grade ≥3 thrombocytopenia. Although no major hemorrhagic events were reported, it is clear that trastuzumab affects the microtubule cytoskeleton of both megakaryocytes and platelets. These findings suggest that thrombocytopenia linked to trastuzumab can be well-tolerated, but it is important to monitor patients closely [41–43].

Neutropenia is a significant hematological side effect that has been observed with pertuzumab treatment. While neutropenia and febrile neutropenia are typically associated with chemotherapy, studies have suggested that pertuzumab use alone may also increase the risk of neutropenia. According to findings from the CLEOPATRA trial, adverse events (AEs) of all grades were reported to be at least 5% more frequent in the pertuzumab group compared to the placebo group. Additionally, febrile neutropenia was observed to be 2% higher in the pertuzumab group. Notably, in the Asian population subset, a significant number of neutropenia and febrile neutropenia events were observed during treatment with docetaxel. However, the incidence of neutropenia decreased significantly after discontinuing docetaxel, and there were no reports of febrile neutropenia among patients. Therefore, it is important to monitor neutrophil counts closely during pertuzumab treatment to ensure timely management of any potential complications [44].

Pembrolizumab is a preferred humanized monoclonal IgG4 kappa anti-PD1 monoclonal antibody utilized for treating breast cancer. Its binding to PD1 does not activate complement or interact with Fc receptors, resulting in a lack of cytotoxic activity. Though non-serious anemia and leukopenia have been linked to pembrolizumab treatment [45].

19.2.2.5 CDK4/6 Inhibitors

In breast cancer, CDK4/6 inhibitors, including palbociclib, ribociclib, and abemaciclib, have emerged as key agents in the treatment of hormone receptor-positive, HER2-negative advanced breast cancer. However, these agents are associated with a spectrum of hematological toxicities that must be recognized and managed to ensure patient safety while maximizing therapeutic efficacy.

The most commonly reported hematological AEs of these inhibitors across studies are neutropenia, leukopenia, and thrombocytopenia. Specifically, neutropenia has been observed in a significant proportion of patients (any grade 74–87%; grade 3–4 26–66%), followed by leukopenia (any grade 32–39%; grade 3–4 20–25%) and thrombocytopenia (any grade 15%; grade 3–4 1.4%). Notably, while neutropenia is a common adverse event, the incidence of febrile neutropenia remains extremely low (0–1.5%), indicating that the risk of infection, while a concern, is not as prevalent as would be expected given the higher rates of neutropenia [46–52].

Management of these toxicities includes close monitoring and appropriate dose adjustments. All patients receiving CDK4/6 inhibitors should have a complete blood count (CBC) at baseline and mid-cycle to closely monitor blood cell counts. For grade 1–2 neutropenia, dose modification is not required and treatment can continue without interruption. For grade 3 neutropenia, a waiting period of 1 week is recommended in the absence of infection or febrile neutropenia. If the neutropenia improves to grade 2 or less, treatment may be resumed at the same dose. However, in the presence of infection or febrile neutropenia, or if neutropenia reaches grade 4, treatment should be interrupted until recovery to grade 2 or less, at which time a dose reduction is recommended [50–52].

Treatment of thrombocytopenia follows a similar principle, withholding treatment for grade 3 (<50,000 to 25,000/mm^3) and grade 4 (<25,000 mm^3) thrombocytopenia until recovery to 50,000/mm^3 and then restarting at a reduced dose. If thrombocytopenia recurs or recovery takes longer than 2 weeks, further dose reductions are warranted. Management of anemia also requires withholding treatment for grade 3 (hemoglobin <8.0 g/dL) and grade 4 (life-threatening; urgent intervention indicated) anemia until improvement to grade 2 (hemoglobin <10.0–8.0 g/dL) or better, followed by dose reduction [50–52]. Packed red cell transfusions may be considered according to institutional protocols.

19.2.2.6 PARP Inhibitors

In the treatment of breast cancer, poly(ADP-ribose) polymerase inhibitors, commonly referred to as PARP inhibitors (PARPi), have emerged as an important therapeutic option, particularly in certain subgroups [53]. These drugs have demonstrated survival benefits in numerous efficacy analyses, both as monotherapy and in combination with other treatments [54, 55]. However, despite their efficacy, safety analyses show consistent concerns regarding hematological toxicities, which are among the most common AEs associated with PARPi treatment. Hematological toxicities, particularly grade 3 and 4 toxicities, have been frequently cited as the most common AEs experienced by patients undergoing PARPi therapy. In clinical observations, the five most common AEs of any grade associated with PARP inhibitors were nausea (64.00%), neutropenia (60.30%), thrombocytopenia (59.20%), anemia (59.17%), and fatigue (51.70%). When considering more severe grade ≥3 AEs, the most common were neutropenia (47.03%), thrombocytopenia (30.32%), anemia (27.56%), leukopenia (14.78%), and fatigue (5.13%) [56]. Specifically, in metastatic breast cancer, hematological AEs accounted for 25% and 75% of all Grade 3–4 AEs for olaparib and talazoparib, respectively, compared to 31% and 41% for physician's choice of chemotherapy [57].

The LUCY trial, a pivotal study evaluating olaparib, is providing important insights into the treatment duration, efficacy, and safety profile of the therapy [58]. Participants in this study received a median total treatment duration of 8.0 months, ranging from 0.2 to 43.3 months. AEs were common and were reported in 85.1% of participants. The majority of AEs observed in the LUCY trial were mild (grade 1 or 2), with nausea, anemia, asthenia, fatigue, and vomiting being the most commonly reported. However, more serious AEs (grade 3+) were reported in 17.6% of participants, mainly consisting of anemia and neutropenia. The discontinuation rate for olaparib due to AEs was 4.3%. Of note, no toxic deaths were reported in the study. Further analysis of olaparib-related AEs through data mining of the U.S. FDA Adverse Event Reporting System is consistent with the results of the clinical trial and cohort study and identified anemia, thrombocytopenia, nausea, and decreased appetite were the most common AEs with a median onset of 61 days after treatment initiation [59].

A retrospective study focused on patient-related risk factors for the development of anemia during olaparib treatment shed light on the incidence and predictors of this condition [60]. With a 32.7% incidence of grade 3+ anemia and a 61.1% incidence of grade 1+ anemia in patients with advanced breast or ovarian cancer, the study highlighted significant associations between low baseline red blood cell count, hematocrit, hemoglobin, and BRCA1/2 mutation with the development of severe anemia. Conversely, higher baseline levels of these blood components were associated with mild anemia, underscoring the importance of the baseline health status of patients in predicting treatment-emergent anemia.

Although these hematological toxicities are significant, they are often managed with dose reductions and rarely require discontinuation, resulting in a relatively low incidence of treatment discontinuation [58]. Nevertheless, these AEs can lead to a decrease in patient quality of life and generate additional costs [61].

19.2.2.7 Chemotherapy

Breast cancer can be treated using a range of chemotherapeutic options. However, some of these options, such as drugs belonging to the anthracycline group, cyclophosphamide, taxanes, 5-fluorouracil, capecitabine, and gemcitabine, are known to have hematologic side effects. This means that they can impact the formation and functions of blood cells, leading to a range of symptoms and complications.

Doxorubicin, a derivative of anthracycline, is a type of chemotherapy agent that can cause several systemic side effects. One of the most concerning effects is bone marrow aplasia, which can lead to microbial infections, delayed healing, and bleeding gums. The main dose-limiting side effect is myelosuppression, which often causes leukopenia, neutropenia, thrombocytopenia, and anemia. The severity of these effects depends on the drug dosage and the bone marrow's regenerative capacity. Typically, myelosuppression reaches its lowest point during the second week of treatment [62].

Cyclophosphamide is classified as an alkylating agent within the oxazaphosporines group. The most common hematotoxic effect is bone marrow suppression associated with cyclophosphamide. Neutropenia, which is typically dose-dependent, is the most frequently observed outcome. Although severe neutropenia is rare in patients receiving low-dose cyclophosphamide, close monitoring is recommended. Thrombocytopenia, leukopenia, and anemia are typical consequences of high-dose cyclophosphamide administration. Patients with normal bone marrow reserve will experience rapid hematological recovery within 2–3 weeks, regardless of the dose of cyclophosphamide [63].

The way in which docetaxel destroys cells is by interfering with microtubule function, which is crucial for cell survival. In addition to this, it also obstructs the antiapoptotic gene Bcl2 and prompts the expression of p27, a chemical that inhibits the cell cycle. The most common dose-limiting side effect associated with docetaxel is myelosuppression, which can lead to neutropenia. However, the most severe manifestation of myelosuppression is febrile neutropenia, which is a critical clinical concern. Febrile neutropenia is a life-threatening condition that may necessitate a reduction in dosage or postponement of planned treatments. Patients who develop febrile neutropenia must be hospitalized due to their higher risk of severe infection. If not managed properly, this clinical situation can result in significant morbidity and mortality [64]. It is recommended to consider primary prophylaxis with G-CSF from the first cycle of therapy if the risk of toxicity is estimated to be 20% or higher, depending on factors such as the patient's characteristics, disease, and treatment regimen. This approach can help reduce the chances of developing neutropenia, especially when an equally effective regimen that does not require growth factor supplementation is not available [65]. To aid in early recognition of febrile neutropenia, a pre-chemotherapy complete blood count should be conducted or more frequent monitoring should be performed based on clinical risk status.

5-FU and 5-fluoro-20-deoxyuridine (FdUrd) are types of chemotherapy agents used to treat various solid tumors. These drugs primarily affect rapidly dividing tissues and can cause toxicity in the body. Myelosuppression is more common when bolus 5-FU is given weekly or with a loading schedule. Granulocytopenia is usually more severe than thrombocytopenia. Anemia can also occur and may require regular blood transfusions during chronic treatment. The effect of erythropoietin on 5-FU-associated anemia is uncertain. A study evaluating long-term treatment with 5-FU combined with cisplatin and leucovorin found evidence of megaloblastic anemia [66].

19.2.2.8 GnRH Agonists (Goserelin, Leuprolide)

Goserelin, an analog of the luteinizing hormone-releasing hormone, effectively inhibits the production of ovarian estrogen in women who are in a pre-or perimenopausal state. In the treatment of hormone-sensitive breast cancer, goserelin has proven to be effective when used alone or in combination with endocrine therapies or chemotherapy. Goserelin is known for its high tolerability, with the primary side effects being associated with ovarian suppression. Unlike chemotherapy, this suppression is potentially reversible. There have been no significant reports of hematotoxicity associated with its use so far [67].

The potential negative effects of leuprolide are mainly due to changes in sex hormone levels experienced during treatment. Unlike estrogens, leuprolide is seldom associated with thromboembolic side effects [68].

19.2.2.9 Treatments Related to Bone Structure (Denosumab, Zoledronic Acid)

Breast cancer often metastasizes to the bone, making it a crucial target for effective therapy. Denosumab, a fully human monoclonal antibody that targets receptor activators of nuclear factor kappa-B ligand (RANKL), has been developed specifically for bone therapy. Overall, denosumab has been well tolerated and its side effects are comparable to those of zoledronic acid [69].

Importantly, studies have not found any hematotoxicity related to denosumab that would negatively impact patient treatment or quality of life [70].

Although there are no specific hematological side effects reported with zoledronic acid, it is known that it may cause a typical systemic acute phase response (AFR) after intravenous administration. After administering zoledronic acid intravenously, the AFR reaches its peak expression between 28 and 36 h and then gradually diminishes within 2–3 days, even with ongoing treatment. The AFR resulting from bisphosphonate usage is caused by the activation of gamma-delta T cells and macrophages, which release proinflammatory cytokines such as IL-6 and tumor necrosis factor α. Fortunately, this AFR is typically benign and self-limiting and can be managed with antipyretics [71].

19.2.3 Thrombotic Events

Malignant diseases are often accompanied by a multitude of complications, and one such complication is thromboembolism. This condition can manifest in various forms, including pulmonary thromboembolism, arterial or venous thrombosis, disseminated intravascular coagulation, nonbacterial thrombotic endocarditis, and migratory thrombophlebitis. These conditions can cause significant harm to the affected individual and require prompt medical attention. Numerous studies have been conducted to examine the relationship between breast malignancies and thrombotic events. According to these studies, the incidence of thrombotic events in patients with breast malignancies is estimated to be approximately 5% [72]. The development of a prothrombotic state in cancer is complex and reflects the interaction of several factors, including activation of fibrinolytic and coagulation systems, cellular mechanisms, and endothelial disruption. Individuals with breast cancer may experience thrombotic events, which are a type of blood clotting disorder. Various factors, including chemotherapy, hormonal therapy, surgery, or central venous catheter, can contribute to this condition. Additionally, nonspecific factors like hemodynamic impairment, abnormal protein metabolism, necrosis, and the formation of acute phase reactants may also play a role in thrombosis activation among this patient group. While the incidence of thrombotic events in breast malignancies is relatively lower than in other solid tumors, it is a potential complication that should not be overlooked and should be monitored closely. In particular, deep vein thrombosis is a common complication in breast cancer cases and should be kept in mind during treatment and management [73].

There are several factors that could potentially indicate a higher risk for thrombotic events in individuals with breast cancer. These include being over the age of 75 (with a hazard ratio of 2.0 compared to those under 45), having a body mass index (BMI) over 25 kg/m^2 (with a hazard ratio 2.92 and a 95% CI of 1.71–5.82), and having three or more comorbidities (with a hazard ratio of 2.9 compared to having none). Additionally, postmenopausal women have a significantly higher risk of VTE during chemotherapy (with a hazard ratio of 2.01 and a 95% CI of 1.09–3.70), as do women who have had a previous mastectomy (with a hazard ratio of 3.57 and a 95% CI of 1.88–6.79) [74]. In addition, the stage of cancer itself is a significant predictor, with a 2-year cumulative incidence hazard ratio of 2.1 for regional breast cancer and 6.3 for metastatic breast cancer, as demonstrated in the California Cancer Registry Study. The British-linked databases study found that the rate of thrombotic events was 6.8 per 1000 person-years for those with local disease, compared to 18.2 per 1000 person-years for those with metastatic breast cancer [75, 76]. Before and after chemotherapy, women who developed VTE consistently showed elevated levels of fibrinogen, D-dimers, TF, and VEGF, according to findings on early hemostatic changes in women receiving chemotherapy [77].

There are two strategies to be considered in the management of breast cancer-related thrombotic events. These are thromboprophylaxis and thrombosis therapy. There exist two primary methods of perioperative thromboprophylaxis: mechanical calf stimulation, which includes compression stockings, venous foot pumps, and compression devices, and pharmacological protection, which includes low molecular weight heparin, unfractionated heparin, and oral anticoagulants. It is noteworthy to mention that pharmacological thromboprophylaxis in breast cancer patients significantly escalates the likelihood of postoperative hematoma and bleeding when compared to mechanical thromboprophylaxis (18% versus 7%). Therefore, mechanical perioperative thromboprophylaxis is generally recommended [78]. It is generally not advised to administer systemic thromboprophylaxis to all patients who are undergoing cytotoxic or hormonal therapy. However, those who have undergone mastectomy and are postmenopausal with a BMI greater than 25 kg/m^2, preexisting coagulation disorders, congenital thrombophilia (such as FV Leiden), a past history of VTE, presence of a long-term central venous catheter, or a combination of these conditions are typically recommended to undergo thromboprophylaxis during chemotherapy [74]. While warfarin, unfractionated heparin, and low-molecular-weight heparin have traditionally been used to treat cancer-associated thrombosis, the advent of direct oral anticoagulants (DOACs) has made treatment and monitoring easier without the need for injection. The American Society of Hematology guidelines now recommend DOACs for the management of breast cancer-related thrombosis. DOACs have been shown to effectively reduce the risk of recurrent thrombosis, and in cases of breast cancer-associated thrombosis, these drugs carry the lowest risk of bleeding compared to other malignancies [79].

19.3 Chronic Hematological Complications

The association between the treatment of breast cancer and the development of secondary cancers has been extensively documented. Cytotoxic regimens in breast cancer especially certain alkylating agents (e.g., melphalan), platinum compounds (e.g., cisplatin), and topoisomerase II inhibitors (e.g., etoposide) heighten the likelihood of developing secondary cancer [80]. Different alkylating agents using in patients with cancer, like cyclophosphamide, pose lower risks compared to others. Conversely, certain drug classes, such as fluoropyrimidines like fluorouracil, do not show any evident association with these risks [81–83]. While there is an established association between radiotherapy and therapy-related myelodysplastic syndrome/acute myeloid leukemia (tMDS/AML), the precise extent of this risk remains uncertain and requires further investigation [84].

Myeloid neoplasms like AML and myelodysplastic syndrome (MDS) may arise as enduring hematological consequences of chemotherapy and radiation treatment in patients with breast cancer [80, 85–87]. Additionally, earlier investigations relying on hospital datasets have documented cases of treatment-induced lymphocytic leukemia and lymphomas [88–91]. Therapy-related acute myeloid leukemia (t-AML) linked to alkylating agents typically emerges 5–7 years post-chemotherapy exposure, often preceded by MDS. Conversely, t-AML tied to topoisomerase II agents tends to manifest with a shorter latency period (under 5 years) and is linked to 11q23 translocation. t-AML carries a grim prognosis, especially in patients with adverse cytogenetic profiles [92]. The incidence rates of therapy-related acute myeloid leukemia (t-AML) and/or MDS post-breast cancer have been documented in various clinical trials and extensive database analyses, ranging from 0.6% to 1.8% [85, 93, 94]. In individuals aged 65 years and older higher rates of patients experienced the development of AML/MDS. Although this figure implies a significantly higher risk among older patients [93].

While numerous clinical trials and observational studies have noted a higher risk of MDS and acute myeloid leukemia after conventional chemotherapies, recent targeted therapies and their potential for developing hematological malignancies remain to be explored.

19.4 Conclusion

Breast cancer represents the predominant form of cancer worldwide, impacting nations at varying levels of development. The necessity for vigilant monitoring of breast cancer and its associated hematological complications is paramount. Acute hematological complications can precipitate severe outcomes. The inherent risks of chemotherapy, encompass both immediate and enduring complications. As a result, routine health monitoring for individuals with breast cancer should include evaluations of hematological profiles throughout every stage of treatment. Healthcare professionals must maintain a vigilant stance regarding potential hematological complications throughout the course of cancer therapy.

References

1. El Masri J, Phadke S. Breast cancer epidemiology and contemporary breast cancer care: a review of the literature and clinical applications. Clin Obstet Gynecol. 2022;65(3):461–81.
2. Terry MB, Colditz GA. Epidemiology and risk factors for breast cancer: 21st century advances, gaps to address through interdisciplinary science. Cold Spring Harb Perspect Med. 2023;13(9):a041317.
3. Katsura C, Ogunmwonyi I, Kankam HK, Saha S. Breast cancer: presentation, investigation and management. Br J Hosp Med. 2022;83(2):1–7.
4. Pelosof LC, Gerber DE. Paraneoplastic syndromes: an approach to diagnosis and treatment. Mayo Clin Proc. 2010;85(9):838–54.
5. Anagnostopoulos GK, Sakorafas GH, Kostopoulos P, Margantinis G, Tsiakos S, Terpos E, et al. Disseminated colon cancer with severe peripheral blood eosinophilia and elevated serum levels of interleukine-2, interleukine-3, interleukine-5, and GM-CSF. J Surg Oncol. 2005;89(4):273–5.
6. Sonoda Y, Arai N, Ogawa M. Humoral regulation of eosinophilopoiesis in vitro: analysis of the targets of interleukin-3, granulocyte/macrophage colony-stimulating factor (GM-CSF), and interleukin-5. Leukemia. 1989;3(1):14–8.
7. Artham S, Chang C-Y, McDonnell DP. Eosinophilia in cancer and its regulation by sex hormones. Trends Endocrinol Metab. 2023;34(1):5–20.
8. Chouliaras K, Tokumaru Y, Asaoka M, Oshi M, Attwood KM, Yoshida K, et al. Prevalence and clinical relevance of tumor-associated tissue eosinophilia (TATE) in breast cancer. Surgery. 2021;169(5):1234–9.
9. Onesti CE, Josse C, Boulet D, Thiry J, Beaumecker B, Bours V, et al. Blood eosinophilic relative count is prognostic for breast cancer and associated with the presence of a tumor at diagnosis and at time of relapse. Onco Targets Ther. 2020;9(1):1761176.
10. Ghebeh H, Elshenawy MA, AlSayed AD, Al-Tweigeri T. Peripheral blood eosinophil count is associated with response to chemoimmunotherapy in metastatic triple-negative breast cancer. Immunotherapy. 2022;14(4):189–99.
11. Inoue T, Minohata J, Tanaka M, Tabuchi T, Morimoto H, Tatsumi Y, et al. A case of granulocyte-colony stimulating factor producing breast cancer that caused rapid progression. Gan To Kagaku Ryoho. 2017;44(12):1257–9.
12. Suzuki K, Ota D, Nishi T, Mori M, Kato T, Takeuchi M, et al. A case of granulocyte-colony stimulating factor-producing spindle cell carcinoma of the breast. Clin Breast Cancer. 2015;15(4):e213–7.
13. Casbon AJ, Reynaud D, Park C, Khuc E, Gan DD, Schepers K, et al. Invasive breast cancer reprograms early myeloid differentiation in the bone marrow to generate immunosuppressive neutrophils. Proc Natl Acad Sci USA. 2015;112(6):E566–75.
14. Zheng C, Xu X, Wu M, Xue L, Zhu J, Xia H, et al. Neutrophils in triple-negative breast cancer: an underestimated player with increasingly recognized importance. Breast Cancer Res. 2023;25(1):88.
15. Kaplan RN, Riba RD, Zacharoulis S, Bramley AH, Vincent L, Costa C, et al. VEGFR1-positive haematopoietic bone marrow progenitors initiate the premetastatic niche. Nature. 2005;438(7069):820–7.
16. Szczerba BM, Castro-Giner F, Vetter M, Krol I, Gkountela S, Landin J, et al. Neutrophils escort circulating tumour cells to enable cell cycle progression. Nature. 2019;566(7745):553–7.
17. Pereira-Veiga T, Schneegans S, Pantel K, Wikman H. Circulating tumor cell-blood cell crosstalk: biology and clinical relevance. Cell Rep. 2022;40(9):111298.
18. Moriyama S, Yano M, Haneda H, Okuda K, Kawano O, Sakane T, et al. Pure red cell aplasia associated with thymoma: a report of a single-center experience. J Thorac Dis. 2018;10(8):5066–72.
19. Mizobuchi S, Yamashiro T, Nonami Y, Yamamoto A, Kume M, Nakaya H, et al. Pure red cell aplasia and myasthenia gravis with thymoma: a case report and review of the literature. Jpn J Clin Oncol. 1998;28(11):696–701.
20. Shen M. A case report of T-LGL leukemia-associated pure red cell aplasia harboring STAT3, TNFAIP3, and KMT2D mutation. Transl Cancer Res. 2023;12(4):1054–9.
21. Korde N, Loeliger K, Simakova O, Zingone A, Childs R, Landgren O, et al. Pure red cell aplasia associated with plasma cell myeloma: does monoclonal protein inhibit erythropoiesis? Blood. 2010;116(21):642.
22. Slater LM, Schlutz MJ, Armentrout SA. Remission of pure red cell aplasia associated with nonthymic malignancy. Cancer. 1979;44(5):1879–81.

23. Harris SJ, Seah J-AA, Barnett F, White SC. Inflammatory breast cancer and secondary Pure Red Cell Aplasia. Acta Oncol. 2011;50(5):727–8.
24. Lobbes H, Lega J-C, Le Guenno G, Ruivard M, Mainbourg S. Treatment strategy for acquired pure red cell aplasia: a systematic review and meta-analysis. Blood Adv. 2023;7(21):6451–65.
25. Gurnari C, Maciejewski JP. How I manage acquired pure red cell aplasia in adults. Blood. 2021;137(15):2001–9.
26. Means RT. Pure red cell aplasia. Blood. 2016;128(21):2504–9.
27. Rajkumar A, Szallasi A. Paraneoplastic thrombocytosis in breast cancer. Anticancer Res. 2013;33(10):4545–6.
28. Harano K, Kogawa T, Wu J, Yuan Y, Cohen EN, Lim B, et al. Thrombocytosis as a prognostic factor in inflammatory breast cancer. Breast Cancer Res Treat. 2017;166(3):819–32.
29. Garmi N, Nasrallah S, Baram Y, Katz A, Koren A, First M, et al. Platelets and breast cancer. Isr Med Assoc J. 2020;22(10):613–7.
30. Stravodimou A, Voutsadakis IA. Pretreatment thrombocytosis as a prognostic factor in metastatic breast cancer. Int J Breast Cancer. 2013;2013:289563.
31. Taucher S, Salat A, Gnant M, Kwasny W, Mlineritsch B, Menzel RC, et al. Impact of pretreatment thrombocytosis on survival in primary breast cancer. Thromb Haemost. 2003;89(6):1098–106.
32. Briest S, Stearns V. Tamoxifen metabolism and its effect on endocrine treatment of breast cancer. Clin Adv Hematol Oncol. 2009;7(3):185–92.
33. Condorelli R, Vaz-Luis I. Managing side effects in adjuvant endocrine therapy for breast cancer. Expert Rev Anticancer Ther. 2018;18(11):1101–12.
34. Mukherjee AG, Wanjari UR, Nagarajan D, et al. Letrozole: pharmacology, toxicity and potential therapeutic effects. Life Sci. 2022;310:121074.
35. Amir E, Seruga B, Niraula S, Carlsson L, Ocana A. Toxicity of adjuvant endocrine therapy in postmenopausal breast cancer patients: a systematic review and meta-analysis. J Natl Cancer Inst. 2011;103(17):1299–309.
36. Robertson JF, Osborne CK, Howell A, Jones SE, Mauriac L, Ellis M, et al. Fulvestrant versus anastrozole for the treatment of advanced breast carcinoma in postmenopausal women: a prospective combined analysis of two multicenter trials. Cancer. 2003;98(2):229–38.
37. Robertson JFR, Bondarenko IM, Trishkina E, Dvorkin M, Panasci L, Manikhas A, et al. Fulvestrant 500 mg versus anastrozole 1 mg for hormone receptor-positive advanced breast cancer (FALCON): an international, randomised, double-blind, phase 3 trial. Lancet. 2016;388(10063):2997–3005.
38. Cheung KL, Robertson JF. Fulvestrant. Expert Opin Investig Drugs. 2002;11(2):303–8.
39. Swain SM, Shastry M, Hamilton E. Targeting HER2-positive breast cancer: advances and future directions. Nat Rev Drug Discov. 2023;22(2):101–26.
40. Dirix LY, Rutten A, Huget P, Dirix M. Trastuzumab emtansine in breast cancer. Expert Opin Biol Ther. 2013;13(4):607–14.
41. Krop IE, Beeram M, Modi S, Jones SF, Holden SN, Yu W, et al. Phase I study of trastuzumab-DM1, an HER2 antibody-drug conjugate, given every 3 weeks to patients with HER2-positive metastatic breast cancer. J Clin Oncol. 2010;28(16):2698–704.
42. Hurvitz SA, Dirix L, Kocsis J, Bianchi GV, Lu J, Vinholes J, et al. Phase II randomized study of trastuzumab emtansine versus trastuzumab plus docetaxel in patients with human epidermal growth factor receptor 2-positive metastatic breast cancer. J Clin Oncol. 2013;31(9):1157–63.
43. Bender BC, Schaedeli-Stark F, Koch R, Joshi A, Chu YW, Rugo H, et al. A population pharmacokinetic/pharmacodynamic model of thrombocytopenia characterizing the effect of trastuzumab emtansine (T-DM1) on platelet counts in patients with HER2-positive metastatic breast cancer. Cancer Chemother Pharmacol. 2012;70(4):591–601.
44. Gao J, Swain SM. Pertuzumab for the treatment of breast cancer: a safety review. Expert Opin Drug Saf. 2016;15(6):853–63.
45. Kwok G, Yau TC, Chiu JW, Tse E, Kwong YL. Pembrolizumab (Keytruda). Hum Vaccin Immunother. 2016;12(11):2777–89.
46. Verma S, Bartlett CH, Schnell P, DeMichele AM, Loi S, Ro J, et al. Palbociclib in combination with fulvestrant in women with hormone receptor-positive/HER2-negative advanced metastatic breast cancer: detailed safety analysis from a multicenter, randomized, placebo-controlled, phase III study (PALOMA-3). Oncologist. 2016;21(10):1165–75.
47. Sledge GW, Toi M, Neven P, Sohn J, Inoue K, Pivot X, et al. MONARCH 2: Abemaciclib in combination with fulvestrant in women with HR+/HER2- advanced breast cancer who had progressed while receiving endocrine therapy. J Clin Oncol. 2017;35(25):2875–84.
48. Finn RS, Crown JP, Ettl J, Schmidt M, Bondarenko IM, Lang I, et al. Efficacy and safety of palbociclib in combination with letrozole as first-line treatment of ER-positive, HER2-negative, advanced breast cancer: expanded analyses of subgroups from the randomized pivotal trial PALOMA-1/TRIO-18. Breast Cancer Res. 2016;18(1):67.
49. O'Shaughnessy J, Petrakova K, Sonke GS, Conte P, Arteaga CL, Cameron DA, et al. Ribociclib plus letrozole versus letrozole alone in patients with de novo HR+, HER2- advanced breast cancer in the randomized MONALEESA-2 trial. Breast Cancer Res Treat. 2018;168(1):127–34.
50. Spring LM, Zangardi ML, Moy B, Bardia A. Clinical management of potential toxicities and drug interactions related to cyclin-dependent kinase 4/6 inhibitors in breast cancer: practical considerations and recommendations. Oncologist. 2017;22(9):1039–48.
51. Thill M, Schmidt M. Management of adverse events during cyclin-dependent kinase 4/6 (CDK4/6)

inhibitor-based treatment in breast cancer. Ther Adv Med Oncol. 2018;10:1758835918793326.
52. Rugo HS, Huober J, Garcia-Saenz JA, Masuda N, Sohn JH, Andre VAM, et al. Management of abemaciclib-associated adverse events in patients with hormone receptor-positive, human epidermal growth factor receptor 2-negative advanced breast cancer: safety analysis of MONARCH 2 and MONARCH 3. Oncologist. 2021;26(1):e53–65.
53. Cortesi L, Rugo HS, Jackisch C. An overview of PARP inhibitors for the treatment of breast cancer. Target Oncol. 2021;16(3):255–82.
54. Zhang M, Yu X, Wang J, Li Y, Cao L. Efficacy and safety of poly (ADP-ribose) polymerase inhibitors therapy for BRCA-mutated breast cancer: a systematic review and meta-analysis. J Cancer Res Ther. 2021;17(7):1672–8.
55. Beas-Lozano EL, Verduzco-Aguirre HC, Gonzalez-Salazar R, Chavarri-Guerra Y. Real-world data in patients with BRCA mutated breast cancer treated with poly (ADP-ribose) polymerase inhibitors. Ecancermedicalscience. 2023;17:1633.
56. Liu X, Wu K, Zheng D, Luo C, Fan Y, Zhong X, et al. Efficacy and safety of PARP inhibitors in advanced or metastatic triple-negative breast cancer: a systematic review and meta-analysis. Front Oncol. 2021;11:742139.
57. Miglietta F, Cinquini M, Dieci MV, Cortesi L, Criscitiello C, Montemurro F, et al. PARP-inhibitors for BRCA1/2-related advanced HER2-negative breast cancer: a meta-analysis and GRADE recommendations by the Italian Association of Medical Oncology. Breast. 2022;66:293–304.
58. Balmana J, Fasching PA, Couch FJ, Delaloge S, Labidi-Galy I, O'Shaughnessy J, et al. Clinical effectiveness and safety of olaparib in BRCA-mutated, HER2-negative metastatic breast cancer in a real-world setting: final analysis of LUCY. Breast Cancer Res Treat. 2024;204(2):237–48.
59. Shu Y, He X, Liu Y, Wu P, Zhang Q. A real-world disproportionality analysis of olaparib: data mining of the public version of FDA adverse event reporting system. Clin Epidemiol. 2022;14:789–802.
60. Tashiro R, Kawazoe H, Mamishin K, Seto K, Udagawa R, Saito Y, et al. Patient-associated risk factors for severe anemia in patients with advanced ovarian or breast cancer receiving olaparib monotherapy: a multicenter retrospective study. Front Oncol. 2022;12:898150.
61. Fan L, Zhang Y, Maguire P, Muston D, Monberg M, Earla JR, et al. Cost comparison of adverse event management among breast and ovarian cancer patients treated with poly (ADP-ribose) polymerase inhibitors: analysis based on phase 3 clinical trials. J Mark Access Health Policy. 2022;10(1):2078474.
62. Carvalho C, Santos RX, Cardoso S, Correia S, Oliveira PJ, Santos MS, et al. Doxorubicin: the good, the bad and the ugly effect. Curr Med Chem. 2009;16(25):3267–85.
63. Emadi A, Jones RJ, Brodsky RA. Cyclophosphamide and cancer: golden anniversary. Nat Rev Clin Oncol. 2009;6(11):638–47.
64. Baker J, Ajani J, Scotte F, Winther D, Martin M, Aapro MS, et al. Docetaxel-related side effects and their management. Eur J Oncol Nurs. 2009;13(1):49–59.
65. Smith TJ, Khatcheressian J, Lyman GH, Ozer H, Armitage JO, Balducci L, et al. 2006 update of recommendations for the use of white blood cell growth factors: an evidence-based clinical practice guideline. J Clin Oncol. 2006;24(19):3187–205.
66. Grem JL. 5-Fluorouracil: forty-plus and still ticking. A review of its preclinical and clinical development. Investig New Drugs. 2000;18(4):299–313.
67. Mitchell H. Goserelin ('Zoladex')–offering patients more choice in early breast cancer. Eur J Oncol Nurs. 2004;8(Suppl 2):S95–S103.
68. Chrisp P, Sorkin EM. Leuprorelin. A review of its pharmacology and therapeutic use in prostatic disorders. Drugs Aging. 1991;1(6):487–509.
69. Drooger JC, van der Padt A, Sleijfer S, Jager A. Denosumab in breast cancer treatment. Eur J Pharmacol. 2013;717(1-3):12–9.
70. Li HS, Lei SY, Li JL, Xing PY, Hao XZ, Xu F, et al. Efficacy and safety of concomitant immunotherapy and denosumab in patients with advanced non-small cell lung cancer carrying bone metastases: a retrospective chart review. Front Immunol. 2022;13:908436.
71. Papapetrou PD. Bisphosphonate-associated adverse events. Hormones. 2009;8(2):96–110.
72. Caine GJ, Stonelake PS, Rea D, Lip GY. Coagulopathic complications in breast cancer. Cancer. 2003;98(8):1578–86.
73. Kirwan CC, Blower EL. Contemporary breast cancer treatment-associated thrombosis. Thromb Res. 2022;213(Suppl 1):S8–S15.
74. Kyriazi V. Breast cancer as an acquired thrombophilic state. J Breast Cancer. 2012;15(2):148–56.
75. Walker AJ, West J, Card TR, Crooks C, Kirwan CC, Grainge MJ. When are breast cancer patients at highest risk of venous thromboembolism? A cohort study using English health care data. Blood. 2016;127(7):849–57.
76. Chew HK, Wun T, Harvey DJ, Zhou H, White RH. Incidence of venous thromboembolism and the impact on survival in breast cancer patients. J Clin Oncol. 2007;25(1):70–6.
77. Kirwan CC, McDowell G, McCollum CN, Kumar S, Byrne GJ. Early changes in the haemostatic and procoagulant systems after chemotherapy for breast cancer. Br J Cancer. 2008;99(7):1000–6.
78. Andtbacka RH, Babiera G, Singletary SE, Hunt KK, Meric-Bernstam F, Feig BW, et al. Incidence and prevention of venous thromboembolism in patients undergoing breast cancer surgery and treated according to clinical pathways. Ann Surg. 2006;243(1):96–101.
79. Middeldorp S, Nieuwlaat R, Baumann Kreuziger L, Coppens M, Houghton D, James AH, et al. American Society of Hematology 2023 guidelines for manage-

ment of venous thromboembolism: thrombophilia testing. Blood Adv. 2023;7(22):7101–38.
80. Morton LM, Dores GM, Schonfeld SJ, Linet MS, Sigel BS, Lam CJK, et al. Association of chemotherapy for solid tumors with development of therapy-related myelodysplastic syndrome or acute myeloid leukemia in the modern era. JAMA Oncol. 2019;5(3):318–25.
81. McNerney ME, Godley LA, Le Beau MM. Therapy-related myeloid neoplasms: when genetics and environment collide. Nat Rev Cancer. 2017;17(9):513–27.
82. Travis LB, Holowaty EJ, Bergfeldt K, Lynch CF, Kohler BA, Wiklund T, et al. Risk of leukemia after platinum-based chemotherapy for ovarian cancer. N Engl J Med. 1999;340(5):351–7.
83. Greene MH, Harris EL, Gershenson DM, Malkasian GD Jr, Melton LJ 3rd, Dembo AJ, et al. Melphalan may be a more potent leukemogen than cyclophosphamide. Ann Intern Med. 1986;105(3):360–7.
84. Radivoyevitch T, Sachs RK, Gale RP, Molenaar RJ, Brenner DJ, Hill BT, et al. Defining AML and MDS second cancer risk dynamics after diagnoses of first cancers treated or not with radiation. Leukemia. 2016;30(2):285–94.
85. Wolff AC, Blackford AL, Visvanathan K, Rugo HS, Moy B, Goldstein LJ, et al. Risk of marrow neoplasms after adjuvant breast cancer therapy: the national comprehensive cancer network experience. J Clin Oncol. 2015;33(4):340–8.
86. Martin MG, Welch JS, Luo J, Ellis MJ, Graubert TA, Walter MJ. Therapy related acute myeloid leukemia in breast cancer survivors, a population-based study. Breast Cancer Res Treat. 2009;118(3):593–8.
87. Beadle G, Baade P, Fritschi L. Acute myeloid leukemia after breast cancer: a population-based comparison with hematological malignancies and other cancers. Ann Oncol. 2009;20(1):103–9.
88. Abdulwahab A, Sykes J, Kamel-Reid S, Chang H, Brandwein JM. Therapy-related acute lymphoblastic leukemia is more frequent than previously recognized and has a poor prognosis. Cancer. 2012;118(16):3962–7.
89. Aldoss I, Dagis A, Palmer J, Forman S, Pullarkat V. Therapy-related ALL: cytogenetic features and hematopoietic cell transplantation outcome. Bone Marrow Transplant. 2015;50(5):746–8.
90. Aldoss I, Stiller T, Tsai NC, Song JY, Cao T, Bandara NA, et al. Therapy-related acute lymphoblastic leukemia has distinct clinical and cytogenetic features compared to de novo acute lymphoblastic leukemia, but outcomes are comparable in transplanted patients. Haematologica. 2018;103(10):1662–8.
91. Krishnan B, Morgan GJ. Non-Hodgkin lymphoma secondary to cancer chemotherapy. Cancer Epidemiol Biomarkers Prev. 2007;16(3):377–80.
92. Schoch C, Kern W, Schnittger S, Hiddemann W, Haferlach T. Karyotype is an independent prognostic parameter in therapy-related acute myeloid leukemia (t-AML): an analysis of 93 patients with t-AML in comparison to 1091 patients with de novo AML. Leukemia. 2004;18(1):120–5.
93. Muss HB, Berry DA, Cirrincione C, Budman DR, Henderson IC, Citron ML, et al. Toxicity of older and younger patients treated with adjuvant chemotherapy for node-positive breast cancer: the Cancer and Leukemia Group B Experience. J Clin Oncol. 2007;25(24):3699–704.
94. Patt DA, Duan Z, Fang S, Hortobagyi GN, Giordano SH. Acute myeloid leukemia after adjuvant breast cancer therapy in older women: understanding risk. J Clin Oncol. 2007;25(25):3871–6.

20 Sexual Dysfunction in Breast Cancer: Managing of Unmet Need of an Important Aspect

Türkan Akbayrak and Gülbala Gülören

20.1 Introduction

The World Health Organization (WHO) defines sexual health as the ability to have pleasurable and safe sexual experiences free from violence, discrimination, and coercion as well as a positive and respectful attitude towards sexual function [1]. Sexual function includes sexual activity without pain or discomfort and sexual response with sexual desire, arousal, plateau, orgasm, and resolution without psychological difficulties [2]. Sexual response also involves physical and emotional changes that occur when a human engages in sexual activity [3].

As stated in the 5th edition of the American Psychiatric Association's (APA) classification system for mental disorders (The Diagnostic and Statistical Manual of Mental Disorders, DSM-V), a woman who has complaints for at least 6 months that cause difficulties in the desire, arousal, or orgasm phases of the sexual response cycle is diagnosed with sexual dysfunction [4]. In DSM-V, female sexual dysfunctions are examined under three headings: sexual interest/arousal disorder, orgasm disorder, and pain in the genitals-pelvis/penetration disorder [4]. WHO describes sexual dysfunction as a common health problem and recommends evaluation, treatment, and, research of this issue due to its negative effects on self-esteem, quality of life, and, sexual relationships [5].

There are many physiological, psychological, biological, and sociocultural factors that play a role in the development, persistence, or exacerbation of sexual dysfunction [6]. Cancer and its treatment are one of the factors that negatively affect sexual activity and the ability to continue healthy sexual function [7]. The sexuality of the women and their partner before the cancer diagnosis, their personalities, upbringing, religious values, culture, and past sexual experiences affect the severity of sexual dysfunction that the person may experience. In addition, the type of surgery, the protocol of the treatment, and the attitude of healthcare professionals can also influence sexual function [8]. Sexual dysfunction is observed in the majority of cancer patients, especially in gynecological and urological cancer patients [9]. It has been reported that 35–50% of cancer patients experience sexual dysfunction as a result of treatment [9]. Despite the high incidence of sexual dysfunction related to cancer treatment, sexual dysfunctions are not sufficiently discussed with patients for various reasons during medical care. However, in one study, cancer patients clearly stated that they would be pleased to receive information on sexual matters [10]. Time

T. Akbayrak
Faculty of Physical Therapy and Rehabilitation, Hacettepe University, Ankara, Turkey

G. Gülören (✉)
Faculty of Health Sciences, Department of Physiotherapy and Rehabilitation, Ordu University, Ordu, Turkey

Y. Bakar, A. Tuğral (eds.), *Managing Side Effects of Breast Cancer Treatment*,
https://doi.org/10.1007/978-3-031-75480-7_20

constraints, lack of training and resources, and religious beliefs are cited as the main barriers to the assessment of sexual function [11]. Educating all members of the medical oncology team, patients, and partners about sexual health is the most effective way to prevent sexual dysfunction after cancer diagnosis and treatment. This requires robust communication between oncology, psychology, psychiatry, urology, gynecology, and pelvic health physiotherapists, and other health professionals in the context of a multidisciplinary team approach [11].

20.2 Sexuality After Breast Cancer as an Unmet Need

Breast cancer accounts for 30% of new cancer diagnoses and the number of breast cancer cases surpassed lung cancer cases in 2020, reaching 2.26 million [12]. Taking into account advances in diagnosis and treatment, it has been reported that the survival rate in early stage breast cancer has reached 76–92% [13]. The current higher survival rates of breast cancer survivors (BCS) have brought the attention of healthcare professionals to the quality of life and sexual life of these women. Sexual problems are a common concern of BCS but are overlooked both in the clinic and in the literature [14]. However, sexuality, which is a sensitive issue, is often neglected in clinical practice. Recently, there has been a focus on strategies that can help patients return to normal life after primary treatment and achieve a better quality of life, including sexuality in BCS [15].

The quality of life of BCS is affected by various factors such as pain, fatigue, lymphedema, fear of recurrence, depression decreased attractiveness, impaired body image, self-esteem, and changes in the view of sexuality [16]. Sexual health, described as physical, mental, emotional, and social well-being, is one of the important parts of quality of life [17]. BCS face the complications of cancer treatment and the effects of treatment methods that can negatively impact their sexual health. A recent meta-analysis shows that sexual dysfunction is commonly reported in BCS, with a prevalence of 73% [15]. However, prevalence estimates vary widely, ranging from 27% to 93% [17–20].

20.2.1 Possible Effects of Breast Cancer Treatment on Sexual Function

Depending on the stage of the cancer, there are various treatment interventions that can have a negative impact on sexual function in many ways. The diagnosis of breast cancer itself can cause depression and helplessness that can reduce or even eliminate interest in sexuality or enjoyment of sexual activities [21]. For all women, the breast is associated with sexual identity and attractiveness. When the breast, which is strongly associated with sexuality, becomes the focal point of a life-threatening disease, it can cause negative emotions in the patient, such as insecurity and frustration [22]. In a study with a qualitative and quantitative design, seven main issues related to sexuality in women with breast cancer were described: decreased sexual frequency, menopausal symptoms, lack of sexual interest, impaired body image, negative effects on marital relationships, misconceptions about sexual function, and the need for professional counseling [23].

20.2.1.1 Breast Cancer Surgery and Sexual Dysfunction

The aim of breast cancer surgery is to completely remove the cancerous tissue within safe limits while preserving the nipple and the existing shape of the breast [16]. Mastectomy is applied for approximately 50% of patients for a variety of reasons, including advanced-stage diagnosis, tumor location, small breast size, and patient preference [16, 19]. Axillary lymph node dissection in conjunction with mastectomy can lead to loss of nipple sensitivity, distortion of breast shape, painful scarring, and lymphedema [24, 25]. For some patients, breast surgery is considered one of the most psychologically devastating treatments, negatively affecting self-esteem, physical attractiveness, femininity, partner relationships, and body image [16].

Surgery can have a direct physical impact on the ability to adequately engage in the various stages of the sexual response cycle (desire, arousal, and orgasm) [26]. Breast cancer surgery also has several indirect effects on sexual function. Uncertainty about whether the surgery will be successful, fear of the surgery itself, and loss of function after surgery can negatively affect sexual function. The loss of the erogenous zone, especially after breast amputation, negatively affects the ability to participate in sexual activities due to reduced sexual arousal [26, 27]. Women who undergo nipple-sparing mastectomy or skin-sparing mastectomy followed by breast reconstruction have been reported to have better psychosocial and sexual function [14]. Studies have reported a trend toward poorer sexual desire outcomes and more symptoms of depression after mastectomy without reconstruction [16, 26, 28]. Breast reconstruction after radical mastectomy can help preserve body image and increase patient self-confidence [28, 29]. Breast reconstruction has a positive effect on quality of life, especially in young patients who are concerned about the deterioration of body image [16]. Although satisfaction with breast appearance increases after reconstruction in BCS, they complain of many changes, including loss of nipple sensation and changes in proprioceptive sensation [7].

20.2.1.2 Chemotherapy and Sexual Dysfunction

Chemotherapy is the standard treatment for many breast cancer patients. Chemotherapy causes significant changes in the body and can also lead to sexual problems [15]. In addition, chemotherapy causes a wide variety of symptoms such as skin changes, hair loss (i.e., alopecia), gastrointestinal symptoms, fatigue, weight imbalance, mucosal damage (i.e., oral mucositis), and bleeding disorders [3, 24]. Chemotherapy-induced early menopause can affect sexual desire and arousal, through direct and indirect effects on the genital area and vasomotor symptoms and sleep disorders, respectively [17]. In addition to breast loss due to mastectomy, various negative effects of cancer treatment, such as hair loss and weight loss due to chemotherapy, cause patients to feel less attractive and cause a decrease in self-confidence [15, 19]. Chemotherapy causes adverse menopausal symptoms such as lack of sexual interest, vaginal dryness, and pain during sexual intercourse, and ultimately leads to decreased frequency of sexual intercourse and decreased intensity of orgasm [30]. Biglia et al. [31] reported that the prevalence of hot flashes in patients receiving breast cancer treatment was highest in patients taking both chemotherapy and hormonal therapy, while vaginal dryness was more common in patients taking chemotherapy alone.

20.2.1.3 Radiotherapy and Sexual Dysfunction

Advances in early diagnosis, surgery, chemotherapy, and radiotherapy contribute to increased survival rates along with the increasing number of cancer survivors [32]. Radiotherapy causes serious problems such as painful dermatitis, burns, increased sensitivity of irradiated skin tissue, fatigue, and insomnia, and negatively affects sexual desire [32, 33]. The mucosa becomes sensitive within a few days after radiotherapy. Skin irritation, dryness, blistering, itching, and peeling may occur. The most common symptom in the early period after radiation is fatigue [33]. The key to the process of sexual dysfunction is thought to be the psychological exhaustion caused by the illness, which can last from diagnosis to the end of treatment [16]. Studies have shown that body image and sexual function are negatively affected after radiotherapy in women with breast cancer [18, 33].

Damage to the skin, the largest erogenous zone of our body, can have a negative effect on sexuality. The impaired appearance of the skin related radiotherapy affects attractiveness. Radiotherapy burns, hyperesthesia, and paresthesia can reduce sexual attraction and desire [34]. Senses of smell and taste can be lost due to radiotherapy or chemotherapy, and the smell of the skin may change due to radiotherapy burns. The smell of tissue decay after radiotherapy can be a reason to separate the bed [21, 34].

20.2.1.4 Hormone Replacement Therapy and Sexual Dysfunction

Most breast cancers are estrogen receptor (ER)-positive, with cancer cells growing in response to estrogen, while approximately 65% are progesterone receptor (PR)-positive, with cancer cells growing in response to progesterone. Antihormonal drugs block estrogen receptors in all tissues of the body, causing symptoms of estrogen withdrawal, which can cause vasomotor symptoms similarly to menopause such as anxiety, depressive mood, atrophy of the urogenital organs, and vaginal dryness, leading to loss of sexual desire, dyspareunia, and arousal disorders [24]. There are studies documenting a strong association between hormone therapy and the prevalence of hot flashes/night sweats and vaginal dryness [31, 35]. The decrease in estrogen level, which is a desired effect of hormone therapy, and the associated changes in serotonin and endorphin levels and thus body temperature, are the primary triggers of hot flash symptoms [35]. In one study, it was reported that hormone therapy has significant side effects on women's quality of life, especially in terms of loss of sexual desire, vaginal dryness, and genito-pelvic pain disorders [36].

Some chemotherapeutic drugs can cause peripheral neuropathy, causing loss of sensation, impaired genital sensation, pins, and needles numbness, and orgasmic problems. In addition, these drugs may affect motor and autonomic nerves, causing urinary and fecal incontinence (especially coital incontinence), and alopecia, all of which may cause women to fear sexual activity through the worsening of physical and body image [14, 37].

20.2.2 Contributing Factors Related to Sexual Dysfunction in Breast Cancer

Sexual function may be affected by medical conditions present in the patient, which can have negative effects on the sexual response cycle [14, 36]. For example, uncontrolled diabetes or neurovascular problems can affect pelvic blood supply and arousal. Cardiovascular diseases can impair sexual function due to vascular problems that can negatively affect sexuality. Moreover, metabolic syndrome and obesity may contribute to sexual problems [24]. Antidepressants and antihypertensive drugs can reduce libido, arousal, and orgasm [38]. Lymphedema, one of the most common complications after breast cancer surgery, is also a visual reminder of breast cancer and is difficult to conceal, negatively affecting body image [39, 40]. Upper extremity swelling and associated changes in appearance have a negative impact on individuals' sexual desire, perceptions of attractiveness, and ability to perform simple daily tasks such as looking in the mirror or buying clothes [24].

Negative effects of cancer treatment, such as amputation of breast tissue due to mastectomy and hair loss due to chemotherapy, undermine patients' identity as women, making them feel less attractive and leading to a loss of self-confidence [15]. Kowalczyk et al. [41], reported that the type of surgical method was the main factor affecting postoperative body image, especially breast defect, and scarring after radical surgery caused a decrease in patient's body image level. Most of the women made comments about their physical appearance after mastectomy such as "strange" and "I feel half of myself" [14, 42].

Body image is a concept used to describe how a person feels about their body [26]. A person's body image is formed through self-observation and observation of others' reactions to their body appearance [29]. It includes not only physical appearance but also one's psychological feelings about "breast integrity" and is recognized as an important determinant of sexual activity [43]. The results of a qualitative study showed that impaired body image in breast cancer survivors can result in higher sexual stress, affecting their intimate relationships and sexual functioning [15]. Because a woman's sexuality includes not only the ability to engage in sexual activity but also feelings about her own body and her ideas about body image and femininity [18]. According to Fang et al. [44], there is a relationship between body image and sexuality, and sexual problems are more common in people with poor body image. It is known that the loss of hair and breasts, which are considered symbols of femininity, causes deterioration of body image after chemotherapy, radiotherapy, and hormonal treatments in women with breast cancer [42]. Body image is impaired by amputation of the breast, hair loss, decreased physical function, weight gain, and lymphedema, and negatively affects sexual function [15].

20.3 Evaluation of Sexual Dysfunction in Women with Breast Cancer

Healthcare professionals should support patients in expressing sexual dysfunction since sexuality is a sensitive, repressed, and private subject and is particularly affected by stereotypes or traditional beliefs. Most health professionals responsible for cancer treatment are not sufficiently informed about the negative effects of cancer treatment on sexual health and are reluctant to discuss this issue with women [33]. To facilitate early detection and improve management strategies of sexual dysfunction, changes in sexual function should be included in the assessment and routine care both before surgery and at different stages during treatment in women with breast cancer [13].

20.3.1 Sexual History

Assessment of sexual disorders should begin with a detailed cancer history, obstetric and gynecologic history, treatment-related myalgias, fatigue, weight change, and sleep disturbance, as well as the presence of vasomotor symptoms, chemotherapy-related weight change, fatigue, and neuropathy [14, 36]. In addition, other medications with known adverse effects on sexual desire or sexual function should be noted. The patient's pelvic musculoskeletal symptoms and limiting factors during sexual activity should be identified. The patient's changing sexual response cycle parameters and pain before and after cancer should be questioned [14]. The American Cancer Society and the American Society of Clinical Oncology (ASCO) recommend regular assessment of sexual function in BCS in their jointly developed Breast Cancer Survivorship Care guidelines [45]. Health professionals can benefit from the questions in Table 20.1 when obtaining information about sexual health in patients with breast cancer:

Administering questionnaires can help assess sexual health problems before and after breast cancer treatment. The Female Sexual Function Index (FSFI) is commonly used in the field of sexual medicine and the assessment of female sexual function for cancer survivors [14, 17, 46]. This self-reported questionnaire is a 19-item assesses female sexual response in 6 different areas (sexual desire, sexual arousal, satisfaction, vaginal lubrication, orgasm, and pain) [47]. Also, the Sexual Activity Questionnaire, the Sexual Adjustment and Body Image Scale, and the Body Image After Breast Cancer Questionnaire are widely used in the evaluation of body image [24, 32].

20.3.2 Physical Examination

Physical examination should include body language, respiratory pattern, and thorax, and musculoskeletal structures extending from the lower thoracic spine to the buttocks and thighs [48]. Patients with sexual dysfunction often have

Table 20.1 Examples of questions when taking sexual history

"Are you sexually active nowadays?" If you are not active, "Does this cause you distress?"
"Most women have sexual difficulties after breast cancer treatment. Have you had any sexual problems since the treatment?"
"What are the factors that negatively affect your sexual activity due to surgery or cancer treatment?"
"Have you experienced any changes in your sexual desire or interest?" If yes, "Does this bother you?"
"Do you have problems with vaginal lubrication during/after intercourse?" "Do you have any other concerns or problems with your sexual health?"

anxious body language, kyphotic posture, superficial and frequent breathing patterns, decreased thoracic and diaphragmatic movements, decreased pelvic joint mobility, and shortened hip and pelvic muscles [6, 49]. In musculoskeletal assessment, it is important to identify common painful and tender points on the body. Evaluation of connective tissue mobility in the thoracolumbar fascia and abdominal, gluteal, and thigh regions, light touch to painful areas or to areas where pain may be reflected from the pelvis, and rolling tests are extremely important in sexual pain disorders [50].

The aim of the pelvic examination is to objectively evaluate the anatomy of the pelvic floor and pelvic organs and to correlate symptoms of sexual dysfunction with anatomical findings. The clinical presentation of external genitalia, mons pubis, perineum, external anal sphincter, redness in the peri-anal area, raised areas, scar tissue, discharge, skin sores, or edema should be recorded. Mucosal integrity, vulvovaginal atrophy, and the presence of birth-related scarring or incision due to episiotomy should be noted. During the observational assessment, voluntary contraction of the pelvic floor muscles should be requested from the patient, and contraction of the bulbospongiosus, bulbocavernosus, ischiocavernosus, and transverse perineal muscles should be evaluated [48].

Digital palpation, either vaginal or anal palpation, is performed to assess the size and position of pelvic floor muscle tissue. It is normal for patients to be anxious during digital palpation. With adequate time to relax, most patients can relax and tolerate a supine pelvic examination. During the digital examination of the normal pelvic floor, the patient will feel a sensation of pressure. However, the examination should not cause pain [14]. Pelvic floor muscle strength can be evaluated by vaginal palpation according to the modified Oxford grading system including the contraction force felt around the physiotherapist's finger, whether there is a palpable elevation of the finger, and the number and duration of contractions. In patients with dyspareunia that prevents penetration, to subjectively test pelvic floor muscle strength, the physiotherapist places the palmar side of the hand on the perineum and tests the inward collapse of the hand during contraction (Fig. 20.1). Assessing the ability to contract and relax the pelvic floor muscles is especially important in problems such as dyspareunia and vaginismus that may be caused by menopause [51]. Evaluation of the contraction/relaxation ability of the pelvic floor muscles can be performed by vaginal pressure measurements, pelvic floor dynamometer, or electromyography (EMG) in addition to digital palpation [52].

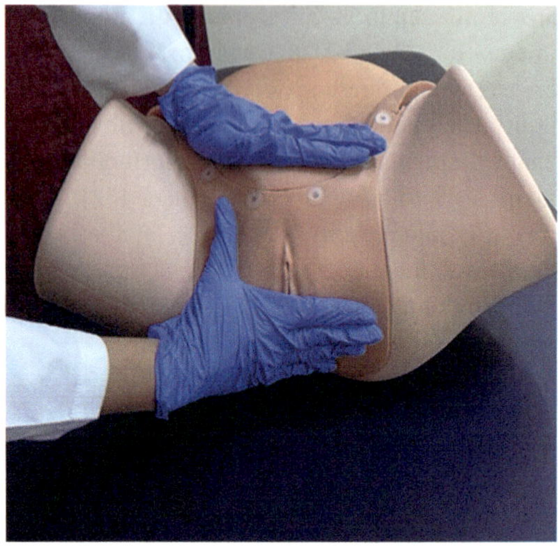

Fig. 20.1 Perineal palpation

20.4 Treatment Approaches of Sexual Dysfunction in Women with Breast Cancer

As women's sexual function is complex, a multidisciplinary team approach is required to manage sexual disorders [29]. Healthcare professionals should provide information about the negative effects of cancer treatment on body image, sexual health, and, fertility, and they should be open about discussing sexuality with patients with breast cancer [15]. In order to develop effective relationship in young couples, the patient's partner should also be involved in the treatment [14].

Since sexual problems are multifactorial in BCS, the first step in treatment is to identify potential factors causing sexual dysfunction [14]. Subsequent treatment approaches include vaginal lubricants and moisturizers for vaginal dryness and dyspareunia, hormone therapy, behavioral therapy, and pelvic floor physiotherapy [28, 50].

20.4.1 Behavior Therapy and Sex Therapy

A clinical practice guideline published by the ASCO recommends receiving psychosocial and sexual counseling to improve sexual function in women with cancer [50]. Psychotherapy, especially cognitive behavioral therapy (CBT), focuses on promoting changes in sexual perceptions and thoughts in women. Cognitive restructuring replaces misperceptions of sexual functioning with more functional, positive cognitions. Furthermore, psychosexual counseling focuses on discussing sexual issues and providing patients with information on psychological and sexuality [22].

20.4.2 Body Image Improvement Approaches

It is known that the decrease in the quality of sexual function of patients after breast cancer surgery is related to the decrease in body image level, and this issue should be included in routine health education, especially for younger breast cancer patients [29]. The deterioration of body image during and after cancer treatment can lead to decreased self-esteem, anxiety, and sadness. To minimize the impact of these changes and for women to accept a new body image, the following strategies may be recommended [22]:

- Use psychoeducational therapy to help improve symptoms and body image.
- Advise patients to wear make-up to make them feel better.
- Advise patients to increase their level of physical activity to improve body image and psychological well-being.

Regular aerobic exercise has been shown to improve body image, cardiorespiratory fitness, body composition, immune function, and fatigue in BCS. Supervised weight training for BCS has also been shown to improve body image, self-esteem, and upper and lower body strength [53]. The functionality of the body and its ability to perform tasks is important for the concept of body image. Therefore, it is hypothesized that an increase in muscle strength may improve body image perception as it will increase functional ability. Therefore, exercise interventions aiming to increase physical strength may improve perceptions of body image in BCS [24]. Weight training twice a week has been reported to positively affect self-perceptions of body image, physical strength, sexuality, personal relationships, and social functioning. It has also been observed that women do exercise to feel good about themselves, not to enhance the attractiveness of a particular body part [24].

20.4.3 Pelvic Floor Rehabilitation

Physiotherapy approaches are considered the first step for pelvic floor dysfunctions in BCS because they are noninvasive and can be combined with other therapies to relieve symptoms and improve function. Physiotherapists usually create a multimodal treatment plan that includes manual therapy techniques, relaxation training, posture training, pain management, pelvic floor rehabilitation, and the use of physical therapy modalities as well as patient education [48].

Pelvic health physiotherapists recognize that sexual dysfunction is a complex problem. At the beginning of treatment, the physiotherapist should carefully assess all possible factors that may contribute to sexual dysfunctions. Pelvic health physiotherapists address patients' sexual function both functionally and psychosocially [6, 48].

20.4.3.1 Patient Education

Patients with pelvic floor dysfunction after breast cancer treatment often have no idea what is causing the sexual changes they are experiencing. Patient education plays an important role in this situation. Patient education includes anatomy and biomechanics of the pelvic floor and genito-pelvic region and pathophysiology of sexual disorders on models or figures (Fig. 20.2). During the pelvic examination, a mirror may be given to increase awareness of the vulvar anatomy of the patient. In addition, patient education includes education on lifestyle changes such as relaxation techniques, stress management, mindfulness, healthy habits for the bowel and bladder, behavioral changes, and sleep hygiene, which are essential for the treatment of factors that may contribute to sexual dysfunction [6].

20.4.3.2 Pelvic Floor Rehabilitation

In pelvic floor rehabilitation, an exercise prescription is prepared according to the condition of the pelvic floor muscles in sexual dysfunction (hypotonic or hypertonic that is appropriate for the patient and consisting of strengthening, relaxation, coordination, and endurance exercises) [52]. Women who experience pain or discomfort during sexual intercourse after breast cancer treatment experience decreased pelvic floor muscle length, excessive increase in muscle tone, weakness in muscle strength, and myofascial pain. Hypoestrogenic state, anxiety, depression, distorted body image, and feelings of exhaustion are among the factors contributing to sexual dysfunction. The goals of pelvic floor rehabilitation are to improve relaxation, and elongation of the genito-pelvic area and to improve the awareness of the pelvic floor muscles. Most commonly, pelvic floor rehabilitation includes treatment approaches such as exercise training for pelvic floor muscles, digital feedback, visual feedback (use of mirrors), and superficial electromyography [6].

20.4.3.3 Dilator Training

Vaginal entry exercises with a finger or dilator are often used to treat women who experience pain during penetration. The aim of these exercises is to stretch the pelvic floor muscles and reduce tissue tension with dilators of various sizes. Dilators can help eliminate myofascial trigger points and lengthen shortened muscle fibers. A person with pain at the vaginal opening can also passively stretch the tissues at the opening

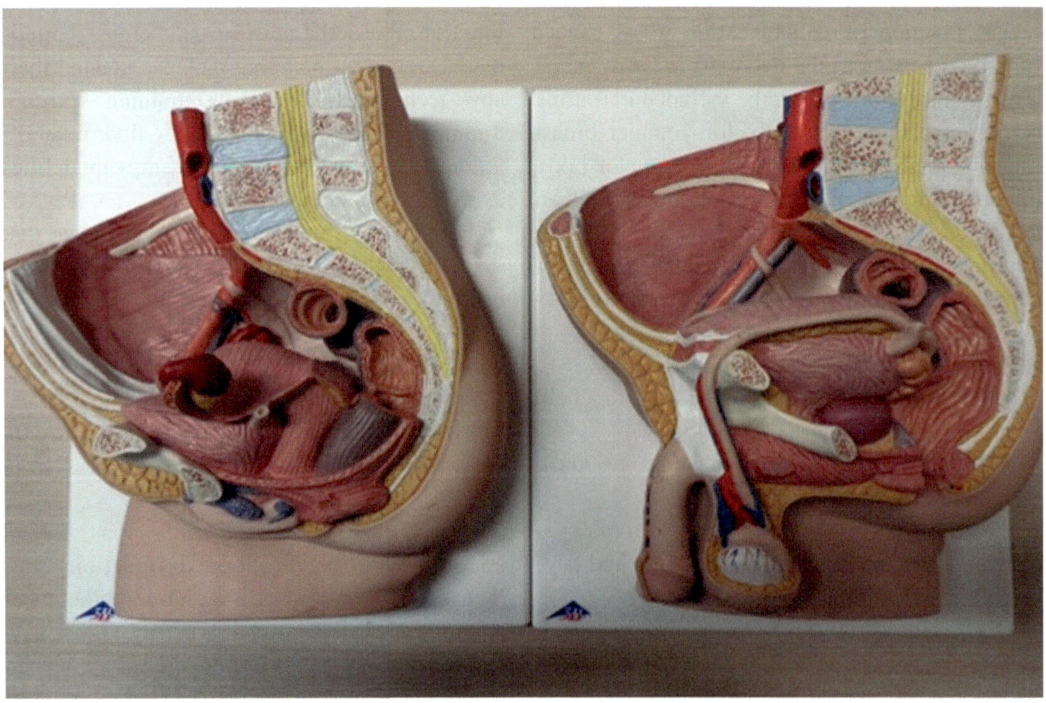

Fig. 20.2 Pelvic models for patient education

with a dilator while applying gradual exposure to an increasing dilator size [14].

20.4.4 Pharmacological Treatment

Pharmacological treatment of sexual dysfunction after breast cancer surgery includes hormonal therapies such as vaginal testosterone designed to reduce the effects of the hypoestrogenic state caused by cancer treatment. In addition, estradiol vaginal ring therapy is also often used to improve the sexual desire and arousal [28]. Topical treatments include moisturizers and lubricants. Specifically perceived discomfort during penetration and vaginal dryness can be improved with topical treatments such as polycarbophil-based moisturizer, compound testosterone cream, pH-balanced lactic acid gel, and vaginal estrogens [3].

20.5 Conclusion

Breast cancer surgery, chemotherapy, radiotherapy, and hormonal treatments cause sexual dysfunction, often remaining a chronic problem for BCS. If treatment of sexual dysfunction is neglected, it can lead to reduced quality of life, depression, and interpersonal conflicts. Treatment of sexual dysfunction in BCS is a multidisciplinary approach that integrates behavioral and sexual therapy, pelvic floor physiotherapy, and pharmacological approaches. Early detection of sexual dysfunction, provision of sexual health counseling as a routine healthcare service to patients and their partners, and prompt holistic treatment will lead to improved sexual health and quality of life.

References

1. WHO. Consolidated guideline on sexual and reproductive health and rights of women living with HIV. Geneva: World Health Organization; 2017.
2. LeVay S, Valente SM, Watson NV. Human sexuality. Cham: Springer; 2006.
3. Gandhi C, Butler E, Pesek S, Kwait R, Edmonson D, Raker C, et al. Sexual dysfunction in breast cancer survivors. Am J Clin Dermatol. 2019;42(6):500–6.
4. Zhang D, Association AP. The diagnostic and statistical manual of mental disorders (DSM-V). Beijing: Peking University Press; 2015.
5. Howes BH, Watson DI, Xu C, Fosh B, Canepa M, Dean NR. Quality of life following total mastectomy with and without reconstruction versus breast-conserving surgery for breast cancer: a case-controlled cohort study. JPRAS. 2016;69(9):1184–91.
6. Bo K, Berghmans B, Morkved S, Van Kampen M. Evidence-based physical therapy for the pelvic floor: bridging science and clinical practice. Amsterdam: Elsevier; 2014.
7. Bober SL, Varela VS. Sexuality in adult cancer survivors: challenges and intervention. J Clin Oncol. 2012;30(30):3712–9.
8. Barton-Burke M, Gustason CJ. Sexuality in women with cancer. Nurs Clin N Am. 2007;42(4):531–54.
9. Katz A, Agrawal LS, Sirohi B. Sexuality after cancer as an unmet need: addressing disparities, achieving equality. ASCO Educ Book. 2022;42:11–7.
10. Shaffer KM, Kennedy E, Glazer JV, Clayton AH, Cohn W, Reese JB, et al. Including partners in discussions of sexual side effects from breast cancer: a qualitative study of survivors, partners, and providers. Support Care Cancer. 2022;30(6):4935–44.
11. Ospina-Serrano AV, Maximiano C, Cantos B, Torrente M, Mendez M, Sanchez JC, et al. Sexual dysfunction in patients with cancer, a challenge in oncology practice: results of the CLARIFY project. Clin Transl Oncol. 2023;26(5):1147–56.
12. Ferlay J, Colombet M, Soerjomataram I, Parkin DM, Piñeros M, Znaor A, Bray F. Cancer statistics for the year 2020: an overview. IJC. 2021;149(4):778–89.
13. Jing L, Zhang C, Li W, Jin F, Wang A. Incidence and severity of sexual dysfunction among women with breast cancer: a meta-analysis based on female sexual function index. Support Care Cancer. 2019;27:1171–80.
14. Vegunta S, Kuhle CL, Vencill JA, Lucas PH, Mussallem DM. Sexual health after a breast cancer diagnosis: addressing a forgotten aspect of survivorship. J Clin Med. 2022;11(22):6723.
15. Yan R, Wang J, Yu J. Association of sexual attitudes with sexual dysfunction and sexual distress among Chinese breast cancer survivors: a cross-sectional study. Support Care Cancer. 2023;31(3):154.
16. Archangelo SCV, Sabino Neto M, Veiga DF, Garcia EB, Ferreira LM. Sexuality, depression and body image after breast reconstruction. Clinics. 2019;74:e883.
17. Smedsland SK, Vandraas KF, Bøhn SK, Dahl AA, Kiserud CE, Brekke M, et al. Sexual activity and functioning in long-term breast cancer survivors; exploring associated factors in a nationwide survey. Breast Cancer Res Treat. 2022;193(1):139–49.

18. Yılmaz M, Gürler H. The relationship between body image and sexuality after surgical treatment in women with breast cancer. JERN. 2020;17(3):244–51.
19. Maleki M, Mardani A, Ghafourifard M, Vaismoradi M. Changes and challenges in sexual life experienced by the husbands of women with breast cancer: a qualitative study. BMC Womens Health. 2022;22(1):326.
20. Che Ya SN, Muhamad R, Mohd Zain N, Zakaria R, Ishak A, Hassan II, et al. Coping strategies for sexual problems and sexual dysfunction amongst Malay women with breast cancer. A qualitative study. Sex Med. 2021;9(3):100336.
21. Reisman Y, Gianotten WL. Cancer, intimacy and sexuality: a practical approach. Cham: Springer; 2017.
22. Miaja M, Platas A, Martinez-Cannon BA. Psychological impact of alterations in sexuality, fertility, and body image in young breast cancer patients and their partners. Rev Investig Clin. 2017;69(4):204–9.
23. Wang F, Chen F, Huo X, Xu R, Wu L, Wang J, Lu C. A neglected issue on sexual well-being following breast cancer diagnosis and treatment among Chinese women. PLoS One. 2013;8(9):e74473.
24. Speck RM, Gross CR, Hormes JM, Ahmed RL, Lytle LA, Hwang W-T, Schmitz KH. Changes in the body image and relationship scale following a one-year strength training trial for breast cancer survivors with or at risk for lymphedema. Breast Cancer Res Treat. 2010;121:421–30.
25. Baran E, Özçakar L, Özgül S, Aksoy S, Akbayrak T. Upper limb sensory evaluations and ultrasonographic skin measurements in breast cancer–related lymphedema receiving complex decongestive physiotherapy. Support Care Cancer. 2021;29:6545–53.
26. Vaziri S, Kashani FL. Sexuality after breast cancer: need for guideline. Iran J Cancer Prev. 2012;5(1):10.
27. Sadovsky R, Basson R, Krychman M, Morales AM, Schover L, Wang R, Incrocci L. Cancer and sexual problems. J Sex Med. 2010;7(1):349–73.
28. Luo F, Link M, Grabenhorst C, Lynn B. Low sexual desire in breast cancer survivors and patients: a review. Sex Med Rev. 2022;10(3):367–75.
29. Du H, Chen C, Yuan F, Hu A, Han J. Correlation analysis of body image level and female sexual dysfunction in young patients with postoperative breast cancer. J Cancer Res Ther. 2022;18(5):1360–71.
30. Qi A, Li Y, Sun H, Jiao H, Liu Y, Chen Y. Incidence and risk factors of sexual dysfunction in young breast cancer survivors. Ann Palliat Med. 2021;10(4):4428–34.
31. Biglia N, Peano E, Sgandurra P, Moggio G, Panuccio E, Migliardi M, et al. Low-dose vaginal estrogens or vaginal moisturizer in breast cancer survivors with urogenital atrophy: a preliminary study. Gynecol Endocrinol. 2010;26(6):404–12.
32. Guedes TSR, de Oliveira NPD, Holanda AM, Reis MA, da Silva CP, Silva BLR, et al. Body image of women submitted to breast cancer treatment. APJCP. 2018;19(6):1487.
33. Chang Y-C, Chang S-R, Chiu S-C. Sexual problems of patients with breast cancer after treatment: a systematic review. Cancer Nurs. 2019;42(5):418–25.
34. Gianotten WL. The various levels of impact. In: Cancer, intimacy and sexuality: a practical approach. Cham: Springer; 2017. p. 27–36.
35. Duijts SF, Stolk-Vos AC, Oldenburg HS, Van Beurden M, Aaronson NK. Characteristics of breast cancer patients who experience menopausal transition due to treatment. Climacteric. 2011;14(3):362–8.
36. Rodrigues-Machado N, Quintana MJ, Gómez-Gómez R, Bonfill-Cosp X. Sexual function in women with breast cancer: an evidence map of observational studies. Int J Environ Res Public Health. 2022;19(21):13976.
37. Farthmann J, Hanjalic-Beck A, Veit J, Rautenberg B, Stickeler E, Erbes T, et al. The impact of chemotherapy for breast cancer on sexual function and health-related quality of life. Support Care Cancer. 2016;24:2603–9.
38. Baumgart J, Nilsson K, Evers AS, Kallak TK, Poromaa IS. Sexual dysfunction in women on adjuvant endocrine therapy after breast cancer. Menopause. 2013;20(2):162–8.
39. Orhan C, Üzelpasaci E, Baran E, Nakip G, Özgül S, Aksoy S, Akbayrak T. The reliability and validity of the Turkish version of the lymphedema life impact scale in patients with breast cancer–related lymphedema. Cancer Nurs. 2020;43(5):375–83.
40. Byrne E, Gaffey J, Hayden L, Daly A, Gallagher P, Dunne S. Body image and cancer-related lymphoedema: a systematic review. Psychooncology. 2023;32(10):1528–38.
41. Kowalczyk R, Nowosielski K, Cedrych I, Krzystanek M, Glogowska I, Streb J, et al. Factors affecting sexual function and body image of early-stage breast cancer survivors in Poland: a short-term observation. Clin Breast Cancer. 2019;19(1):e30–9.
42. Parton CM, Ussher JM, Perz J. Women's construction of embodiment and the abject sexual body after cancer. Qual Health Res. 2016;26(4):490–503.
43. Dahlbäck C, Manjer J, Rehn M, Ringberg A. Determinants for patient satisfaction regarding aesthetic outcome and skin sensitivity after breast-conserving surgery. World J Surg Oncol. 2016;14:1–11.
44. Fang S-Y, Lin Y-C, Chen T-C, Lin C-Y. Impact of marital coping on the relationship between body image and sexuality among breast cancer survivors. Support Care Cancer. 2015;23:2551–9.
45. Runowicz CD, Leach CR, Henry NL, Henry KS, Mackey HT, Cowens-Alvarado RL, et al. American cancer society/American society of clinical oncology breast cancer survivorship care guideline. CA Cancer J Clin. 2016;66(1):43–73.
46. Nakip G, Gürşen C, Baran E, Üzelpasaci E, Çinar GN, Özgül S, et al. Psychometric properties of the Turkish version of the pregnancy sexual response inventory. Arch Gynecol Obstet. 2021;304:101–7.

47. Bartula I, Sherman KA. the female sexual functioning index (FSFI): evaluation of acceptability, reliability, and validity in women with breast cancer. Support Care Cancer. 2015;23:2633–41.
48. FitzGerald M, Kotarinos R. Rehabilitation of the short pelvic floor. I: background and patient evaluation. Int Urogynecol J Pelvic Floor Dysfunct. 2003;14:261–8.
49. da Conceição TMA, Da Roza T, dos Santos KM, da Luz SCT, da Luz CM. Pelvic floor muscles contraction and sexual function are associated with hormonal treatment in women after breast cancer? Man Ther Posturol Rehab J. 2017;15:4.
50. Seav SM, Dominick SA, Stepanyuk B, Gorman JR, Chingos DT, Ehren JL, et al. Management of sexual dysfunction in breast cancer survivors: a systematic review. Womens Midlife Health. 2015;1:1–27.
51. Long B, Bojko A. Cancer and genito-pelvic pain. In: Female sexual pain disorders: evaluation and management. Hoboken: Wiley; 2020. p. 349–58.
52. Orhan C, Akbayrak T, Özgül S, Baran E, Üzelpasaci E, Nakip G, et al. Effects of vaginal tampon training added to pelvic floor muscle training in women with stress urinary incontinence: randomized controlled trial. Int Urogynecol J. 2019;30:219–29.
53. Schmitz KH, Ahmed RL, Hannan PJ, Yee D. Safety and efficacy of weight training in recent breast cancer survivors to alter body composition, insulin, and insulin-like growth factor axis proteins. Cancer Epidemiol Biomarkers Prev. 2005;14(7):1672–80.

21 Cognitive Problems and Management in Breast Cancer

Yagmur Cam

Advances in early diagnosis and treatment of breast cancer (BC) have resulted in a significant increase in survival rates [1, 2]. Thanks to these developments, cancer has moved away from its identity as an incurable disease [3]. Nowadays, the issue that has gained importance in treatment success is the effect of late and long-term symptoms related to cancer and cancer treatment on the quality of life (QoL) [2]. One of the most common complaints of breast cancer survivors (BCS) during the diagnosis and treatment process is cognitive problems that significantly affect their functionality in daily life [4]. All cognitive problems seen after the cancer itself and cancer treatment are referred to as cancer-related cognitive impairment (CRCI).

CRCI causes significant long-term problems in a large percentage of BCS [5]. In a longitudinal study, CRCI was observed in approximately 30% of cancer patients before treatment, 75% during treatment, and 35% months or years after completion of treatment [6]. In BC, approximately 75% of women report CRCI [7, 8]. The cognitive domains most commonly affected in BC patients are attention, concentration, information processing speed, working memory, cognitive flexibility, executive function, learning, psychomotor ability, visual-spatial ability, language, multitasking, and word finding [9–11]. These cognitive problems are variable for each patient and can be mild or severe, temporary or permanent, stable or progressive [12].

Many BCS state that CRCI is the issue that they are most affected by after cancer treatment [7, 8]. CRCI may occur in BC patients due to the cancer itself or systemic cancer treatment. Also, CRCI symptoms can persist for years after patients' treatment ends [10]. From this perspective, CRCI can be described as a serious issue that can affect the social and professional lives of BCS in the long term [7, 8]. Therefore, understanding and evaluating the impact of CRCI on BCS' life and functionality and providing the necessary management has critical importance for their cognitive health [13].

21.1 Breast Cancer Itself is Sufficient to Cause Cognitive Impairment

Cancer patients face many symptoms such as depression, anxiety, stress, fear, and sleep disturbance after diagnosis. These symptoms can negatively affect cognitive functions such as memory, concentration, processing speed, and language [8, 14]. Psychological distress and fatigue caused by the cancer itself may cause a decrease in cognitive performance and impairment of the neuro-

Y. Cam (✉)
Department of Physiotherapy and Rehabilitation, Faculty of Health Sciences, Izmir Demokrasi University, Izmir, Turkey
e-mail: yagmur.cam@idu.edu.tr

Y. Bakar, A. Tuğral (eds.), *Managing Side Effects of Breast Cancer Treatment*,
https://doi.org/10.1007/978-3-031-75480-7_21

plasticity mechanism in BCS [15–17]. This decline in cognitive performance has been associated with cancer-related stress, similar to that observed in post-traumatic stress disorder [17].

21.1.1 Aging: The Natural End of Every Human Being

The aging factor, along with symptoms such as depression, fatigue, and sleep disturbance, also has a negative impact on CRCI in BCS [8, 11]. Average life expectancy has increased with improvements in health and the geriatric population has increased in the world. It is predicted that in the next 10 years, 75% of the cancer survivors in the United States will be individuals over 65 years old. The increase in cancer survival as a result of advanced and individualized treatment methods has brought an increase in the population of geriatric cancer survivors [18].

Along with the aging process, oxidative stress causes unrepairable damage to the DNA of central nervous system (CNS) neurons. This may partially explain cognitive problems in a healthy aging process [19]. In a study [20], more oxidative DNA damage and lower gray matter density were detected in BCS after 6 years of completion of chemotherapy treatment than in the healthy group, and it was concluded that there may be cognitive impairment due to unrepaired neuronal damage. This effect of chemotherapy caused a pathophysiological process similar to the normal aging process in the patient. From this perspective, when the pathophysiological process that develops with healthy aging, additional health problems, cancer itself, and the negative effects of cancer treatments come together, cancer survival in the geriatric population may cause serious problems in the long term, such as a decline in cognitive functions [8, 19] and QoL [18].

21.1.2 Genetic Factors: Inheritance from Ancestors

The most important identified genes associated with BC are BRCA1 and BRCA2. The BRCA1 gene is also thought to be associated with cognitive impairment. A study found that BRCA1 protein levels were reduced in the brains of people diagnosed with Alzheimer's disease and mice that developed a form of the disease [21].

In some patients, the blood–brain barrier may be genetically more permeable or there may be inadequacy in detoxification mechanisms. These genetic factors may affect neural repair capacity, the effectiveness of drugs used in cancer treatment, and neurotransmitter activity. It is thought that alteration in DNA repair mechanisms and neurotoxicity may predispose to both cancer and neurodegenerative conditions [22].

Regarding polymorphisms of genes involved in repair processes, there are some studies suggesting that polymorphic expression of both apolipoprotein E (ApoE) and catechol-o-methyltransferase (COMT) may increase the impairment of cognitive functions in cancer patients. Studies have found that the polymorphism of ApoE expression is closely related to retrospective and prospective memory deficits [23], and the processing speed of patients with ApoE4 is significantly slower [24]. It has been determined that BC patients with the ApoE genotype may have significant problems in the areas of executive function, attention, language function, memory, and visual learning [25].

21.2 Cognitive Impairments Hidden Behind Innocent-Looking Agents: The Reality of Chemotherapy in Breast Cancer

Although chemotherapy is lifesaving in cancer treatment, the incidence of cognitive problems in the short and long term after treatment varies between 20% and 70% [26, 27]. Both during and after chemotherapy, patients have difficulty concentrating and memory. They express this as a mental slowing and the inability to multitask as much as they could before the cancer diagnosis. This condition is referred to as "chemobrain" or "chemofog." These patients experience mild to moderate difficulties in cognitive functions [27, 28].

The most affected cognitive functions after chemotherapy are decision making, executive function, information processing speed, memory, attention, concentration, language, and visuospatial function [13, 26, 29]. Although cognitive complaints partially decrease in BC patients 6 months after chemotherapy, the patient cannot fully return to the pre-treatment cognitive level [30]. Cognitive problems may begin immediately following chemotherapy, or they may have a later onset [29] and may last up to 20 years following treatment [31]. When chemotherapy was compared with other treatment modalities in cancer survivors 5 years after completion of treatment, neuropsychological test results after standard-dose chemotherapy were found to be worse than those after surgery and radiotherapy [29]. This short- and long-term impairment in cognitive functions may cause difficulties in patients' psychological well-being and performing activities of daily life [28].

Many mechanisms have been proposed for how chemotherapy affects cognitive functions. Factors causing CRCI can be grouped as oxidative stress, direct damage to DNA and nervous system structures, cytokines, and inflammatory responses [8, 32].

21.2.1 Oxidative Stress and DNA Damage

The increase in oxidative stress levels and DNA damage in the CNS with chemotherapy is one of the mechanisms of CRCI. Higher levels of oxidative stress of DNA after chemotherapy cause DNA destruction or abnormal expression [33, 34]. The mutation rate in mitochondrial DNA increases significantly. Studies [35, 36] have found that cisplatin causes mitochondrial DNA damage and reduces ATP production by 70%. In a study conducted in rats [37], single- and double-stranded DNA breaks in brain cells after chemotherapy were found to be associated with a decrease in cognitive functions.

21.2.2 Central Nervous System Damage

Oxidative stress in the brain increases with chemotherapy and cell damage increases. Accompanied by DNA damage, breaks in the DNA chains are observed [38]. The aging and weakening of CNS cells are accelerated [33, 34, 38]. Healthy proliferating cells increase apoptosis by changing their own repair mechanisms, and damage is observed in neural precursor cells [39]. As a result, regional changes in brain activity and structural and functional damage occur in the brain [40]. Also, this condition causes disruption in the blood–brain barrier and the integration of transport mechanisms [38]. It is thought that toxic effects on neural progenitor cells and changes in brain structure and function may be the underlying mechanism of cognitive impairment [39].

Studies [31, 41] have found a decrease in gray and white matter in the brains of BC patients a few months/years after chemotherapy. Decrease in metabolic activity in the gyrus precentalis and Broca's area [42], a decrease in cerebral blood flow in some regions of the frontal cortex and cerebellum 5–10 years after chemotherapy [43], and structural and functional changes in many regions of the brain, including the temporal cortex [44]. Also, volume reduction in the hippocampus and white matter and damage to their connections have been detected in BC patients after adjuvant chemotherapy [45, 46].

21.2.3 Inflammatory Cytokines: By the Power of Interleukins and TNF-α

Inflammation is an important mechanism in the pathogenesis of CRCI. In BC patients, high levels of inflammatory cytokines are observed during chemotherapy, shortly after chemotherapy, and up to 5 years later [46–48]. Proinflammatory cytokines such as interleukin (IL)-1, IL-6, and tumor necrosis factor-α (TNF-α) change the permeability of the blood–brain barrier and increase the access of chemotherapeutic agents to the CNS [38]. Chemotherapy drugs, which often cannot pass the blood–brain barrier due to their molecular size, can indirectly cause neuroinflammation and neurotoxicity in the brain through pro-inflammatory cytokines [49, 50].

It is thought that higher levels of inflammatory cytokines may be associated with cognitive dysfunctions in BC patients [49, 50]. Severe cognitive impairments have been detected in BC patients with higher levels of IL1-β and IL-6 after chemotherapy [46]. A relationship has been found between inflammatory cytokines and impairment in different cognitive domains such as psychomotor speed [47] and memory [46, 48] in BC patients.

Neuronal damage may also be linked to a pro-inflammatory cytokine process that can be triggered by chemotherapy as well as cancer-related psychological stress [51]. Chronic stress can increase glucocorticoid levels as a result of hypothalamic–pituitary–adrenal axis dysregulation [52], and with this increase, structural and functional damage can occur in the brain [53].

21.3 Hormone Therapy and Cognitive Impairment in Breast Cancer: The Only Arena That Estrogen Cannot Win

Estrogen receptors are located in the hippocampus, which is essential for cognitive processes such as learning, memory, and emotional status [54, 55]. Estrogen increases synapse formation and synaptic branching density in the hippocampus [56, 57] and affects dopaminergic, serotonergic, glutamatergic, noradrenergic, and cholinergic neurotransmitter systems in the brain [58]. Estradiol, an estrogen hormone, plays a neuroprotective role by showing an antioxidative effect against oxidative stress in traumatic brain injury and neurodegenerative diseases [59].

Verbal memory [60], verbal attention [61], psychomotor efficiency, concentration [62], and global cognitive function [61, 63] were found better in women exposed to more estrogen. Although increased estrogen exposure appears to be cognitively beneficial for women, it is a factor that increases the risk of BC [64].

Hormone therapy is the standard treatment for 70% of estrogen receptor-positive (ER+) BC patients [65]. With hormone therapy, estrogen binding to estrogen receptors on BC cells is prevented or estrogen levels are reduced [59]. Considering the neuroprotective properties of estradiol in the brain, it is possible that CRCI may occur as a result of decreased estrogen levels in the body with hormone therapy [59]. However, agents used in hormone therapy can cause synaptic dysregulation, synapse, and neuron losses in the hippocampus [66, 67]. In studies [68, 69], women with BC who received chemotherapy and hormone therapy were found to be at higher risk for the development of cognitive impairment than women who only received chemotherapy or did not receive any systemic treatment.

21.4 Living with Cancer-Related Cognitive Impairment in Breast Cancer: Beyond Physical Health

After cancer treatment, some symptoms such as fatigue, pain, lymphedema, anxiety, depression, and cognitive impairment may become chronic in BCS. These symptoms may cause some functional difficulties in the long term, which will affect patients' participation in daily life activities, performance, and social roles in life. Many BC patients have stated that cognitive problems are more challenging than the physical side effects of cancer and cancer treatment [7].

CRCI can seriously affect patients' social and occupational functionality, preventing them from performing normal daily activities and reducing their QoL [70, 71]. Even in simple task performance, compensating for a mild cognitive problem caused by CRCI can increase cognitive load [72]. Also, BC patients may face a decrease in their ability to work due to CRCI [73], and they have difficulty returning to work and maintaining employment [72].

21.5 How Should We Assess Cancer-Related Cognitive Impairment in Breast Cancer?

For cancer survivors, cognitive change caused by cancer and/or cancer treatment is a serious problem that needs to be considered [74]. Clinically, CRCI is considered one of the most persistent late effects of cancer treatment. CRCI is a difficult condition to manage for both patients and clinicians [75]. In addition, it may remain unclear whether the cognitive problems expressed by patients after cancer treatments are due to the cancer itself, cancer treatment, or another disease the patient had before [11]. Due to the physical symptoms of cancer, patients are often unaware of cognitive changes. These findings are the most important factor showing the importance of cognitive evaluation before cancer treatment. For the effective management of CRCI, which has a multidimensional nature [9], the patient should be evaluated with clinically accurate evaluation methods at each stage of the cancer treatment [76].

CRCI can be evaluated with objective neuropsychological tests and patient self-reported questionnaires. Although there is a weak correlation between neuropsychological tests and patient self-reported questionnaires [77, 78] and controversy continues, both are important assessment methods used in the clinic.

21.5.1 Neuropsychological Tests

Neuropsychological tests are objective and gold-standard methods for assessing cognitive impairments but are difficult to perform [79] and may not be sensitive to detect mild cognitive impairment in cancer survivors [76]. Neuropsychological tests recommended by the International Cognition and Cancer Task Force (ICCTF) in the evaluation of CRCI are the Hopkins Verbal Learning Test-Revised (HVLT-R), the Trail Making Test (TMT), and the Controlled Oral Word Association Test (COWAT) [79]. In systematic reviews and clinical studies addressing the assessment of CRCI in BC patients [80–83], the cognitive domains and neuropsychological tests evaluated are as follows:

Executive function: Stroop Color and Word Test; Controlled Oral Word Association Test (COWAT); Fepsy Visual Searching Test; Fepsy Binary Choice Test.

Attention: Trail Making Test—Part A; The Rapid Visual Information Processing Test; Paced Auditory Serial Addition Test (PASAT); Wechsler Adult Intelligence Scale-Third Version (WAIS-III) Digit Span.

Spatial function: Wechsler Adult Intelligence Scale-Third Version (WAIS-III) Block Design; Rey–Osterrieth Complex Figure Test.

Verbal function: Wide Range Achievement Test-Fourth Edition (WRAT-4) Reading Subtest; Boston Naming Test; Controlled Oral Word Association Test (COWAT).

Verbal learning and memory: Hopkins Verbal Learning and Memory Test—revised; Verbal Recognition Memory (VRM) Test; Rey Auditory Verbal Learning Test (RAVLT).

Visual memory: Rey–Osterrieth Complex Figure Test; Fepsy Visual Reaction Test.

Psychomotor function: Wechsler Adult Intelligence Scale-Third Version (WAIS-III) Digit Symbol; Trail Making Test—Part A and B.

Motor speed and function: Grooved Peg Board Test; Fepsy Finger Tapping Task; Fepsy Binary Choice Test.

Thanks to developing technology, neuropsychological tests have been converted into computer-based versions and have become easier to administer in a shorter time. CogState, which evaluates psychomotor speed, manual dexterity, learning, memory, and executive function, and the Cambridge Neuropsychological Test Automated Battery (CANTAB), a semi-automatic computerized assessment method that evaluates multiple cognitive domains, are examples of these methods [84, 85].

21.5.2 Patient Self-Reported Questionnaires

Patient self-reported questionnaires are easy to apply, practical, and can provide insight into the patient's QoL. Despite the possibility of potential self-report bias in the evaluation [11], the fact that the patient's CRCI-related complaints cannot be detected through neuropsychological tests makes patient self-reported questionnaires important [76].

The patient self-reported questionnaires designed specifically for cancer survivors and most used to evaluate CRCI are the Functional Assessment of Cancer Therapy-Cognitive Function (FACT-Cog) and the European Organization for Research and Treatment of Cancer-QoL Questionnaire-Core 30-Cognitive Functioning (EORTC-QLQ-C30-CF). These questionnaires primarily focus on global cognitive functioning. Cognitive Symptom Checklist-Work-21 (CSC-W21) is also used to evaluate work-related cognitive problems in BC patients.

The Functional Assessment of Cancer Therapy-Cognitive Function (FACT-Cog) Version 3 The 37-item and 5-point Likert type (0: Several times a day—4: Never) FACT-Cog questionnaire is a part of the Functional Assessment of Chronic Illness Therapy (FACIT) collection [86]. This questionnaire is designed to evaluate improvements in QoL and cognitive performance. This measure focuses on the discernible disruptions to function and ability in the several domains that are specific to perceived cognitive functioning [87]. Perceived cognitive impairments (PCI), perceived cognitive abilities, the impact of perceived cognitive impairment on QoL, and comments from others on cognitive function are the four subscales that make up the FACT-Cog. Better self-reported cognitive functioning is indicated by higher values [88]. FACT-Cog has also been found to be valid and reliable in BC and several types of cancer [88, 89].

The European Organization for Research and Treatment of Cancer-QoL Questionnaire-Core 30 (EORTC-QLQ-C30) This 30-item questionnaire is commonly used for evaluating cancer patients' QoL and overall perceived health status [90]. Two items of EORTC-QLQ-C30 focuses on cognitive functioning with a 4-point Likert system (1: None—4: A lot): *"Have you had difficulty in concentrating on things, like reading a newspaper or watching television?"* and *"Have you had difficulty remembering things?"*. The higher scores indicate worse cognitive functioning [90, 91]. The validity and reliability of EORTC-QLQ-C30 have been demonstrated in BC patients [92].

Cognitive Symptom Checklist-Work-21 (CSC-W21) This is a generic self-reported questionnaire that is designed to be used for cognitive problems experienced in functional tasks. It has five domains (attention/concentration, memory, visual processing, language, and executive function) [93] and consists of 100 items indicating whether the patient believes the item is a problem/not a problem. Based on the CSC-100, the 21-item version (CSC-W21) was developed and validated in working BCS to reduce the measurement burden [94]. Higher scores indicate worse cognitive performance and thus greater work-related cognitive limitations. CSC-W21 is validated with BCS [94, 95].

21.6 How Can We Manage the Cancer-Related Cognitive Impairment in Breast Cancer?

Although evidence on effective intervention strategies is limited, management of CRCI in BC patients is mainly provided by pharmacological treatment, cognitive training, and exercise.

21.6.1 Pharmacological Treatment

Pharmacological interventions in CRCI management aim to reduce inflammation and oxidative stress but they have limited success [13, 96]. In a randomized placebo-controlled study in which acetylcholinesterase inhibitors

(AChEI) were used in the treatment of CRCI in BC survivors, improvement was observed in the group using AChEI [97]. Modafinil is also a medical treatment that reduces severe fatigue in cancer patients [98]. Psychomotor speed and visual information processing showed some improvement 4.5 hours after modafinil usage compared with placebo in patients with advanced cancer [99].

21.6.2 Cognitive Training

It is necessary to provide BCS with CRCI with efficient therapies to improve cognitive function. Occupational therapy, which focuses on improving cognitive function, was recognized as a first-line intervention for cognitive impairment in cancer survivors by the National Comprehensive Cancer Network (NCCN) guidelines [100]. After reviewing evidence-based therapies for cancer and CRCI, the Oncology Nursing Society recommended cognitive training as a probable effective intervention [101]. Furthermore, studies of cognitive rehabilitation in BCS indicated that the most promising interventions for BCS are cognitive training programs that target attention, memory, and processing speed [102]. Computer-based cognitive exercises target specific cognitive domains such as attention, memory, processing speed, or executive functionality. These exercises have the ability to improve cognitive functions with the principle of motor learning when repeated many times [103].

Kesler et al. [104] conducted home-based, online cognitive training targeting executive functions in BCS receiving chemotherapy. After the 12-week program, the patients were evaluated with neurocognitive and self-reported evaluation methods. Improvements in cognitive flexibility, processing speed, verbal fluency, and executive behavior were observed in BCS who received cognitive training compared to the control group.

In the study of Yao et al. [105], a cognitive intervention called "CALM (Managing Cancer and Living Meaningfully)" was applied to female BCS who experienced cognitive disorders due to chemotherapy. In this psychological intervention, practices were applied in a comfortable and quiet environment, accompanied by soothing background music, in areas such as symptom management, communication, changes in relationships with the social environment, spirituality, sense of meaning and purpose, preparing for the future, maintaining hope, and facing death. As a result of the 12-week training, a significant improvement was observed in the FACT-Cog-PCI score. Also, a positive correlation was found between the amplitude of low-frequency fluctuations (ALFF) value in the hippocampus, which is detected in MRI findings and has an important place in cognitive functions, and the FACT-Cog-PCI score. Differences in signal strength in different brain regions of BCS were observed after the CALM intervention. This demonstrated that CALM intervention could improve cognitive functions by modulating the activation or inhibition of signals in brain regions and highlights the importance of the hippocampus in cognitive management.

Ferguson et al. [106] performed a cognitive training called "Memory and Attention Adaptation Training (MAAT)" for BCS with cognitive impairment via video conferencing for 8 weeks. MAAT is a cognitive behavioral therapy method that includes awareness, stress, memory, self-awareness, self-regulation, cognitive compensatory strategies, and verbal-auditory coding in situations at risk. This memory and attention adaptation training emphasizes the activation of adaptive behavioral changes in work life, home life, and social activity to compensate for cognitive difficulties. As a result of the study, a significant difference was detected in the FACT-Cog PCI score, processing speed, QoL, and anxiety related to cognitive problems in the MAAT group compared to the control group. In another study [107], in which MAAT was applied to BC patients with cognitive impairment due to chemotherapy and complaints about memory and attention, it was found that the patients' QoL, memory, attention, concentration and language skills, and executive functions were improved. MAAT was interpreted as helpful in improving cognitive functions.

Mihuta et al. [108] implemented a web-based cognitive rehabilitation program based on cognitive behavioral therapy principles in female BCS. The "Responding to Cognitive Concerns (ReCog)" program included practices, questions, and homework related to psychoeducation, relaxation, strategy training, aging, health, cancer, cognitive function, memory, attention, fatigue, and emotions. As a result of the 12-week program, fatigue perceived cognitive impairment and memory problems decreased and the QoL increased in BCS.

In the psychoeducation-based cognitive rehabilitation intervention called "Haze" conducted by Myers et al. [109] via teleconference for BCS, the patient was taught cognitive strategies for depression, anxiety and stress management, relaxation techniques, mindfulness meditation, increasing attention, improving memory, problem solving, and social support. In addition, the homework was given to the patients who keep a cognitive change diary, relaxation exercises, mindfulness meditation, and exercises, which they had to practice for at least 15 minutes a day. As a result of the study, QoL, perceived cognitive ability, perceived cognitive function increased, and perceived cognitive impairment decreased in BCS.

21.6.3 Exercise: The Most Powerful Key of Physiotherapists

Exercise is an effective nonpharmacological intervention to reduce cognitive problems after BC treatment [110]. Many interventions as cognitive rehabilitation approaches target the consequences of cognitive decline. Exercise training may affect its underlying mechanisms [111]. The molecular mechanisms that underlie the relationship between exercise and cognition in cancer survivors remain unknown. Numerous routes were identified about which exercise may improve brain functioning by research on humans and animal models [112–114].

Though no consistent effects have been discovered, systematic studies suggested that exercise may have an impact on TNF-α [115], C-reactive protein (CRP) [116], IL-2, IL-6, and IL-8 after chemotherapy. As of right now, the mechanism that appears to be most strongly supported by data is that exercise raises neurotrophic factor levels, which then favorably impact neurogenesis [117]. Brain-derived neurotrophic factor (BDNF), a biomarker of brain health, is one of the important mechanisms [113, 114].

Since BDNF is controlled by cytokines and insulin, exercise is one of the main mechanisms thought to indirectly affect cognitive functions by affecting these metabolic components [118]. The findings of a meta-analysis [119] suggested that aerobic exercise increased BDNF levels at rest. In addition, exercise increases cerebral blood flow in the anterior cingulate region, and it is linked to improved memory function [120]. Research on rodents [111] has demonstrated that exercise training can help various biological processes disrupted by chemotherapy, most notably neurogenesis in the hippocampus, which is crucial for memory and learning.

Although the evidence is inconsistent, new research has revealed the presence of "muscle–brain crosstalk," a phenomenon that may provide insight into the potential effects of exercise on brain health. Because muscle cells have a high metabolic activity, they can produce and release substances known as myokines that have autocrine, paracrine, and endocrine effects when muscles contract repeatedly [121]. Myokines can reorganize various pathways that have neuroprotective and anti-inflammatory effects [122]. In addition, myokines increase the release of neurotrophins and growth factors (such as BDNF, VEGF (vascular endothelial growth factor), and IGF-1 (insulin-like growth factor)), which are known to be involved in neuronal plasticity [123], enhance mitochondrial biogenesis and antioxidant capacities [124], angiogenic processes, and vascular function [125].

A Closer Outlook of the Association Between Exercise and CRCI Hartman and colleagues [118] evaluated the effect of a 3-month physical activity intervention on neuropsychological outcomes and cognitive concerns in BCS with cognitive impairment. The exercise group did

150 minutes of moderate-to-vigorous physical activity per week. This group was contacted via telephone during the second and sixth weeks. They were asked to increase their activity via e-mail every 3 days. Also, recommendations for being more active in social life, personalized exercise, and motivation videos were sent via e-mail. As a result of the study, there was a positive correlation between physical activity and cognitive functions in BCS.

Gentry et al. [126] evaluated the effect of moderate-intensity aerobic exercise on cognitive function in postmenopausal BC patients receiving aromatase inhibitor therapy. The patients performed aerobic exercise for 10–15 minutes, 3 days/week for the first 2 weeks, at 60–75% of their maximum heart rate, and then increased the duration to 45–60 minutes, 3 days/week. Each exercise session included 5–10 minute warm-up and cool-down periods. The exercise was modified according to the patient. It was concluded that exercise improves physical and cognitive functions, increases QoL reduces fatigue, and has a positive effect on cancer prognosis in BC patients.

Gokal et al. [127] evaluated whether physical activity protects and maintains cognitive function and psychosocial well-being in BC patients receiving chemotherapy. After 2 cycles of chemotherapy, the intervention group did a moderate-intensity walking program of at least 150 minutes a week, starting from 10 minutes/day, and gradually increasing to 30 minutes, for 12 weeks. As a result of the study, improvements were achieved in memory, attention, visual-spatial skills, cognitive function, fatigue, anxiety, depression, mood, and self-confidence in BC patients.

Koevoets et al. [128] investigated the effect of exercise on cognitive function in BCS after chemotherapy, including participants who had been 2–4 years after their cancer diagnosis and who did less than 150 minutes of moderate-to-high intensity physical activity per week. Participants were randomly divided into exercise and control groups. The control group maintained their usual physical activity levels. An individual program was applied to the exercise group, including 2 hours of supervised aerobic and strength training per week, and 2 hours of moderate-intensity Nordic power walking, which can be done individually or in groups, supervised by a physiotherapist for a total of 6 months. The intensity of the supervised program increased as the program progressed, including high-intensity interval training starting at week 10. Exercises were recorded by the participants in their exercise diaries, and two-thirds of the participants attended ≥80% of the exercise sessions. As a result, self-reported physical, mental, general fatigue, and depression decreased, and motivation, cognitive function level, physical fitness, and QoL increased in BC patients with cognitive problems who underwent chemotherapy. In particular, physical fitness improved significantly compared to patients in the control group. It was concluded that exercise has a positive effect on cognitive function, specifically in patients with higher levels of fatigue.

Wei et al. [129] investigated the effect of Baduanjin, a mind-body therapy, on cognitive functions in BC patients receiving chemotherapy. The patients did 5 times/week for 3 months, each session lasting 30 minutes. The program is determined as 2-minute stretching, inhalation–exhalation, two sets of 12-minute Baduanjin sessions, and a 2-minute muscle relaxation exercise, respectively. Before the first cycle of chemotherapy, patients had the first session in the hospital and then followed the exercises via video at home. Participants kept exercise diaries and were interviewed via WeChat twice a week. The study showed that low-intensity exercise may help prevent cognitive impairment and improve attention in BC patients receiving chemotherapy.

Yoga is a particularly considerable exercise intervention in BCS to improve cognitive function. Yoga can be easily modified for BCS who may be experiencing common physical symptoms such as pain or fatigue by using mild physical activity, breathing techniques, and meditation [130]. In BCS, yoga may additionally decrease inflammation [131]. Derry et al. [132] evaluated the effect of yoga on cognitive problems in BCS in a randomized controlled trial. The intervention group received Hatha Yoga twice a week for 12 weeks, each session lasting 90 minutes.

Participants also received brochures and a yoga video about poses and breathing exercises. Participants recorded yoga classes and yoga practice times in their diaries. As a result, fewer cognitive problems, stress, fatigue, and better sleep quality were reported in the intervention group. These findings showed that yoga positively affects cognitive functions in female BCS.

Exercise is shown as a safe and useful treatment for several side effects of cancer treatments, including fatigue, psychological distress, functional decline, and unfavorable changes in body composition [133]. However, after receiving a diagnosis, the majority of BC patients tend to decrease their physical activity, which raises the possibility of neurodegeneration as a result of both cancer and physical inactivity [134]. Because exercise programs may be individualized for each patient, it is becoming increasingly relevant for the maintenance of brain health in BCS [135]. Prescribing exercise specifically for the improvement of cognitive functions in BCS remains one of the most important issues among exercise guidelines in this population [136].

References

1. DeSantis CE, Ma J, Gaudet MM, Newman LA, Miller KD, Goding Sauer A, Jemal A, Siegel RL. Breast cancer statistics, 2019. CA Cancer J Clin. 2019;69(6):438–51. https://doi.org/10.3322/caac.21583.
2. Von Ah D, Habermann B, Carpenter JS, Schneider BL. Impact of perceived cognitive impairment in breast cancer survivors. Eur J Oncol Nurs. 2013;17(2):236–41. https://doi.org/10.1016/j.ejon.2012.06.002.
3. So WKW, Law BMH, Ng MSN, He X, Chan DNS, Chan CWH, McCarthy AL. Symptom clusters experienced by breast cancer patients at various treatment stages: A systematic review. Cancer Med. 2021;10(8):2531–65. https://doi.org/10.1002/cam4.3794.
4. Schagen SB, Klein M, Reijneveld JC, Brain E, Deprez S, Joly F, Scherwath A, Schrauwen W, Wefel JS. Monitoring and optimising cognitive function in cancer patients: present knowledge and future directions. EJC Suppl. 2014;12(1):29–40. https://doi.org/10.1016/j.ejcsup.2014.03.003.
5. Dyk KV, Crespi CM, Petersen L, Ganz PA. Identifying cancer-related cognitive impairment using the FACT-cog perceived cognitive impairment. JNCI Cancer Spectr. 2019;4(1):pkz099. https://doi.org/10.1093/jncics/pkz099.
6. Janelsins MC, Kohli S, Mohile SG, Usuki K, Ahles TA, Morrow GR. An update on cancer- and chemotherapy-related cognitive dysfunction: current status. Semin Oncol. 2011;38(3):431–8. https://doi.org/10.1053/j.seminoncol.2011.03.014.
7. Boykoff N, Moieni M, Subramanian SK. Confronting chemobrain: an in-depth look at survivors' reports of impact on work, social networks, and health care response. J Cancer Surviv. 2009;3(4):223–32. https://doi.org/10.1007/s11764-009-0098-x.
8. Janelsins MC, Kesler SR, Ahles TA, Morrow GR. Prevalence, mechanisms, and management of cancer-related cognitive impairment. Int Rev Psychiatry. 2014;26(1):102–13. https://doi.org/10.3109/09540261.2013.864260.
9. Jansen C, Miaskowski C, Dodd M, Dowling G, Kramer J. Potential mechanisms for chemotherapy-induced impairments in cognitive function. Oncol Nurs Forum. 2005;32(6):1151–63. https://doi.org/10.1188/05.ONF.1151-1163.
10. Ahles TA, Root JC. Cognitive effects of cancer and cancer treatments. Annu Rev Clin Psychol. 2018;14:425–51. https://doi.org/10.1146/annurev-clinpsy-050817-084903.
11. Ahles TA, Saykin AJ, McDonald BC, Li Y, Furstenberg CT, Hanscom BS, Mulrooney TJ, Schwartz GN, Kaufman PA. Longitudinal assessment of cognitive changes associated with adjuvant treatment for breast cancer: impact of age and cognitive reserve. J Clin Oncol. 2010;28(29):4434–40. https://doi.org/10.1200/JCO.2009.27.0827.
12. Schagen SB, Hamburger HL, Muller MJ, Boogerd W, van Dam FS. Neurophysiological evaluation of late effects of adjuvant high-dose chemotherapy on cognitive function. J Neuro-Oncol. 2001;51(2):159–65. https://doi.org/10.1023/a:1010635229762.
13. Ahles TA, Root JC, Ryan EL. Cancer-and cancer treatment-associated cognitive change: an update on the state of the science. J Clin Oncol. 2012;30(30):3675–86. https://doi.org/10.1200/JCO.2012.43.0116.
14. Starkweather AR, Lyon DE, Elswick RK Jr, Montpetit AJ, Conley Y, McCain NL. A conceptual model of psychoneurological symptom cluster variation in women with breast cancer: bringing nursing research to personalized medicine. Curr Pharmacogenomics Person Med. 2013;11(3):224–30. https://doi.org/10.2174/18756921113119990004.
15. Hermelink K. Chemotherapy and cognitive function in breast cancer patients: the so-called chemo brain. J Natl Cancer Inst Monogr. 2015;2015(51):67–9. https://doi.org/10.1093/jncimonographs/lgv009.
16. Andreotti C, Root JC, Ahles TA, McEwen BS, Compas BE. Cancer, coping, and cognition: a model for the role of stress reactivity in cancer-related cog-

nitive decline. Psychooncology. 2015;24(6):617–23. https://doi.org/10.1002/pon.3683.
17. Hermelink K, Bühner M, Sckopke P, Neufeld F, Kaste J, Voigt V, Münzel K, Wuerstlein R, Ditsch N, Hellerhoff K, Rjosk-Dendorfer D, Braun M, von Koch FE, Härtl K, Hasmüller S, Bauerfeind I, Debus G, Herschbach P, Mahner S, Harbeck N. Chemotherapy and post-traumatic stress in the causation of cognitive dysfunction in breast cancer patients. J Natl Cancer Inst. 2017;109(10) https://doi.org/10.1093/jnci/djx057.
18. Churchill NW, Strother SC. PHYCAA+: an optimized, adaptive procedure for measuring and controlling physiological noise in BOLD fMRI. NeuroImage. 2013;82:306–25. https://doi.org/10.1016/j.neuroimage.2013.05.102.
19. Bluethmann SM, Mariotto AB, Rowland JH. Anticipating the "silver tsunami": prevalence trajectories and comorbidity burden among older cancer survivors in the United States. Cancer Epidemiol Biomarkers Prev. 2016;25(7):1029–36. https://doi.org/10.1158/1055-9965.EPI-16-0133.
20. Conroy SK, McDonald BC, Smith DJ, Moser LR, West JD, Kamendulis LM, Klaunig JE, Champion VL, Unverzagt FW, Saykin AJ. Alterations in brain structure and function in breast cancer survivors: effect of post-chemotherapy interval and relation to oxidative DNA damage. Breast Cancer Res Treat. 2013;137(2):493–502. https://doi.org/10.1007/s10549-012-2385-x.
21. Suberbielle E, Djukic B, Evans M, Kim DH, Taneja P, Wang X, Finucane M, Knox J, Ho K, Devidze N, Masliah E, Mucke L. DNA repair factor BRCA1 depletion occurs in Alzheimer brains and impairs cognitive function in mice. Nat Commun. 2015;6:8897. https://doi.org/10.1038/ncomms9897.
22. Ongnok B, Chattipakorn N, Chattipakorn SC. Doxorubicin and cisplatin induced cognitive impairment: the possible mechanisms and interventions. Exp Neurol. 2020;324:113118. https://doi.org/10.1016/j.expneurol.2019.113118.
23. Dongés B, Haupt LM, Lea RA, Chan RC, Shum DH, Griffiths LR. Role of the apolipoprotein E and catechol-O-methyltransferase genes in prospective and retrospective memory traits. Gene. 2012;506(1):135–40. https://doi.org/10.1016/j.gene.2012.06.067.
24. Harrison RA, Rao V, Kesler SR. The association of genetic polymorphisms with neuroconnectivity in breast cancer patients. Sci Rep. 2021;11(1):6169. https://doi.org/10.1038/s41598-021-85768-4.
25. Koleck TA, Bender CM, Sereika SM, Ahrendt G, Jankowitz RC, McGuire KP, Ryan CM, Conley YP. Apolipoprotein E genotype and cognitive function in postmenopausal women with early-stage breast cancer. Oncol Nurs Forum. 2014;41(6):E313–25. https://doi.org/10.1188/14.ONF.E313-E325.
26. Wefel JS, Schagen SB. Chemotherapy-related cognitive dysfunction. Curr Neurol Neurosci Rep. 2012;12(3):267–75. https://doi.org/10.1007/s11910-012-0264-9.
27. Bernstein LJ, McCreath GA, Komeylian Z, Rich JB. Cognitive impairment in breast cancer survivors treated with chemotherapy depends on control group type and cognitive domains assessed: A multilevel meta-analysis. Neurosci Biobehav Rev. 2017;83:417–28. https://doi.org/10.1016/j.neubiorev.2017.10.028.
28. Pullens MJ, De Vries J, Roukema JA. Subjective cognitive dysfunction in breast cancer patients: a systematic review. Psychooncology. 2010;19(11):1127–38. https://doi.org/10.1002/pon.1673.
29. Ahles TA, Saykin AJ, Furstenberg CT, Cole B, Mott LA, Skalla K, Whedon MB, Bivens S, Mitchell T, Greenberg ER, Silberfarb PM. Neuropsychologic impact of standard-dose systemic chemotherapy in long-term survivors of breast cancer and lymphoma. J Clin Oncol. 2002;20(2):485–93. https://doi.org/10.1200/JCO.2002.20.2.485.
30. Janelsins MC, Heckler CE, Peppone LJ, Kamen C, Mustian KM, Mohile SG, Magnuson A, Kleckner IR, Guido JJ, Young KL, Conlin AK, Weiselberg LR, Mitchell JW, Ambrosone CA, Ahles TA, Morrow GR. Cognitive complaints in survivors of breast cancer after chemotherapy compared with age-matched controls: an analysis from a nationwide, multicenter. Prospective Longitudinal Study J Clin Oncol. 2017;35(5):506–14. https://doi.org/10.1200/JCO.2016.68.5826.
31. Koppelmans V, Breteler MM, Boogerd W, Seynaeve C, Gundy C, Schagen SB. Neuropsychological performance in survivors of breast cancer more than 20 years after adjuvant chemotherapy. J Clin Oncol. 2012;30(10):1080–6. https://doi.org/10.1200/JCO.2011.37.0189.
32. Bagnall-Moreau C, Chaudhry S, Salas-Ramirez K, Ahles T, Hubbard K. Chemotherapy-induced cognitive impairment is associated with increased inflammation and oxidative damage in the hippocampus. Mol Neurobiol. 2019;56(10):7159–72. https://doi.org/10.1007/s12035-019-1589-z.
33. Atukeren P, Yavuz B, Soydinc HO, Purisa S, Camlica H, Gumustas MK, Balcioglu I. Variations in systemic biomarkers of oxidative/nitrosative stress and DNA damage before and during the consequent two cycles of chemotherapy in breast cancer patients. Clin Chem Lab Med. 2010;48(10):1487–95. https://doi.org/10.1515/CCLM.2010.249.
34. Asakawa H, Koizumi H, Koike A, Takahashi M, Wu W, Iwase H, Fukuda M, Ohta T. Prediction of breast cancer sensitivity to neoadjuvant chemotherapy based on status of DNA damage repair proteins. Breast Cancer Res. 2010;12(2):R17. https://doi.org/10.1186/bcr2486.
35. Kruidering M, Van de Water B, de Heer E, Mulder GJ, Nagelkerke JF. Cisplatin-induced nephrotoxicity in porcine proximal tubular cells: mitochondrial dysfunction by inhibition of complexes I to

IV of the respiratory chain. J Pharmacol Exp Ther. 1997;280(2):638–49.
36. Marullo R, Werner E, Degtyareva N, Moore B, Altavilla G, Ramalingam SS, Doetsch PW. Cisplatin induces a mitochondrial-ROS response that contributes to cytotoxicity depending on mitochondrial redox status and bioenergetic functions. PLoS One. 2013;8(11):e81162. https://doi.org/10.1371/journal.pone.0081162.
37. Krynetskiy E, Krynetskaia N, Rihawi D, Wieczerzak K, Ciummo V, Walker E. Establishing a model for assessing DNA damage in murine brain cells as a molecular marker of chemotherapy-associated cognitive impairment. Life Sci. 2013;93(17):605–10. https://doi.org/10.1016/j.lfs.2013.03.013.
38. Tangpong J, Cole MP, Sultana R, Estus S, Vore M, St Clair W, Ratanachaiyavong S, St Clair DK, Butterfield DA. Adriamycin-mediated nitration of manganese superoxide dismutase in the central nervous system: insight into the mechanism of chemobrain. J Neurochem. 2007;100(1):191–201. https://doi.org/10.1111/j.1471-4159.2006.04179.x.
39. Seigers R, Schagen SB, Van Tellingen O, Dietrich J. Chemotherapy-related cognitive dysfunction: current animal studies and future directions. Brain Imaging Behav. 2013;7(4):453–9. https://doi.org/10.1007/s11682-013-9250-3.
40. Pomykala KL, de Ruiter MB, Deprez S, McDonald BC, Silverman DH. Integrating imaging findings in evaluating the post-chemotherapy brain. Brain Imaging Behav. 2013;7(4):436–52. https://doi.org/10.1007/s11682-013-9239-y.
41. de Ruiter MB, Reneman L, Boogerd W, Veltman DJ, Caan M, Douaud G, Lavini C, Linn SC, Boven E, van Dam FS, Schagen SB. Late effects of high-dose adjuvant chemotherapy on white and gray matter in breast cancer survivors: converging results from multimodal magnetic resonance imaging. Hum Brain Mapp. 2012;33(12):2971–83. https://doi.org/10.1002/hbm.21422.
42. Silverman DH, Castellon SA, Abraham L, Dy CJ, Pio BS, Ganz PA. Abnormal regional brain metabolism in breast cancer survivors after adjuvant chemotherapy is associated with cognitive changes. Proc Am Soc Clin Oncol. 2003;22:12.
43. Silverman DH, Dy CJ, Castellon SA, Lai J, Pio BS, Abraham L, Waddell K, Petersen L, Phelps ME, Ganz PA. Altered frontocortical, cerebellar, and basal ganglia activity in adjuvant-treated breast cancer survivors 5-10 years after chemotherapy. Breast Cancer Res Treat. 2007;103(3):303–11. https://doi.org/10.1007/s10549-006-9380-z.
44. Kaiser J, Bledowski C, Dietrich J. Neural correlates of chemotherapy-related cognitive impairment. Cortex. 2014;54:33–50. https://doi.org/10.1016/j.cortex.2014.01.010.
45. Inagaki M, Yoshikawa E, Matsuoka Y, Sugawara Y, Nakano T, Akechi T, Wada N, Imoto S, Murakami K, Uchitomi Y. Smaller regional volumes of brain gray and white matter demonstrated in breast cancer survivors exposed to adjuvant chemotherapy. Cancer. 2007;109(1):146–56. https://doi.org/10.1002/cncr.22368.
46. Kesler S, Janelsins M, Koovakkattu D, Palesh O, Mustian K, Morrow G, Dhabhar FS. Reduced hippocampal volume and verbal memory performance associated with interleukin-6 and tumor necrosis factor-alpha levels in chemotherapy-treated breast cancer survivors. Brain Behav Immun. 2013;30(Suppl(0)):S109–16. https://doi.org/10.1016/j.bbi.2012.05.017.
47. Cheung YT, Ng T, Shwe M, Ho HK, Foo KM, Cham MT, Lee JA, Fan G, Tan YP, Yong WS, Madhukumar P, Loo SK, Ang SF, Wong M, Chay WY, Ooi WS, Dent RA, Yap YS, Ng R, Chan A. Association of proinflammatory cytokines and chemotherapy-associated cognitive impairment in breast cancer patients: a multi-centered, prospective, cohort study. Ann Oncol. 2015;26(7):1446–51. https://doi.org/10.1093/annonc/mdv206.
48. Pomykala KL, Ganz PA, Bower JE, Kwan L, Castellon SA, Mallam S, Cheng I, Ahn R, Breen EC, Irwin MR, Silverman DH. The association between pro-inflammatory cytokines, regional cerebral metabolism, and cognitive complaints following adjuvant chemotherapy for breast cancer. Brain Imaging Behav. 2013;7(4):511–23. https://doi.org/10.1007/s11682-013-9243-2.
49. Ahles TA, Saykin AJ. Candidate mechanisms for chemotherapy-induced cognitive changes. Nat Rev Cancer. 2007;7(3):192–201. https://doi.org/10.1038/nrc2073.
50. Janelsins MC, Mustian KM, Palesh OG, Mohile SG, Peppone LJ, Sprod LK, Heckler CE, Roscoe JA, Katz AW, Williams JP, Morrow GR. Differential expression of cytokines in breast cancer patients receiving different chemotherapies: implications for cognitive impairment research. Support Care Cancer. 2012;20(4):831–9. https://doi.org/10.1007/s00520-011-1158-0.
51. Chandrashekara S, Jayashree K, Veeranna HB, Vadiraj HS, Ramesh MN, Shobha A, Sarvanan Y, Vikram YK. Effects of anxiety on TNF-alpha levels during psychological stress. J Psychosom Res. 2007;63(1):65–9. https://doi.org/10.1016/j.jpsychores.2007.03.001.
52. Wiedenmayer CP, Bansal R, Anderson GM, Zhu H, Amat J, Whiteman R, Peterson BS. Cortisol levels and hippocampus volumes in healthy preadolescent children. Biol Psychiatry. 2006;60(8):856–61. https://doi.org/10.1016/j.biopsych.2006.02.011.
53. Sapolsky RM. Glucocorticoids and hippocampal atrophy in neuropsychiatric disorders. Arch Gen Psychiatry. 2000;57(10):925–35. https://doi.org/10.1001/archpsyc.57.10.925.
54. Behl C, Moosmann B. Neuroprotektive Aktivitäten von Estrogen. Nachr Chem. 2001;49(3):332–6.
55. Wenderlein JM. Aromatasehemmer riskant für das Gehirn? Geburtsh Frauenheilk. 2005;65(02):144–8. https://doi.org/10.1055/s-2004-830483.

56. Foy MR. 17beta-estradiol: effect on CA1 hippocampal synaptic plasticity. Neurobiol Learn Mem. 2001;76(3):239–52. https://doi.org/10.1006/nlme.2001.4018.
57. Eberling JL, Wu C, Tong-Turnbeaugh R, Jagust WJ. Estrogen- and tamoxifen-associated effects on brain structure and function. NeuroImage. 2004;21(1):364–71. https://doi.org/10.1016/j.neuroimage.2003.08.037.
58. Riecher-Rösler A. Östrogene und Psychopharmaka. Östrogene in der Psychiatrie—Psychopharmaka in der Gynäkologie. 2015;2:403–8.
59. Buwalda B, Schagen SB. Is basic research providing answers if adjuvant anti-estrogen treatment of breast cancer can induce cognitive impairment? Life Sci. 2013;93(17):581–8. https://doi.org/10.1016/j.lfs.2012.12.012.
60. Henderson VW, Guthrie JR, Dudley EC, Burger HG, Dennerstein L. Estrogen exposures and memory at midlife: a population-based study of women. Neurology. 2003;60(8):1369–71. https://doi.org/10.1212/01.wnl.0000059413.75888.be.
61. Smith CA, McCleary CA, Murdock GA, Wilshire TW, Buckwalter DK, Bretsky P, Marmol L, Gorsuch RL, Buckwalter JG. Lifelong estrogen exposure and cognitive performance in elderly women. Brain Cogn. 1999;39(3):203–18. https://doi.org/10.1006/brcg.1999.1078.
62. Ryan J, Carrière I, Scali J, Ritchie K, Ancelin ML. Life-time estrogen exposure and cognitive functioning in later life. Psychoneuroendocrinology. 2009;34(2):287–98. https://doi.org/10.1016/j.psyneuen.2008.09.008.
63. Heys M, Jiang C, Cheng KK, Zhang W, Au Yeung SL, Lam TH, Leung GM, Schooling CM. Life long endogenous estrogen exposure and later adulthood cognitive function in a population of naturally postmenopausal women from Southern China: the Guangzhou Biobank Cohort Study. Psychoneuroendocrinology. 2011;36(6):864–73. https://doi.org/10.1016/j.psyneuen.2010.11.009.
64. American Cancer Society. What are the risk factors for breast cancer? Available at: https://www.cancer.org/cancer/types/breast-cancer/risk-and-prevention.html . Accessed 17 Mar 2024.
65. Chlebowski RT, Kim J, Haque R. Adherence to endocrine therapy in breast cancer adjuvant and prevention settings. Cancer Prev Res (Phila). 2014;7(4):378–87. https://doi.org/10.1158/1940-6207.CAPR-13-0389.
66. Zhou L, Fester L, von Blittersdorff B, Hassu B, Nogens H, Prange-Kiel J, Jarry H, Wegscheider K, Rune GM. Aromatase inhibitors induce spine synapse loss in the hippocampus of ovariectomized mice. Endocrinology. 2010;151(3):1153–60. https://doi.org/10.1210/en.2009-0254.
67. Nobakht M, Najafzadeh N, Kordestani SB. Effects of tamoxifen on morphological and ultrastructural aspects of developing hippocampus of rat. Iran Biomed J. 2009;13(4):237–43.
68. Bender CM, Sereika SM, Berga SL, Vogel VG, Brufsky AM, Paraska KK, Ryan CM. Cognitive impairment associated with adjuvant therapy in breast cancer. Psychooncology. 2006;15(5):422–30. https://doi.org/10.1002/pon.964.
69. Castellon SA, Ganz PA, Bower JE, Petersen L, Abraham L, Greendale GA. Neurocognitive performance in breast cancer survivors exposed to adjuvant chemotherapy and tamoxifen. J Clin Exp Neuropsychol. 2004;26(7):955–69. https://doi.org/10.1080/13803390490510905.
70. Craig CD, Monk BJ, Farley JH, Chase DM. Cognitive impairment in gynecologic cancers: a systematic review of current approaches to diagnosis and treatment. Support Care Cancer. 2014;22(1):279–87. https://doi.org/10.1007/s00520-013-2029-7.
71. Wefel JS, Kesler SR, Noll KR, Schagen SB. Clinical characteristics, pathophysiology, and management of noncentral nervous system cancer-related cognitive impairment in adults. CA Cancer J Clin. 2015;65(2):123–38. https://doi.org/10.3322/caac.21258.
72. Munir F, Burrows J, Yarker J, Kalawsky K, Bains M. Women's perceptions of chemotherapy-induced cognitive side affects on work ability: a focus group study. J Clin Nurs. 2010;19(9–10):1362–70. https://doi.org/10.1111/j.1365-2702.2009.03006.x.
73. Von Ah D, Storey S, Crouch A. Relationship between self-reported cognitive function and work-related outcomes in breast cancer survivors. J Cancer Surviv. 2018;12(2):246–55. https://doi.org/10.1007/s11764-017-0664-6.
74. Bender CM, Thelen BD. Cancer and cognitive changes: the complexity of the problem. Semin Oncol Nurs. 2013;29(4):232–7. https://doi.org/10.1016/j.soncn.2013.08.003.
75. LoBiondo-Wood G, Brown CG, Knobf MT, Lyon D, Mallory G, Mitchell SA, Von Ah D, Wesmiller S, Fellman B. Priorities for oncology nursing research: the 2013 national survey. Oncol Nurs Forum. 2014;41(1):67–76. https://doi.org/10.1188/14.ONF.67-76.
76. Lange M, Joly F, Vardy J, Ahles T, Dubois M, Tron L, Winocur G, De Ruiter MB, Castel H. Cancer-related cognitive impairment: an update on state of the art, detection, and management strategies in cancer survivors. Ann Oncol. 2019;30(12):1925–40. https://doi.org/10.1093/annonc/mdz410.
77. Hutchinson AD, Hosking JR, Kichenadasse G, Mattiske JK, Wilson C. Objective and subjective cognitive impairment following chemotherapy for cancer: a systematic review. Cancer Treat Rev. 2012;38(7):926–34. https://doi.org/10.1016/j.ctrv.2012.05.002.
78. Dhillon HM, Tannock IF, Pond GR, Renton C, Rourke SB, Vardy JL. Perceived cognitive impairment in people with colorectal cancer who do and do not receive chemotherapy. J Cancer Surviv. 2018;12(2):178–85. https://doi.org/10.1007/s11764-017-0656-6.

79. Wefel JS, Vardy J, Ahles T, Schagen SB. International Cognition and Cancer Task Force recommendations to harmonise studies of cognitive function in patients with cancer. Lancet Oncol. 2011;12(7):703–8. https://doi.org/10.1016/S1470-2045(10)70294-1.
80. Hurria A, Lachs M. Is cognitive dysfunction a complication of adjuvant chemotherapy in the older patient with breast cancer? Breast Cancer Res Treat. 2007;103(3):259–68. https://doi.org/10.1007/s10549-006-9383-9.
81. Janelsins MC, Heckler CE, Peppone LJ, Ahles TA, Mohile SG, Mustian KM, Palesh O, O'Mara AM, Minasian LM, Williams AM, Magnuson A, Geer J, Dakhil SR, Hopkins JO, Morrow GR. Longitudinal trajectory and characterization of cancer-related cognitive impairment in a nationwide cohort study. J Clin Oncol. 2018;36(32):JCO2018786624. https://doi.org/10.1200/JCO.2018.78.6624.
82. Janelsins MC, Lei L, Netherby-Winslow C, Kleckner AS, Kerns S, Gilmore N, Belcher E, Thompson BD, Werner ZA, Hopkins JO, Long J, Cole S, Culakova E. Relationships between cytokines and cognitive function from pre- to post-chemotherapy in patients with breast cancer. J Neuroimmunol. 2022;362:577769. https://doi.org/10.1016/j.jneuroim.2021.577769.
83. van Dam FS, Schagen SB, Muller MJ, Boogerd W, vd Wall E, Droogleever Fortuyn ME, Rodenhuis S. Impairment of cognitive function in women receiving adjuvant treatment for high-risk breast cancer: high-dose versus standard-dose chemotherapy. J Natl Cancer Inst. 1998;90(3):210–8. https://doi.org/10.1093/jnci/90.3.210.
84. Collie A, Darekar A, Weissgerber G, Toh MK, Snyder PJ, Maruff P, Huggins JP. Cognitive testing in early-phase clinical trials: development of a rapid computerized test battery and application in a simulated Phase I study. Contemp Clin Trials. 2007;28(4):391–400. https://doi.org/10.1016/j.cct.2006.10.010.
85. Fray PJ, Robbins TW. CANTAB battery: proposed utility in neurotoxicology. Neurotoxicol Teratol. 1996;18(4):499–504. https://doi.org/10.1016/0892-0362(96)00027-x.
86. Webster K, Cella D, Yost K. The Functional Assessment of Chronic Illness Therapy (FACIT) measurement system: properties, applications, and interpretation. Health Qual Life Outcomes. 2003;1:79. https://doi.org/10.1186/1477-7525-1-79.
87. Park JH, Bae SH, Jung YS, Jung YM. The psychometric properties of the Korean version of the functional assessment of cancer therapy-cognitive (FACT-Cog) in Korean patients with breast cancer. Support Care Cancer. 2015;23(9):2695–703. https://doi.org/10.1007/s00520-015-2632-x.
88. Wagner LI, Sweet J, Butt Z, Lai J, Cella D. Measuring patient selfreported cognitive function: development of the functional assessment of Cancer therapy–cognitive function instrument. J Support Oncol. 2009;7:W32–9.
89. Cheung YT, Lim SR, Shwe M, Tan YP, Chan A. Psychometric properties and measurement equivalence of the English and Chinese versions of the functional assessment of cancer therapy-cognitive in Asian patients with breast cancer. Value Health. 2013;16(6):1001–13. https://doi.org/10.1016/j.jval.2013.06.017.
90. Aaronson NK, Ahmedzai S, Bergman B, Bullinger M, Cull A, Duez NJ, Filiberti A, Flechtner H, Fleishman SB, de Haes JC, et al. The European Organization for Research and Treatment of Cancer QLQ-C30: a quality-of-life instrument for use in international clinical trials in oncology. J Natl Cancer Inst. 1993;85(5):365–76. https://doi.org/10.1093/jnci/85.5.365.
91. Fayers P, Aaronson N, Bjordal K, Grønvold M, Curran D, Bottomley A. EORTC QLQ-C30 scoring manual. Brussels: European Organisation for Research and Treatment of Cancer; 2001.
92. Luckett T, King MT, Butow PN, Oguchi M, Rankin N, Price MA, Hackl NA, Heading G. Choosing between the EORTC QLQ-C30 and FACT-G for measuring health-related quality of life in cancer clinical research: issues, evidence and recommendations. Ann Oncol. 2011;22(10):2179–90. https://doi.org/10.1093/annonc/mdq721.
93. O'Hara C, Harrell M, Bellingrath E, Lisicia K. Cognitive symptom checklists: clinician's guide. Lutz (FL): Psychological Assessment Resources, Inc; 1993.
94. Ottati A, Feuerstein M. Brief self-report measure of work-related cognitive limitations in breast cancer survivors. J Cancer Surviv. 2013;7(2):262–73. https://doi.org/10.1007/s11764-013-0275-9.
95. Cheng AS, Zeng Y, Feuerstein M. Validation of the Chinese version of the Cognitive Symptom Checklist-Work-21 in breast cancer survivors. J Occup Rehabil. 2015;25(4):685–95. https://doi.org/10.1007/s10926-015-9576-3.
96. Fardell JE, Vardy J, Johnston IN, Winocur G. Chemotherapy and cognitive impairment: treatment options. Clin Pharmacol Ther. 2011;90(3):366–76. https://doi.org/10.1038/clpt.2011.112.
97. Lawrence JA, Griffin L, Balcueva EP, Groteluschen DL, Samuel TA, Lesser GJ, Naughton MJ, Case LD, Shaw EG, Rapp SR. A study of donepezil in female breast cancer survivors with self-reported cognitive dysfunction 1 to 5 years following adjuvant chemotherapy. J Cancer Surviv. 2016;10(1):176–84. https://doi.org/10.1007/s11764-015-0463-x.
98. Jean-Pierre P, Morrow GR, Roscoe JA, Heckler C, Mohile S, Janelsins M, Peppone L, Hemstad A, Esparaz BT, Hopkins JO. A phase 3 randomized, placebo-controlled, double-blind, clinical trial of the effect of modafinil on cancer-related fatigue among 631 patients receiving chemotherapy: a University of Rochester Cancer Center Community Clinical Oncology Program Research base study. Cancer.

2010;116(14):3513–20. https://doi.org/10.1002/cncr.25083.

99. Lundorff LE, Jønsson BH, Sjøgren P. Modafinil for attentional and psychomotor dysfunction in advanced cancer: a double-blind, randomised, crossover trial. Palliat Med. 2009;23(8):731–8. https://doi.org/10.1177/0269216309106872.
100. Denlinger CS, Ligibel JA, Are M, Baker KS, Demark-Wahnefried W, Friedman DL, Goldman M, Jones L, King A, Ku GH, Kvale E, Langbaum TS, Leonardi-Warren K, McCabe MS, Melisko M, Montoya JG, Mooney K, Morgan MA, Moslehi JJ, O'Connor T, Overholser L, Paskett ED, Raza M, Syrjala KL, Urba SG, Wakabayashi MT, Zee P, McMillian NR, Freedman-Cass DA. National Comprehensive Cancer Network. Survivorship: cognitive function, version 1.2014. J Natl Compr Cancer Netw. 2014;12(7):976–86. https://doi.org/10.6004/jnccn.2014.0094.
101. Von Ah D, Jansen CE, Allen DH. Evidence-based interventions for cancer- and treatment-related cognitive impairment. Clin J Oncol Nurs. 2014;18(Suppl):17–25. https://doi.org/10.1188/14.CJON.S3.17-25.
102. Morean DF, O'Dwyer L, Cherney LR. Therapies for cognitive deficits associated with chemotherapy for breast cancer: A systematic review of objective outcomes. Arch Phys Med Rehabil. 2015;96(10):1880–97. https://doi.org/10.1016/j.apmr.2015.05.012.
103. Conklin HM, Ogg RJ, Ashford JM, Scoggins MA, Zou P, Clark KN, Martin-Elbahesh K, Hardy KK, Merchant TE, Jeha S, Huang L, Zhang H. Computerized cognitive training for amelioration of cognitive late effects among childhood cancer survivors: A randomized controlled trial. J Clin Oncol. 2015;33(33):3894–902. https://doi.org/10.1200/JCO.2015.61.6672.
104. Kesler S, Hadi Hosseini SM, Heckler C, Janelsins M, Palesh O, Mustian K, Morrow G. Cognitive training for improving executive function in chemotherapy-treated breast cancer survivors. Clin Breast Cancer. 2013;13(4):299–306. https://doi.org/10.1016/j.clbc.2013.02.004.
105. Yao S, Zhu Q, Zhang Q, Cai Y, Liu S, Pang L, Jing Y, Yin X, Cheng H. Managing Cancer and Living Meaningfully (CALM) alleviates chemotherapy related cognitive impairment (CRCI) in breast cancer survivors: A pilot study based on resting-state fMRI. Cancer Med. 2023;12(15):16231–42. https://doi.org/10.1002/cam4.6285.
106. Ferguson RJ, Sigmon ST, Pritchard AJ, LaBrie SL, Goetze RE, Fink CM, Garrett AM. A randomized trial of videoconference-delivered cognitive behavioral therapy for survivors of breast cancer with self-reported cognitive dysfunction. Cancer. 2016;122(11):1782–91. https://doi.org/10.1002/cncr.29891.
107. Ferguson RJ, Ahles TA, Saykin AJ, McDonald BC, Furstenberg CT, Cole BF, Mott LA. Cognitive-behavioral management of chemotherapy-related cognitive change. Psychooncology. 2007;16(8):772–7. https://doi.org/10.1002/pon.1133.
108. Mihuta ME, Green HJ, Shum DHK. Web-based cognitive rehabilitation for survivors of adult cancer: A randomised controlled trial. Psychooncology. 2018;27(4):1172–9. https://doi.org/10.1002/pon.4615.
109. Myers JS, Cook-Wiens G, Baynes R, Jo MY, Bailey C, Krigel S, Klemp J, Asher A. Emerging from the haze: a multicenter, controlled pilot study of a multidimensional, psychoeducation-based cognitive rehabilitation intervention for breast cancer survivors delivered with telehealth conferencing. Arch Phys Med Rehabil. 2020;101(6):948–59. https://doi.org/10.1016/j.apmr.2020.01.021.
110. Myers JS, Erickson KI, Sereika SM, Bender CM. Exercise as an intervention to mitigate decreased cognitive function from cancer and cancer treatment: an integrative review. Cancer Nurs. 2018;41(4):327–43. https://doi.org/10.1097/NCC.0000000000000549.
111. Liu PZ, Nusslock R. Exercise-mediated neurogenesis in the hippocampus via BDNF. Front Neurosci. 2018;12:52. https://doi.org/10.3389/fnins.2018.00052.
112. Voss MW, Nagamatsu LS, Liu-Ambrose T, Kramer AF. Exercise, brain, and cognition across the life span. J Appl Physiol (1985). 2011;111(5):1505–13. https://doi.org/10.1152/japplphysiol.00210.2011.
113. Gomez-Pinilla F, Vaynman S, Ying Z. Brain-derived neurotrophic factor functions as a metabotrophin to mediate the effects of exercise on cognition. Eur J Neurosci. 2008;28(11):2278–87. https://doi.org/10.1111/j.1460-9568.2008.06524.x.
114. Baker LD, Frank LL, Foster-Schubert K, Green PS, Wilkinson CW, McTiernan A, Plymate SR, Fishel MA, Watson GS, Cholerton BA, Duncan GE, Mehta PD, Craft S. Effects of aerobic exercise on mild cognitive impairment: a controlled trial. Arch Neurol. 2010;67(1):71–9. https://doi.org/10.1001/archneurol.2009.307.
115. Meneses-Echávez JF, Correa-Bautista JE, González-Jiménez E, Schmidt Río-Valle J, Elkins MR, Lobelo F, Ramírez-Vélez R. The effect of exercise training on mediators of inflammation in breast cancer survivors: a systematic review with meta-analysis. Cancer Epidemiol Biomarkers Prev. 2016;25(7):1009–17. https://doi.org/10.1158/1055-9965.EPI-15-1061.
116. Kang DW, Lee J, Suh SH, Ligibel J, Courneya KS, Jeon JY. Effects of exercise on insulin, IGF Axis, Adipocytokines, and inflammatory markers in breast cancer survivors: A systematic review and meta-analysis. Cancer Epidemiol Biomarkers Prev. 2017;26(3):355–65. https://doi.org/10.1158/1055-9965.EPI-16-0602.
117. Knaepen K, Goekint M, Heyman EM, Meeusen R. Neuroplasticity – exercise-induced response of peripheral brain-derived neurotrophic factor: a sys-

tematic review of experimental studies in human subjects. Sports Med. 2010;40(9):765–801. https://doi.org/10.2165/11534530-000000000-00000.
118. Hartman SJ, Natarajan L, Palmer BW, Parker B, Patterson RE, Sears DD. Impact of increasing physical activity on cognitive functioning in breast cancer survivors: rationale and study design of Memory & Motion. Contemp Clin Trials. 2015;45(Pt B):371–6. https://doi.org/10.1016/j.cct.2015.09.021.
119. Dinoff A, Herrmann N, Swardfager W, Liu CS, Sherman C, Chan S, Lanctôt KL. The effect of exercise training on resting concentrations of peripheral Brain-Derived Neurotrophic Factor (BDNF): a meta-analysis. PLoS One. 2016;11(9):e0163037. https://doi.org/10.1371/journal.pone.0163037.
120. Chapman SB, Aslan S, Spence JS, Defina LF, Keebler MW, Didehbani N, Lu H. Shorter term aerobic exercise improves brain, cognition, and cardiovascular fitness in aging. Front Aging Neurosci. 2013;5:75. https://doi.org/10.3389/fnagi.2013.00075.
121. Pedersen BK. Physical activity and muscle-brain crosstalk. Nat Rev Endocrinol. 2019;15(7):383–92. https://doi.org/10.1038/s41574-019-0174-x.
122. Gleeson M, Bishop NC, Stensel DJ, Lindley MR, Mastana SS, Nimmo MA. The anti-inflammatory effects of exercise: mechanisms and implications for the prevention and treatment of disease. Nat Rev Immunol. 2011;11(9):607–15. https://doi.org/10.1038/nri3041.
123. Skriver K, Roig M, Lundbye-Jensen J, Pingel J, Helge JW, Kiens B, Nielsen JB. Acute exercise improves motor memory: exploring potential biomarkers. Neurobiol Learn Mem. 2014;116:46–58. https://doi.org/10.1016/j.nlm.2014.08.004.
124. Burtscher J, Millet GP, Place N, Kayser B, Zanou N. The muscle-brain axis and neurodegenerative diseases: the key role of mitochondria in exercise-induced neuroprotection. Int J Mol Sci. 2021;22(12):6479. https://doi.org/10.3390/ijms22126479.
125. Ainslie PN, Cotter JD, George KP, Lucas S, Murrell C, Shave R, Thomas KN, Williams MJ, Atkinson G. Elevation in cerebral blood flow velocity with aerobic fitness throughout healthy human ageing. J Physiol. 2008;586(16):4005–10. https://doi.org/10.1113/jphysiol.2008.158279.
126. Gentry AL, Erickson KI, Sereika SM, Casillo FE, Crisafio ME, Donahue PT, Grove GA, Marsland AL, Watt JC, Bender CM. Protocol for Exercise Program in Cancer and Cognition (EPICC): A randomized controlled trial of the effects of aerobic exercise on cognitive function in postmenopausal women with breast cancer receiving aromatase inhibitor therapy. Contemp Clin Trials. 2018;67:109–15. https://doi.org/10.1016/j.cct.2018.02.012.
127. Gokal K, Munir F, Wallis D, Ahmed S, Boiangiu I, Kancherla K. Can physical activity help to maintain cognitive functioning and psychosocial well-being among breast cancer patients treated with chemotherapy? A randomised controlled trial: study protocol. BMC Public Health. 2015;15:414. https://doi.org/10.1186/s12889-015-1751-0.
128. Koevoets EW, Schagen SB, de Ruiter MB, Geerlings MI, Witlox L, van der Wall E, Stuiver MM, Sonke GS, Velthuis MJ, Jobsen JJ, Menke-Pluijmers MBE, Göker E, van der Pol CC, Bos MEMM, Tick LW, van Holsteijn NA, van der Palen J, May AM, Monninkhof EM, PAM study group. Effect of physical exercise on cognitive function after chemotherapy in patients with breast cancer: a randomized controlled trial (PAM study). Breast Cancer Res. 2022;24(1):36. https://doi.org/10.1186/s13058-022-01530-2.
129. Wei XL, Yuan RZ, Jin YM, Li S, Wang MY, Jiang JT, Wu CQ, Li KP. Effect of Baduanjin exercise intervention on cognitive function and quality of life in women with breast cancer receiving chemotherapy: study protocol of a randomized controlled trial. Trials. 2021;22(1):405. https://doi.org/10.1186/s13063-021-05355-w.
130. Bower JE, Garet D, Sternlieb B, Ganz PA, Irwin MR, Olmstead R, Greendale G. Yoga for persistent fatigue in breast cancer survivors: a randomized controlled trial. Cancer. 2012;118(15):3766–75. https://doi.org/10.1002/cncr.26702.
131. Kiecolt-Glaser JK, Bennett JM, Andridge R, Peng J, Shapiro CL, Malarkey WB, Emery CF, Layman R, Mrozek EE, Glaser R. Yoga's impact on inflammation, mood, and fatigue in breast cancer survivors: a randomized controlled trial. J Clin Oncol. 2014;32(10):1040–9. https://doi.org/10.1200/JCO.2013.51.8860.
132. Derry HM, Jaremka LM, Bennett JM, Peng J, Andridge R, Shapiro C, Malarkey WB, Emery CF, Layman R, Mrozek E, Glaser R, Kiecolt-Glaser JK. Yoga and self-reported cognitive problems in breast cancer survivors: a randomized controlled trial. Psychooncology. 2015;24(8):958–66. https://doi.org/10.1002/pon.3707.
133. Schmitz KH, Courneya KS, Matthews C, Demark-Wahnefried W, Galvão DA, Pinto BM, Irwin ML, Wolin KY, Segal RJ, Lucia A, Schneider CM, von Gruenigen VE, Schwartz AL, American College of Sports Medicine. American College of Sports Medicine roundtable on exercise guidelines for cancer survivors. Med Sci Sports Exerc. 2010;42(7):1409–26. https://doi.org/10.1249/MSS.0b013e3181e0c112.
134. Schmitz KH, Campbell AM, Stuiver MM, Pinto BM, Schwartz AL, Morris GS, Ligibel JA, Cheville A, Galvão DA, Alfano CM, Patel AV, Hue T, Gerber LH, Sallis R, Gusani NJ, Stout NL, Chan L, Flowers F, Doyle C, Helmrich S, Bain W, Sokolof J, Winters-Stone KM, Campbell KL, Matthews CE. Exercise is medicine in oncology: engaging clinicians to help patients move through cancer. CA Cancer J Clin. 2019;69(6):468–84. https://doi.org/10.3322/caac.21579.

135. Stout NL, Baima J, Swisher AK, Winters-Stone KM, Welsh J. A systematic review of exercise systematic reviews in the cancer literature (2005-2017). PM R. 2017;9(9S2):S347–84. https://doi.org/10.1016/j.pmrj.2017.07.074.
136. Campbell KL, Winters-Stone KM, Wiskemann J, May AM, Schwartz AL, Courneya KS, Zucker DS, Matthews CE, Ligibel JA, Gerber LH, Morris GS, Patel AV, Hue TF, Perna FM, Schmitz KH. Exercise guidelines for cancer survivors: consensus statement from international multidisciplinary roundtable. Med Sci Sports Exerc. 2019;51(11):2375–90. https://doi.org/10.1249/MSS.0000000000002116.

22 Psychosocial Perspective in Breast Cancer: From Diagnosis to Survivorship

Elif Deniz Kaçmaz

22.1 Introduction

The rising survival rate of breast cancer, attributable to early diagnosis and effective treatment methods, is becoming increasingly apparent. With extended survival times, issues pertaining to diagnosis and treatment are coming into sharper focus [1]. From the moment of cancer diagnosis to the journey of survival, patients often face numerous psychosocial challenges, which can have a lasting impact on their lives [2]. During this process, patients experience a spectrum of emotional and behavioral reactions, ranging from mild emotional symptoms to psychiatric disorders [3].

It has been noted that factors such as young age, low income, educational level, and history of mental illness, as well as experiences of pain and insomnia, can predispose breast cancer patients to mental health issues [4]. Nearly 99% of breast cancer patients are female [5]. It is well-recognized that breast cancer alone impacts women's mental well-being differently from other types of cancer. Because breasts are attributed to the feminine characteristics and sexuality in women, the diagnosis and treatment of breast cancer can threaten their sense of femininity and can give additional psychosocial challenges [6, 7].

E. D. Kaçmaz (✉)
Faculty of Health Sciences, Department of Nursing, İzmir Bakircay University, İzmir, Türkiye

In addition to the physical challenges common to all types of cancer, breast cancer can lead to psychological, social, and existential issues for an individual [7]. From the moment of cancer diagnosis to the journey of survival, individuals may display a range of emotional and behavioral responses. Some of these reactions are aimed at adaptation [6]. The occurrence and intensity of psychosocial issues can vary among breast cancer patients, influenced by factors such as the signs and symptoms of the disease, treatment methods, prior experiences with the illness, age, available support systems, cultural context, and coping abilities [7, 8]. While significant reductions in psychological distress are usually observed in many patients within one year after completion of treatment, approximately one-quarter of breast cancer patients still can experience psychological challenges associated with diagnosis and treatment [9]. Psychosocial problems can create a fertile ground for the development of psychological disorders [3]. Therefore, it is necessary to detect psychosocial reactions before they reach pathological levels and to provide the necessary intervention. The most common psychosocial problems in breast cancer patients are depression, anxiety, anger, hopelessness, and fear [1, 8]. Moreover, breast cancer patients often experience numerous psychosocial challenges related to self-perception, physical adjustment, family, and social dynamics, as well as profes-

Y. Bakar, A. Tuğral (eds.), *Managing Side Effects of Breast Cancer Treatment*,
https://doi.org/10.1007/978-3-031-75480-7_22

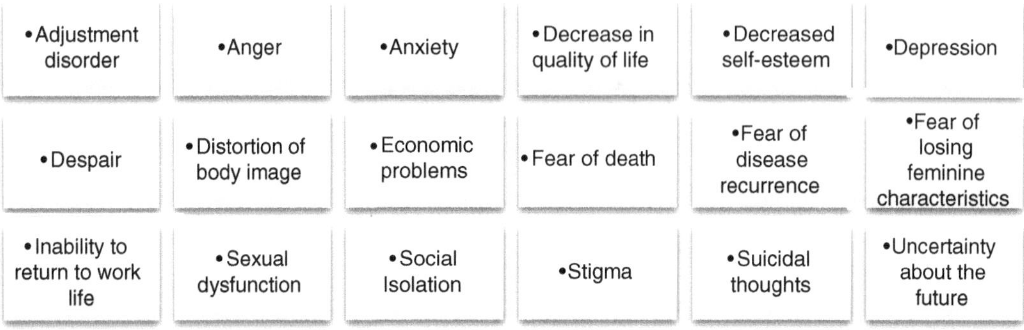
•Adjustment disorder
•Anger
•Anxiety
•Decrease in quality of life
•Decreased self-esteem
•Depression
•Despair
•Distortion of body image
•Economic problems
•Fear of death
•Fear of disease recurrence
•Fear of losing feminine characteristics
•Inability to return to work life
•Sexual dysfunction
•Social Isolation
•Stigma
•Suicidal thoughts
•Uncertainty about the future

Fig. 22.1 Psychosocial problems that can be seen in breast cancer patients from diagnosis to survival. Created by the author

sional and economic concerns [8]. Psychosocial problems and contributing factors that can be seen in breast cancer patients from diagnosis to survival are shown in Fig. 22.1.

In this chapter, the psychosocial perspective of breast cancer is discussed, from diagnosis to survivorship.

22.2 Psychosocial Effects of Being Diagnosed with Breast Cancer

Receiving a cancer diagnosis is perceived as a devastation and causes a crisis that disrupts psychological balance [6]. Being diagnosed with breast cancer is inherently stressful and can have negative impacts on mental health, treatment decisions, and prognosis [10]. Cancer, often viewed as a chronic disease with improved survival rates, still evokes fears of suffering and mortality. The meaning that patients attach to cancer and how they perceive the disease affect their psychosocial adaptation [7, 11].

Reactions that occur after a cancer diagnosis vary from person to person [2, 8]. Elisabeth Kübler Ross described the five stages of emotional and behavioral reactions that occur in cancer as follows: [8, 12].

1. Shock and Denial: In the first stage, a shock reaction often occurs. It is the phase when the patient and their relatives are so confused that they do not know what to say or how to act after receiving the diagnosis. At this stage, denial of the truth, anxiety caused by the truth, and feelings of helplessness are defense mechanisms. The patient uses the expressions like "This cannot be true" or "This cannot happen to me." Denial occurs via ignoring the disease.
2. Anger: It is the individual's reaction to the experience of loss, which includes feeling resentment, anger, and blaming external factors. Due to the inability to control the experience of loss, the previous expression "This cannot happen to me" changed to "Why me?". The individual tries to find the causes of the disease. The anger experienced may be directed at others or oneself.
3. Bargaining: At this stage, the individual believes that she/he will be successful in preventing the inevitable by agreeing with the higher power. They are the secret oaths of an individual with a higher power. This stage is useful for a person with a terminal illness because she/he attempts to gain control over his/her situation. A bargain of a cancer patient is "If my test results come back clear, I'll do a favor."
4. Depression: In an individual with a fatal disease such as cancer, feelings of denial and anger disappear during the treatment process. Feelings of guilt and sadness due to losses can lead to depression. Anxiety also increases with depression. At this stage, the individual

may frequently use the phrase "leave me alone."
5. Acceptance: At this stage, the individual does not feel angry or depressed but accepts the facts. He/she can direct his/her energy and spiritual power to his/her new life. At this stage, the individual uses expressions such as "we will all die one day." Individuals diagnosed with cancer may experience these periods sequentially, while some phases may not occur for everyone [12].

In a study conducted with women diagnosed with breast cancer, cognitive factors such as shock, denial, and sadness were observed during the diagnosis process. Emotional responses such as fear, loneliness, anger, and guilt were also noted. Additionally, participants exhibited behavioral reactions such as crying, seeking social support, and praying. Interpersonal reactions included isolating oneself, attempting not to upset family members, and concealing their emotions [13]. In studies conducted with breast cancer patients, it is stated that the most common psychological problems are depression, anxiety, and adjustment disorder [8]. Anxiety is characterized by tension and worry, while depression manifests as a depressed mood, thinking slow, and loss of interest. Patients with depression are at higher risk for suicide than those with anxiety. Depression and anxiety can lead to insomnia. Anxiety is characterized by difficulty in falling asleep, while depression is characterized by early waking. Anxiety and depression in breast cancer patients have been found to have negative effects on recurrence and mortality rates [14]. In patients diagnosed with breast cancer, other factors that create a risk for psychopathology, including demographic and socioeconomic factors, disease-related factors, psychiatric history, and medical comorbidity, need to be taken into account [13]. It is noted that pretreatment care programs, informational support, participation in social support groups, and the adoption of individual effective coping strategies can assist in reducing distress levels related to treatment [15].

22.3 Psychosocial Effects of Breast Cancer Treatment

Breast cancer treatment includes surgical treatment, chemotherapy, radiotherapy, and hormone therapy, depending on the type and clinical status of the cancer [5]. In a study involving women undergoing treatment for breast cancer, various cognitive, emotional, behavioral, and interpersonal reactions were observed. Cognitive factors included denial, while emotional responses encompassed anger, sadness, pain, fear, pessimism, emptiness, worry, and anxiety. Behavioral reactions included insomnia, social withdrawal, and efforts to avoid upsetting relatives. Additionally, interpersonal reactions such as avoidance and social withdrawal were noted [15]. Psychosocial problems arising from breast cancer treatment negatively affect the well-being of patients [1].

Curative surgery is used as one of the main treatment steps, depending on the stage of breast cancer. It is accepted that the deterioration in body shape caused by surgery will affect the psychological state of patients and lead to depressive symptoms. Mastectomy, a common surgical procedure in breast cancer treatment, leads to a significant alteration in the external appearance of women [13]. Surgical interventions performed during the treatment process cause anxiety in patients. While the first factor that causes this anxiety in most patients is the life-threatening nature of the disease, the second factor is related to the external appearance [6]. Loss of an organ and change in body image can have devastating consequences for patients. Surgical interventions during the treatment process lead to physical changes that affect self-esteem, sexual functions, and identity [15]. Mastectomy, along with the feeling of loss of a feminine symbol, negatively affects the person's self-confidence, body image, and mental health [6]. A woman's reaction to losing her breast is determined by the value of the woman's self-concept and the values of the society she lives in. In a society where the breast symbolizes femininity, sexuality, and motherhood, it is unsurprising that the loss of a breast negatively impacts self-esteem and body image [7, 16]. The effect of breast cancer treatment on the female body negatively affects sexuality and close relationships [17]. In a study, it was found that after breast surgery, especially in women receiving chemotherapy treatment, sexual reluctance causes problems with the partner and changes in body image [18]. When comparing the quality of life outcomes between breast-conserving surgery and mastectomy, breast-conserving surgery tends to be superior in terms of body image and role function [19]. In another study, half of the patients underwent mastectomy, while the other half underwent preventive breast surgery. The study concluded that patients who underwent mastectomy experienced negative impacts on body image and sexual dysfunction [16]. However, a systematic review shows that there is no significant difference between total mastectomy, breast-conserving surgery, and breast reconstruction in terms of depressive symptoms occurring in breast cancer patients one year after surgery. This situation might have been associated with being diagnosed with breast cancer rather than the devastating effect of the surgical treatment [13]. The significance of breast loss for the patient plays a crucial role in determining their psychological response to surgery [20].

Treatments for breast cancer can cause severe side effects. Radiotherapy, chemotherapy, and hormone therapy can cause symptoms such as fatigue, pain, and nausea, causing changes in the individual's social and family roles [21]. Chemotherapy and hormone therapy can lead to ovarian deficiency, early menopause, hormonal disruption, and issues with sexual function as potential side effects. These side effects also affect fertility and cause physical and psychosocial problems, especially in women who desire to have children [8]. Alopecia (loss of hair, eyebrows, and eyelashes) and weight loss are common side effects of treatment. They can negatively impact patients' well-being by causing anxiety, depression, and deterioration in body image [22]. Depending on the treatment, depression is more common in breast cancer than other types of cancer due to the decrease in estrogen levels and the early onset of menopause [1]. Depression experienced during the treatment process negatively affects treatment compliance [23]. Although some side effects of chemotherapy are common among breast cancer patients, the frequency and severity of symptoms vary individually. Negative psychosocial effects specific to chemotherapy treatment also arise from patients' side effect experiences [19]. Chemotherapy has negative effects on the physical, psychological, and social functionality of breast cancer patients [20]. The cognitive functions of patients receiving chemotherapy are also changed and this condition is called chemotherapy-related cognitive impairment (CRCI). This condition characterized by symptoms such as memory impairment and lack of concentration during daily-life activities is also referred to as "chemo-brain". It has been noted that depression, anxiety, and other psychological factors can have a negative impact on cognitive functions in the development of chemo-brain [21].

Long-lasting physical side effects caused by breast cancer treatment cause psychosocial problems in patients [8]. One of the most common symptoms associated with breast cancer treatment is fatigue. Studies have found that most patients experience chronic fatigue [17]. Breast cancer causes negative psychosocial effects that affect roles and responsibilities within the family [6]. During the breast cancer continuum, family members serve as crucial sources of support. However, they also face their own psychosocial challenges alongside the patient. It is reported that family members or caregivers frequently experience feelings of anxiety, uncertainty, and helplessness. Children may experience different fears and anxiety depending on their development period. Additionally, the fact that hereditary characteristics of breast cancer can cause concerns for family members [7, 8]. Research shows that the patient's spouse has a lower quality of life than other family members [19]. One of the most important determinants of the mental and sexual health of women diagnosed with breast cancer is the quality of their relationship with their partner [20]. During the treatment process, some patients develop closer relationships with their family members, while others avoid interpersonal relationships. During cancer treatment, patients may have to leave work due to the side effects of the treatment. This can lead to economic difficulties for patients [8].

22.4 Psychosocial Effects After Breast Cancer Treatment

The increase in survival rates of breast cancer affects individuals both positively and negatively [23]. In cancer survivors, attention should be given not only to physical disabilities but also to psychosocial issues that may arise, such as sexual problems, changes in work and social roles, concerns about the future, and alterations in body image [17]. For many patients, every check-up and examination after treatment can cause anxiety. The most important experienced threat by patients immediately after treatment is the fear of cancer recurrence [6, 7]. A recent meta-review examining the psychosocial experiences of breast cancer survivors revealed a range of psychological symptoms in addition to physiological ones such as pain and lymphedema. These include uncertainty about the future, fear of death, depression, adjustment disorder, decreased quality of life, anxiety, anger, hopelessness, social isolation, and decreased self-esteem. Moreover, psychological issues concerning body image deterioration, menopausal symptoms, sexual problems, and fertility concerns persist among survivors [24]. The risk of depression is high both during breast cancer treatment and in the post-treatment period [7]. Since depression and anxiety levels may change throughout the treatment process, regular screening should be performed during post-treatment follow-ups [14]. Many survivors experience anxiety about returning to work and social relationships. Additionally, the mandatory isolation required during the treatment process to mitigate the risk of infection has a negative impact on the psychological well-being of patients. Limitations and stigma cause breast cancer survivors to isolate themselves and reduce social support [24]. Stigmatization prevents return to work and social life. A study showed that stigma in breast cancer has a positive relationship with the type of surgery, employment status, depression, and delays in seeking help. In the same study, it was found that stigma was negatively correlated with age, education, income, quality of life, social support, self-efficacy, and psychological adjustment [25].

With the growing number of breast cancer patients surviving after diagnosis, the emphasis on post-treatment quality of life has become increasingly significant [20]. Breast cancer survivors continue to face challenges and require interventions to cope with them [19]. After receiving a diagnosis, breast cancer patients live with this diagnosis for the rest of their lives. After completion of primary treatments, the patient is regularly monitored with tests [7]. Receiving a chronic and death-related diagnosis causes the person to re-evaluate his/her life and priorities [26]. In addition to the negative effects experienced during the breast cancer survival period, individuals may also undergo positive changes such as finding meaning in life, developing empathy, enhancing spirituality, adopting healthier lifestyle habits, strengthening relationships, and experiencing post-traumatic growth [23].

22.5 Psychosocial Adjustment and Coping in Breast Cancer Patients from Diagnosis to Survivorship

Various emotional and behavioral reactions may occur in a person diagnosed with cancer, starting from the diagnosis phase and throughout the treatment stages. It is not right to consider all these reactions as psychopathological or to accept all of them as normal. Psychological responses are normal for adaptation and coping purposes. At this point, adaptive reactions may occur, as well as maladaptive behaviors [8]. As with all cancers, breast cancer patients must cope with many physical and psychosocial symptoms that affect their quality of life [1]. Factors that alleviate the psychosocial burden of breast cancer patients include coping styles, information preferences, social support, and pretreatment mental state. Studies on psychosocial interventions showed that social support, cognitive therapy, and supportive information have positive effects [9]. As psychosocially supportive interventions:

- In the pre-treatment period, Patients should be informed about treatment options, given the opportunity to express their feelings and thoughts, and guided to join support groups for themselves and their families.
- During the treatment process, Information should be given about the treatment implemented and possible side effects, the fears and concerns of the patient and their relatives should be reduced, and their integration into social life should be supported.
- In the posttreatment period, their concerns about the recurrence of the disease should be discussed, their existential and spiritual needs should be evaluated, and they should be supported to meet with patients experiencing similar problems [8].

Breast cancer survivors need psychosocial support from their families, partners, friends, other breast cancer survivors, and healthcare professionals [24]. Appropriate coping and adaptation to the disease are very important in facing chronic diseases [22]. Coping with breast cancer is an important issue in the adaptation process of survivors [2]. Breast cancer patients can effectively cope with the psychosocial problems they experience due to cancer, with or without psychological help [7]. Studies show that coping strategies can affect the treatment outcomes and survival rates of breast cancer patients [26]. Patients can adopt positive or negative coping strategies. Positive coping is associated with emotional support, acceptance, and cognitive restructuring. Negative coping includes avoidance, denial, and wishful thinking. The coping method of a person depends on their values, goals, resources, and demands of the situation [27]. In a systematic review, coping was found to be an important predictor of post-traumatic growth [28]. Coping has two basic functions. The first is problem-focused coping and the other is emotion-focused coping. In problem-focused coping, the individual focuses on the problem that causes distress, while in emotion-focused coping, it is used to regulate stressful emotions [28]. The coping strategies used by breast cancer patients at different stages of the disease can vary [2]. In a study examining the coping skills of women with breast cancer during chemotherapy, it was found that women resorted to behavioral and emotional coping strategies. While behavioral coping is used to gain a greater sense of control over disease-related symptoms and the recovery process, it has been found that patients use emotional coping strategies to reduce emotional distress and anxiety [28]. In a systematic review investigating coping strategies among patients diagnosed with breast cancer, it was found that individuals most commonly employed strategies such as seeking social support, utilizing problem- or emotion-focused coping, and engaging in religious/spiritual practices, as well as utilizing avoidance and distraction techniques [2]. It was stated that most survivors use spirituality to cope with breast cancer and its impact on their lives [24]. Spirituality is a universal tool that provides relief during stressful times and it is an effective coping method for long-term survival [8]. In a study, the effectiveness of spirituality and religion in the survival process of women with breast cancer was emphasized, particularly in navigating the crisis phase triggered by diagnosis. It was noted that prayer played a significant role in helping them cope with [29]. It is stated that religious coping is an important determinant of posttraumatic growth during treatment [26]. Patients have to cope with many problems, from problems such as incompatibility and depression that occur in the early stages of breast cancer to complex treatments and obstacles encountered in the survival process. Psychological resilience is an important concept in the coping process. Many breast cancer patients develop resilience to the disease. Resilience is defined as the individual's stability in maintaining functionality during and after exposure to stressful life events [27]. Increasing the resilience of patients supports their adaptation to cancer-related adversities [26].

Psychiatric evaluation has an important place in the prognosis of breast cancer and patients' compliance with treatment [3]. Psychological support should also be continued for breast cancer survivors. The purpose of psychological support in cancer is to help the individual gain strength to cope with the disease and the problems caused by the disease and to make sense of experiencing the disease [7]. One of the primary responsibilities of healthcare professionals in supporting individuals coping with breast cancer is to assess patients with a holistic approach and aid them in navigating their disease experiences. This includes assisting patients in finding meaning in their lives when they feel overwhelmed by their illness and helping to fill gaps in their strength and knowledge. It is important to request psychiatric consultations in this process [8]. Notably, individuals diagnosed with breast cancer may tend to hide the disease in the beginning, and patients with a higher perception of stigma have more negative attitudes toward receiving psychological support [30].

Psychosocial care provided by health professionals to breast cancer patients should address the needs of the patient and their family [27]. Cancer is considered a family disease rather than an individual disease [22]. Cancer diagnosis is a process that involves emotional problems for both the patient and her family. Spousal support of patients with breast cancer affects patients' quality of life, anxiety, and coping levels [25]. Relatives of patients diagnosed with breast cancer may also experience various psychological problems. The challenges faced by spouses are often linked to changes in roles and responsibilities within the household, as well as feelings of inadequacy and helplessness when confronted with the physical, psychological, and social difficulties experienced by the patient [7]. While cancer-related stress decreases in couples with a high marital harmony, couples who cannot receive counseling for the problems experienced during the treatment process cannot cope with the process effectively [25]. A study found that as partner harmony and perceived social support are increase, depression, sexual dysfunction, and anxiety decrease [31].

Psychological interventions have been shown to mitigate the stressful consequences of breast cancer diagnosis and treatment. It has been found that interventions such as cognitive behavioral therapy, mindfulness techniques, coping therapy, psychoeducation, spiritual-religious counseling, social interventions like family therapy, and complementary approaches such as acupuncture can enhance the coping skills of patients diagnosed with breast cancer [32]. A meta-analysis study confirms the effectiveness of cognitive behavioral therapies and psychoeducation in reducing anxiety and depression and improving mood and quality of life in women with breast cancer [33]. Health professionals need to create training, support, and consultancy activities in line with the psychosocial needs of the patients and their families, taking into consideration the educational background they have. Breast cancer patients who are evaluated holistically will be able to cope effectively with this difficult process [24]. It is stated that cognitive interventions, meditation, and psychoeducation programs are effective in reducing negative emotions and increasing the quality of life of breast cancer patients [29]. Psychoeducation is a process that includes receiving information, providing information, discussing concerns, problem solving, coping skills training, expressing emotions, and social support. A recent meta-analysis study emphasizes that psychoeducation is an important tool in reducing anxiety and improving the quality of life in breast cancer [27]. Another meta-analysis study showed that cognitive behavioral interventions such as relaxation training and interpersonal skills training can reduce stress, anxiety, depression, avoidance, and negative mood in patients treated for breast cancer [29].

Despite the negative psychosocial effects of being diagnosed with a chronic disease, experiences of struggling with the disease can also have positive results [34, 35]. After a traumatic event, there may be positive changes in a person's views about him/herself and his/her relationships. This positive change is defined as posttraumatic growth [35]. Post-traumatic growth is associated with posttraumatic life events and the positive outcomes of individuals' coping processes.

Patients are able to rearrange their priorities by leaving aside the unimportant details of life. They may find empowerment in being able to assert their desires and preferences, and they can forge deeper connections with their loved ones as a result [26]. In addition to the negative effects of breast cancer and its treatment, studies have been conducted describing posttraumatic growth in patients [24, 35]. In breast cancer patients, intervention programs that predict posttraumatic growth and include functional coping strategies need to be integrated into the treatment process [35]. In order for individuals diagnosed with breast cancer to cope with the psychosocial problems they experience, social support and the development of effective coping strategies, as well as the emergence of posttraumatic growth can facilitate adaptation to the disease process [26].

22.6 Conclusion

Breast cancer causes many psychosocial difficulties in patients, from the initial diagnosis to survival. In addition to individual difficulties, these problems are generally related to family, sexuality, social relations, and working life. To alleviate the psychosocial burdens experienced by patients, the needs of patients should be determined through education and consultancy services, and supportive interventions should be planned for patients during the survival process. The aims of psychological support given to patients in the posttreatment period are to reduce psychological morbidity, increase quality of life by ensuring compliance, reduce psychiatric symptoms such as anxiety and depression, ensure participation in treatment, support patients to express their emotions, ensure the participation of patients and their relatives in the treatment process, and provide information on social support resources. The treatment process for breast cancer patients should be managed by a multidisciplinary team employing a holistic approach. The aim is to educate individuals about available social support resources. It is essential to offer timely and readily accessible psychosocial support to breast cancer survivors.

References

1. Eti Aslan F, Özdemir AE. Psychosocial problems and nursing approaches in breast cancer diseases. In: Uzun Ö, editor. Breast cancer and nursing care. 1st ed. Ankara: Turkiye Klinikleri; 2019. p. 51–4.
2. Mehrabi E, Hajian S, Simbar M, Hoshyari M, Zayeri F. Coping response following a diagnosis of breast cancer: a systematic review. Electron Physician. 2015;7(8):1575–83.
3. İzci F, İlgün AS, Fındıklı E, Özmen V. Psychiatric symptoms and psychosocial problems in patients with breast cancer. J Breast Heal. 2016;12(3):94–101.
4. Tsaras K, Papathanasiou IV, Mitsi D, Veneti A, Kelesi M, Zyga S, et al. Assessment of depression and anxiety in breast cancer patients: prevalence and associated factors. Asian Pac J Cancer Prev. 2018;19(6):1661–9.
5. World Health Organization. Breast cancer [Internet]. 2024. Available from: https://www.who.int/news-room/fact-sheets/detail/breast-cancer.
6. Tünel M, Vural A, Evlice YE, Tamam L. Psychiatric problems in patients with breast cancer. Arch Med Rev J. 2012;21(3):189–219.
7. Işık I. Psychosocial problems of breast cancer patients in the post-treatment period and supportive nursing interventions. J Educ Res Nurs. 2014;11(3):58–64.
8. Babacan GA. Psychosocial Issius in breast cancer and supportive interventions. J Breast Heal. 2006;2(3):108–14.
9. Kumar K, Mattoo S. Psychosocial aspects of breast cancer. In: Mazumdar A, Kaushik R, editors. Breast cancer. Singapore: Springer; 2022. p. 567–75.
10. Fortin J, Leblanc M, Elgbeili G, Cordova MJ, Marin M-F, Brunet A. The mental health impacts of receiving a breast cancer diagnosis: a meta-analysis. Br J Cancer. 2021;125:1582–92.
11. Güleç G, Büyükkınacı A. Cancer and psychiatric disorders. Curr Approaches Psychiatry. 2011;3(2):343–67.
12. Shehenaz İ, Mardiana M, Jamilah HAK, Mariam AD. The role of 'stage theory of bereavement', 'Dual Process Model (DPM)' and spirituality in dealing with grief during illness experience in cancer patients. IIUM J Hum Sci. 2023;5(1):51–64.
13. Zhang C, Hu G, Biskup E, Qiu X, Zhang H, Zhang H. Depression induced by total mastectomy, breast conserving surgery and breast reconstruction: a systematic review and meta-analysis. World J Surg [Internet]. 2018;42(7):2076–85. Available from: https://doi.org/10.1007/s00268-018-4477-1.

14. Wang X, Wang N, Zhong L, Wang S, Zheng Y, Yang B, et al. Prognostic value of depression and anxiety on breast cancer recurrence and mortality : a systematic review and meta-analysis of 282, 203 patients. Mol Psychiatry [Internet]. 2020;25:3186–97. Available from: https://doi.org/10.1038/s41380-020-00865-6.
15. Liu L, Wu Y, Cong W, Hu M, Li X, Zhou C. Experience of women with breast cancer undergoing chemotherapy : a systematic review of qualitative research. Qual Life Res [Internet]. 2021;30(5):1249–65. Available from: https://doi.org/10.1007/s11136-020-02754-5.
16. Denizgil T, Sönmez İ. Comparison of self esteem, body image, sexual satisfaction and sexual experiences between women who had mastectomy or breast conserving surgery for breast carcinoma. New Symp. 2015;53(3):17–25.
17. Kıyak M, Özkaraman A. Post-cancer life: requirements of survivors. Izmir Katip Çelebi Univ Fac Heal Sci J. 2022;7(1):99–104.
18. Taylan S, Kolaç N. The self image and sexual adaptation of women undering breast cancer surgery. Androl Bul. 2021;23(1):163–9.
19. Li Y, Guo J, Sui Y, Chen B, Li D, Jiang J. Quality of life in patients with breast cancer following breast conservation surgery: a systematic review and meta-analysis. J Healthc Eng. 2022;2022:3877984.
20. Özkan S, Alçalar N. Psychological reactions to surgical treatment in breast cancer. J Breast Heal. 2009;5(2):60–4.
21. Gho S, Steele J, Jones S, Munro B. Selfreported side effects of breast cancer treatment: a crosssectional study of incidence, associations, and the influence of exercise. Cancer Causes Control. 2013;24:517–28.
22. Bahar A, Ovayolu Ö, Ovayolu N. Common symptoms of oncology patients and nursing management. Erciyes Univ J Heal Sci. 2019;6(2):42–58.
23. Şengül İnan F, Üstün B. Biopsychosocial changes in post-treatment period of breast cancer. J Breast Heal. 2013;9:48–51.
24. King R, Stafford L, Butow P, Giunta S, Laidsaar-Powell R. Psychosocial experiences of breast cancer survivors: a meta – review. J Cancer Surviv [Internet]. 2024;18:84–123. Available from: https://doi.org/10.1007/s11764-023-01336-x.
25. Tang W, Yusuf A, Jia K, Iskandar YHP, Manganting E, Mo X, et al. Correlates of stigma for patients with breast cancer : a systematic review and meta – analysis. Support Care Cancer [Internet]. 2023;31:55. Available from: https://doi.org/10.1007/s00520-022-07506-4.
26. Babayiğit A. Breast cancer, coping strategies and post-cancer growth: a case presentation. J Soc Humanit Adm Sci. 2023;6(2):257–78.
27. Yıldız G, Hiçdurmaz D. An overlooked group in the psychosocial care in breast cancer: spouses. Curr Approaches Psychiatry. 2019;11(2):239–47.
28. Elsheshtawy E, Abo-Elez W, Ashour H, Farouk O, El zaafarany M. Coping strategies in Egyptian ladies with breast cancer. Breast cancer basic. Clin Res. 2014;8:97–102.
29. Hajian S, Mehrabi E, Simbar M, Houshyari M. Coping strategies and experiences in women with a primary breast cancer diagnosis. Asian Pac J Cancer Prev. 2017;18(1):215–24.
30. Dönmez A, Avcı A. Determining the variables affecting the status of psychological help in cancer diagnosed individuals. J Ege Univ Nurs Fac. 2023;39(3):325–31.
31. Duran K, Sarandöl A. Investigation of the effects of spousal adjustment and social support level on mental health, self-esteem and sexual function in patients diagnosed with breast cancer. J Uludağ Univ Med Fac. 2022;48(3):349–55.
32. Samami E, Elyasi F, Nasab NM, Shojaee L, Zaboli E, Shahhosseini Z. Coping strategies-oriented interventions in breast cancer women: a systematic scoping review of the quantitative evidence. Iran J psychiatry. Behav Sci. 2020;14(2):e99884.
33. Guarino A, Polini C, Forte G, Favieri F, Boncompagni I, Casagrande M. The effectiveness of psychological treatments in women with breast cancer: a systematic review and meta-analysis. J Clin Med. 2020;9:209.
34. Jansen L, Hoffmeister M, Chang-Claude J, Brenner H, Arndt V. Benefit finding and post-traumatic growth in long-term colorectal cancer survivors: prevalence, determinants, and associations with quality of life. Br J Cancer. 2011;105(8):1158–65.
35. Yastıbaş C, Yılmaz Karaman İG. Breast cancer and post-traumatic growth: a systematic review. Curr Approaches Psychiatry. 2021;13(3):490–510.

23 Auditory/Vestibular Problems and Their Management After Systemic Chemotherapy in Breast Cancer

Burak Öztürk

Ototoxicity refers to the harmful effects of certain substances on the ear, specifically structures of hearing or vestibular system, leading to hearing loss, tinnitus, dizziness, or balance problems. The Ototoxicity Working Group of Pharmaceutical Interventions for Hearing Loss has provided a clear definition of ototoxicity. It refers to the damage caused to the inner ear, specifically affecting the cochlear and vestibular structures, as well as sensory function. This damage is a result of exposure to certain pharmaceuticals, chemicals, and/or ionizing radiation. Although ototoxicity usually affects the inner ear, it can also impact central auditory pathways and is, thus, considered neurotoxic [1]. Common ototoxic substances include certain medications (such as aminoglycosides, chemotherapeutic agents, loop diuretics, salicylates, and antimalarial drugs) as well as environmental chemicals like heavy metals and solvents. The most common drugs related to ototoxicity are listed in Table 23.1.

Anticancer chemotherapy drugs are used for a variety of cancers, such as breast cancer, prostate cancer, and cancers involving the cervical region [2]. A well-known side effect related to a subset of antineoplastic therapy is ototoxicity. These therapies include radiation, platinum chemotherapy, and surgery that involves the ear and auditory nerve. In cancer patients, supportive care medications including loop diuretics and aminoglycoside antibiotics may also exacerbate ototoxicity [3]. Some factors related to the individual (e.g., older age, renal dysfunction, and previous history of hearing loss) or the treatment applied (e.g., dose and duration of the drug, using additional ototoxic drugs simultaneously) make patients more prone to ototoxic effects [4].

Although cisplatin-based chemotherapeutic drugs (e.g., cisplatin and carboplatin) are well known to have an ototoxic effect [5], there is limited information in the literature about the ototoxic effect of taxane antineoplastic drugs, particularly docetaxel. Docetaxel is a highly significant anti-microtubule medication that is widely utilized in the treatment of various types of solid tumors, particularly breast cancer. As a key component of chemotherapy regimens, docetaxel continues to be an important option for patients and healthcare providers. In the literature, few studies have reported that ototoxicity may develop due to the use of docetaxel agent alone [6]. However, there are studies in the literature reporting the existence of patients with hearing loss as a result of the use of cisplatin and docetaxel together [7].

The pathophysiologic mechanism underlying aminoglycoside- and platinum-induced ototoxicity is related to the accumulation of harmful levels of reactive oxygen species within the inner

B. Öztürk (✉)
Faculty of Health Sciences, Department of Audiology, İzmir Bakircay University, İzmir, Türkiye
e-mail: burak.ozturk@bakircay.edu.tr

Y. Bakar, A. Tuğral (eds.), *Managing Side Effects of Breast Cancer Treatment*,
https://doi.org/10.1007/978-3-031-75480-7_23

Table 23.1 Common ototoxic drugs and their effects on hearing

<table>
<tr><th>Type of drug</th><th>Type of hearing loss</th><th>Permanent/ Temporary</th></tr>
<tr><td>Aminoglycoside antibiotics</td><td>Sensorineural</td><td rowspan="2">Permanent hearing loss</td></tr>
<tr><td>Cancer chemotherapeutics</td><td>Sensorineural</td></tr>
<tr><td>Loop diuretics</td><td>Sensorineural</td><td rowspan="3">Temporary hearing loss that returns to normal soon after the medication treatment is terminated.</td></tr>
<tr><td>Salicylates</td><td>Sensorineural</td></tr>
<tr><td>Antimalarial drugs</td><td>Sensorineural</td></tr>
</table>

ear. This leads to the loss of cochlear hair cells and damage to the spiral ganglion and stria vascularis cells [8]. Changes in fluid and electrolyte concentrations in the inner ear are thought to be linked to the ototoxicity of loop diuretics. These changes may cause cochlear tissue edema and an associated reduction in endocochlear potential [9]. A potential ototoxic mechanism associated with docetaxel administration has not yet been reported. The toxic effect of paclitaxel has been reported to cause degeneration in nerve fibers by disrupting axon transport in nerves. Therefore, toxic exposure occurs in auditory nerve fibers and spiral ganglion cells rather than in the outer hair cells, resulting in sensorineural hearing loss [10]. Although the potential ototoxic mechanism of docetaxel has not yet been reported in the literature, it is thought to be similar to paclitaxel [6].

23.1 Symptoms Related to Cochleotoxicity

The majority of ototoxic medications impact the inner ear's vestibular and cochlear systems. Nonetheless, some medications are comparatively more vestibulotoxic and others more cochleotoxic. Clinical manifestations of ototoxicity typically include hearing loss, tinnitus, and vestibular dysfunction [11].

Ototoxic medications damage the stria vascularis and cochlear hair cells, which results in hearing loss. The hearing loss is usually bilateral and symmetrical. The outer hair cells are usually affected before the inner hair cells. In the early stages of ototoxic damage, the basal part of the cochlea is typically affected first, which results in high-frequency hearing loss. If the ototoxic medication is continued ototoxic damage progresses toward the apical part of the cochlea, involving gradually lower frequencies. Tinnitus typically precedes or coexists with hearing loss. Additionally, the tinnitus is usually continuous and has a high pitch. Vertigo and nystagmus are two signs of vestibulotoxicity. Patients experiencing vestibular system dysfunction may experience general disequilibrium or unsteadiness [11–13].

23.2 Basic Audiological Principles of Ototoxicity Monitoring

Audiological monitoring for ototoxicity serves the purpose of assessing and managing potential hearing loss and balance issues caused by exposure to ototoxic medications or chemicals. This monitoring involves regular hearing tests and assessments to detect any changes in hearing sensitivity or balance function. By identifying early signs of ototoxicity, healthcare providers can adjust medication dosages or explore alternative treatment options to minimize the risk of permanent inner ear damage. Additionally, audiological monitoring allows for the implementation of interventions such as hearing aids or vestibular rehabilitation to support patients who suffer from ototoxicity-related symptoms. Overall, the goal of audiological monitoring for ototoxicity is to preserve and protect the patient's auditory and vestibular function while undergoing treatments that might have harmful side effects [14–16].

23.3 Assessment of Ototoxicity-Related Hearing Loss

Currently, the three main approaches to audiologic monitoring for ototoxicity are the basic audiologic assessment, high-frequency audiometry (HFA), and otoacoustic emissions (OAEs). These approaches can be used separately or in combination. It is important to conduct a baseline evaluation before administering any ototoxic drugs so that later results can be compared meaningfully [14]. The timing for conducting the baseline evaluation is largely influenced by the specific drugs being administered to the patient [16]. Prior to or within 72 hours of the first treatment dose, it is recommended to conduct a baseline audiometric evaluation for patients receiving aminoglycosides [17]. This is an important step to ensure the monitoring of potential hearing-related side effects associated with the medication. For patients who are undergoing platinum-based chemotherapy, it is important to conduct baseline tests within a week before the initial treatment, and no later than 24 hours after the treatment. This will help in monitoring and assessing the patient's response to the chemotherapy [16]. It has been suggested that before administering cisplatin, it is crucial to conduct baseline testing for hearing to assess any potential marked hearing loss that may occur following a single administration of the drug [18–19].

The basic audiologic assessment is an important component of most ototoxicity monitoring programs, but it may not identify the early ototoxic changes detected by HFA and OAEs. However, it evaluates patients' hearing in the speech frequency range for communication, measures their speech recognition skills, and examines whether a conductive component is a contributing factor to any hearing loss or change in hearing over time [15]. Pure tone audiometry is a diagnostic test used to assess a person's hearing ability across different frequencies from 250 to 8000 Hz. During the test, the individual is presented with tones at varying pitches and indicates when the sound is heard. This evaluation assists in identifying the faintest sounds detectable at different frequencies, essential for evaluating hearing impairment and deciding on appropriate treatment. Audiologists use pure tone audiometry to identify the type and degree of hearing loss, as well as to monitor changes in hearing over time. If there is a significant increase in air-conduction thresholds, it may be necessary to undergo a comprehensive audiological evaluation. This is important because a decrease in hearing could be due to middle ear involvement, so immittance or bone-conduction testing should be conducted to differentiate between sensorineural and conductive hearing loss. Word recognition testing should be included in basic audiological assessment [16].

HFA has become a widely used tool in ototoxicity monitoring programs. It involves testing air-conduction thresholds for frequencies between 8 kHz and 20 kHz, similar to conventional frequency range testing. Because the basal turn or high-frequency region of the cochlea is often affected first by ototoxic changes, HFA is effective in detecting aminoglycoside-induced or cisplatin-induced ototoxicity before changes appear in the conventional frequency range [17–18].

OAEs are another option for monitoring ototoxicity. OAEs are low-intensity acoustic vibrations that are produced by the inner ear and measured in the ear canal with a sensitive microphone [20]. OAEs can be classified into various types depending on their specific characteristics. The most common types include spontaneous otoacoustic emissions (SOAEs), which occur without any external stimulation; transient otoacoustic emissions (TOAEs), which are elicited by brief acoustic stimuli; and distortion product otoacoustic emissions (DPOAEs), which result from the interaction of two pure tones within the cochlea. Although SOAEs are not widely used clinically, each type of OAE provides valuable information about the function of the auditory system, and they are often used in clinical settings to assess hearing sensitivity and cochlear function [21].

OAEs are a useful tool for monitoring ototoxicity. They are a noninvasive and objective way to assess the function of the cochlea, making them a valuable option for detecting early signs of hearing damage caused by ototoxic drugs or other factors. It is important to note that both HFA and TOAE and DPOAE responses are capable of detecting ototoxicity at an early stage, even before changes in hearing thresholds in the conventional frequency range occur. This early detection provides physicians and patients with the opportunity to adjust treatment protocols before any permanent changes in the speech frequency range take place. This proactive approach can help mitigate potential long-term effects on hearing and overall quality of life [22]. Although changes in both TOAEs and DPOAEs before hearing thresholds in the conventional frequency range occur, DPOAEs may provide an earlier indication of changes in hearing thresholds compared to TOAEs due to their ability to measure at higher frequencies and being more sensitive to the cochlear frequency areas first affected [23, 24]. OAEs have a significant limitation as they are inconsistently detectable in individuals with conductive hearing loss. This implies that OAE testing may not be the most suitable approach for evaluating hearing function in individuals with this type of hearing impairment [25]. Furthermore, OAEs may present challenges in patients with hearing impairment, especially in the elderly, as there may be either no responses or limited responses that can be used for monitoring purposes [26, 27].

HFA has a clear advantage over OAEs because of its well-established significant change criteria, which provide excellent specificity and sensitivity in testing [16]. Several change criteria have been suggested for interpreting OAEs, indicating the significance of potential changes [28] but none yet have universal acceptance [14].

Following the initial evaluation, subsequent assessments will typically only include pure tone air-conduction threshold tests if there is no observed change in the hearing threshold. However, if a significant change is detected, it is important to repeat the entire basic audiologic assessment. Various ototoxicity grading systems are presently being employed to evaluate ototoxic changes. The American Speech-Language-Hearing Association (ASHA) has published the most widely used and validated criteria for determining ototoxic threshold shift. These criteria are essential for accurately assessing the impact of ototoxicity on individuals and guiding appropriate interventions. Significant ototoxic change is determined by meeting one of the following three criteria: (1) a decrease of 20 dB or more at any single test frequency, (2) a decrease of 10 dB or more at any two adjacent frequencies, or (3) a loss of response at three consecutive frequencies where responses were previously obtained. Changes are always calculated based on initial measurements and should be verified through retesting, usually within 24 hours [16].

Following the end of chemotherapy, the patient should still be seen. It's crucial to perform long-term audiologic monitoring to identify whether hearing loss is progressive or stable. Testing for follow-up should begin immediately and continue for three, six, and a year following the completion of therapy. Weekly monitoring should be implemented until the hearing stabilizes if any of these tests reveal a decline in hearing sensitivity. A comprehensive audiological assessment is advised if hearing stabilizes at a level that is noticeably worse than what was observed during baseline testing. Frequent monitoring and early identification permit early intervention as appropriate [16, 29].

23.4 Management of Ototoxicity-Related Hearing Loss

Effective communication is a critical quality of life concern for patients with life-threatening illnesses and ototoxic medication treatment is necessary. Early detection of ototoxic damage can enhance treatment results by slowing the progression of hearing loss and by providing counseling and rehabilitation [29].

23.5 Hearing Aids

Hearing aids can be a helpful solution for individuals experiencing ototoxicity. Hearing aids are designed to amplify sounds and improve speech clarity, making it easier for individuals with ototoxicity to hear and understand conversations. It's important to note that while hearing aids can amplify speech sounds, they cannot fully restore normal hearing.

Table 23.2 Disadvantages, advantages, and indication criteria of common hearing aid styles

Style of hearing instrument	Indication criteria	Disadvantages	Advantages
Behind-the-ear (BTE) hearing aids	Mild to profound hearing loss No restrictions due to ear canal size	Larger than others (cosmetic concerns) Ear molds need to be remade periodically	Comfortable to wear. Easy to clean. Easy to operate. Fewer feedback problems
Open fitting style BTE hearing aids	Mild to moderate-to-severe hearing loss No restrictions due to ear canal volume	Ear tips will have to be changed periodically	Comfortable to wear. Own voice sounds more natural.
Receiver-in-canal (RIC) style BTE hearing aids	Mild to moderate-to-severe hearing loss No restrictions due to ear canal volume	Ear molds need to be remade periodically. -because the receiver is in the ear canal, they are more prone to failure than traditional type BTEs.	Fewer feedback problems It can be exceptionally discrete even for severe to profound losses
In-the-canal (ITC) hearing aids	Moderate-severe hearing loss Minimal restrictions due to ear canal size Good hand dexterity and motor skills	More susceptible to ear wax damage Feedback problems More prone to repairs	Good cosmetics Comfortable to wear
Completely-in-canal (CIC) hearing aids	Mild to moderate-to-severe hearing loss Sufficient ear canal size Good hand dexterity and motor skills	Most prone to repairs Occlusion can be a significant problem. Feedback problems	Good cosmetics Comfortable to wear

There are many styles of hearing aids available, including behind-the-ear aids (BTE), open fit, in-the-canal (ITE), and completely-in-the-canal (CIC) models. Each style offers its own set of benefits and considerations, so it's important to work with a hearing care professional to determine which style is best suited for a patient's individual needs (see Table 23.2). BTE hearing aids are worn behind the ear and are suitable for a wide range of hearing loss. ITE hearing aids are custom-made to fit within the outer portion of the ear, making them less visible. CIC hearing aids are nearly invisible as they fit completely inside the ear canal, while RIC hearing aids have a small device that sits behind the ear and a receiver inside the ear canal. With so many options available, it's essential to consider factors such as comfort, visibility, and specific hearing requirements when choosing a hearing aid style. The advancements in digital technology have led to enhanced programmability and more sophisticated speech-processing capabilities in the latest models. With increased programmability and advanced speech processing, digital devices are becoming more versatile and powerful, paving the way for exciting developments in areas such as artificial intelligence, virtual assistants, and communication technology [30–31].

23.6 Cochlear Implants

A cochlear implant can be a beneficial alternative for patients with severe to profound hearing loss who are unable to benefit from hearing aids [32]. Cochlear implants are electronic devices that can provide individuals with severe to profound hearing loss the ability to perceive sound by directly stimulating the auditory nerve [33]. This technology can bypass the damaged parts of the inner ear and provide improved hearing capabilities for patients suffering from ototoxicity. Furthermore, it has been demonstrated that cochlear implants greatly enhance speech comprehension and general quality of life for individuals with ototoxicity-related hearing loss [34]. Therefore, cochlear implants can be a valuable approach for addressing the challenges associated with ototoxicity [3].

Hybrid cochlear implants, another option for the management of hearing loss, are a type of hearing device that puts together the characteristics of both traditional cochlear implants and hearing aids. They are intended for individuals who need amplification for high-frequency sounds but also have some residual low-frequency hearing. When compared to traditional cochlear implants alone, this technology improves speech understanding in noisy environments. For individuals with steeply sloping high-frequency sensorineural hearing loss typically seen following exposure to ototoxic agents-hybrid cochlear implants offer a special solution that provides a more natural hearing experience. [35].

23.7 Assistive Listening Devices

In addition to hearing aids, assistive devices such as FM systems can also greatly improve the quality of life for individuals with hearing loss. These devices work in conjunction with hearing aids to provide enhanced auditory support in difficult listening environments, allowing individuals to better communicate and engage in daily activities. Telephone amplifiers, vibrating alarm clocks, TV closed-caption decoders, inexpensive personal hand-held or body-borne amplifiers, visual alarm systems, and telephone devices for the deaf (TDDs) are further nonwearable equipment that aids the hearing-impaired listener [36].

23.8 Symptoms Related to Vestibulotoxicity

Vestibular ototoxicity typically results in a simultaneous and symmetric loss of vestibular function in both ears. This can lead to symptoms and signs such as ataxia, oscillopsia, unsteadiness, difficulty with motion, and a feeling of dizziness or imbalance. Interestingly, individuals affected by this condition do not usually experience vertigo. This absence of vertigo may be due to the fact that damage to both vestibular systems does not cause significant differences in electrical activity in the brainstem, or because the bilateral slow process allows for some level of compensatory adjustment within the central mechanism [37]. The blurring of vision that happens when a patient moves their head is another issue for those with bilateral vestibular dysfunction. Even after completing a series of gaze stabilization exercises, oscillopsia is a complaint reported by about 70% of patients with bilateral vestibular loss [38].

23.9 Assessment of Ototoxicity-Related Vestibular Loss

Rotatory chair testing (RCT) is accepted as the gold standard test for bilateral vestibular loss. This is because, in contrast to the caloric test, which evaluates only the extremely low frequencies, and the vHIT test, which evaluates only the high frequencies, it examines responses ranging from high to low frequencies (i.e., high to low acceleration). The equipment required for successfully executing RCT is expensive, hence its availability is primarily limited to major centers [39].

The caloric portion of videonystagmography (VNG) is sensitive to bilateral vestibular impairment. Because warm and cool water caloric testing delivers a thermal stimulus, which is typically described that corresponds to an oscillation frequency of 0.003 Hz, it is commonly referred to as a "low-frequency test," which explains its sensitivity for bilateral vestibular loss [40].

The vHIT has several advantages including its ability to evaluate all six semicircular canals, speed of performance, and relative difficulty in changing with medicine or uncooperative patients. Additionally, the equipment costs considerably less than the rotatory chair device. Nevertheless, because the vHIT test is not intended to detect low-frequency vestibular responses (in the vHIT, 2.5 Hz is the primary stimulation frequency), it is not as sensitive as the RCT [41].

There are currently two different kinds of vestibular evoked myogenic potentials (VEMPs) available. The first is cervical VEMP (cVEMP), mostly reflecting the sacculo-collic reflex and recorded in the sternocleidomastoid muscle. The other is ocular VEMP (oVEMP), which primarily represents the utriculo-ocular reflex and is often recorded from the obliquus inferior muscle [42]. VEMPs can assist in differentiating between disorders with incomplete lesions, such as bilateral vestibular neuritis, and disorders affecting the entire inner ear, such as gentamicin ototoxicity, which can cause bilateral vestibular loss [39].

While sensitive to bilateral vestibular loss, computerized dynamic posturography lacks specificity since it cannot differentiate bilateral vestibular loss from a number of significant and more prevalent neurological causes of imbalance such as ataxia from cerebellar lesions [39].

Individuals who have been exposed to ototoxic substances should also be closely monitored in order to ensure early detection and intervention for any potential vestibular damage. However, there are no widely accepted guidelines for monitoring vestibular function before, during, or after exposure to potentially ototoxic drugs. This is partly due to the high cost of the required laboratory equipment. Moreover, patients receiving ototoxic medications may be too unwell to undergo comprehensive testing [43].

23.10 Management of Ototoxicity-Related Vestibular Loss

Different etiologies including ototoxicity can cause bilateral vestibular hypofunction. The main concerns of patients with bilateral vestibular loss are balance and gait problems. Vestibular rehabilitation has been shown to be effective in improving postural stability and reducing the sense of disequilibrium for individuals with bilateral vestibular loss. Additionally, it can enhance visual acuity during head movements, allowing people with bilateral vestibular loss to regain a sense of normalcy in their daily lives [44, 45].

Vestibular rehabilitation is a crucial element of any program designed to address vestibular ototoxicity. Vestibular rehabilitation is a specialized form of exercise-based therapy aimed at alleviating both primary and secondary symptoms of vestibular disorders. The vestibular rehabilitation program typically includes a combination of gaze stabilization, habituation, and postural stabilization exercises. Each exercise plays a crucial role in the overall rehabilitation process, helping individuals regain their vestibular function and improve their quality of life. Activities of daily living, gait, and endurance exercises should be added to the rehabilitation program [46].

Gaze stability exercises are designed using the principles of vestibular-ocular reflex adaptation and substitution. These exercises are often known as adaptation and substitution exercises. Adaptation exercises involve making long-term changes in the neuronal response to head movements. The ultimate aim is to alleviate symptoms and restore normal gaze and postural stability. The purpose of adaptation exercises is to create long-term alterations in the vestibular system's neural response to a specific error signal, known as retinal slip. The ultimate goals of these exercises are to minimize visual blurring during head movements, enhance postural stability, and alleviate symptoms associated with vestibular dysfunction. Substitution exercises are designed to help patients develop alternative strategies to compensate for any loss or impairment of their vestibular function. These exercises aim to enhance gaze stability while moving the head. Gaze stability exercises are essential for patients with a lack of vestibulo-ocular reflex function, such as those with bilateral vestibular loss (e.g., vestibulotoxicity). These exercises help improve the patient's ability to maintain visual focus and stability, which can greatly impact their daily activities and quality of life. Habituation exercises involve gradually exposing individuals to the stimuli that trigger their symptoms to reduce their sensitivity over time [38, 47]. Habituation refers to the process of becoming accustomed to a specific stimulus that causes dizziness through repeated exposure. This systematic repetition of provocative movements can lead to a significant decrease in symptoms and an overall improvement in well-being. Cawthorne and Cooksey developed the first exercise program based on habituation in the 1940's [48, 49]. In addition, these programs often incorporate specific exercises to improve coordination and stability while walking or engaging in various daily activities. These exercises are designed to enhance overall balance and gait function, promoting better mobility and reducing the risk of falls. Balance and gait training exercises focus on using visual and somatosensory cues to compensate for the lack of vestibular function. These exercises aim to improve stability and coordination by training the body to rely on alternative sensory inputs [38, 50].

There is no specific vestibular rehabilitation program designed for patients with ototoxicity-related vestibular loss. Treatment approaches are tailored according to the findings of the vestibular assessment, the patient's symptoms and concerns, initial assessment before therapy, and the patient's overall health and physical capabilities. The primary goals of this therapy include reducing symptoms and functional limitations, improving mobility and self-sufficiency, and lowering the likelihood of falls and harm. Examples of exercises that can be included in the vestibular rehabilitation program of patients with vestibular problems due to vestibulotoxicity are reported in Table 23.3.

The issues to be considered when creating a vestibular rehabilitation program are as follows:

Table 23.3 Some exercises to improve gaze stability, postüral stability, and gait

A piece of paper with writing on it (foveal target) is glued to the wall at a distance that the patient can read. The patient turns his head slightly to the right and left while continuing to look at the paper. The same exercise is repeated by moving the head up and down. This exercise can be performed 3 times a day for 1 minute at the beginning. Duration, frequency, and speed of head movements should be increased over time.
Two targets with a distance between them are placed in front of the patient. It is important that both targets are in the line of sight. The patient first looks at the target with his eyes and then turns his head toward the target. Then it performs the same operation by looking at the other target. Duration, frequency, and speed of head movements should be increased over time.
A target is placed in front of the patient. After looking at the target, the patient closes his eyes and turns his head. Meanwhile, he imagines that he is still looking toward the target. When he opens his eyes, the fact that he is looking towards the target will mean that the exercise is done correctly.
The patient stands on a hard surface with his eyes open and his feet shoulder-width apart. To make the exercise difficult, the patient can close his eyes, bring his feet closer, or stand on a soft surface. Exercises that include eye–head movements can also be added.
In the acute phase, the patient should be encouraged to walk. To make the exercise more difficult, head movements should be added, or the patient may be asked to count the days of the week while walking, asked to walk on a narrower surface/on a soft surface, or asked to turn around while walking, or asked to walk outdoors, for example in a shopping mall.

1. Therapy should be started as early as possible. Some researchers have shown that early vestibular exercises lead to reduced symptoms and improved postural stability [51, 52].
2. Eye–head movements should be included in the exercise program for habituation and adaptation to take place.
3. Exercises should be for brief periods in the beginning but gradually extended over time depending on the general health status of the patient.
4. The frequency and difficulty of the exercises should be increased over time (either from session to session or within a session).
5. The speed of head movements should be increased gradually.
6. The exercises should be planned to be performed in a variety of positions and activities (e.g., head movements exercises can be performed first while sitting, then standing, and finally walking.)
7. The rehabilitation program should initially be planned to include visual and/or somatosensory input, but these inputs should be reduced over time (e.g., balance exercises can be performed with eyes open and then eyes closed.).
8. Exercises may initially cause symptoms to increase. The patient should be encouraged to continue with exercises.
9. The patient should be informed that the recovery process will take time.

10. Exercises should be performed within the functional limits of the patient.
11. As the rehabilitation process progresses, exercises should be performed using distracting stimuli (e.g., mental tasks such as counting by twos up to 100).

23.11 Conclusion

Systemic chemotherapy is one of the most important parts of breast cancer treatment, but drugs with side effects must be used to eliminate the potentially life-threatening risk. There is a substantial concern regarding the possibility of inner ear damage caused by toxic agents in cancer patients receiving treatment with medications (e.g., chemotherapy) that could result in hearing loss and/or vestibular loss. It is vital to understand that the level of damage is not definite, highlighting the significance of monitoring both auditory and vestibular function throughout and after the use of ototoxic medications in treatment. Early detection of damage due to ototoxicity is a necessary prerequisite for early intervention. In breast cancer patients who develop inner ear damage due to chemotherapy, auditory and/or vestibular rehabilitation should be started at an early stage in order to maintain the patient's communication skills, manage vestibular loss-related symptoms, and improve overall quality of life.

References

1. Steyger PS. Mechanisms of Ototoxicity & Otoprotection. Otolaryngol Clin N Am. 2021;54(6):1101. https://doi.org/10.1016/j.otc.2021.08.007.
2. Paken J, Govender CD, Sewram V. Research protocol: Cisplatin-associated ototoxicity amongst patients receiving cancer chemotherapy and the feasibility of an audiological monitoring program. BMC Womens Health. 2017;17(129):129. https://doi.org/10.1186/s12905-017-0486-8.
3. Landier W. Ototoxicity and cancer therapy. Cancer. 2016;122(11):1647–58. https://doi.org/10.1002/cncr.29779.
4. Roland PS, Rutka JA, editors. Ototoxicity. Hamilton, London: BC Decker Inc.; 2004.
5. Jamesdaniel S, Coling D, Hinduja S, Ding D, Li J, Cassidy L, Seigel GM, Qu J, Salvi R. Cisplatin-induced ototoxicity is mediated by nitroxidative modification of cochlear proteins characterized by nitration of Lmo4. J Biol Chem. 2012;287(22):18674–86. https://doi.org/10.1074/jbc.M111.297960.
6. Xuan L, et al. Ototoxicity in patients with invasive ductal breast cancer who were treated with docetaxel: report of two cases. Cancer Biol Ther. 2020;21(11):990–3.
7. Ridwelski K, Gebauer T, Fahlke J, Kröning H, Kettner E, Meyer F, Eichelmann K, Lippert H. Combination chemotherapy with docetaxel and cisplatin for locally advanced and metastatic gastric cancer. Ann Oncol. 2001;12(1):47–51. https://doi.org/10.1023/A:1008328501128.
8. Gratton MA, Smyth BJ. Ototoxicity of platinum compounds. In: Roland PS, Rutka JA, editors. Ototoxicity. Hamilton, London: BC Decker Inc.; 2004.
9. Rybak LP. Ototoxicity of loop diuretics. Otolaryngol Clin N Am. 1993;26:829–44.
10. Dong Y, Ding D, Jiang H, Shi J, Salvi R, Roth JA. Ototoxicity of paclitaxel in rat cochlear organotypic cultures. Toxicol Appl Pharm. 2014;280(3):526–33. https://doi.org/10.1016/j.taap.2014.08.022.
11. Gelfand SA. Essentials of audiology. New York: Thieme Medical Publishers, Inc; 2009.
12. Kramer S, Brown DK. Audiology science to practise. San Diego: Plural Publishing, Inc; 2019.
13. Musiek FE, Baran JA, Shinn JB, Jones RA. Disorders of the auditory system. San Diego: Plural Publishing, Inc; 2012.
14. Campbell KCM. Audiologic monitoring for Ototoxicity. In: Roland PS, Rutka JA, editors. Ototoxicity. Hamilton, London: BC Decker Inc.; 2004.
15. Campbell KCM, Durrant JD. Audiologic monitoring for ototoxicity. Otolaryngol Clin N Am. 1993;26:903–14.
16. American Speech-Language-Hearing Association (ASHA). Guidelines for the audiologic management of individuals receiving cochleotoxic drug therapy. ASHA. 1994;36(suppl 12):11–9.
17. Fausti SA, Henry JA, Schaffer HI, Olson DJ, Frey RH, McDonald WJ. High-frequency audiometric monitoring for early detection of aminoglycoside ototoxicity. J Infect Dis. 1992;165:1026–32.
18. Fausti SA, Henry JA, Schaffer HI, Olson DJ, Frey RH, Bagby GC. High-frequency monitoring for early detection of cisplatin ototoxicity. Arch Otolaryngol Head Neck Surg. 1993;119:661–8.
19. Durrant JD, Rodgers G, Meyers EN, Johnson JT. Hearing loss risk factor for cisplatin ototoxicity? Observations. Am J Otol. 1990;11:375–7.
20. Dhar S, Hall JW. Otoacoustic emissions: principles, procedures, and protocols. San Diego: Plural Publishing, Inc; 2012.
21. Katz J, Chasin M, English K, Hood LJ, Tillery KL. Handbook of clinical audiology. Wolters Kluwer Health; 2015.

22. Lonsbury-Martin BL, Martin GK. Evoked otoacoustic emissions as objective screeners for ototoxicity. Semin Hear. 2001;22:377–91.
23. Zorowka PG, Schmitt HJ, Gutjahr P. Evoked otoacoustic emissions and pure tone threshold audiometry in patients receiving cisplatinum therapy. Int J Pediatr Otorhinolaryngol. 1993;25:73–80.
24. Mulheran M, Degg C. Comparison of distortion product OAE generation between a group requiring frequent gentamicin therapy and control subjects. Br J Audiol. 1997;31:5–9.
25. Kreitmayer C, Marcrum SC, Picou EM, Steffens T, Kummer P. Subclinical conductive hearing loss significantly reduces otoacoustic emission amplitude: implications for test performance. Int J Pediatr Otorhinolaryngol. 2019 Aug;123:195–201.
26. Suckfüll M, Schneewei S, Dreher A, Schorn K. Evaluation of TEOAE and DPOAE measurements for the assessment of auditory thresholds in sensorineural hearing loss. Acta Otolaryngol. 1996;116:528–33.
27. Stover L, Norton SJ. The effects of aging on oto-acoustic emissions. J Acoust Soc Am. 1993;94:2670–81.
28. Katbamna B, Homnick DN, Marks JH. Effects of chronic tobramycin treatment on distortion product otoacoustic emissions. Ear Hear. 1999;20:393–402.
29. Konrad-Martin D, Helt WJ, Reavis KM, Gordon JS, Coleman LL, Bratt GW, Fausti SA. Ototoxicity: early detection and monitoring. The ASHA Leader Archieve. 2005;10(7):1–14.
30. Dillon H. Hearing aids. New York: Thieme Medical Publishers, Inc; 2012.
31. Mueller HG, Ricketts T, Bentler R. Modern hearing aids pre-fitting testing and selection considerations. San Diego: Plural Publishing, Inc; 2014.
32. Iseli C, Buchman CA. Management of children with severe, severe-profound, and profound sensorineural hearing loss. Otolaryngol Clin N Am. 2015;48(6):995–1010.
33. Naples JG, Ruckenstein MJ. Cochlear implant. Otolaryngol Clin N Am. 2020 Feb;53(1):87–102.
34. Schvartz-Leyzac KC, Colesa DJ, Swiderski DL, Raphael Y, Pfingst BE. Cochlear health and Cochlear-implant function. J Assoc Res Otolaryngol. 2023 Feb;24(1):5–29.
35. Woodson EA, Reiss LA, Turner CW, Gfeller K, Gantz BJ. The hybrid cochlear implant: a review. Adv Otorhinolaryngol. 2010;67:125–34.
36. Compton CL. Assistive devices. Semin Hear. 1989;10(1):31–41.
37. Kisilevsky VE, Tomlinson RD, Ranalli PJ, Prepageran N. Monitoring vestibular ototoxicity. In: Roland PS, Rutka JA, editors. Ototoxicity. Hamilton, London: BC Decker Inc.; 2004.
38. Herdman SJ, Clendaniel RA, editors. Vestibular rehabilitation. 4th ed. Philadelphia: FA Davis Co.; 2014.
39. Hain TC, Cherchi M, Yacovino DA. Bilateral vestibular weakness. Front Neurol. 2018;9:344–58.
40. Goncalves DU, Felipe L, Lima TM. Interpretation and use of caloric testing. Braz J Otorhinolaryngol. 2008;74:440–6.
41. McGarvie LA, MacDougall HG, Halmagyi GM, Burgess AM, Weber KP, Curthoys IS. The video head impulse test (vHIT) of semicircular canal function—age-dependent normative values of VOR gain in healthy subjects. Front Neurol. 2015;6:154.
42. Murofushi T. Clinical application of vestibular evoked myogenic potential (VEMP). Auris Nasus Larynx. 2016 Aug;43(4):367–76.
43. Handelsman JA. Vestibulotoxicity: strategies for clinical diagnosis and rehabilitation. Int J Audiol. 2018;57:S69–77.
44. Brown KE, Whitney SL, Wrisley DM, Furman JM. Physical therapy outcomes for persons with bilateral vestibular loss. Laryngoscope. 2001;111:1812.
45. Herdman SJ, Hall CD, Schubert M, Das VE, Tusa RJ. Recovery of dynamic visual acuity in patients with bilateral vestibular hypofunction. Arch Otolaryngol Head Neck Surg. 2007;133(4):383.
46. Hall CD, Herdman SJ, Whitney SL, Cass SP, Clendaniel RA, Fife TD, Furman JM, Getchius TSD, Goebel JA, Shepard NT, Woodhouse SN. Vestibular rehabilitation for peripheral vestibular hypofunction: an evidence-based clinical practice guideline. The American Physical Therapy Association Neurology Section. 2016;40(2):124–55.
47. Herdman SJ. Vestibular rehabilitation. Curr Opin Neurol. 2013;26(1):96–101.
48. Cawthorne T. The physiological basis for head exercises. J Chart Soc Physiother. 1944;30:106.
49. Cooksey FS. Rehabilitation in vestibular injuries. Pro Royal Soc Med. 1946;39:273.
50. Desmond A. Vestibular function: evaluation and treatment. New York: Thieme Medical Publishers, Inc; 2004.
51. Vereeck L, Wuyts FL, Truijen S, De Valck C, Van de Heyning PH. The effect of early customized vestibular rehabilitation on balance after acoustic neuroma resection. Clin Rehabil. 2008;22(8):698.
52. Teggi R, Caldirola D, Fabiano B, Recanati P, Bussi M. Rehabilitation after acute vestibular disorders. J Laryngol Otol. 2009;123(4):397.

Sleep Problems and Management of Breast Cancer

24

Songül Çağlar

24.1 Sleep Problems in Breast Cancer Patients During Treatment

Sleep disorder is one of the most significant problems of breast cancer patients [1]. These disorders are common among breast cancer patients and are determinants of life quality [2, 3]. There are various physiological and psychological reasons why sleep disorders are common in patients with breast cancer. Anxiety experienced before chemotherapy, fatigue, and perceived stress during the treatment process are circumstances that trigger sleep disorders in patients [4]. In a study conducted with breast cancer patients receiving chemotherapy, the determination of a relationship between the patient's depression and anxiety and their sleep quality also supports this information [1].

Although sleep disorders are generally more common in women with breast cancer who receive chemotherapy or radiotherapy, it is difficult to draw a clear conclusion about surgical treatment and hormonal treatment [5, 6]. Circadian rhythm disorder occurs in women during chemotherapy treatment [7]. In addition, chemotherapy treatment is associated with anxiety, which causes disruption of sleep patterns in patients undergoing chemotherapy [8]. Nevertheless, breast cancer patients with lymphedema may experience various sleep disorders depending on the management of lymphedema [9]. Sleep problems in cancer patients receiving hormone therapy (aromatase inhibitors, etc.) can occur due to drug-induced menopausal symptoms, and approximately 94% of breast cancer survivors may experience one or more side effects, including sleep disorders, during or after endocrine therapy [10].

Sleep quality deteriorates in many breast cancer patients, whether metastasized or not [11, 12]. According to the results of a meta-analysis study, the global prevalence of poor sleep quality in breast cancer patients was identified as 62% [13]. It means that almost one in every two women with breast cancer has poor sleep quality.

24.2 Sleep Problems in Breast Cancer Patients After Treatment

Insomnia may be considered an independent risk factor for future depression in females who survive breast cancer [14]. Sleep can impact the quality of life (QoL) during cancer treatment, and symptoms related to poor sleep may worsen. Insomnia may lead to severe and undesirable consequences for individuals. The adverse

S. Çağlar (✉)
Faculty of Health Sciences, Department of Nursing, Bolu Abant İzzet Baysal University, Bolu, Turkey

Y. Bakar, A. Tuğral (eds.), *Managing Side Effects of Breast Cancer Treatment*,
https://doi.org/10.1007/978-3-031-75480-7_24

impacts of cancer-related insomnia (CRI) include depression, anxiety, fatigue, aggressive pain, impaired immune function, reduced quality of life, and even increased cancer-related deaths [12].

Sleep disorders may continue after completion of breast cancer treatment finishes and may even be more common in some people [15]. Temporary sleep problems can become permanent in approximately 60% of patients who are undergoing chemotherapy [16]. The results of a planned cross-sectional study show that sleep problems gradually increase during breast cancer treatment, and when the treatment finishes, this rate gradually increases compared to both during and before treatment [17]. Younger age, lower education level, lower income, obesity, and lymphedema may be risk factors for experiencing sleep disorders after treatment [15].

Excessive subjective insomnia may occur in many breast cancer survivors, and some breast cancer survivors need sleep improvement interventions more than others [11]. Sleep problems continue to be frequent in breast cancer patients even after completion of chemotherapy [18]. Cancer-related sleep problems may continue for the first three years or even longer after completion of treatment [10, 19, 20]. Therefore, to improve the quality of life of patients, these patients should be followed closely for sleep problems for at least three years after treatment. Also, it should be taken due precautions because sleep problems can closely affect survival by causing circadian disruption and immune and metabolic disorders [16]. Insomnia has a significant impact on cancer patients' QoL [3]. It was shown that it has been reported. That better sleep efficiency and fewer sleep disruptions are essential independent prognostic factors in women with advanced breast cancer [16]. Addressing physical symptoms (e.g., vasomotor symptoms and pain) and providing education about behavioral, social, environmental, and medical factors that affect sleep can significantly improve the quality of life of breast cancer survivors [11]. Therefore, early diagnosis and appropriate management of sleep disorders are vital to improve the quality of life and survival of breast cancer patients [3].

24.3 Diagnosis and Detection of Sleep Disorders in Breast Cancer Patients

24.3.1 Insomnia

The most frequently studied sleep disorder in breast cancer patients is insomnia [14]. Its prevalence varies between 3% and 32% [6]. The frequency, severity, and pattern of insomnia symptoms may vary between different types of cancer and treatment regimens. It does not come across a standard assessment tool that is used routinely to evaluate insomnia in the literature [21]. The first attempt at assessing insomnia is a structured clinical interview. During the interview, all significant factors that may interfere with sleep are covered, including nighttime symptoms (type, frequency, and duration), daytime symptoms (degree of sleepiness and extent of daytime consequences), presence of comorbid conditions (mental or medical or other sleep disorder), and the patient's daytime lifestyle (e.g., substance use, work schedule, school, social activities, light exposure, eating habits, exercise, and preferred bedtime and wake-up times), need to be evaluated [22]. In addition, the use of questionnaires and scales that have been validated and reliable can help healthcare professionals when diagnosing sleep disorders. The Insomnia Severity Index (ISI) for insomnia is a 7-item questionnaire assessing the perceived severity of insomnia over the past two weeks. The scale evaluates difficulty in falling asleep, maintaining sleep, and frequency of early morning awakenings, alongside the degree of dissatisfaction with current sleep [23]. A clinical cutoff score of 8 provides maximum sensitivity and specificity for detecting sleep difficulties (score 8–14 = Possible Insomnia) [21]. Another measurement tool that can be used for insomnia is the Women's Health Initiative Insomnia Rating Scale (WHIIRS). However, this tool was primarily developed to assess the insomnia status of postmenopausal women. WHIIRS, a short five-item scale, requires individuals to rate their sleep quality and the frequency of experiencing particular sleep problems and is suitable for either research or clinical use [24]. After the evaluation with ISI and WHIIRS subjective measurement tools for insomnia, a more detailed examination can be performed with Polysomnography or Actigraphy if it is supposed to be used [21, 25]. However, evaluation can be made using both subjective and objective sleep tools together.

24.3.2 Obstructive Sleep Apnea

The prevalence of obstructive sleep apnea (OSA) is high, especially in postmenopausal women with breast cancer. Since OSA may affect the quality of life and surgical risks, it is significant to perform screening on these people and to provide the necessary intervention if detected [26]. In a study conducted with women hospitalized with the diagnosis of primary breast cancer, the most common sleep problem was determined to be OSA (70.5%). Additionally, patients with sleep disorders were found to be more likely to experience complications than those without [27]. The gold standard for the diagnosis of OSA is polysomnography in cancer patients [19]. However, along with polysomnography, the High STOP-Bang score can be used as a subjective measuring tool [19, 26]. The STOP-Bang questionnaire is a measurement tool used to screen patients for OSA [28]. It is a scoring model consisting of eight questions and scored based on Yes/No answers (score: 1/0). Therefore, scores range from 0 to 8. A score of ≥3 indicates high sensitivity in detecting OSA: 93% and 100% for moderate and severe OSA, respectively [28].

24.3.3 Poor Sleep Quality

Level of depression and duration of cancer are critical determinants of sleep quality [3]. Sleep quality tends to decrease gradually throughout breast cancer treatment [29]. Therefore, the sleep quality of patients should be evaluated at least three times: before, during, and after treatment. In addition, patients' sleep quality and depression situation should also be assessed, as they are related. The Pittsburgh Sleep Quality Index (PSQI) can be considered the gold standard for quality of sleep. It is seen that PSQI is used most frequently in studies [1, 18, 21]. The scale, developed in 1998, consists of seven components (sleep disorder, onset latency, sleep duration, sleep disorder, sleep efficiency, general sleep quality, daytime dysfunction, and use of sleeping medication). A global score ranging between 0 and 21 is also calculated. Since each score results from a subjective sleep complaint, higher scores indicate worse sleep quality [30]. The PSQI has good reliability and validity and is widely used in general medical and psychiatric studies. An overall score of ≥5 indicates poor sleep quality. It has been recommended that the cut-off score for breast cancer patients be 8 [31].

24.3.4 Excessive Daytime Sleepiness (EDS)

According to a meta-analysis study, the prevalence of EDS is 24% in breast cancer patients [13]. This rate shows that even if the patient does not complain, the clinician should screen the patient for EDS. Epworth Sleepiness Scale (ESS) is a simple self-report scale used to evaluate daytime sleepiness [19, 32]. Total values range from 2 to 10, with scores >14 indicating prominent levels of daytime sleepiness. It is often preferred to measure sleepiness in breast cancer patients [19, 33]. The scale asks the participant to rate the likelihood of falling asleep in various situations, such as reading a book, watching television, sitting still in a public place, or driving in a car. A study in which breast cancer patients were followed up before surgery and for six months following surgery showed that although there was a slight increase in women's daytime sleepiness for up to three months before surgery, followed by a gradual decrease, it kept going for a long time

[34]. However, sleepiness was evaluated with the DS sub-dimension of the General Sleep Disturbance Scale in the study (GSDS) [34].

24.4 Interventions to Manage Sleep Problems in Breast Cancer Patients During and After Treatment

It is common among breast cancer survivors to use medications to manage sleep problems. However, this situation may also bring with it various health risks. In a study conducted with approximately 22,000 women who survived breast cancer, it was determined that the risk of fracture increased with the use of sleeping pills [35]. Therefore, choosing non-pharmacological methods instead of pharmacological remedies may be more appropriate in the management of sleep problems of these patients. Developing sleep quality can increase compliance with treatments, improve patients' quality of life, and prevent complications in patients with hormone-related cancer.

24.4.1 Exercises

Both physical and mind-body exercises are essential interventions to improve personal sleep quality in breast cancer patients [36]. A supervised exercise practice may improve the sleep quality of female breast cancer survivors by reducing sleep disorders and daytime dysfunction symptoms [37]. However, uncontrolled exercises may not be efficient in improving sleep quality. Breast cancer patients can get positive results in their sleep quality when they plan exercise using mobile applications. However, there are few resources to support this in the literature. As a result of a mixed design study conducted by Zhu et al. [38]. With seventeen women receiving radiotherapy and chemotherapy, it was found that the application called "Yun Dong RuKang" was efficient in improving the sleep quality of women.

24.5 Physical Exercises

24.5.1 Progressive Relaxation Exercises

Progressive relaxation exercises are self-performed exercises aimed at reducing tension in the body. During exercise, large muscle groups are systematically tensed and relaxed in the body. These exercises can help cancer patients gain a positive life by changing mental processes and behavior to control expected or unexpected symptoms during the disease process [39]. According to studies, progressive relaxation exercises are efficient for improving sleep quality in breast cancer patients.

24.5.2 Endurance Exercises

According to a systematic review, endurance training in combination with resistance training significantly improves sleep quality. Endurance training combined with resistance training has been shown to achieve superior sleep quality results compared to stretching exercises [40].

24.5.3 Pilates

Regular physical exercise is a significant complementary treatment method to the clinical treatment of breast cancer, which reduces the adverse effects of treatment with adjuvant hormone therapy [41]. Considering the pre- or postoperative lifestyles of women with breast cancer, Pilates exercise may be a complementary intervention in addition to standard treatment [42]. There is evidence that Pilates improves sleep quality in healthy adults [43]. Furthermore, Pilates practices are a secure way for breast cancer patients [41]. In a randomized controlled study conducted by Leite et al. [44], it was determined that the sleep quality of women who did mat Pilates for six months increased.

24.5.4 Dance

Cultural dances may also be beneficial in managing sleep problems in women receiving breast cancer treatment. It was determined that women in dance practice experienced less fatigue and sleep problems at the end of the intervention in a randomized controlled study of 16-week dance practice with Chinese women receiving adjuvant chemotherapy [45]. In another study in which a 6-week tango program was applied, it was determined that there was an improvement of nearly 10% in the sleep quality of 50 breast cancer patients [46]. This benefit was even more significant in women who were on endocrine therapy, were obese, or had no previous dance experience [46]. However, there are also some studies where dance is not efficient. In a nonrandomized clinical study involving 21 breast cancer survivors, a 12-week mixed dance intervention was determined to have no impact on sleep quality [47].

24.6 Mind–Body Exercises

24.6.1 Yoga

Yoga consists of practices involving physical movements (asana), special breathing techniques (pranayama), and deep concentration (meditation). These practices increase the innate immune response, interrupt inflammation, and thus prevent the emergence of chronic diseases [48]. Originating in India, yoga has been practiced for more than five thousand years and is now considered an effective method for improving health alongside preventing and managing diseases [48, 49]. Numerous studies have demonstrated that yoga is particularly effective on the endocrine system and hormonal balance [49]. Yoga and meditation regulate neurotransmitters, neuropeptides, hormones, and cytokines that mediate interactions between the central nervous and the immune system [48]. Also, the release of the hormone melatonin is affected positively by yoga practices [49]. Especially, people who practice pranayama may experience an increase in their blood melatonin levels. Yoga can be considered a sufficient practice for sleep and related disorders as it reduces stress and supports the release of melatonin [48, 50]. It was determined that yoga was beneficial in managing the sleep problems of women with sleep problems [51]. There are also many studies investigating the relationship between yoga and cancer-related fatigue and sleep quality in patients with breast cancer [52, 53]. According to a recent meta-analysis, yoga can positively affect sleep quality by relieving fatigue and improving negative emotions among breast cancer survivors [53]. However, to obtain positive results in sleep quality, an intervention period of at least 6–8 weeks should be taken into consideration, and during the yoga exercise process, consultation with a doctor or professional health trainer should be taken into account, depending on their condition, to ensure that their physical condition is suitable for yoga exercise [53].

24.7 Psychological Interventions

Sleep disorders may be associated with anxiety and depression in cancer patients [1]. Therefore, psychological interventions are effective in managing both the psychological problems and sleep disorders of these people.

24.7.1 Cognitive Behavioral Therapy

Cognitive behavioral therapy (CBT) is among the non-pharmacological interventions used to cope with medical side effects, improve quality of life, and reduce emotional distress in cancer patients [54]. The use of CBTs in recent years, especially in the treatment of insomnia, has led to the development of CBT-I, a cognitive behavioral therapy for insomnia [21]. Cognitive behavioral therapies can be applied together with bright light treatment as a combination [55, 56]. CBT can contribute to sleep quality, especially by affecting general dysfunctional sleep beliefs [56].

24.7.2 Mindfulness

Mindfulness can be considered for insomnia treatment after cognitive behavioral therapy [21]. For mindfulness practice to improve personal sleep quality, it should be planned two or more times a week for more than three months, and the total intervention duration should be more than 24 hours [57]. In a study conducted with active breast cancer patients receiving chemotherapy, the intervention group was administered an online mindfulness-based stress reduction intervention consisting of four two-hour sessions for four weeks. At the end of the experiment, it was determined that the sleep quality of the intervention group increased at the end of the intervention, and it was preserved for two months [58].

24.8 Complementary and Supportive Therapies

24.8.1 Acupuncture

Acupuncture is a holistic method that addresses multiple symptoms and side effects in a single therapy. Acupuncture is a modality of traditional Chinese medicine (TCM). Acupuncture involves the insertion of thin, disposable, sterile needles into acupuncture points that access channels to balance the body's essential energy. Acupuncture is especially effective for managing insomnia associated with chemotherapy. Thus, it may reduce the use of sleep medications in breast cancer patients [59].

24.8.2 Aromatherapy

24.8.2.1 Lavender Oil

Lavender oil is considered a preferred, reliable, non-pharmaceutical application to improve sleep quality and make it easier to fall asleep. Lavender is often favored as inhalation aromatherapy in cancer patients [60]. However, it is difficult to say that lavender oil has a significant benefit on the sleep quality of breast cancer patients. Studies generally indicate that it does not improve sleep quality compared to regular care [61]. According to a randomized controlled study, in the microvascular breast reconstruction setting, lavender oil did not have any side effects or complications and did not provide a measurable advantage on anxiety and sleep measures compared to the control group [62]. In this sense, it can be used for breast cancer survivors if desired.

24.8.2.2 Ayurveda

Ayurveda is a holistic approach that is customizable to the individual through a range of therapies, including special diets, massages, and herbs. In a case study, it was determined that the sleep quality of a patient with breast cancer increased after a 14-week Ayurveda application [63]. However, based on the results of this study conducted on a single person, it is not proper to comment that Ayurveda will increase sleep quality. More randomized controlled studies with larger sample groups are needed to clearly reveal the effects of Ayurveda on sleep quality and insomnia.

24.8.3 Pharmacotherapy

24.8.3.1 Hypnotics

For the treatment of insomnia, the "z-drugs" zopiclone, zolpidem, eszopiclone, and zaleplon were introduced in the 1980s [64]. While hypnotics remain the most commonly prescribed treatment for insomnia, their use should be limited to ≤2 weeks [21]. Studies reporting safe use are generally in this range [65]. The effect of triazolam was measured in three consecutive evenings. For this reason, it is unclear what side effects will occur if used for longer than this period. Also, patients who are given sedative–hypnotic drugs during adjuvant chemotherapy for breast cancer are at risk of becoming long-term users of these drugs after the chemotherapy has ended.

24.8.4 Melatonin Replacement Therapy

Low levels of serum melatonin closely affect the sleep quality of breast cancer patients. In a study conducted with 45 breast cancer patients between the ages of 25 and 65, a relationship was found between melatonin level and sleep quality [66]. Therefore, melatonin supplementation may be considered in patients with low melatonin levels. Various treatments and strategies, including melatonin supplementation, have been proposed to improve breast cancer patients' sleep and quality of life. Melatonin may be a good option for managing sleep problems in cancer patients and cancer survivors where appropriate non-pharmacological options are limited [21]. Melatonin [N-acetyl-5-methoxytryptamine] is a hormone synthesized and secreted by the pineal gland mainly at night. Melatonin, which helps regulate sleep patterns and circadian rhythms, functions in oncostatic, hypnotic, immune regulation, reproduction, puberty timing, mood disorders, and transplantation with its antioxidant, anti-stimulating, and anti-inflammatory effects [67]. Although melatonin deficiency is also associated with the development of breast cancer, it can be said that it is a significant factor that should be included in post-cancer treatment planning. According to a systematic review, melatonin supplementation was determined to have a moderate effect on improving sleep quality in breast cancer patients. Pooled data from studies on melatonin supplementation indicate that melatonin administration may alleviate sleep problems associated with treatments in breast cancer patients [68]. Although there is no clear information on the daily melatonin level, it is usually used as 2–20 mg [21].

24.8.5 Phototherapy

24.8.5.1 Bright Light Therapy

Bright light therapy is effective in reducing common symptoms experienced by individuals with cancer, such as fatigue, and improves patients' quality of life [69]. Additionally, it improves the circadian rhythm [7]. Bright light therapy is a form of treatment that leads to an improvement in mood and, accordingly, an improvement in depressive symptoms, has a regulatory effect on circadian rhythm, increases the impact of antidepressant drugs, and leads to progress in sleep quality [70]. Bright light therapy improves sleep quality in breast cancer patients both during chemotherapy and at the end of treatment. Studies show that bright light therapy should take at least 30 minutes to obtain positive results in sleep quality [7, 71]. It was determined that 30 minutes of light therapy a day for 21 days in women receiving chemotherapy led to shorter sleep latency, longer total sleep time, and higher sleep efficiency [69]. Although bright light therapy applied in the morning hours is effective on sleep quality, people's chronotype should be considered when planning treatment. This kind of planning can increase the effect of the treatment. A dichromatically adapted light therapy appears to provide significant improvement in fatigue and sleep disturbance in women who survive 1 to 3 years after completion of chemotherapy and/or radiation therapy for stage I to III breast cancer [72].

References

1. El Kherchi O, Aquil A, Elkhoudri N, Guerroumi M, El Azmaoui N, Mouallif M, et al. Relationship between sleep quality and anxiety-depressive disorders in Moroccan Women with breast cancer: A cross-sectional study. Iran J Public Health. 2023;52(7):1457–65.
2. Elamin N, Althebity N, Alkhamisi TA, Al-Foheidi M. Sleep quality and psychological disorders in breast cancer female patients receiving radiotherapy at a tertiary oncology center in West Saudi Arabia. Support Care Cancer. 2024;32(3):163.
3. Perrier J, Duivon M, Clochon P, Rehel S, Doidy F, Grellard JM, et al. Sleep macro- and microstructure in breast cancer survivors. Sci Rep. 2022;12(1):2557.
4. Yang GS, Starkweather AR, Lynch Kelly D, Meegan T, Byon HD, Lyon DE. Longitudinal analysis of sleep disturbance in breast cancer survivors. Nurs Res. 2022;71(3):177.
5. Costa AR, Fontes F, Pereira S, Gonçalves M, Azevedo A, Lunet N. Impact of breast cancer treatments on sleep disturbances—A systematic review. Breast. 2014;23(6):697–709.
6. Van Onselen C, Cooper BA, Lee K, Dunn L, Aouizerat BE, West C, et al. Identification of distinct subgroups of breast cancer patients based on self-reported changes in sleep disturbance. Support Care Cancer. 2012;20(10):2611–9.
7. Neikrug AB, Rissling M, Trofimenko V, Liu L, Natarajan L, Lawton S, et al. Bright light therapy protects women from circadian rhythm desynchronization during chemotherapy for breast cancer. Behav Sleep Med. 2012;10(3):202–16.

8. Ilham R, Satriana A, Mulfiyanti D. The relationship between anxiety levels and sleep patterns of breast cancer patients who undergo chemotherapy in the operating room Tenriawaru Bone Hospital. Asian J Healthy Sci. 2024;3(1):22–33.
9. Bock K, Peltzer J, Liu W, Colgrove Y, Smirnova I, Siengsukon C. Sleep quality and lymphedema in breast cancer survivors: a mixed method analysis. J Cancer Surviv. 2024; https://doi.org/10.1007/s11764-023-01516-9.
10. Li H, Schlaeger JM, Patil CL, Danciu O, Chen Z, Lif N, et al. Feasibility of implementing acupuncture in medically underserved breast cancer survivors (FAB): A protocol. Contemp Clin Trials. 2024;136:107387.
11. Emre N, Yılmaz S. Sleep quality, mental health, and quality of life in women with breast cancer. Indian J Cancer [Internet]. 2024;61:299.
12. Yarosh RA, Jackson CL, Anderson C, Nichols HB, Sandler DP. Sleep disturbances among cancer survivors. Cancer Epidemiol. 2023;87:102471.
13. Cheng WH, Teo RH, Cheng LJ, Lau Y, Lau ST. Global prevalence of sleep disturbances among breast cancer survivors: A systematic review with meta-analysis. Sleep Health. 2023;9(5):704–16.
14. Leysen L, Lahousse A, Nijs J, Adriaenssens N, Mairesse O, Ivakhnov S, et al. Prevalence and risk factors of sleep disturbances in breast cancersurvivors: systematic review and meta-analyses. Support Care Cancer. 2019;27(12):4401–33.
15. Gonzalez BD, Eisel SL, Qin B, Llanos AAM, Savard J, Hoogland AI, et al. Prevalence, risk factors, and trajectories of sleep disturbance in a cohort of African-American breast cancer survivors. Support Care Cancer. 2021;29(5):2761–70.
16. Palesh O, Aldridge-Gerry A, Ulusakarya A, Ortiz-Tudela E, Capuron L, Innominato PF. Sleep disruption in breast cancer patients and survivors. J Natl Compr Cancer Netw. 2013;11(12):1523–30.
17. Zhu W, Li W, Gao J, Wang L, Guo J, Yang H. Factors associated with the sleep disturbances of people with breast cancer during chemotherapy in China: A cross-sectional study. Nurs Open. 2023;10(8):5453–61.
18. Ertaş H, Caner B, Oyucu Orhan S, Ocak B, Çubukçu E. Evaluation of the frequency of sleep disorders, depression and anxiety in patients with early-stage breast cancer: cross-sectional study. Turk Klin J Med Sci. 2023;43(3):314–22.
19. Subramanian H, Trivedi R, Fuchsova V, Elder E, Brand A, Howle J, et al. Follow-up assessment of sleep-related symptoms in patients after treatment for cancer: responses to continuous positive airway pressure treatment for co-morbid obstructive sleep apnoea. Sleep Breath Schlaf Atm. 2023;28:725.
20. Beverly Hery CM, Janse SA, Van Zee KJ, Naftalis EZ, Paskett ED, Naughton MJ. Factors associated with insomnia symptoms over three years among premenopausal women with breast cancer. Breast Cancer Res Treat. 2023;202(1):155–65.
21. Grassi L, Zachariae R, Caruso R, Palagini L, Campos-Ródenas R, Riba MB, et al. Insomnia in adult patients with cancer: ESMO Clinical Practice Guideline. ESMO Open. 2023;8(6):102047.
22. Palagini L, Manni R, Aguglia E, Amore M, Brugnoli R, Girardi P, et al. Expert opinions and consensus recommendations for the evaluation and management of insomnia in clinical practice: joint statements of five Italian scientific societies. Front Psych. 2020;11:558.
23. Bastien CH, Vallières A, Morin CM. Validation of the insomnia severity index as an outcome measure for insomnia research. Sleep Med. 2001;2(4):297–307.
24. Shahid A, Wilkinson K, Marcu S, Shapiro CM. Women's Health Initiative Insomnia Rating Scale (WHIIRS). In: Shahid A, Wilkinson K, Marcu S, Shapiro CM, editors. STOP, THAT and One Hundred Other Sleep Scales [Internet]. Springer New York: New York, NY; 2011.
25. Vasbinder A, Zaslavsky O, Heckbert SR, Thompson H, Cheng RK, Saquib N, et al. Associations of health-related quality of life and sleep disturbance with cardiovascular disease risk in postmenopausal breast cancer survivors. Cancer Nurs. 2023;46(6):E355–64.
26. Madut A, Fuchsova V, Man H, Askar S, Trivedi R, Elder E, et al. Increased prevalence of obstructive sleep apnea in women diagnosed with endometrial or breast cancer. PLoS One. 2021;16(4):e0249099.
27. Vin-Raviv N, Akinyemiju TF, Galea S, Bovbjerg DH. Sleep disorder diagnoses and clinical outcomes among hospitalized breast cancer patients: a nationwide inpatient sample study. Support Care Cancer. 2018;26(6):1833–40.
28. Chung F, Subramanyam R, Liao P, Sasaki E, Shapiro C, Sun Y. High STOP-Bang score indicates a high probability of obstructive sleep apnoea. Br J Anaesth Mayıs. 2012;108(5):768–75.
29. Chang WP, Chang YP. Meta-analysis of changes in sleep quality of women with breast cancer before and after therapy. Breast Care. 2019;15(3):227–35.
30. Buysse DJ, Reynolds CF, Monk TH, Berman SR, Kupfer DJ. The Pittsburgh sleep quality index: A new instrument for psychiatric practice and research. Psychiatry Res. 1989;28(2):193–213.
31. Carpenter JS, Andrykowski MA. Psychometric evaluation of the Pittsburgh sleep quality index. J Psychosom Res. 1998;45(1):5–13.
32. Johns MW. A new method for measuring daytime sleepiness: the Epworth sleepiness scale. Sleep. 1991;14(6):540–5.
33. Henneghan AM, Carter P, Stuifbergan A, Parmelee B, Kesler S. Relationships between self-reported sleep quality components and cognitive functioning in breast cancer survivors up to 10 years following chemotherapy. Psychooncology. 2018;27(8):1937–43.
34. Van Onselen C, Paul SM, Lee K, Dunn L, Aouizerat BE, West C, et al. Trajectories of sleep disturbance and daytime sleepiness in women before and after surgery for breast cancer. J Pain Symptom Manag. 2013;45(2):244–60.
35. Haque R, Chlebowski RT, Chen L. Sleep medication use and risk of fractures in breast cancer survivors. Breast Cancer Res Treat. 2021;190(3):541–8.

36. Rogers LQ, Courneya KS, Oster RA, Anton PM, Phillips S, Ehlers DK, et al. Physical activity intervention benefits persist months post-intervention: randomized trial in breast cancer survivors. J Cancer Surviv Res Pract. 2023;17(6):1834–46.
37. de Moura Ferraz Barbosa MP, de Jesus NT, Bergmann A, da Silva Alves Gomes VM, Sacomori C, Dantas D. Efficacy of supervised exercise on sleep of women who survived breast cancer: a systematic review with meta-analysis. J Cancer Surviv. 2024.
38. Zhu J, Niu H, Lu D, Li Y, Ding M. Research on the applicability of an exercise rehabilitation app aiming to improve the mental and physical health of breast cancer patients in the post-operative period. Front Psychol. 2023;14:1126284.
39. Kirca K, Kutlutürkan S. Application of progressive relaxation exercises in cancer and treatment process. Adıyaman Üniversitesi Sağlık Bilim Derg. 2020;6(2):258–67.
40. Hasan F, Tu YK, Lin CC, Yuliana LT, Romadlon DS, Chiu HY. Exercise regimens for improved sleep quality in adult breast cancer survivors: systematic review and network meta-analysis. BMJ Support Palliat Care. 2023;13(4):393–400.
41. Leite B, de Bem FT, Boing L, de Azevedo C, Guimarães A. Can belly dance and mat Pilates be effective for range of motion, self-esteem, and depressive symptoms of breast cancer women? Complement Ther Clin Pract. 2021;45:101483.
42. Espíndula RC, Nadas GB, da Rosa MI, Foster C, de Araújo FC, Grande AJ. Pilates for breast cancer: A systematic review and meta-analysis. Rev Assoc Médica Bras. 2017;63:1006–12.
43. Chen Z, Ye X, Shen Z, Chen G, Chen W, He T, et al. Effect of Pilates on sleep quality: A systematic review and meta-analysis of randomized controlled trials. Front Neurol. 2020;11:1–7.
44. Leite B, Andreatta Denig L, Boing L, de Bem FT, de Azevedo C, Guimarães A. Effects of Pilates method on quality of life, fatigue and sleep quality among breast cancer women receiving hormone therapy—two-arm randomized clinical trial. J Bodyw Mov Ther. 2024;37:18–24.
45. He X, Ng MSN, Choi KC, So WKW. Effects of a 16-week dance intervention on the symptom cluster of fatigue-sleep disturbance-depression and quality of life among patients with breast cancer undergoing adjuvant chemotherapy: A randomized controlled trial. Int J Nurs Stud. 2022;133:104317.
46. Schad F, Rieser T, Becker S, Groß J, Matthes H, Oei SL, et al. Efficacy of tango Argentino for cancer-associated fatigue and quality of life in breast cancer survivors: A randomized controlled trial. Cancers. 2023;15(11):2920.
47. Hiansdt JS, Boing L, Sperandio FF, de Bem FT, de Azevedo C, Guimarães A. The influence of 12-week dance intervention on sleep quality and pain among women with breast cancer—pilot study of a non-randomized clinical trial. J Bodyw Mov Ther. 2021;26:43–8.
48. Madan S, Sembhi J, Khurana N, Makkar K, Byati P. Yoga for preventive health: a holistic approach. Am J Lifestyle Med. 2023;17(3):418–23.
49. Mahajan A. Role of yoga in hormonal homeostasis. Int J Clin Exp Physiol. 2014;1(3):173.
50. Panjwani U, Dudani S, Wadhwa M. Sleep, cognition, and yoga. Int J Yoga. 2021;14(2):100–8.
51. Wang WL, Chen KH, Pan YC, Yang SN, Chan YY. The effect of yoga on sleep quality and insomnia in women with sleep problems: a systematic review and meta-analysis. BMC Psychiatry. 2020;20(1):195.
52. Rao RM, Vadiraja H, Nagaratna R, Gopinath KS, Patil S, Diwakar RB, et al. Effect of yoga on sleep quality and neuroendocrine immune response in metastatic breast cancer patients. Indian J Palliat Care. 2017;23(3):253–60.
53. Hou L, Wang J, Mao M, Zhang Z, Liu D, Gao S, et al. Effect of yoga on cancer-related fatigue in patients with breast cancer: A systematic review and meta-analysis. Medicine (Baltimore). 2024;103(1):e36468.
54. Tunç A. Effectiveness of cognitive behavioral therapies in women with breast cancer: a systematic review. Current Approaches in Psychiatry. 2021;13(1):34–51.
55. Bean HR, Diggens J, Ftanou M, Alexander M, Stafford L, Bei B, et al. Light enhanced cognitive behavioral therapy for insomnia and fatigue during chemotherapy for breast cancer: a randomized controlled trial. Sleep. 2022;45(3):zsab246.
56. Maccora J, Bean HR, Diggens J, Ftanou M, Alexander M, Lu Q, et al. Mechanisms of cognitive behavioral therapy and light therapy for cancer-related insomnia: a randomized clinical trial during chemotherapy for breast cancer. Behav Sleep Med. 2023;21(3):227–41.
57. Yang J, Du Y, Shen H, Ren S, Liu Z, Zheng D, et al. Mindfulness-based movement intervention to improve sleep quality: a meta-analysis and moderator analysis of randomized clinical trials. Int J Environ Res Public Health. 2022;19(16):10284.
58. Yegane ZA, Nasiri A, Sahranavard S, Sebzari AR. Effect of online mindfulness-based stress reduction intervention on sleep quality of breast cancer patients. Mod Care J. 2024;21(1):2.
59. Zhang J, Qin Z, So TH, Chang TY, Yang S, Chen H, et al. Acupuncture for chemotherapy-associated insomnia in breast cancer patients: an assessor-participant blinded, randomized, sham-controlled trial. Breast Cancer Res. 2023;25(1):49.
60. Mardani A, Maleki M, Hanifi N, Borghei Y, Vaismoradi M. A systematic review of the effect of lavender on cancer complications. Complement Ther Med. 2022;67:102836.
61. Tamaki K, Fukuyama AK, Terukina S, Kamada Y, Uehara K, Arakaki M, et al. Randomized trial of aromatherapy versus conventional care for breast cancer patients during perioperative periods. Breast Cancer Res Treat. 2017;162(3):523–31.
62. Shammas RL, Marks CE, Broadwater G, Le E, Glener AD, Sergesketter AR, et al. The effect of lavender oil on perioperative pain, anxiety, depression, and sleep after microvascular breast reconstruction: A prospec-

tive, single-blinded, randomized. Controlled Trial J Reconstr Microsurg. 2021;37(6):530–40.
63. Arathi P, Sreejith K, Pavithran K, Soman D. Integrative management of insomnia during cancer chemotherapy: a case report. J Ayurveda Integr Med. 2024;15(1):100899.
64. Stranks EK, Crowe SF. The acute cognitive effects of zopiclone, zolpidem, zaleplon, and eszopiclone: A systematic review and meta-analysis. J Clin Exp Neuropsychol. 2014;36(7):691–700.
65. Jacobsen PB, Massie MJ, Kinne DW, Holland JC. Hypnotic efficacy and safety of triazolam administered during the postoperative period. Gen Hosp Psychiatry. 1994;16(6):419–25.
66. Zaki NF, Sabri YM, Farouk O, Abdelfatah A, Spence DW, Bahammam AS, vd. Depressive symptoms, sleep profiles and serum melatonin levels in a sample of breast cancer patients. Nat Sci Sleep. 2020;12:135–49.
67. Ahmad SB, Ali A, Bilal M, Rashid SM, Wani AB, Bhat RR, et al. Melatonin and health: insights of melatonin action, biological functions, and associated disorders. Cell Mol Neurobiol. 2023;43(6):2437–58.
68. Seo K, Kim JH, Han D. Effects of melatonin supplementation on sleep quality in breast cancer patients: A systematic review and meta-analysis. Healthcare. 2023;11(5):675.
69. Wu HS, Gao F, Davis JE, Given CW. Effects of chronotype-tailored bright light intervention on post-treatment symptoms and quality of life in breast cancer survivors. Support Care Cancer. 2023;31(12):705.
70. Güzel Özdemir P, Yılmaz E, Selvi Y, Boysan M. Bright light treatment in psychiatry. Curr Approaches Psychiatry. 2017;9(2):177.
71. Rissling M, Liu L, Youngstedt SD, Trofimenko V, Natarajan L, Neikrug AB, et al. Preventing sleep disruption with bright light therapy during chemotherapy for breast cancer: A phase II randomized controlled trial. Front Neurosci. 2022;16:815872.
72. Wu HS, Gao F, Yan L, Given C. Evaluating chronotypically tailored light therapy for breast cancer survivors: preliminary findings on fatigue and disrupted sleep. Chronobiol Int. 2022;39(2):221–32.

Fertility Problems in Breast Cancer Survivorship: Special Focus on Younger Breast Cancer Survivors

25

Serpil Abalı Çetin

25.1 Introduction

Fertility plays an important role in the continuation of human life and young adulthood is the most favorable period for having biological children. However, in younger cancer survivors, reproductive function is often adversely affected by the devastating impact of cancer itself and the side effects caused by multimodal cancer treatments. Therefore, fertility potential is a particular concern among younger cancer patients (15–39 years) [1].

Younger breast cancer survivors often face unique challenges when it comes to fertility issues. First, those who are young at the time of diagnosis (< 40 years) are genetically predisposed to more aggressive tumors [2] and probably have a poorer prognosis and more extensive treatment protocols [3]. Second, a diagnosis of breast cancer at reproductive age can affect important life goals, such as establishing close relationships and having children [4]. In addition, younger women are more sensitive to hormonal changes caused by cancer treatment. For this reason, they are generally more concerned about body image, especially in the postoperative period, and therefore, they might face sexual desire problems [5, 6].

It is well known that both cancer and related multimodal treatment, whether through chemotherapy, radiotherapy, hormone therapy, or surgery, can adversely affect reproductive function [7–10]. Chemotherapy and radiotherapy have direct adverse effects on ovarian function [8] and can be affected by endocrine therapy [11, 12] directly or indirectly through impairment of ovarian function [11–14], and all components of the reproductive system can also be affected by surgery.

Population-based data show that women are 38% less likely to become pregnant after cancer diagnosis and over the course of treatment [15]. In addition to effects related to fertility and sexual health, it is becoming increasingly clear that endocrine deficiency has multiple side effects and indeed reduces life expectancy [16, 17]. The quality of life (QoL) of survivors is significantly affected by these side effects and can be of central importance when considering both the medical and psychosocial well-being of women with breast cancer [8, 18].

25.2 Fertility Problems

Individuals diagnosed with breast cancer at a young age (15–39) are part of an important population in terms of both the biology of cancer and

S. A. Çetin (✉)
Faculty of Health Sciences, Department of Women's Health Nursing, Izmir Bakircay University, İzmir, Türkiye
e-mail: serpil.cetin@bakircay.edu.tr

Y. Bakar, A. Tuğral (eds.), *Managing Side Effects of Breast Cancer Treatment*,
https://doi.org/10.1007/978-3-031-75480-7_25

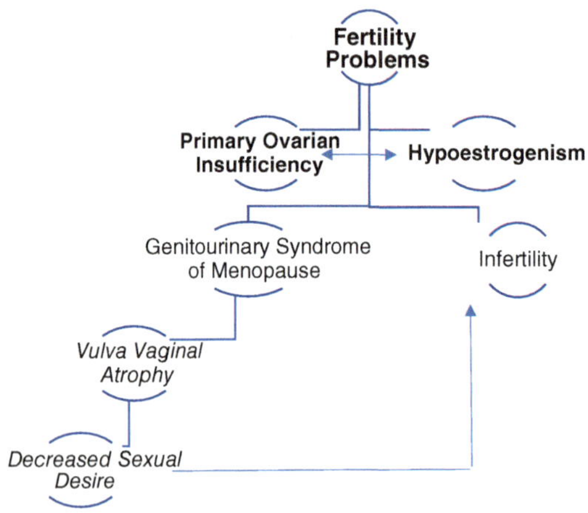

Fig. 25.1 Fertility problems in breast cancer survivorship

the way of experience during their cancer journey. This age range covers an important period of the reproductive period when key events in a woman's life can occur. Survival rates in breast cancer have recently increased thanks to advances in diagnosis and treatments. However, especially, chemotherapy and radiotherapy treatments may result in primary ovarian insufficiency/hypoestrogenism and genitourinary syndrome of menopause. Infertility (Fig. 25.1), which develops due to all these cumulative side effects, indicates that it is more difficult to have children for breast cancer survivors [19].

25.3 Primary Ovarian Insufficiency and Hypoestrogenism

Approximately 17% to 29% of all breast cancers are diagnosed before the average age of menopause (51 years) [20–22]. For women who were diagnosed with breast cancer in this period, multimodal treatments often impair ovarian function and the physiological effects of estrogen [23]. Natural menopause is a gradual decline in estrogen levels, whereas treatment causes a sudden drop in estrogen levels and severe symptoms.

Younger women with treatment-induced early menopause are at increased risk for various long-term health consequences of hypoestrogenism, including various systemic diseases (cardiovascular disease, diseases of the musculoskeletal system, etc.). In younger breast cancer survivors (YBCS) iatrogenic primary ovarian insufficiency (POI) and subsequent hypoestrogenism can occur by multiple mechanisms [24].

Due to the limited number of follicles in the ovaries and their coexistence at different stages of development, there are several pathophysiological mechanisms of treatment-induced POI as follows:

"Accelerated" Maturation of the Ovarian Follicle Chemotherapy agents stimulate the initiation of apoptosis of mature, functional ovarian follicles and suppress the negative feedback of estrogen and Anti-Mullerian Hormone (AMH) in the gonadotropic cells of the anterior pituitary. Elevated gonadotropins accelerate the maturation of follicles, which undergo apoptosis due to systematic chemotherapy. Thus, ovarian follicle accumulation is gradually depleted [25–28].

Direct Immobilized Follicle DNA Damage Chemotherapeutics such as alkylating agents and doxorubicin can accelerate the cross-link formation in the DNA of non-dividing, immobilized oocytes. DNA strand breaks then accumulate, activating pro-apoptotic intracellular pathways. Affected ovarian follicles undergo apoptosis [29].

Impairment of Ovarian Vascularization Chemotherapy can compromise ovarian vasculature and the functionality of the stroma. Local vascular spasm, which reduces ovarian blood flow, and fibrosis in the ovarian cortex, which affects blood vessel formation, can impair ovarian follicle formation [30].

Hypoestrogenism or low estrogen levels can occur in breast cancer survivors (BCS) for various reasons. Breast cancer treatments such as chemotherapy, hormonal therapies (e.g., tamoxifen, aromatase inhibitors), and surgical removal of the ovaries (oophorectomy) can all lead to low estrogen levels. Low estrogen levels are associated with early menopausal symptoms, adverse sexual health, and reduced fertility [24, 31].

25.4 Genitourinary Syndrome of Menopause

Genitourinary syndrome of menopause (GSM) refers to a large number of symptoms (genital, urinary, sexual symptoms, etc.) that develop in women as a result of menopause and age-related structural and functional changes in urogenital tissues [32]. Vaginal dryness, burning, dyspareunia, and itching are the clinical signs of vulvovaginal atrophy (VVA), the genital component of GSM [33]. Many factors have been reported to determine the clinical presentation of VVA. Even iatrogenic reduction in androgen levels due to age may play a role in the clinical course of GSM [34].

The decrease/withdrawal of estrogen after menopause triggers changes such as decreased cervical gland secretions, decreased vascularity, tissue damage, loss of elasticity, and increased pH. The glycogen content of the vaginal mucosa decreases. Lactobacilli, which convert glycogen to lactic acid, decrease to maintain the vaginal pH in the range of 3.5–4.5. This decrease increases the vaginal pH (5.0–7.5). This pH environment becomes favorable for pathogenic microorganisms to cause infection. This makes the woman more susceptible to vaginal infections [35].

Although VVA is not life-threatening, its adverse effects might have a profound negative impact on quality of life (QoL) when combined with symptoms such as early menopause and sexual reluctance problems [36]. Due to the nature of life, women of all ages strive to maintain their sexual function and improve their quality of sexual life and sexual satisfaction [37, 38]. In addition, loss of fertility caused by early menopause and physiological symptoms such as night sweats, hot flashes, vaginal dryness, and weight gain are among the problems that need to be solved. These problems can be particularly distressing for young women; they can negatively affect both health-related and psychosocial quality of life [39]. All these symptoms and problems indirectly lead to loss of fertility.

The diagnosis of GSM is a clinical diagnosis based on medical anamnesis and physical examination. Lubricants, soaps, non-cotton panties, and spermicides should generally be questioned for potential irritants that may cause discomfort in the genitourinary area. Antiestrogen drugs or a history of oophorectomy, radiation, or chemotherapy increase the suspicion of GSM, especially in premenopausal women. Over-the-counter irritants such as soap, detergent, and wet wipes should be evaluated for urogenital contact. Urogenital irritants (such as caffeine and alcohol) should also be taken into consideration and the volume and time of fluid intake should be discussed. Health professionals should be able to counsel perimenopausal women on the management of symptoms of GSM [40].

Physical examination findings include thin and pale external genitalia, especially the vulva. The pubic ears are reduced and the labia majora and labia minora are fused due to fat loss. Fusion may occur in the clitoral hood. There may be red urethral cartilage at the entrance of the urethra. Posterior fissures may be present in the introitus. Prolonged VVA may result in introital constriction, which may result in pain and/or tearing during sexual activity and/or speculum examination. The vaginal dome may shorten. There may be yellow, sticky, and foul-smelling discharge in the vaginal secretion.

It is very important to review existing medical problems, medications, and dermatological diseases for the differential diagnosis of GSM. Any suspicious or non-healing lesion should be evaluated in more detail and a biopsy should be performed if necessary [41].

The diagnosis of GSM can be supported by tests such as vaginal pH and vaginal maturation index. After exclusion of infection or bleeding, a vaginal pH above 5 is suggestive of VVA. The increasing awareness of quality of life problems in BCSs has made GSM an important issue that needs to be more widely recognized by health professionals. The aim of GSM and/or VVA treatment is to determine the severity of symptoms and the degree of discomfort to provide individualized treatment [23, 40, 41]. Current treatments for GSM include both non-hormonal treatments (over-the-counter local treatments such as vaginal moisturizers and lubricants) and hormonal treatments (local or systemic hormone therapy). According to international guidelines, the first-line treatment of mild-to-moderate GSM

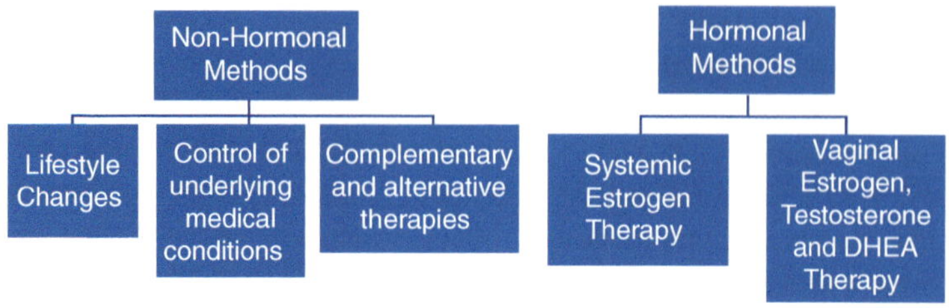

Fig. 25.2 Management of genitourinary syndrome of menopause

is non-hormonal therapies. Therefore, the American Society of Clinical Oncology (ASCO)/ American Cancer Society (ACS) [40–42] guidelines recommend non-hormonal therapies (water/ silicone-based vaginal lubricant and/or moisturizer) for mild to moderate symptoms and pharmacological treatment (local hormonal therapy) for severe signs or symptoms [23, 41, 42] for the management of menopause (Fig. 25.2).

25.5 Infertility

25.5.1 Definition

When the major events in a woman's life occur in the context of the reproductive period, spans the age range of 15–39 years. Therefore, young women aged 15–39 years when diagnosed with BC are part of a unique population in terms of both the biology of their cancer and the way they experience their cancer journey [43]. This is because YBCS may experience infertility because of the depletion of the limited ovarian reserve due to cancer treatment, impaired hypothalamic-pituitary-ovarian function, and/or uterine injury. In the literature, more infertility and fewer live births have been reported in YBCS women compared to women without cancer and between those who are childhood cancer survivors [43].

25.6 Effect of Breast Cancer Treatments on Infertility

25.6.1 Chemotherapy

Breast cancer often has aggressive biological characteristics in younger women. Therefore, systemic chemotherapy characterized by gonadotoxic effects is implemented [43]. Chemotherapy is directly toxic as it destroys the ovarian follicles [44–47] and may cause temporary or permanent amenorrhea. In addition, even if a woman regains a regular menstrual cycle after treatment, it may result in early menopause as part of the loss of ovarian reserve [46]. The effect of chemotherapy on fertility depends on the ovarian reserve, the type and dose of chemotherapy, and the age of the patient. For instance, BC patients undergoing oncological treatment at an older age (> 40) are at greater risk of POI, defined as early menopause, than younger (≤ 40) patients. Another important factor is the type of treatment, dose, and duration of the chemotherapeutic agent. In terms of POI, alkylating agents are considered to have the highest gonadotoxic effect; anthracycline-based and taxane-based therapies are considered to have medium-low risk, and agents such as fluorouracil or methotrexate are considered to have the least gonadotoxic effect [48, 49].

25.6.2 Endocrine Therapy (ET)

Endocrine therapy has indirect effects on infertility. First, endocrine therapy may impair ovulation and endometrial function, which may further lead to fertility disorders, including an increased risk of transient amenorrhea in some women. In addition, pregnancy during endocrine therapy is contraindicated as it may cause congenital anomalies. The risk of age-related infertility would increase, especially if endocrine therapy is continued for 5 years or longer [50].

In women with hormone receptor positive (HR+) BC, adjuvant ET is implemented for up to 10 years after diagnosis, and (neo)adjuvant therapy is recommended if necessary. Adjuvant ET options for premenopausal women include tamoxifen (5–10 years) ovarian function suppressors (OFS) (5 years), tamoxifen plus OFS, and aromatase inhibitor for 5 years [51].

25.6.3 Immunotherapy

Information on the risk of amenorrhea associated with immunotherapy treatment, tyrosine kinase inhibitors, or anti-human epidermal growth factor receptor 2 (HER-2) agents is very limited [52]. However, stimulation of the immune system, which facilitates the immune system of the body against cancer cells in this type of treatment, may adversely affect sexuality as it may cause fatigue, dryness of mucous membranes, cold-like symptoms, and changes in body image [53].

25.6.4 Radiotherapy

In the treatment of cancers other than breast cancer, radiation may reduce fertility by causing ovarian failure, damaging the structure and function of the endometrium, or disrupting the hypothalamic-pituitary-gonadal axis. Locoregional and total breast irradiation for BC treatment has minimal effect on ovarian reserves and fertility. However, doses delivered through internal scatter, external scatter, and radiation leakage during breast irradiation may affect the ovaries and uterus by reaching the urogenital system [52].

25.6.5 Reproductive Concerns

Although the potential of having children is preserved after breast cancer treatment, concerns about infertility can cause serious psychological distress. When false beliefs and perceptions about fertility potential arise, unplanned pregnancies and/or wrong reproductive decisions may occur [54].

Women all over the world tend to postpone childbearing for professional and cultural reasons. Therefore, women may not have completed their family planning when they are diagnosed with BC [23]. However, studies indicated that more than 85% of YBCS have a strong desire to have children [55, 56]. Thus, there is significant concern about treatment-related infertility in many younger women with BC [23]. Gorman et al. [57] reported that patients' reproductive concerns during cancer survivorship have six main components: fertility potential, disclosure of fertility status to partner, child health, personal health, acceptance, and achieving pregnancy. In addition to their potential impact on psychological status, these reproductive concerns can affect all phases of medical treatment, including decision-making in treatment protocol and treatment adherence [58].

A previous study found that 29% of breast cancer patients' treatment decisions were influenced by concerns about their fertility. For example, since ET should last at least 5 years for women with HR-positive BC, women who desire to become pregnant do not start or discontinue ET before the treatment process is fully completed. Reproductive concerns have also been associated with psychological health in cancer patients [59].

25.7 Evaluation of Infertility

The menstrual cycle is the first condition evaluated in the assessment of infertility. However, although the presence or absence of menstruation is an indicator of ovarian reserve and activity, regular menstruation may continue in case of dramatically reduced ovarian reserve. In this case, POI cannot be excluded.

Follicle-stimulating hormone (FSH) measurement is the well-known common diagnostic test for POI. Women with diminished ovarian reserve who continue to menstruate may show an elevated FSH level at the onset of POI and, therefore, they need to be followed up at frequent intervals [60, 61].

Measurement of anti-Mullerian hormone (AMH) has an important role in the assessment of normal menopause or ovarian reserve after cancer treatment [61]. Measurement of AMH not only allows assessment of ovarian reserve during diagnosis but also shows the effect of interventions to improve ovarian function after treatment [62].

Analysis of the number of antral follicles by transvaginal ultrasonography (TVU) is an important method to assess the reserve of each ovary. However, the application of TVU requires specialized skills and there are often inconsistencies between experts. Thus, this should be considered in fertility counseling [63].

25.8 Management of Infertility

It is important to address the gonadotoxicity of anticancer therapy for newly diagnosed BC women of reproductive age during fertility counseling. Since many younger women might not have completed their family processes/planning when they are diagnosed with BC [7, 64].

To eliminate the risk of chemotherapy-induced fertility impairment, oocyte/embryo freezing for controlled ovarian stimulation (COS) before initiation of chemotherapy should be the standard of care for younger women [65].

ASCO guidelines recommend that women of reproductive age whose fertility may be affected by cancer treatment should be offered fertility preservation options as soon as possible after cancer diagnosis [66].

25.9 Approaches to Preserve Ovarian Function

25.9.1 Ovarian Suppression with GnRHa (Gonadotropin-Releasing Hormone Agonists)

GnRH agonists can show activity more than a hundred thousand times compared to endogenous GnRH and secreted LH and FSH from the pituitary gland. While the half-life of natural GnRH is quite short, GnRH agonists, whose effect can last for 10–14 days after binding to the receptor, gonadotropin secretion is increased first for 3–6 days then rapidly decreases the binding capacity of GnRH receptors. As a result, the amount and release of pituitary FSH and LH decreases. In IVF (İn-Vitro Fertilization) cycles, inhibition of maturation of the leading follicle by fluctuating LH levels and sudden LH peak results in failure in the cycle. In long-term use, GnRH analogs stimulate ovarian follicle development with exogenous FSH but suppress pituitary LH [65, 66].

25.9.2 Oocyte Cryopreservation

Cryopreservation is a combination of chemical events that allow cells and tissues to be stored for a long time at sub-zero temperatures. There are two different cryopreservation techniques: "slow freezing," which was widely used in previous years, and "vitrification," which has been widely used today. Although successful results were obtained with the slow freezing method in previous years, its use has decreased considerably due to the difficulty of clinical application and low success rates in comparison with fresh oocytes. The vitrification method, which uses higher concentrations of cryoprotectants, reduces the risk of crystal formation and can be applied very quickly and practically, has taken its place in clinical applications with higher success rates [67]. Although there is ample evidence in the literature regarding the success of oocyte cryopreservation as a means of fertility preservation in younger cancer patients, data specific to breast cancer are very limited. Some evidence suggests that success in oocyte cryopreservation is reduced in BC patients carrying BRCA pathogenic gene variants. Nonetheless, the controversy regarding this method in BC patients with BRCA mutations is still ongoing [68].

25.9.3 Embryo Cryopreservation

Although embryo cryopreservation is recognized as the most effective option for fertility preservation in women with BC, it is necessary to delay anti-cancer therapies for up to 6 weeks for proper endometrial implantation. This may delay the systemic treatment. In YBCS, special attention should be paid to embryo transfer of preserved embryos. Some treatment protocols recommend that women who have been successfully treated for BC should wait at least 2 years to monitor for possible early recurrences before attempting to become pregnant [66, 67].

25.9.4 Cryopreservation of the Ovarian Cortex

This method, which has been recognized as one of the methods for fertility preservation according to the American Society for Reproductive Medicine and the Society for Assisted Reproductive Technologies, is based on the principle of preserving ovarian tissue by cryopreservation without the need for ovarian stimulation. Thus, both fertility and hormonal production can be preserved. It is especially suitable for puberty/premenarche adolescents diagnosed with malignancy and patients in need of urgent cancer treatment. When transplantation is decided, the dissolved ovarian tissue can be re-implanted to its original site in the pelvic cavity or an alternative site (abdominal wall or forearm) [68].

25.9.5 Ovarian Stem Cells (OSCs)

It is a potentially safe method for fertility preservation in HR-positive BC. It is a method that allows the future use of stem cells obtained from the ovarian cortex in vitro. This method is also suitable for women with primary infertility. OSCs can be easily recovered by small surgical approaches, such as laparoscopy or mini-laparotomy, regardless of the status of the menstrual cycle. In younger women with BC, this method is an accurate method that allows the selection of the best oocytes/eggs to be fertilized after the cancer is fully cured [66, 67, 69].

25.10 Conclusion

The journey of young breast cancer survivors involves the complex interplay between fertility preservation, survival, and quality of life. While advances in medical technology offer options for fertility preservation (egg or embryo cryopreservation), both physiological and psychological factors are often limiting. The long-term effects of cancer treatment on fertility emphasize the need for comprehensive support and information for young survivors.

Oncofertility counseling is a popular concept that enables patients to be informed about the options they have to lead a normal life and have children after the end of cancer treatment. To have a better chance against infertility, a multidisciplinary approach should be adopted, and appropriate treatment planning with free/affordable access to resources and information. Rapid fertility counseling of breast cancer survivorship programs can help to ensure that all young women who are likely to lose their fertility due to gonadotoxic chemotherapy treatment are counseled about the lasting effects of treatment and increase the likelihood of having children after treatment. Providing personalized care plans, education about fertility preservation options, and access to financial assistance could significantly improve the well-being of young breast cancer survivors. Future research should focus on developing more accessible and cost-effective fertility preservation options, as well as exploring the impact of fertility-related decisions on survival outcomes. Ultimately, by addressing the unique challenges faced by young breast cancer survivors, we can improve their quality of life and enable them to make informed choices about their fertility and survival.

References

1. Ussher JM, Perz J, Australian Cancer and Fertility Study Team (ACFST). The threat of biographical disruption: the gendered construction and experience of infertility following cancer for women and men.

BMC Cancer. 2018;18:1–7. https://doi.org/10.1186/s12885-018-4172-5.
2. Anders CK, Hsu DS, Broadwater G, Acharya CR, Foekens JA, Zhang Y, Wang Y, Marcom PK, Marks JR, Febbo PG, Nevins JR, Potti A, Blackwell KL. Young age at diagnosis correlates with worse prognosis and defines a subset of breast cancers with shared patterns of gene expression. J Clin Oncol. 2008;26(20):3324–30. https://doi.org/10.1200/JCO.2007.14.2471.
3. Fredholm H, Eaker S, Frisell J, Holmberg L, Fredriksson I, Lindman H. Breast cancer in young women: poor survival despite intensive treatment. PLoS One. 2009;4(11):1–9. https://doi.org/10.1371/journal.pone.0007695.
4. Duffy C, Allen S. Medical and psychosocial aspects of fertility after cancer. Cancer J. 2009;15(1):27–33. https://doi.org/10.1097/PPO.0b013e3181976602.
5. Burwell SR, Case LD, Kaelin C, Avis NE. Sexual problems in younger women after breast cancer surgery. J Clin Oncol. 2006;24(18):2815–21. https://doi.org/10.1200/JCO.2005.04.2499.
6. Stead ML. Sexual dysfunction after treatment for gynaecologic and breast malignancies. Curr Opin Obstet Gynecol. 2003;15(1):57–61.
7. Lambertini M, Peccatori FA, Demeestere I, Amant F, Wyns C, Stukenborg JB, Paluch-Shimon S, Halaska MJ, Uzan C, Meissner J, von Wolff M, Anderson RA, Jordan K, Guidelines ESMO, Committee. Fertility preservation and post-treatment pregnancies in post-pubertal cancer patients: ESMO Clinical Practice Guidelines†. Ann Oncol. 2020;31(12):1664–78. https://doi.org/10.1016/j.annonc.2020.09.006.
8. Jacobs LA, Pucci DA. Adult survivors of childhood cancer: the medical and psychosocial late effects of cancer treatment and the impact on sexual and reproductive health. J Sex Med. 2013;10(Suppl 1):120–6. https://doi.org/10.1111/jsm.12050.
9. van Dorp W, Haupt R, Anderson RA, Mulder RL, van den Heuvel-Eibrink MM, van Dulmen-den BE, Su HI, Winther JF, Hudson MM, Levine JM, Wallace WH. Reproductive function and outcomes in female survivors of childhood, adolescent, and young adult cancer: a review. J Clin Oncol. 2018;36(21):2169–80. https://doi.org/10.1200/JCO.2017.76.34.
10. Skinner R, Mulder RL, Kremer LC, Hudson MM, Constine LS, Bardi E, Boekhout A, Borgmann-Staudt A, Brown MC, Cohn R, Dirksen U, Giwercman A, Ishiguro H, Jahnukainen K, Kenney LB, Loonen JJ, Meacham L, Neggers S, Nussey S, Petersen C, Shnorhavorian M, van den Heuvel-Eibrink MM, van Santen HM, Wallace WH, Green DM. Recommendations for gonadotoxicity surveillance in male childhood, adolescent, and young adult cancer survivors: a report from the International Late Effects of Childhood Cancer Guideline Harmonization Group. Lancet Oncol. 2017;18(2):e75. https://doi.org/10.1016/S1470-2045(17)30026-8.
11. Lester J, Pahouja G, Andersen B, Lustberg M. Atrophic vaginitis in breast cancer survivors: a difficult survivorship issue. J Personalized Med. 2015;5(2):50–66. https://doi.org/10.3390/jpm5020050.
12. Bakkum-Gamez JN, Laughlin SK, Jensen JR, Akogyeram CO, Pruthi S. Challenges in the gynecologic care of premenopausal women with breast cancer. Mayo Clin Proc. 2011;86(3):229–40. https://doi.org/10.4065/mcp.2010.0794.
13. Critchley HOD, Wallace WHB. Impact of cancer treatment on uterine function. JNCI Monographs. 2005;2005(34):64–8. https://doi.org/10.1093/jncimonographs/lgi022.
14. Lambertini M, Goldrat O, Clatot F, Demeestere I, Awada A. Controversies about fertility and pregnancy issues in young breast cancer patients: current state of the art. Curr Opin Oncol. 2017;29(4):243–52. https://doi.org/10.1097/CCO.0000000000000380.
15. Anderson RA, Brewster DH, Wood R, Nowell S, Fischbacher C, Kelsey TW, Wallace WHB. The impact of cancer on subsequent chance of pregnancy: a population-based analysis. Hum Reprod. 2018;33(7):1281–90. https://doi.org/10.1093/humrep/dey216.
16. ESHRE Guideline Group on Good Practice in IVF Labs, De los Santos MJ, Apter S, Coticchio G, Debrock S, Lundin K, Plancha CE, Prados F, Rienzi L, Verheyen G, Woodward B, Vermeulen N. Revised guidelines for good practice in IVF laboratories (2015). Hum Reprod. 2016;31(4):685–6. https://doi.org/10.1093/humrep/dew016.
17. Araujo AB, Dixon JM, Suarez EA, Murad MH, Guey LT, Wittert GA. Clinical review: endogenous testosterone and mortality in men: a systematic review and meta-analysis. J Clin Endocrinol Metab. 2011;96(10):3007–19. https://doi.org/10.1210/jc.2011-1137.
18. Peate M, Meiser B, Hickey M, Friedlander M. The fertility-related concerns, needs and preferences of younger women with breast cancer: a systematic review. Breast Canc Res Treat. 2009;116(2):215–23. https://doi.org/10.1007/s10549-009-0401-6.
19. Johnson RH, Anders CK, Litton JK, Ruddy KJ, Bleyer A. Breast cancer in adolescents and young adults. Pediatr Blood Cancer. 2018;65(12):e27397. https://doi.org/10.1002/pbc.27397.
20. International Agency for Research on Cancer. Estimated number of new cases in 2020, worldwide, females, ages 0–49 (Excl. NMSC). n.d. Available: https://gco.iarc.fr/today/online-analysistable.
21. Ljungman L, Ahlgren J, Petersson LM, Flynn KE, Weinfurt K, Gorman JR, Wettergren L, Lampic C. Sexual dysfunction and reproductive concerns in young women with breast cancer: type, prevalence, and predictors of problems. Psycho-Oncology. 2018;27(12):2770–7. https://doi.org/10.1002/pon.4886.
22. Ferlay J, Colombet M, Soerjomataram I, Parkin DM, Piñeros M, Znaor A, Bray F. Cancer statistics for the year 2020: An overview. Int J Cancer. 2021;149:778. https://doi.org/10.1002/ijc.33588.

23. O'Sullivan CC, Ruddy KJ. Management of potential long-term toxicities in breast cancer patients. Curr Breast Cancer Rep. 2016;8:183–92. https://doi.org/10.1007/s12609-016-0229-0.
24. Esch M. Treatment-induced ovarian insufficiency and early menopause in breast cancer survivors. Clin J Oncol Nurs. 2023;27(1):7–12.
25. Cui W, Stern C, Hickey M, Goldblatt F, Anazodo A, Stevenson WS, Phillips KA. Preventing ovarian failure associated with chemotherapy. Med J Aust. 2018;209(9):412–6. https://doi.org/10.5694/mja18.00190.
26. Roness H, Kashi O, Meirow D. Prevention of chemotherapy-induced ovarian damage. Fertil Steril. 2016;105(1):20–9. https://doi.org/10.1016/j.fertnstert.2015.11.043.
27. Kalich-Philosoph L, Roness H, Carmely A, Fishel-Bartal M, Ligumsky H, Paglin S, Wolf I, Kanety H, Sredni B, Meirow D. Cyclophosphamide triggers follicle activation and "burnout"; AS101 prevents follicle loss and preserves fertility. Sci Transl Med. 2013;5(185):185ra62. https://doi.org/10.1126/scitranslmed.3005402.
28. Adhikari D, Liu K. Molecular mechanisms underlying the activation of mammalian primordial follicles. Endocr Rev. 2009;30(5):438–64. https://doi.org/10.1210/er.2008-0048.
29. Bedoschi G, Navarro PA, Oktay K. Chemotherapy-induced damage to ovary: mechanisms and clinical impact. Future Oncol. 2016;12(20):2333–44. https://doi.org/10.2217/fon-2016-0176.
30. Mauri D, Gazouli I, Zarkavelis G, Papadaki A, Mavroeidis L, Gkoura S, Ntellas P, Amylidi AL, Tsali L, Kampletsas E. Chemotherapy associated ovarian failure. Front Endocrinol (Lausanne). 2020;11:572388. https://doi.org/10.3389/fendo.2020.572388.
31. Franzoi MA, Agostinetto E, Perachino M, Del Mastro L, de Azambuja E, Vaz-Luis I, Partridge AH, Lambertini M. Evidence-based approaches for the management of side-effects of adjuvant endocrine therapy in patients with breast cancer. Lancet Oncol. 2021;22(7):e303–13. https://doi.org/10.1016/S1470-2045(20)30666-5.
32. Shifren JL. Genitourinary syndrome of menopause. Clin Obstet Gynecol. 2018;61(3):508–16. https://doi.org/10.1097/GRF.0000000000000380.
33. Portman DJ, Gass ML, Vulvovaginal Atrophy Terminology Consensus Conference Panel. Genitourinary syndrome of menopause: new terminology for vulvovaginal atrophy from the International Society for the Study of Women's Sexual Health and the North American Menopause Society. Menopause. 2014;21(10):1063–8. https://doi.org/10.1097/GME.0000000000000329.
34. Simon JA, Goldstein I, Kim NN, Davis SR, Kellogg-Spadt S, Lowenstein L, Pinkerton JV, Stuenkel CA, Traish AM, Archer DF, Bachmann G, Goldstein AT, Nappi RE, Vignozzi L. The rolc of androgens in the treatment of genitourinary syndrome of menopause (GSM): International Society for the Study of Women's Sexual Health (ISSWSH) expert consensus panel review. Menopause. 2018;25(7):837–47. https://doi.org/10.1097/GME.0000000000001138.
35. Cucinella L, Tiranini L, Cassani C, Martella S, Nappi RE. Genitourinary syndrome of menopause in breast cancer survivors: current perspectives on the role of laser therapy. Int J Women's Health. 2023;15:1261–82. https://doi.org/10.2147/IJWH.S414509. PMID: 37576184; PMCID: PMC10422970.
36. Rosenberg SM, Partridge AH. Premature menopause in young breast cancer: effects on quality of life and treatment interventions. J Thorac Dis. 2013;5(Suppl 1):55–61. https://doi.org/10.3978/j.issn.2072-1439.2013.06.20].
37. Krychman M. Impact of vaginal atrophy on quality of life and sexuality. Obstet Gyncol Manage. 2010;22:S14–9.
38. Kingsberg S, Kellogg S, Krychman M. Treating dyspareunia caused by vaginal atrophy: a review of treatment options using vaginal estrogen therapy. Int J Women's Health. 2010;1:105–11. https://doi.org/10.2147/ijwh.s4872.
39. Lubián López DM. Management of genitourinary syndrome of menopause in breast cancer survivors: an update. World J Clin Oncol. 2022;13(2):71–100. https://doi.org/10.5306/wjco.v13.i2.71. PMID: 35316932; PMCID: PMC8894268.
40. Gandhi J, Chen A, Dagur G, Suh Y, Smith N, Cali B, Khan SA. Genitourinary syndrome of menopause: an overview of clinical manifestations, pathophysiology, etiology, evaluation, and management. Am J Obstet Gynecol. 2016;215(6):704–11. https://doi.org/10.1016/j.ajog.2016.07.045.
41. Phillips NA, Bachmann GA. The genitourinary syndrome of menopause. Menopause. 2021;28(5):579–88. https://doi.org/10.1097/GME.0000000000001728.
42. Qi W, Li H, Wang C, Li H, Fan A, Han C, Xue F. The effect of pathophysiological changes in the vaginal milieu on the signs and symptoms of genitourinary syndrome of menopause (GSM). Menopause. 2020;28(1):102–8. https://doi.org/10.1097/GME.0000000000001644.
43. Velez MP, Richardson H, Baxter NN, Chad McClintock E, Greenblatt RB, Green M. Risk of infertility in female adolescents and young adults with cancer: a population-based cohort study. Human Reprod. 2021;36(7):1981–8. https://doi.org/10.1093/humrep/deab036.
44. Soleimani R, Heytens E, Darzynkiewicz Z, Oktay K. Mechanisms of chemotherapy-induced human ovarian aging: double strand DNA breaks and microvascular compromise. Aging (Albany NY). 2011;3(8):782–93. https://doi.org/10.18632/aging.100363.
45. Ruddy KJ, Partridge AH. The uniquc reproductive concerns of young women with breast cancer. Adv Exp Med Biol. 2012;732:77–87.

46. Partridge AH, Gelber S, Peppercorn J, et al. Fertility and menopausal outcomes in young breast cancer survivors. Clin Breast Cancer. 2008;8:65–9.
47. Hulvat MC, Jeruss JS. Fertility preservation options for young women with breast cancer. Curr Opin Obstet Gynecol. 2011;23:174–82.
48. Beck-Peccoz P, Persani L. Premature ovarian failure. Orphanet J Rare Dis. 2006;1:1–5.
49. Vriens IJ, De Bie AJ, Aarts MJ, de Boer M, van Hellemond IE, Roijen JH, van Golde RJ, Voogd AC, Tjan-Heijnen VC. The correlation of age with chemotherapy-induced ovarian function failure in breast cancer patients. Oncotarget. 2017;8(7):11372–9. https://doi.org/10.18632/oncotarget.14532.
50. Trivers KF, Fink AK, Partridge AH, Oktay K, Ginsburg ES, Li C, Pollack LA. Estimates of young breast cancer survivors at risk for infertility in the U.S. Oncologist. 2014;19(8):814–22. https://doi.org/10.1634/theoncologist.2014-0016.
51. Francis PA, Pagani O, Fleming GF, et al. Tailoring adjuvant endocrine therapy for premenopausal breast cancer. N Engl J Med. 2018;379(2):122–37.
52. McCray DK, Simpson AB, Flyckt R, Liu Y, O'Rourke C, Crowe JP, Grobmyer SR, Moore HC, Valente SA. Fertility in women of reproductive age after breast cancer treatment: practice patterns and outcomes. Ann Surg Oncol. 2016;23(10):3175–81. https://doi.org/10.1245/s10434-016-5308.
53. Moragón S, Di Liello R, Bermejo B. Fertility and breast cancer: a literature review of counseling, preservation options and outcomes. Crit Rev Oncol Hematol. 2021;166:103461. https://doi.org/10.1016/j.critrevonc.2021.103461.
54. Din HN, Singh-Carlson S, Corliss HL, Hartman SJ, Strong D, Madanat H, Su HI. Perceived and objective fertility risk among female survivors of adolescent and young adult cancer. JAMA Netw Open. 2023;6(10):e2337245. https://doi.org/10.1001/jamanetworkopen.2023.37245.
55. Korte E, Schilling R, Balcerek M, Byrne J, Dirksen U, Herrmann G, Kepak T, Klco-Brosius S, Kruseova J, Kunstreich M, Langer T, Panasiuk A, Stefanowicz J, Strauß G, Wiegele K, Borgmann-Staudt A. Fertility-related wishes and concerns of adolescent cancer patients and their parents. J Adolesc Young Adult Oncol. 2020;9(1):55–62. https://doi.org/10.1089/jayao.2019.0064.
56. Ellis SJ, Wakefield CE, McLoone JK, Robertson EG, Cohn RJ. Fertility concerns among child and adolescent cancer survivors and their parents: a qualitative analysis. J Psychosoc Oncol. 2016;34(5):347–62. https://doi.org/10.1080/07347332.2016.1196806.
57. Gorman JR, Su HI, Pierce JP, Roberts SC, Dominick SA, Malcarne VL. A multidimensional scale to measure the reproductive concerns of young adult female cancer survivors. J Cancer Surviv. 2014;8(2):218–28. https://doi.org/10.1007/s11764-013-0333-3.
58. Logan S, Perz J, Ussher JM, Peate M, Anazodo A. Systematic review of fertility-related psychological distress in cancer patients: informing on an improved model of care. Psychooncology. 2019;28(1):22–30. https://doi.org/10.1002/pon.4927.
59. Xie J, Sun Q, Duan Y, Cheng Q, Luo X, Zhou Y, Liu X, Xiao P, Cheng ASK. Reproductive concerns among adolescent and young adult cancer survivors: a scoping review of current research situations. Cancer Med. 2022;11(18):3508–17. https://doi.org/10.1002/cam4.4708. Epub 2022 Mar 24.
60. European Society for Human Reproduction and Embryology (ESHRE) Guideline Group on POI, Webber L, Davies M, Anderson R, Bartlett J, Braat D, Cartwright B, Cifkova R, de Muinck Keizer-Schrama S, Hogervorst E, Janse F, Liao L, Vlaisavljevic V, Zillikens C, Vermeulen N. ESHRE guideline: management of women with premature ovarian insufficiency. Hum Reprod. 2016;31(5):926–37. https://doi.org/10.1093/humrep/dew027.
61. Anderson RA, Clatot F, Demeestere I, Lambertini M, Morgan A, Nelson SM, Peccatori F, Cameron D. Cancer survivorship: reproductive health outcomes should be included in standard toxicity assessments. Eur J Cancer. 2021;144:310–6. https://doi.org/10.1016/j.ejca.2020.11.032.
62. Anderson RA, Mansi J, Coleman RE, Adamson DJA, Leonard RCF. The utility of anti-Müllerian hormone in the diagnosis and prediction of loss of ovarian function following chemotherapy for early breast cancer. Eur J Cancer. 2017;87:58–64. https://doi.org/10.1016/j.ejca.2017.10.001.
63. Coelho Neto MA, Ludwin A, Borrell A, Benacerraf B, Dewailly D, da Silva CF, Condous G, Alcazar JL, Jokubkiene L, Guerriero S, Van den Bosch T, Martins WP. Counting ovarian antral follicles by ultrasound: a practical guide. Ultrasound Obstet Gynecol. 2018;51(1):10–20. https://doi.org/10.1002/uog.18945.
64. ESHRE Guideline Group on Female Fertility Preservation, Anderson RA, Amant F, Braat D, D'Angelo A, de Sousa C, Lopes SM, Demeestere I, Dwek S, Frith L, Lambertini M, Maslin C, Moura-Ramos M, Nogueira D, Rodriguez-Wallberg K, Vermeulen N. ESHRE guideline: female fertility preservation. Hum Reprod Open. 2020;2020(4):hoaa052. https://doi.org/10.1093/hropen/hoaa052.
65. Arecco L, Blondeaux E, Bruzzone M, Ceppi M, Latocca MM, Marrocco C, Boutros A, Spagnolo F, Razeti MG, Favero D, Spinaci S, Condorelli M, Massarotti C, Goldrat O, Del Mastro L, Demeestere I, Lambertini M. Safety of fertility preservation techniques before and after anticancer treatments in young women with breast cancer: a systematic review and meta-analysis. Hum Reprod. 2022;37(5):954–68. https://doi.org/10.1093/humrep/deac035.

66. Warner E, Glass K, Foong S, Sandwith E. Update on fertility preservation for younger women with breast cancer. CMAJ. 2020;192(35):E1003–9.
67. Silvestris E, Dellino M, Cafforio P, Paradiso AV, Cormio G, D'Oronzo S. Breast cancer: an update on treatment-related infertility. J Cancer Res Clin Oncol. 2020;146(3):647–57. https://doi.org/10.1007/s00432-020-03136-7.
68. Boutas I, Kontogeorgi A, Koufopoulos N, Dimas DT, Sitara K, Kalantaridou SN, Dimitrakakis C. Breast cancer and fertility preservation in young female patients: a systematic review of the literature. Clin Pract. 2023;13(6):1413–26. https://doi.org/10.3390/clinpract13060127.
69. Oktay K, Harvey BE, Partridge AH, Quinn GP, Reinecke J, Taylor HS, Wallace WH, Wang ET, Loren AW. Fertility preservation in patients with cancer: ASCO clinical practice guideline update. J Clin Oncol. 2018;36:1994–2001.

Financial Toxicity and Employment: Experienced Drawbacks for Back to Work

26

Mustafa Orhan and Ümit Çıraklı

26.1 Introduction

The goal of cancer treatment has always been to strike a compromise between the benefits of therapies intended to cure, manage or stop the progression of potentially fatal illnesses and their inherent toxicity. A fundamental component of oncology practice is evaluating the risks associated with an intervention, fully disclosing them to patients and effectively managing them [1]. With the advancement of advanced diagnostic techniques and treatment modalities, breast cancer patients are seeing improvements in their life expectancy and clinical outcomes but face a huge medical financial burden in the process [2]. Cancer care, which creates a significant financial burden on health systems, accounts for approximately 5% of total health expenditure in OECD countries [3] According to the Agency for Healthcare Research and Quality; direct medical costs for cancer, including all healthcare expenditures in the United States in 2020, is $172 billion [4]. According to global cancer statistics published by the International Agency for Research on Cancer in 2020; Breast cancer has surpassed lung cancer and has become the leader in global cancer incidence, showing a rapidly increasing trend every year. Approximately 2.3 million new cases of breast cancer were diagnosed in 2020 [1].

Increasing cancer incidence, long-term survival and high costs of new drugs and technologies indicate that these expenditures will increase further in the coming years [3]. Analysing the potential economic costs of cancer types for 2020–2050, the economic burden of breast cancer ($2.0 trillion) is estimated to be the largest after tracheal, bronchial and lung (TBL) cancer ($3.9 trillion) and colon and rectal cancer ($2.8 trillion) [5]. When analysing costs per capita, it becomes evident that the diagnosis stage substantially impacts costs. An analysis of female cancer patients in the United States in 2010 found the mean expenditure per individual during the 12 months following a breast cancer diagnosis. Based on this study, the average expenses per patient within a year of being diagnosed with breast cancer were $60,637, $82,121, $129,387 and $134,682 for stages 0, I/II, III and IV of the disease, respectively. This indicates that an early diagnosis can decrease the prospective cost by around 50% [6]. Since cancer is now considered a chronic disease with prolonged and sometimes recurrent treatment processes, expenditures are rapidly increasing [7]. Research shows that cancer patients spend more out-of-pocket during this period than their demographic peers without a cancer diagnosis or patients with other chronic

M. Orhan (✉) · Ü. Çıraklı
Faculty of Health Sciences, Health Management Department, İzmir Bakırçay University, Izmir, Turkey
e-mail: m.orhan@bakircay.edu.tr; umit.cirakli@bakircay.edu.tr

Y. Bakar, A. Tuğral (eds.), *Managing Side Effects of Breast Cancer Treatment*,
https://doi.org/10.1007/978-3-031-75480-7_26

conditions [8, 9]. With increasing concerns about costs, the concept of risk, which was previously used only in relation to the vital functions of cancer, has now gained importance in a different dimension. This dimension is called financial toxicity (FT) [10].

26.2 Financial Toxicity

FT is defined as 'the unintended and unforeseen objective financial burden and subjective financial distress that cancer patients experience as a result of their treatment' [11]. In another definition, the perspective is broader: '*FT refers to the financial burden and distress faced by patients and family members as a result of cancer treatment*' [12]. This term, which corresponds to the financial burden of receiving cancer treatment, describes people with high out-of-pocket medical expenses, resulting in a lower quality of life and reduced utilisation of health services. In this sense, neutropenia is very similar to treatment-related toxicities such as nausea, vomiting, insomnia or depression [13]. Patients face higher out-of-pocket health expenditures, while treatment decisions are often made without **considering these costs.** The adverse effects of out-of-pocket health expenditures are referred to as a form of treatment-related toxicity or FT [14]. Although there are many methods for measuring FT, the ratio of the amount of expenditures to income, scales measuring individuals' perceptions and data from various databases and surveys created by researchers are commonly used [15]. FT has a broader meaning than similar terms, such as financial burden, financial hardship, financial distress, financial or economic stress, strain and financial difficulty [12]. This covers direct treatment costs that must be paid for out of pocket and indirect factors that can raise the cost of cancer, like time, travel and job changes [10].

Essentially, FT, which occurs when the financial impact of a patient's care exceeds the patient's available resources [16], includes both the objective financial burden and subjective financial distress caused by cancer disease and treatment [11]. The direct and indirect expenses of cancer therapy, which rise with time after diagnosis, are the source of the objective financial burden. Indirect costs from treatment and ancillary services to enhance quality of life are also included, in addition to 'out-of-pocket' expenditures or the direct costs of care not covered by insurance and any care to avoid problems. Subjective financial distress results from the higher costs associated with the illness and the decline in quality of life [11]. It describes how the patient feels about the financial situation of the household since the cancer diagnosis and includes all negative emotions and disturbing experiences [17, 18]. Therefore, the term FT comprehensively refers to the unpredictable, unpredictable, tangibly measurable financial impact (objective financial burden) and financial anxiety and discomfort (subjective financial distress) that not only patients but also their families experience, distinguishing it from other toxicities that arise during cancer diagnosis and treatment [19]. In addition, patients may make significant changes in their lives. They can reduce their hobbies, nutrition and clothing expenses. They may not even be able to cope with FT. Of greater concern, there is also evidence that it may reduce patients' adherence to medications and medical appointments, and thus their expenses related to cancer treatment [14]. A systematic review conducted by Longo and Fitch [20] examined the relationship between cancer types and FT. The three most frequently examined cancers were breast, colorectal and prostate cancer. It was also stated that breast cancer ranked first in terms of income loss and travel expenses. Through collaborative efforts between stakeholders and health systems, we can further increase access to screening and treatment and thereby accelerate progress against breast cancer mortality [21].

26.3 Health System and Financial Toxicity

The relationship between undesirable job changes and FT in healthcare systems can be explained in part by the link between employment and health insurance [15]. The number of insured patients is increasing, but due to increased cost-sharing, insured patients are burdened with paying more out-of-pocket for cancer treatment. This leads to an increase in underinsured cancer patients [15]. In many countries, health financing and health insurance are closely related to each other. The role of health insurance is vital for cancer patients. Patients who have private health insurance and the associated paid leave face fewer difficulties related to FT. In a situation where the loss of a job occurs, a sustainable health insurance is also can be lost [15]. Those who are uninsured are more vulnerable to the risk of FT. In addition to the relationship between employment and health insurance, the contribution of the social security system is also very important. The coverage (who is covered), depth (which services are covered) and height (proportion of the costs covered) of the social security system are important determinants of FT [15, 22, 23]. Strategies for coping with FT vary from individual to individual and healthcare system. While some health systems distribute the cancer-related financial burdens related to cancer to the society with the understanding of solidarity required by the system, they minimise the out-of-pocket expenses for individuals who have health insurance. Some systems individualize the risks and leave the potential effects on individuals to their responsibilities.

In Japan, there is a general public health insurance system in which every citizen or foreign resident is obliged to join the national health insurance, which covers 70% of health care costs. However, the remaining 30% of healthcare costs must be covered by patients. The system includes some measures against FT. For example, it reduces the amount of mandatory health insurance costs for patients over 75 years of age, yet there is also a upper limit on high-cost medical expenses for them. However, research shows that cancer patients in Japan are also exposed to FT. Many patients use their savings or borrow to cope with the additional cost of the treatment. These financial difficulties persist even after patients have completed their primary treatment. Therefore, FT in Japan's healthcare system is often caused by income-based factors and is emerging as a long-term problem [24].

The United States has a unique health system model among many highly industrialised countries [25]. While other developed nations have universal health insurance programs in which the government plays a central role, the healthcare system of the United States is financed by a complex network of public and private insurance programs for those without universal health insurance coverage. Since 2010, more than 20 million Americans are now covered by universal health insurance with the Affordable Care of Act. However, cancer care, in particular, is the fastest growing component of U.S. healthcare costs, and these costs are being shared with patients by third-party payers. This can lead to severe FT and financial problems for patients following the treatment. The U.S. Healthcare System is a system, where the cost of treatment for most patients is not known in advance, which can lead to unexpected medical bills after treatment that can surprise patients and can cause severe financial hardship [26].

Italy has a public health system, so patients do not have to pay directly costs for cancer diagnosis and treatment, unlike the U.S. Patients in Italy are not directly responsible for the costs of their cancer diagnosis and treatment because the country has a public health care system. Since 1978, general taxes have been the primary funding source for the National Health Service, which is the model used to construct the Italian healthcare system [27]. However, some services (such as specialised outpatient and inpatient services, specialised medicines and home health care) may not be covered by free healthcare, and patients may have to pay for these services [28]. There are also additional burdens associated with access to healthcare services. For example, patients who have to receive treatment in a remote location generally face additional costs, such as travel and accommodation costs [27]. This suggests that patients may face unexpected financial burdens due to accessibility to healthcare. In Italy, despite having a public insurance system, studies are showing that cancer patients experience financial difficulties. For example, according to the results of a clinical trial in 16-center consisting of 3670 patients diagnosed with lung, breast or ovarian cancer, 26% of patients reported financial difficulties. The study also highlighted that financial difficulties were significantly associated with poor quality of life [28].

With the increasing prevalence of FT, it has become remarkably crucial for the healthcare systems of many developed countries. This is driven by several factors in healthcare systems, including the rising costs of new cancer treatments [29], increasing health-related debt of patients and their families in certain countries [30], and factors affecting the labour force participation of patients [31] and their caregivers [32]. As a result, patients and their families usually struggle with financial problems due to FT, regardless of the financial protection they have.

26.4 Cancer and Employment

Cancer negatively affects individuals' ability to work, thereby patients are forced to reduce their working hours or to leave their jobs. Many patients struggle to re-enter the workforce even after treatment, although they are more likely to be unable to work due to poor health, which is specifically characterised by missing more days of work, sick leaves [33].

Receiving a cancer diagnosis and starting treatment significantly affects the working status and working capacity of individuals. Forty percent of those diagnosed with cancer cannot fully return to work after their treatment [34]. Those who cannot return to their jobs have a negative impact on their financial situation and quality of life as they move away from both employment and social life [34]. This can lead to a vicious cycle in which direct and indirect healthcare expenses are increased due to the impact of unemployment contributes further to FT by reducing individual savings. Increased healthcare costs due to cancer and loss of employment can have an impact even years after a cancer diagnosis [35]. More broadly, cancer survivors often face challenges in maintaining employment, potential job loss, restrictions on the nature or scope of their work, as well as job lock-in situations where advancement opportunities or job transitions are blocked due to concerns about potential changes in health insurance. In addition, there is a trend towards high cost-sharing burdens, particularly in the healthcare framework of the United States, which collectively contributes to the phenomenon known as FT [15].

According to the data of the Korean National Health Insurance between 2001 and 2006, the devastating effect of cancer on employment was observed. Within 1 year of their cancer diagnosis, 25.9% of cancer patients lost their jobs, and nearly half of the patients lost their jobs within 5 years of their cancer diagnosis. Only about 30% of cancer survivors can return to work after completion of their cancer treatment [36]. The prejudices of employers, which are on the other side of the coin in employment, also have an essential place. Those who have to leave their jobs due to cancer might have problems to start a new job due to the social stigma associated with cancer and negative attitudes towards cancer patients. According to a study conducted in Korea, more than half of the society believes that cancer patients' ability to work will decrease even if they undergo a successful treatment process, and 23.5% of the study participants stated that they do not want to work with cancer patients. In a study conducted in Australia in which the relationship between cancer diagnosis and employment was studied, 25.2% of participants worked full-time before diagnosis, 16.8% worked part-time and 58% were not employed before diagnosis. Around 32.7% of participants who were employed before their cancer diagnosis reported that there was no significant change in their employment status due to their cancer diagnosis. In general, changes in employment situations associated with the diagnosis of cancer included reduction of working hours, early retirement and resignation or unemployment [37]. In another study conducted by Nekhlyudov and Walker [38] in the United States, nearly two-thirds of cancer patients reported that they had changed their work life. These changes included measures such as taking long-term paid leave, taking unpaid leave, switching to flexible working arrangements, changing working hours and changing jobs. Most of these changes took place during treatment. Some of the participants made a career change that included changing their retirement date. Around a quarter of respondents reported that cancer was a barrier to their physical, mental or work productivity at work. Around 42% of respondents reported experiencing a change in their work life. While these approaches are quite strict for breast cancer, colorectal cancer and lung cancer, they are more flexible for those with prostate cancer and melanoma.

26.5 Conclusion

When the challenges of FT in the process of return to work are evaluated process and discussed in this chapter are evaluated, it is seen that breast cancer patients face a significant set of barriers in the context of back to work. Although FT has been addressed in different ways in diverse health systems, both objective financial burden and subjective financial distress are seen in these patient groups. Factors such as cancer treatment costs and job loss during the treatment process can negatively affect patients' financial situation, making it difficult for them to return to work. Moreover, job changes and reduced work capacity may prevent patients from remaining employed and returning to work.

In this context, understanding the relationship between FT and employment is critical for the development of health policies and social security systems. The development of financial support mechanisms and workplace adjustment programs to facilitate post-treatment return to work can encourage cancer patients to re-enter the workforce. There is a need to examine and improve how health policies should respond to the financial needs of breast cancer patients and the return to work process. In particular, it is essential to identify the FT and difficulties in returning to work faced by breast cancer patients due to the increasing number of new patients diagnosed with breast cancer annually. In this context, how cancer treatment costs, job loss and other financial challenges affect patients' return to work should be examined in detail, as well as the impact of financial support mechanisms, workplace adjustment programs and health policies to facilitate return to work. These efforts can improve the health and economic well-being of both individuals and society. In conclusion, reducing FT and supporting the return to work process are essential steps to improve the quality of life of cancer patients and contribute to their social participation.

References

1. Sung H, Ferlay J, Siegel RL, Laversanne M, Soerjomataram I, Jemal A, et al. Global cancer statistics 2020: GLOBOCAN estimates of incidence and mortality worldwide for 36 cancers in 185 countries. CA Cancer J Clin. 2021;71(3):209–49.
2. Zheng A, Zhu Y, Wang Y, Liu F, Jin F, Zang S, et al. Assessment of medical expenditure for patients with breast cancer in China: evidence from current curative expenditure by system of health accounts 2011. Value Health. 2022;25(1):77–83.
3. OECD. Cancer Care: Assuring Quality to Improve Survival. 2013.
4. Agency for Healthcare Research and Quality. Total expenditure in millions by condition, United States, 2020. Medical Expenditure Panel Survey. 2023.
5. Chen S, Cao Z, Prettner K, Kuhn M, Yang J, Jiao L, et al. Estimates and projections of the global economic cost of 29 cancers in 204 countries and territories from 2020 to 2050. JAMA Oncol. 2023;9(4):465–72.
6. Blumen H, Fitch K, Polkus V. Comparison of treatment costs for breast cancer, by tumor stage and type of service. Am Health Drug Benefits. 2016;9(1):23.
7. Meeker CR, Wong Y-N, Egleston BL, Hall MJ, Plimack ER, Martin LP, et al. Distress and financial distress in adults with cancer: an age-based analysis. J Natl Compr Cancer Netw. 2017;15(10):1224–33.
8. Langa KM, Fendrick AM, Chernew ME, Kabeto MU, Paisley KL, Hayman JA. Out-of-pocket health-care expenditures among older Americans with cancer. Value Health. 2004;7(2):186–94.
9. Bernard DS, Farr SL, Fang Z. National estimates of out-of-pocket health care expenditure burdens among nonelderly adults with cancer: 2001 to 2008. J Clin Oncol. 2011;29(20):2821.
10. Abrams HR, Durbin S, Huang CX, Johnson SF, Nayak RK, Zahner GJ, et al. Financial toxicity in cancer care: origins, impact, and solutions. Transl Behav Med. 2021;11(11):2043–54.
11. Carrera P, Yousuf ZS. Financial toxicity. In: The MASCC textbook of cancer supportive care and survivorship. Springer; 2018. p. 127–43.

12. Gordon LG, Merollini KM, Lowe A, Chan RJ. Financial toxicity-what it is and how to measure it. Cancer Forum. 2017;41(2):30.
13. Gordon LG, Merollini KM, Lowe A, Chan RJ. A systematic review of financial toxicity among cancer survivors: we can't pay the co-pay. Patient. 2017;10:295–309.
14. Zafar SY, Peppercorn JM, Schrag D, Taylor DH, Goetzinger AM, Zhong X, et al. The financial toxicity of cancer treatment: a pilot study assessing out-of-pocket expenses and the insured cancer patient's experience. Oncologist. 2013;18(4):381–90.
15. Mols F, Tomalin B, Pearce A, Kaambwa B, Koczwara B. Financial toxicity and employment status in cancer survivors. A systematic literature review. Support Care Cancer. 2020;28:5693–708.
16. McDermott C. Financial toxicity: a common but rarely discussed treatment side effect. Ann Am Thorac Soc. 2017;14(12):1750–2.
17. Carrera PM, Kantarjian HM, Blinder VS. The financial burden and distress of patients with cancer: understanding and stepping-up action on the financial toxicity of cancer treatment. CA Cancer J Clin. 2018;68(2):153–65.
18. Sharp L, Timmons A. The financial impact of a cancer diagnosis. 2010.
19. Ürek D. Kanser Hastalarında Finansal Toksisite Düzeyinin Sağlıkla İlgili Yaşam Kalitesi ve Tedaviye Uyum Üzerindeki Etkileri. Department of Health Management. Ankara, Hacettepe University, PhD; 2021.
20. Longo CJ, Fitch MI, Banfield L, Hanly P, Yabroff KR, Sharp L. Financial toxicity associated with a cancer diagnosis in publicly funded healthcare countries: a systematic review. Support Care Cancer. 2020;28:4645–65.
21. Giaquinto AN, Sung H, Miller KD, Kramer JL, Newman LA, Minihan A, et al. Breast cancer statistics, 2022. CA Cancer J Clin. 2022;72(6):524–41.
22. Pearce A, Tomalin B, Kaambwa B, Horevoorts N, Duijts S, Mols F, et al. Financial toxicity is more than costs of care: the relationship between employment and financial toxicity in long-term cancer survivors. J Cancer Surviv. 2019;13:10–20.
23. World Health Organization. Health systems financing: the path to universal coverage. (No Title); 2010.
24. Honda K, Gyawali B, Ando M, Kumanishi R, Kato K, Sugiyama K, et al. Prospective survey of financial toxicity measured by the comprehensive score for financial toxicity in Japanese patients with cancer. J Glob Oncol. 2019;5:1–8.
25. Department for Professional Employees (DPE) Research Department. The U.S. health care system: an international perspective. Washington, DC; 2016. Available from: https://www.dpeaflcio.org/factsheets/the-us-health-care-system-an-international-perspective.
26. Honda K, Gyawali B, Ando M, Sugiyama K, Mitani S, Masuishi T, et al. A prospective survey of comprehensive score for financial toxicity in Japanese cancer patients: report on a pilot study. Ecancermedicalscience. 2018;12:12.
27. De Vita F, Greco G, Sperti E, Zichi C, Caglio A, Gamba T, et al. Patient-reported financial toxicity within the Italian public healthcare system: a single center cross-sectional analysis in patients with cancer. Ann Oncol. 2022;2:94.
28. Perrone F, Jommi C, Di Maio M, Gimigliano A, Gridelli C, Pignata S, et al. The association of financial difficulties with clinical outcomes in cancer patients: secondary analysis of 16 academic prospective clinical trials conducted in Italy. Ann Oncol. 2016;27(12):2224–9.
29. Tran G, Zafar SY. Financial toxicity and implications for cancer care in the era of molecular and immune therapies. Ann Transl Med. 2018;6(9):166.
30. Reeves A, McKee M, Basu S, Stuckler D. The political economy of austerity and healthcare: cross-national analysis of expenditure changes in 27 European nations 1995–2011. Health Policy. 2014;115(1):1–8.
31. Torp S, Nielsen RA, Gudbergsson SB, Dahl AA. Worksite adjustments and work ability among employed cancer survivors. Support Care Cancer. 2012;20:2149–56.
32. Swanberg JE. Making it work: informal caregiving, cancer, and employment. J Psychosoc Oncol. 2006;24(3):1–18.
33. Michigan Cancer Consortium. Financial navigation for people undergoing cancer treatment. Available online at: michigancancer. https://navectis.com/wp-content/uploads/2020/02/FinancialNavigationReport_FinalAccessible20183.pdf.
34. Mehnert A. Employment and work-related issues in cancer survivors. Crit Rev Oncol Hematol. 2011;77(2):109–30.
35. Guy GP Jr, Ekwueme DU, Yabroff KR, Dowling EC, Li C, Rodriguez JL, et al. Economic burden of cancer survivorship among adults in the United States. J Clin Oncol. 2013;31(30):3749.
36. Park J-H, Park E-C, Park J-H, Kim S-G, Lee S-Y. Job loss and re-employment of cancer patients in Korean employees: a nationwide retrospective cohort study. J Clin Oncol. 2008;26:1302.
37. Paul C, Boyes A, Hall A, Bisquera A, Miller A, O'Brien L. The impact of cancer diagnosis and treatment on employment, income, treatment decisions and financial assistance and their relationship to socioeconomic and disease factors. Support Care Cancer. 2016;24:4739–46.
38. Nekhlyudov L, Walker R, Ziebell R, Rabin B, Nutt S, Chubak J. Cancer survivors' experiences with insurance, finances, and employment: results from a multisite study. J Cancer Surviv. 2016;10:1104–11.

Body Image and Body Awareness in Breast Cancer: The Role of Imagination

27

Naciye Vardar Yagli and Aydan Asli Aksel Uylar

27.1 Body Image in Breast Cancer

Breast cancer is diagnosed in a significant number of women every year. Various factors have been identified in terms of the increased risk of breast cancer, including age, age of menopause, family history, obesity, nulliparity, and physical inactivity [1]. However, the most important risk factor is age. In 2022, breast cancer affected 2.3 million women and caused 670,000 deaths, according to the World Health Organization [2]. Survival rates of breast cancer are increasing thanks to advances in treatment. However, 25% of breast cancer survivors will continue to experience at least one physical or psychological symptom every day [3].

The processes of diagnosis and treatment of breast cancer affect women physically and psychologically [4]. Although the disease history and treatments received by women diagnosed with breast cancer can be different, treatment-related side effects are usually observed [5]. The impact of these side effects can be observed in many areas, especially in body image. Body image can negatively be affected by hair loss, weight gain or weight loss, lymphedema, breast loss or deformity, postural problems, and shoulder joint limitation in breast cancer [6].

N. V. Yagli (✉) · A. A. A. Uylar
Faculty of Physical Therapy and Rehabilitation, Hacettepe University, Ankara, Turkey
e-mail: naciye@hacettepe.edu.tr; aydanaksel@hacettepe.edu.tr

The extent to which the disturbance in body image depends on the individual's concern about body image [7]. Body image is a multidimensional concept that refers to an individuals' internal representation of their external appearance, encompassing perceptual, behavioral, affective, cognitive, and attitudinal aspects [8]. The perceptual dimension is related to the accuracy of body size compared to the actual size, the behavioral dimension is related to compensatory behaviors, the affective dimension is related to feelings associated with the body, the cognitive dimension is related to beauty perception about the body and attitudinal dimension is related to the subjective satisfaction of the body [8]. There are some factors concerning all these dimensions.

27.2 Factors Affecting Body Image in Breast Cancer

Factors affecting body image can be discussed specifically on breast deformities, weight changes, skin changes, and hair loss in breast cancer [4].

27.3 What Happens in the Body After Chemotherapy?

Women are often interested in their appearance and weight. Cancer-related weight loss or weight gain is also common in this disease. According to

Y. Bakar, A. Tuğral (eds.), *Managing Side Effects of Breast Cancer Treatment*,
https://doi.org/10.1007/978-3-031-75480-7_27

the studies, weight change has a negative impact on the quality of life, self-esteem, and joy of life of women with breast cancer. The main causes of weight gain are physical inactivity, chemotherapy, and increased calorie intake. Sarcopenic obesity with no increase in lean body weight develops secondary to chemotherapy [4]. Conversely, individuals undergoing chemotherapy may experience symptoms such as nausea, vomiting, and loss of appetite, which can result in significant weight loss [9].

Alopecia is the most unpleasant side effect of chemotherapy which is experienced with 65% of cancer patients [10]. Because hair represents itself as a characteristic of gender, sexual attractiveness, and beauty in many cultures, while its absence or lack may imply the loss of attractiveness and death. Hair loss also damages the perception of body image [4].

The need to wear a headscarf or wig due to alopecia might be evidence of this. Along with hair, eyebrows, eyelashes, and nose hair also fall out. Eyelashes protect the eyes and nasal hairs protect the upper respiratory tract against infections, and in their absence, individuals become more vulnerable to external airway pathogens [9].

27.4 What Happens in the Body After Radiotherapy?

During the treatment process, the size, location, and characteristics of the tumor are taken into consideration to decide whether the patient needs radiotherapy or not [11]. A recent study suggests that radiotherapy for breast cancer has long-term effects on body image [12].

Breast tissue and surrounding tissues exposed to radiation appear to affect the body image negatively in the long term due to adverse reactions that might occur [11]. In addition, skin changes such as burns, edema, irritation, radiation scars, and upper extremity limitation after radiation therapy can also affect body image [9, 13].

One study compared patients with breast reconstruction with and without radiation and found that women who received radiation therapy reported lower breast satisfaction and decreased quality of life [14]. According to a study of 4451 women with a 5-year follow-up, 40% of patients reported moderate or obvious changes in breast tissue after radiotherapy, and at least one-third of patients reported arm and shoulder pain. However, disturbance in body image tends to decrease over time [15].

27.5 What Happens in the Body After Endocrine Therapy?

Women with breast cancer benefit from endocrine therapies as part of their chemopreventive treatment. Side effects such as hot flashes and weight gain are also seen during endocrine therapy [16]. If hormone therapy is used in addition to the main treatment, the individual's menopausal symptom-suppressing hormone medication must be stopped. This will bring back the menopausal symptoms. The individual begins to live with these symptoms until the end of hormone therapy, and perhaps longer [9].

Hormone therapies bring menopause forward and cause infertility in premenopausal women. Loss of attraction at an early age, low self-esteem, and the burden of not being able to have children put a psychological strain on individuals [9]. However, no clear relationship has yet been found between endocrine therapy and body image [9].

27.6 What Happens in the Body After Breast Cancer Surgery?

One of the side effects of breast cancer treatments is disorders in the perception of body image after surgical removal of breast cancer. Losing a breast, tissue damage, and breast deformities are the most important issues that negatively affect body image in breast cancer survivors [8]. The breast is seen as a symbol of femininity, motherhood, and sexuality, and deterioration in body image and decrease in self-esteem are observed after surgical operation of the breast. Especially mastectomy surgeries negatively affect body image, feelings of femininity, and sexuality. In the literature, it is stated that 15–30% of body image deterioration occurs after breast cancer surgeries. Negative effects on body image lead to anxiety, depression, and social isolation [17]. Unilateral or bilateral total mastectomy surgeries have been found to be associated with an increase in loss of femininity, fertility, sexuality, and problems with the partner [18].

Postural changes seen after unilateral mastectomy are quite common and affect body image. Scoliotic changes, scapula asymmetry, and shoulder and pelvis inequality have been observed after unilateral mastectomy compared to breast-conserving surgery and breast reconstruction [19]. These compensatory changes bring pain and indirectly affect the quality of life of individuals. Early rehabilitation is important to prevent postural changes and their complications after unilateral mastectomy [19].

Sexual health, which is an important part of the quality of life, is affected by body image disorders. Problems in sexual life in breast cancer can reach up to 70% [20]. In addition, young and sexually active women show worse perceptions of body image and poorer psychosocial adjustment after treatment because they attribute more importance to their appearance [21]. According to a study, it was found that breast reconstruction after mastectomy was associated with improvements in sexual function and body image [20].

Despite all the negative perceptions, some patients also attribute a higher value to the well-being achieved with mastectomy and believe that mastectomy will not have only negative effects. Contrary to social norms, these patients see the breast as part of the disease and see themselves from a new perspective [22].

Axillary lymph node dissection (ALND) is associated with postoperative complications such as decreased range of motion of the upper extremity and lymphedema. Lymphedema, which is seen between 20 and 35% after this surgical intervention, negatively affects patients from the perspectives both aesthetically and functionally [13]. The decreased shoulder abduction seen in breast cancer patients after ALND contributes to postoperative upper limb dysfunction [23]. According to a review of 9 studies with 977 participants, lymphedema has a greater negative impact on body image in individuals who experience pain, and sensory and functional differences [3]. This clearly suggests that body image perception is not only influenced by psychological factors.

27.7 Impact of Other Factors on Body Image

Body mass index, age, physical activity level, and relationship status of the individual are also effective on body image [11]. Struggling with physical limitations, decreased self-esteem, and less perception of attractiveness at a young age affects body image more than older individuals [9].

According to research, it has been determined that patients who are included in the decision-making mechanisms about their treatment are able to better manage the results of their treatment. This means that they can cope better with changes in their bodies [9].

Studies emphasize the need to include the male partner in the management process of the disease. Including the spouse in psychosocial interventions will provide social support to the patient. In addition, the cancer diagnosis and treatment process not only affects the patient but also affects her partner, children, and family [24]. The male partner must be ready for a change in gender roles, such as doing housework or taking care of children. One should know and understand that cancer-specific fatigue is different from normal fatigue, that forgetfulness may be common, and that pain and loss of libido may also occur. This understanding alone can reduce the stress experienced by women [24].

The change in body image is also influenced by the change in personal identity during the disease. Changes in the body affect the individual's mood and beliefs as much as they affect the body. The challenges of the pathophysiology of the disease and treatment side effects can have a negative impact on one's psychology [9].

The perception of a positive body image has been found to be closely associated with an individual's self-efficacy in coping with a diagnosis of breast cancer and its treatment [21]. The issue of body image is considered to be a crucial aspect of the quality of life for cancer survivors, as highlighted by the reasons mentioned above [8]. Body image assessment should be included in the follow-up processes of all women after breast cancer surgeries and counseling should be provided.

27.8 Assessment of Body Image

In this section, body image evaluation methods will be discussed. Since body image is a subjective perception of a patient's appearance, it can be evaluated by subjective methods such as questionnaires [25]. Some of these evaluation methods emphasize different aspects of body image, which is a multidimensional concept, while others evaluate it in a general concept. Again, some are breast cancer-specific questionnaires, while others are for the general population.

27.8.1 53-Item Body Image After Breast Cancer Questionnaire (BIBCQ)

The BIBCQ evaluates body image in breast cancer patients across six dimensions, body stigma, namely vulnerability, limitations, transparency, body concerns, and arm concerns. BIBCQ includes a total of 53 questions, and higher scores indicate a negative perception of body image [26].

27.8.2 Body Image Self-Rating Questionnaire for Breast Cancer (BISQ-BC)

The BISQ-BC contains 26 items with subitems on behavior change related to body image, role changes, psychological change, sexual activity change, and social change. Questions are scored on a 5-point Likert scale. High scores reflect worse body image perception [27].

27.8.3 Body Acceptance Scale for Women with Breast Cancer (BAS-BC)

Another body image questionnaire developed specifically for breast cancer is BAS-BC. It evaluates the positive body image perception of an individual with positive questions with 6 subheadings and 17 items: encountering, adaptation, return to daily life, understanding, successful transition, and leap into the future [28].

27.8.4 Breast Impact of Treatment Scale (BITS)

This 13-item scale measures the stress related to body change after—mastectomy or that causes less body change, such as segmental mastectomy. The BITS scale offers a 4-point rating scale of 0,1,3, and 5 in its items. Higher scores out of a total score of 65 indicate more body change stress [29].

27.8.5 The European Organization for Research and Treatment of Cancer Breast Cancer Module (EORTC QLQ-BR23)

The EORTC QLQ-BR23 questionnaire has been specifically designed for breast cancer patients and is comprised of 23 items that are categorized into subheadings of body image, sexuality, arm symptoms, breast symptoms, and side effects of the systemic treatment. The body image subheading includes items such as feeling physically less attractive, difficulty looking at oneself naked, feeling less feminine, and body dissatisfaction. Patients are required to consider their last week while scoring the items of EORTC-BR23. Higher scores indicate better body image. A significant change is indicated by a score difference of 20 points or more [11].

27.8.6 The 10-Item Body Image Scale (BIS)

The BIS scale is a general scale that can be used in all cancer patients to measure body image in emotional, behavioral, and cognitive aspects. Patients score each item between 0 and 3 on 10 questions. The total score is obtained by summing the scores given to the questions and as the scores increase, the perception of body image deteriorates [30].

27.8.7 Body Image Screener for Cancer Reconstruction (BICR)

The BICR begins with a short paragraph stating that patients undergoing reconstructive surgery may have concerns about their appearance. It consists of 4 questions that question current and future concerns, thoughts, and avoidance and can be used in all cancer patients [31].

27.8.8 Body Image and Relationship Scale (BIRS)

The BIRS questionnaire is a 32-item scale scored on a 5-point Likert scale. High scores indicate poor body image [21].

27.8.9 Body Dysmorphic Disorder Examination (BDDE)

The BDDE instrument is a questionnaire that assesses dissatisfaction with a body part. The 34-item questionnaire is also used to diagnose body dysmorphic disorders. A score of 66 and above out of a total of 168 points indicates that the individual is not satisfied with her appearance [20].

27.8.10 Sexual Adjustment and Body Image Scale (SABIS)

The SABIS, developed specifically for breast cancer to assess body image and sexual dysfunction, consists of two scales, the body image scale and the sexual adjustment scale. The Body Image Scale is divided into two sections, prior body image and post body image, while the sexual adjustment scale is divided into three sections, prior sexual adjustment, sexual importance of the breasts, and impact on sexual functioning. A total of 28 items are scored on a 5-point Likert scale. Each item has an additional "not applicable" response option [32].

27.8.11 Body Satisfaction Scale (BSS)

The BSS scale consists of 25 questions scored on a 5-point Likert scale. The items question the individual's appearance concerns and weight-related concerns. As the score increases, satisfaction increases and weight anxiety decreases [33].

27.8.12 Multidimensional Body-Self Relations Questionnaire (MBSRQ)

MSBRQ is a multidimensional self-reported questionnaire with a total of 69 items. The subheadings are appearance orientation, appearance evaluation, fitness orientation, fitness evaluation, health orientation, health evaluation, overweight preoccupation, illness orientation, self-classified weight, and body area satisfaction scale. In cases where appearance-related body image is investigated, the subscale of the MBSRQ-Appearance Scales, which includes 5 of the above subscales, is preferred. It can be used in adolescents and adults aged 15 years and older [34].

27.8.13 Body Image Avoidance Questionnaire (BIAQ)

The BIAQ is a behavioral avoidance scale. It is based on the individual's avoidance of events that may increase dissatisfaction with body image. It consists of a total of 19 items with 4 subheadings: clothing, social activities, restriction, and care. The individual scores between 0 and 5 for each item This questionnaire helps health professionals to understand patients' body image concerns by assessing behavioral avoidance in more than one aspect [35].

27.8.14 Body Appreciation Scale (BAS)

The 10-item BAS measures positive views of body appreciation and body image. Items are scored on a 5-point Likert scale. Higher scores indicate favorable body image and body appreciation [36].

27.9 Body Awareness in Breast Cancer

Treatment options for breast cancer negatively affect the patient's self-perception and body awareness, as well as their body image [37]. Body awareness is a concept that aims to focus on and be aware of internal sensations regarding the body [38]. Proprioception and interoception are subjective perceptions that can be influenced by mental processes [39]. Interoception is defined as the sensation of the physiological states of all tissues. It provides the body's connection with the world and internal adaptation to the changing environment. Therefore, it is closely related to body awareness [40].

Awareness is focusing on the moment, and body awareness is being aware of the body at the moment. Body awareness therapy, yoga, Tai Chi, massage, breathing therapies, body-focused psychotherapy, awareness-based therapy and meditations, and mind–body association practices have been used for years to increase body awareness [38]. According to a study conducted on 29 women with breast cancer, an increase in body awareness was observed in individuals who participated in a mindfulness program [41]. Differently, in a study phototherapy intervention aiming to increase self-awareness was investigated in breast cancer. The phototherapy intervention used in this study is to create a poster as a collage from photographs to improve the individual's body image and self-awareness. After this 16-week intervention, an improvement was observed in the individuals' self-esteem and emotional status [37].

27.10 Intervention for Body Image and Body Awareness in Breast Cancer

Reducing the side effects and complications of standard cancer treatments such as radiotherapy, chemotherapy, and surgery by associated conditions such as alopecia, weight gain/loss, upper limb movement limitation, lymphedema, and neuropathy affect the quality of life and body image of the individuals [13, 23].

In the literature, there are many cognitive, behavioral, and psychosocial interventions that aim to reduce psychological distress and improve body image in breast cancer patients. In addition, interventions that encourage physical activity are also cognitively beneficial as they may reduce treatment complications [13]. However, in addition to these, pretreatment patient education and shared decision-making mechanisms after determining expectations may also facilitate the patient's treatment process. Treatment options and their potential effects on body image change should be discussed before treatment [13].

27.10.1 Physical Activity-Based Interventions

The multicomponent concept of prehabilitation includes targeted components that aim to bring the individual to the best possible physical and psychological levels until the treatment begins. Including individuals in a pretreatment rehabilitation program is an intervention that can serve to improve treatment outcomes and reduce complications, thereby improving posttreatment bodily well-being and body image. Prehabilitation includes patient education, exercise training, nutritional support, and psychological support. Prehabilitation allows patients to have more of a say during the course of treatment and reduces anxiety levels. Pretreatment rehabilitation improves cardiovascular fitness, leading to recovery faster, and fewer complications after treatment [23]. Breast cancer patients who were more physically active before surgery reported an 85% faster recovery at 3 weeks after surgery [42]. Although the concept of prehabilitation is mostly considered in patients in whom surgery is planned, its effects should continue to be investigated on patients in the preparation phase of chemotherapy and radiotherapy [23].

In a study, breast cancer patients who had been treated with chemotherapy or radiotherapy for at least 4 weeks were included in a 10-week exercise training program twice a week. The exercise program consisted of gymnastics, walking, jogging, movement games, and relaxation exercises. According to the results, patients in the intervention group showed improvement in depression, anxiety, and body image [43].

Resistance exercise training is known to improve body image by changing subjective perceptions and making one feel fit. Researchers wondered whether the same was true in breast cancer patients. In the studies included in a review examining this issue, resistance training was applied 2–3 days a week for at least 8 weeks. According to this review, resistance exercise training is an intervention that contributes to body image in breast cancer [44].

Dance is a type of psychotherapeutic physical activity that encourages movement, providing a connection between body and mind. It allows the expression of existing emotions. According to a systematic review, dance therapy appears to be effective in reducing the side effects of multimodal treatment of breast cancer [45].

27.10.2 Cognitive-Based Interventions

Cognitive behavioral therapy (CBT) is an approach used in the regulation of body image perception in cancer diagnosis and treatment processes. It is a targeted intervention that focuses on changing thoughts and behaviors [13]. In a study, weekly 2-h sessions of CBT for 7 weeks led to improvements in body esteem, weight and shape anxiety, acceptance of age-related changes in appearance, and self-esteem in breast cancer survivors. A CBT-based body image intervention was developed in collaboration with health professionals called "Set Your Body Free" [46].

Mindfulness-based mind–body alliance interventions are used to improve body image perception in breast cancer [5]. Mindfulness is defined as the awareness of the event or situation based on the main focus. With mindfulness training, the individual tries to accept the consciousness of the present moment and the experience as it is. In breast cancer patients who were subjected to mindfulness training consisting of body scanning techniques, yoga, and meditation, mindfulness training was found to be beneficial in reducing negative thoughts about body image after the training. Additionally, the mindfulness program was found to be effective in reducing negative feelings and thoughts [41].

In a 2020 study, individuals who underwent breast cancer surgery performed a 12-week Qigong Mind-Body Exercise Program. In this intervention, in which no adverse events occurred, improvements were observed in the patients' pain intensity, symptoms of anxiety and depression, stress level, self-esteem, shoulder range of motion, and quality of life. Qigong Mind-Body Exercise Program includes upper body stretching and strengthening exercises based on correct posture, diaphragmatic breathing, and body awareness [47].

Relaxation, mental images, and spirituality intervention (RIME), a biopsychosocial model, is an intervention that includes relaxation, mental images, and spirituality. In a study conducted on women with breast cancer who underwent mastectomy, there were significant improvements in self-esteem and quality of life after RIME [48].

Web-based online writing applications were also investigated whether they can reduce body image problems. This activity aims to reduce the patient's body image problems by focusing on a single session of self-compassion for the changing body. This session was repeated after 1 week, 1 month, and 3 months. Patients showed 88% compliance with this intervention and improved perceptions of their body image, body appreciation, and self-compassion [49].

Acceptance and commitment therapy, which is a continuation of cognitive behavioral therapies, is reported to reduce psychological pain, anxiety, and depression symptoms. A study included a total of 31 breast cancer patients reported an improved body image and quality of sexual life with acceptance and commitment therapy [50].

27.10.3 Breast Reconstruction After Breast Cancer Surgery

Meeting the body image expectations of these patients continues to be difficult due to body dissatisfaction, psychological distress, and social and sexual dysfunctions. Breast reconstruction is one of the procedures used to regain body image satisfaction [51].

In breast reconstruction, implants or autologous tissues are used to create a new breast. Muscle skin flaps such as transverse rectus abdominis and latissimus dorsi flaps have more cosmetic results than non-autologous ones [52]. This procedure can be performed urgently or on a delayed basis. Immediate reconstruction is carried out during mastectomy, while delayed reconstruction is performed after the mastectomy wound has healed. Occasionally, a healthy breast may also be included in this surgery to achieve symmetry in size and shape. In cases where reconstruction is difficult or not possible, patients also use external breast prostheses to achieve a normal breast appearance [53].

A study of 30 women with breast cancer who underwent breast reconstruction combined with mastectomy found that they showed better sexual function, better body image, and fewer depressive symptoms than those without breast reconstruction [20].

Despite the known benefits, 25% of women who undergo breast reconstruction cannot accept breast implants [51]. Although it gives most women a sense of normalcy again, unnatural appearance, feeling unnatural and decreased sensation can be among the reasons for this situation [52]. A meta-analysis suggests that women who have breast-conserving surgery have better body image than those who have breast reconstruction. This shows the importance of preserving the breast [52]. A 2018 study also reported that breast-conserving therapies were associated with higher breast satisfaction than mastectomy and breast reconstruction [54].

Follow-up of the patient is important in terms of complications and side effects that may occur after reconstruction. After this surgical procedure, physiotherapy and rehabilitation with a physiotherapist will be beneficial to maintaining shoulder patency, healing the donor tissue, regaining muscle strength, returning to activities of daily living, and adapting to the new body [53].

27.11 The Role of Imagination

Imagination is the retrieval of information about the appearance of an object from long-term memory for processing. This shows that imagination is closely related to visual and memory processes [55]. Imagination encourages individuals to imagine thoughts and behaviors to improve their coping strategies and gain a different perspective. Verbal instructions are given to individuals to direct them to visual and auditory sensations that will have a positive effect during the sessions [56]. Media that use guided imagery instead of a health professional are also used. In one study, a CD was prepared for guided imaging and this CD was checked by psychiatrists. The CD included guidance on visualization, relaxation, and deep breathing exercises [57]. This mind–body intervention is often used as an adjunct to another treatment method [56].

Relaxation and visualization therapy encourages the patient to visualize and imagine the desired outcome is known as a relaxation technique that includes meditation and deep breathing exercises. The 20-minute sessions are designed with guided imagery. This therapy has been investigated in the context of stress, anxiety, depression, lymphocyte, and salivary cortisol levels in patients with breast cancer receiving radiotherapy. Patients were requested to visualize the immune system attacking the tumor, and they were also told to visualize a completely healthy breast tissue. Patients continued this practice twice a day at home. Although cortisol and lymphocyte levels did not change with this intervention, it was effective in reducing psychological distress [58].

Yoga is a mind–body exercise with similar effects to aerobic exercise in addition to meditation content. Good mood and reduced fatigue are the main expected results of yoga. In 52 breast cancer patients, improvement in general well-being, physical and mental functioning, emotional, cognitive, and social functioning was observed after 6 weeks of yoga training [59]. In a study examining the effect of yoga on quality of life and anxiety in breast cancer, it was found that yoga reduced stress and anxiety levels by helping to relax [60]. Guided imagery and meditation support the individual physically and emotionally during yoga, in addition to strengthening the unity of mind and body [61]. Guided imagery is known to reduce stress and anxiety levels in breast cancer [56]. It reduces perceived pain sensation when applied during treatment [62].

In addition to the effects mentioned above, imagination is used today to reduce body dissatisfaction. A study published in 2022 reported that imagery is a promising option for changing negative perceptions of the body [63]. According to a randomized controlled trial conducted in 2023, guided imaginary application improved a healthy lifestyle and quality of life in breast cancer [64]. An intervention called "Restoring Body Image After Cancer (REBIC)" used guided imagery to address body image issues. After 1 year, patients experienced lower body image concerns compared to the control group [65].

Current literature focuses on alternative interventions to improve body awareness and body image perception. Virtual reality, which allows the illusion of a full body experience in a virtual world, is used to increase body awareness. Advanced human/computer interfaces can improve individuals' ability to receive and manage sensations [66]. The individual can feel a virtual and real body simultaneously. The belonging sense of a virtual body offers the individual an opportunity to position and define their own body and recognize his/her inner senses. Virtual reality applications can improve symptom control in breast cancer by increasing internal sensory awareness with visual support and can enable socialization by reducing anxiety and body shame [66].

27.12 Self-Esteem in Breast Cancer

Self-esteem is closely associated with an individual's self-confidence and self-satisfaction. The breast cancer diagnosis and treatment process brings with it many physical and psychological difficulties. Changes in physical appearance caused by surgery, chemotherapy, and radiotherapy can cause anxiety, depression, and low self-confidence [67]. Moreover, the importance of self-esteem in returning to normal life has been demonstrated [68]. Therefore, self-esteem is an important issue in breast cancer. Various questionnaires are used to measure self-esteem in breast cancer.

27.12.1 Rosenberg Self-Esteem Scale (RSES)

The RSES contains 10 items, each scored on a 4-point Likert scale. As the total score increases, the individual's self-esteem increases. The total score is 40 [67].

27.12.2 The Single-Item Self-Esteem Scale (SISE)

The SISE scale consists of a single item, "I have high self-esteem", scored on a 7-point Likert-type scale. A high score indicates high self-esteem [46].

27.13 Summary

Breast cancer continues to cause mortality and morbidity every year. Diagnosis and treatment processes affect patients both physically and psychologically. Chemotherapy, radiotherapy, hormone therapy, and surgery are the standard treatments for breast cancer. Treatments have both positive and negative effects, which vary from person to person. Influence on body image and body awareness is one of them. To date, various interventions have aimed to improve body image perception before, during, and after treatments. These interventions show improvements in body awareness and body image by changing the patient's perspective, regulating sensory inputs, and providing psychological support with a holistic approach. In addition, physical therapy and rehabilitation programs implemented by physiotherapists increase the physical activity level of the patient and have a positive effect on body image and self-esteem. Imagination and its underlying mechanisms continue to be investigated to improve body image and body awareness in breast cancer survivors.

References

1. Sung H, Ferlay J, Siegel RL, Laversanne M, Soerjomataram I, Jemal A, et al. Global cancer statistics 2020: GLOBOCAN estimates of incidence and mortality worldwide for 36 cancers in 185 countries. CA Cancer J Clin. 2021;71(3):209–49.
2. WHO. Breast cancer 2024. https://www.who.int/newsroom/fact-sheets/detail/breast-cancer#:~:text=In%20 2022%2C%20there%20were%202.3,increasing%20 rates%20in%20later%20life.
3. Byrne E, Gaffey J, Hayden L, Daly A, Gallagher P, Dunne S. Body image and cancer-related lymphoedema: a systematic review. Psychooncology. 2023;32(10):1528–38.
4. Helms RL, O'Hea EL, Corso M. Body image issues in women with breast cancer. Psychol Health Med. 2008;13(3):313–25.
5. Brunet J, Price J, Baillot A, Dann E, Vani MF. Feasibility and acceptability of study methods and psychosocial interventions for body image among women diagnosed with breast cancer: a systematic review and narrative synthesis. Psychooncology. 2024;33(1):e6278.
6. Morales-Sanchez L, Luque-Ribelles V, Gil-Olarte P, Ruiz-Gonzalez P, Guil R. Enhancing self-esteem and body image of breast cancer women through interventions: a systematic review. Int J Environ Res Public Health. 2021;18(4):1640.
7. Carver CS, Pozo-Kaderman C, Price AA, Noriega V, Harris SD, Derhagopian RP, et al. Concern about aspects of body image and adjustment to early stage breast cancer. Psychosom Med. 1998;60(2):168–74.
8. Brunet J, Sabiston CM, Burke S. Surviving breast cancer: women's experiences with their changed bodies. Body Image. 2013;10(3):344–51.
9. Kołodziejczyk A, Pawłowski T. Negative body image in breast cancer patients. Adv Clin Exp Med. 2019;28(8):1137–42.
10. Wikramanayake TC, Haberland NI, Akhundlu A, Laboy Nieves A, Miteva M. Prevention and treatment of chemotherapy-induced alopecia: what is available and what is coming? Curr Oncol. 2023;30(4):3609–26.
11. Afshar-Bakshloo M, Albers S, Richter C, Berninger O, Blohmer J-U, Roehle R, et al. How breast cancer therapies impact body image—real-world data from a prospective cohort study collecting patient-reported outcomes. BMC Cancer. 2023;23(1):705.
12. Schmitz KH, Speck RM, Rye SA, DiSipio T, Hayes SC. Prevalence of breast cancer treatment sequelae over 6 years of follow-up: the pulling through study. Cancer. 2012;118(8 Suppl):2217–25.
13. Fiser C, Crystal JS, Tevis SE, Kesmodel S, Rojas KE. Treatment and survivorship interventions to prevent poor body image outcomes in breast cancer survivors. Breast Cancer (Dove Med Press). 2021;13:701–9.
14. Albornoz CR, Matros E, McCarthy CM, Klassen A, Cano SJ, Alderman AK, et al. Implant breast reconstruction and radiation: a multicenter analysis of long-term health-related quality of life and satisfaction. Ann Surg Oncol. 2014;21(7):2159–64.
15. Hopwood P, Haviland JS, Sumo G, Mills J, Bliss JM, Yarnold JR. Comparison of patient-reported breast, arm, and shoulder symptoms and body image after radiotherapy for early breast cancer: 5-year follow-up in the randomised standardisation of breast radiotherapy (START) trials. Lancet. 2010;11(3):231–40.
16. Przezdziecki A, Sherman KA, Baillie A, Taylor A, Foley E, Stalgis-Bilinski K. My changed body: breast cancer, body image, distress and self-compassion. Psychooncology. 2013;22(8):1872–9.
17. TTaylan S, Kolaç N. The self image and sexual adaptation of women undering breast cancer surgery. Androl Bul. 2021;23:163–9.
18. Paterson CL, Lengacher CA, Donovan KA, Kip KE, Tofthagen CS. Body image in younger breast cancer survivors: a systematic review. Cancer Nurs. 2016;39(1):E39–58.
19. Liu R, Xie H, Wang Y, Wang Q, Xie X, Zhang X. Impact of unilateral mastectomy on body posture: a prospective longitudinal observational study. Asia Pac J Oncol Nurs. 2024;11(2):100336.

20. Archangelo SCV, Sabino Neto M, Veiga DF, Garcia EB, Ferreira LM. Sexuality, depression and body image after breast reconstruction. Clinics. 2019;74:e883.
21. Hormes JM, Lytle LA, Gross CR, Ahmed RL, Troxel AB, Schmitz KH. The body image and relationships scale: development and validation of a measure of body image in female breast cancer survivors. J Clin Oncol. 2008;26(8):1269–74.
22. Sun L, Ang E, Ang WHD, Lopez V. Losing the breast: a meta-synthesis of the impact in women breast cancer survivors. Psychooncology. 2018;27(2):376–85.
23. Santa Mina D, Brahmbhatt P, Lopez C, Baima J, Gillis C, Trachtenberg L, et al. The case for prehabilitation prior to breast cancer treatment. PM R. 2017;9(9S2):S305–S16.
24. Akpor OA, Kolawole ER, Olorunfemi O, Oduyemi RO. Breast cancer and body image: the roles of the male partner. J Intern Med. 2023;11(2):65–9.
25. Brunet J, Price J. A scoping review of measures used to assess body image in women with breast cancer. Psychooncology. 2021;30(5):669–80.
26. Liu Y, Liu W, Ma Y, Yang X, Zhou H, Zhang T, et al. Research on body image cognition, social support and illness perception in breast cancer patients with different surgical methods. Front Psychol. 2022;13:931679.
27. Zhu F, Zhang W, Liu C, Qiang W, Lu Q. Association of self-compassion and body image disturbance among young breast cancer patients: mediating effect of body surveillance and body shame. Asia Pac J Oncol Nurs. 2023;10(4):100199.
28. Ahn J, Suh EE. Body acceptance scale for women with breast cancer: development and validation of a measurement. Semin Oncol Nurs. 2023;39(5):151486.
29. Frierson GM, Thiel DL, Andersen BL. Body change stress for women with breast cancer: the breast-impact of treatment scale. Ann Behav Med. 2006;32(1):77–81.
30. Melissant HC, Neijenhuijs KI, Jansen F, Aaronson NK, Groenvold M, Holzner B, et al. A systematic review of the measurement properties of the body image scale (BIS) in cancer patients. Support Care Cancer. 2018;26(6):1715–26.
31. Fingeret MC, Nipomnick S, Guindani M, Baumann D, Hanasono M, Crosby M. Body image screening for cancer patients undergoing reconstructive surgery. Psychooncology. 2014;23(8):898–905.
32. Dalton EJ, Rasmussen VN, Classen CC, Grumann M, Palesh OG, Zarcone J, et al. Sexual adjustment and body image scale (SABIS): a new measure for breast cancer patients. Breast J. 2009;15(3):287–90.
33. Prates ACL, Freitas-Junior R, Prates MFO, Veloso MF, Barros NM. Influence of body image in women undergoing treatment for breast cancer. Rev Bras Ginecol Obstet. 2017;39(4):175–83.
34. Thompson JK, Schaefer LM, Thomas F. Cash: a multidimensional innovator in the measurement of body image; some lessons learned and some lessons for the future of the field. Body Image. 2019;31:198–203.
35. Lydecker J. Body image avoidance questionnaire (BIAQ). In: Wade T, editor. Encyclopedia of feeding and eating: disorders. Cham: Springer; 2015.
36. Zarate D, Marmara J, Potoczny C, Hosking W, Stavropoulos V. Body appreciation scale (BAS-2): measurement invariance across genders and item response theory examination. BMC Psychol. 2021;9(1):114.
37. Marafante G, Ferri C, Giuffredi I, Bidin L. Image and self-esteem: a photo-therapy program to improve body image, increase self-awareness and the expression of emotions in breast cancer patients. A pilot study. Ann Oncol. 2017;28:28.
38. Mehling WE, Wrubel J, Daubenmier JJ, Price CJ, Kerr CE, Silow T, et al. Body awareness: a phenomenological inquiry into the common ground of mind-body therapies. Philos Ethics Humanit Med. 2011;6:6.
39. Mehling WE, Gopisetty V, Daubenmier J, Price CJ, Hecht FM, Stewart A. Body awareness: construct and self-report measures. PLoS One. 2009;4(5):e5614.
40. Grabauskaite A, Baranauskas M, Griskova-Bulanova I. Interoception and gender: what aspects should we pay attention to? Conscious Cogn. 2017;48:129–37.
41. Pintado S, Andrade S. Randomized controlled trial of mindfulness program to enhance body image in patients with breast cancer. Eur J Integr Med. 2017;12:147–52.
42. Nilsson H, Angeras U, Bock D, Borjesson M, Onerup A, Fagevik Olsen M, et al. Is preoperative physical activity related to post-surgery recovery? A cohort study of patients with breast cancer. BMJ Open. 2016;6(1):e007997.
43. Mehnert A, Veers S, Howaldt D, Braumann KM, Koch U, Schulz KH. Effects of a physical exercise rehabilitation group program on anxiety, depression, body image, and health-related quality of life among breast cancer patients. Onkologie. 2011;34(5):248–53.
44. Effa CJ, Dolgoy ND, McNeely ML. Resistance exercise and art therapy on body image in breast cancer: a scoping review. Womens Health Rep. 2020;1(1):424–35.
45. Silva da Costa N, Alves da Silva AS, de Melo-Neto JS. Effects of dance therapy in women with breast cancer: a systematic review protocol. PLoS One. 2022;17(6):e0257948.
46. Lewis-Smith H, Diedrichs PC, Harcourt D. A pilot study of a body image intervention for breast cancer survivors. Body Image. 2018;27:21–31.
47. Osypiuk K, Ligibel J, Giobbie-Hurder A, Vergara-Diaz G, Bonato P, Quinn R, et al. Qigong mind-body exercise as a biopsychosocial therapy for persistent post-surgical pain in breast cancer: a pilot study. Integr Cancer Ther. 2020;19:1534735419893766.
48. Elias AC, Ricci MD, Rodriguez LH, Pinto SD, Giglio JS, Baracat EC. The biopsychosocial spiritual model applied to the treatment of women with breast cancer, through RIME intervention (relaxation, mental images, spirituality). Complement Ther Clin Pract. 2015;21(1):1–6.

49. Sherman KA, Przezdziecki A, Alcorso J, Kilby CJ, Elder E, Boyages J, et al. Reducing body image-related distress in women with breast cancer using a structured online writing exercise: results from the my changed body randomized controlled trial. J Clin Oncol. 2018;36(19):1930–40.
50. Tunc E, Sevcan Orak O, Iseri O. The effect of acceptance and commitment therapy-based psychoeducation on body image, quality of sexual life, and dyadic adjustment of women after breast cancer surgery. Oncol Nurs Forum. 2023;50(5):599–609.
51. Zhao W, Chong YY, Chien WT. Effectiveness of cognitive-based interventions for improving body image of patients having breast cancer: a systematic review and meta-analysis. Asia Pac J Oncol Nurs. 2023;10(4):100213.
52. Fang SY, Shu BC, Chang YJ. The effect of breast reconstruction surgery on body image among women after mastectomy: a meta-analysis. Breast Cancer Res Treat. 2013;137(1):13–21.
53. NCI. Breast Reconstruction After Mastectomy. 2017. https://www.cancer.gov/types/breast/reconstruction-fact-sheet#:~:text=Breasts%20can%20be%20rebuilt%20using,used%20to%20rebuild%20the%20breast.
54. Lagendijk M, van Egdom LSE, van Veen FEE, Vos EL, Mureau MAM, van Leeuwen N, et al. Patient-reported outcome measures may add value in breast cancer surgery. Ann Surg Oncol. 2018;25(12):3563–71.
55. Ganis G, Schendan HE. Visual imagery. Wiley Interdiscip Rev Cogn Sci. 2011;2(3):239–52.
56. Sinha MK, Barman A, Goyal M, Patra S. Progressive muscle relaxation and guided imagery in breast cancer: a systematic review and meta-analysis of randomised controlled trials. Indian J Palliat Care. 2021;27(2):336–44.
57. Chen SF, Wang HH, Yang HY, Chung UL. Effect of relaxation with guided imagery on the physical and psychological symptoms of breast cancer patients undergoing chemotherapy. Iran Red Crescent Med J. 2015;17(11):e31277.
58. Nunes DF, Rodriguez AL, da Silva HF, Luz C, Braga Filho AP, Muller MC, et al. Relaxation and guided imagery program in patients with breast cancer undergoing radiotherapy is not associated with neuroimmunomodulatory effects. J Psychosom Res. 2007;63(6):647–55.
59. Vardar Yagli N, Sener G, Arikan H, Saglam M, Inal Ince D, Savci S, et al. Do yoga and aerobic exercise training have impact on functional capacity, fatigue, peripheral muscle strength, and quality of life in breast cancer survivors? Integr Cancer Ther. 2015;14(2):125–32.
60. Ulger O, Yagli NV. Effects of yoga on the quality of life in cancer patients. Complement Ther Clin Pract. 2010;16(2):60–3.
61. Gimbel MA. Yoga, meditation, and imagery: clinical applications. Nurse Pract Forum. 1998;9(4):243–55.
62. Saleh A, Bachtiar SM, Sjattar EL, Abrar EA. The effectiveness of technical guided imagery on pain intensity decreasing in breast cancer patients. Enferm Clin. 2020;30:45–8.
63. Ghaderi A, Welch E, Zha C, Holmes EA. Imagery rescripting for reducing body image dissatisfaction: a randomized controlled trial. Cogn Ther Res. 2022;46(4):721–34.
64. Ata G, Kılıç D, Yıldırım D. The effect of guided imagery based on health promotion model on quality of life in breast cancer patients: a randomized controlled study. Res Sq. 2023.
65. Viale PH. Breast cancer and body image issues. J Adv Pract Oncol. 2018;9(4):375–6.
66. Sebri V, Durosini I, Strika M, Pizzoli SFM, Mazzocco K, Pravettoni G. Virtual reality for the promotion of interoception awareness and body image in breast cancer survivors: a study protocol. Front Psychol. 2023;14:1165905.
67. Tsai PL, Kuo TT, Ku CH, Liao GS, Lin CK, Pan HH. Self-esteem as a predictor of mental adjustment in patients with breast cancer. Int J Environ Res Public Health. 2021;18(23):12588.
68. Mustian KM, Katula JA, Gill DL, Roscoe JA, Lang D, Murphy K. Tai chi Chuan, health-related quality of life and self-esteem: a randomized trial with breast cancer survivors. Support Care Cancer. 2004;12(12):871–6.

Quality of Life in Breast Cancer Patients

28

Derya Çinar and Aslıhan Öztürk Çetin

28.1 Quality of Life

The World Health Organization (WHO) defines quality of life (QOL) as "an individual's relationships, goals, expectations, norms and concerns within his or her culture and value system" [1]. QOL is a concept that expresses how an individual feels and is able to carry out daily activities and should be considered as a whole with biophysiological, psychological, sociocultural, and socioeconomic dimensions [1–3].

Cancer is a chronic disease that negatively affects the QOL of patients with cancer [4]. Assessment of QOL is an important prognostic factor in the management of the potential side effects of cancer [2, 5]. Besides, QOL has critical importance at all stages of cancer, such as cancer diagnosis, treatment, palliative care, and survival [1]. Assessment of QOL of cancer patients is also an important predictive factor for the survival of patients. Therefore, it is important to evaluate QOL and factors affecting QOL in cancer diagnosis, treatment, and survival process [6]. In the literature, it has been reported that patients with breast cancer have low physical, mental, and emotional quality of life. On the other hand, it has been reported that patients with hematological malignancy have a lower QOL than patients with breast cancer. In addition, it has been highlighted that QoL is also negatively affected in patients with bone metastases and those with high symptom severity [7]. Yet, age is a well-known prognostic factor in cancer patients, it has been reported that younger patients have a lower QOL in terms of social functioning than older patients [8].

28.2 Breast Cancer and Quality of Life

The increasing incidence of breast cancer has put the concept of QOL of breast cancer patients on the agenda, aiming to help improve survival through the development of early diagnosis and effective treatments [6]. It has been reported that sociodemographic and clinical characteristics of women with breast cancer affect their level of QOL. These characteristics include sociodemographic characteristics such as age, marital status, education level, employment status, having children, social support, financial support, spousal support, and clinical characteristics such as side effects of anticancer treatments, symptom burden, and cancer stage, as well as including various medical and psychosocial factors [9, 10].

Studies have shown that younger women with breast cancer and those without young children have higher QOL levels than older women and

D. Çinar (✉) · A. Öztürk Çetin
Nursing Department, Faculty of Health Science, Izmir Bakırcay University, Izmir, Turkey
e-mail: derya.cinar@bakircay.edu.tr; aslihan.ozturk@bakircay.edu.tr

Y. Bakar, A. Tuğral (eds.), *Managing Side Effects of Breast Cancer Treatment*,
https://doi.org/10.1007/978-3-031-75480-7_28

those with young children [11]. On the other hand, women with breast cancer aged 50 years and older are reported to have a better QOL, and better emotional and physical functioning levels [12]. It has been reported that the QOL of breast cancer patients with low educational levels worsens after breast cancer treatment [13]. In addition, patients' perception of social support is also thought to be related to QOL. It is observed that people with strong social support have a higher level of QOL [14]. Studies reported that the QOL levels of patients do not differ in terms of the type of surgical intervention applied to patients with breast cancer. It has been reported that body image perceptions and sexual functioning of patients who underwent mastectomy were negatively affected compared to patients who underwent breast-conserving surgery [11]. It has also been highlighted that breast cancer patients who receive chemotherapy have a lower QOL than those who receive hormone therapy alone [6]. Factors such as pain, fatigue, and menopausal symptoms that are common in people with breast cancer can affect the QOL [13]. Research has shown that people with advanced breast cancer have poorer physical, sexual, and social functioning than those with early disease [12, 15].

Addressing the physical, social, functional, and emotional well-being levels of breast cancer patients with a holistic approach during the disease and treatment process increases treatment compliance and the chance of treatment success [2].

28.3 Physical Well-Being in Patients with Breast Cancer

The QOL of breast cancer patients can be directly impacted by the severity of physical symptoms they may experience, as well as the associated problems [9, 16]. Symptoms such as fatigue, pain, nausea, vomiting, dysphagia, alopecia, diarrhea, constipation, hot flashes, depression, and anxiety, which can develop as a result of the disease and treatment, can affect patients' QOL [9, 16]. Fatigue is a common symptom reported by breast cancer survivors. Research has shown that the majority (99%) of breast cancer patients report fatigue during adjuvant chemotherapy, and this may reduce physical functioning and QOL [9, 17]. It is emphasized that due to the diagnosis of breast cancer and related problems such as fatigue, weakness, and alopecia, patients are avoiding to participate in social activities, cannot enter the community comfortably due to the risk of infection, cannot eat what they want and thereby their QOL is affected due to the uncertainty they experience [9, 18]. A study reported that there was a correlation between fatigue and depressive symptoms in patients with breast cancer [4], that approximately 50% of patients experienced pain at all stages of breast cancer, and that 60–90% of patients with advanced breast cancer experienced pain [19]. It has been shown that 30%–80% of patients with breast cancer experience treatment-related nausea and vomiting, and when it cannot be controlled, it negatively affects the psychosocial status, family relationships, and QOL of patients [18]. In addition, the decrease in daily living activity performances of patients due to breast cancer treatment leads to a decrease in functional and physical well-being and greatly affects the QOL. Regardless of the cancer diagnosis, the loss of a breast after surgery makes it difficult for the individual to adapt to the new body appearance that occurs against his/her will. In addition, in patients who develop lymphedema after mastectomy, movement disorders are reported to cause a decrease in QOL and simultaneously affect aesthetic anxiety and social isolation [20]. It is explained that 30% of patients with breast cancer develop alopecia due to the side effects of cytotoxic agents during systemic chemotherapy, although it is a reversible symptom within 4–6 weeks after treatment, it causes anxiety, depression, low self-esteem, and decreased physical well-being of patients [7]. It has been reported that some patients refuse treatment due to fear of alopecia and terminate the treatment, thus their QOL is negatively affected [8]. It has been emphasized that high self-efficacy level in breast cancer patients is associated with an increase in self-care behaviors and a decrease in physical and psychological symptoms, which is associated with poor QOL after treatment [13]. In this manner, it reveals the need to implement interventions to improve the QOL of patients diagnosed with breast cancer during and after treatment and in case of the recurrence of the disease [16].

28.4 Emotional Well-Being in Patients with Breast Cancer

The diagnosis and treatment of breast cancer are considered to be a stressful process for patients [19]. Emotions such as sadness, anger, fear, hopelessness, guilt, helplessness, abandonment, and fear of death are commonly observed in breast cancer patients [17]. In addition, patients' reactions to the disease may increase depression and anxiety and can affect their QOL during and after treatment. In a meta-analysis, the incidence of depression in breast cancer patients ranged from 1.5% to 46% [13, 21]. In addition, some studies have reported that posttraumatic stress disorder (PTSD) occurs in 30% of breast cancer patients, and about 80% of patients experience one or more symptoms of PTSD [22]. In addition, mood changes are among other psychological problems that can be frequently seen in patients with breast cancer. Fear and anxiety about the recurrence of the disease continue to affect the daily lives of patients with breast cancer [21]. Most of the patients with breast cancer express that they feel intense anxiety due to uncertainty and lack of control over the disease [15]. These problems brought about by the disease itself and the consequences of related treatments may negatively affect the QOL of patients. Especially in women who underwent a mastectomy, the loss of a breast may cause patients to experience more intense distress and anxiety [9]. Breast cancer patients state that they feel less feminine and attractive, they are uncomfortable with weight gain, and their body perception and appearance have changed [15]. Patients' methods of coping with stress and their perceived social support are important factors in the experienced psychological problems. It has been found that patients who use more effective and functional coping strategies and have stronger social support have lower levels of anxiety and depression [18]. Untreated anxiety and depression make it difficult for patients to cope with stressful situations both during and after treatment and may negatively affect their social relationships and enjoyment of life [23]. It is emphasized that the type of surgical intervention applied in the treatment of the disease, family history of cancer, and some sociodemographic characteristics have different effects on the anxiety and depression levels of patients. In a study, it was reported that low socioeconomic level was a risk factor for increased anxiety, and family history of breast cancer and mastectomy were also risk factors for increased depression in patients with early-stage breast cancer [24]. Stress, anxiety, depression, and sexual problems experienced by breast cancer patients have been reported to reduce their QOL. Psychosocial intervention programs such as psychoeducation, cognitive behavioral therapy, social support, and mindfulness-based stress reduction have been shown to be effective in improving the QoL of breast cancer patients [14, 25]. Although breast cancer is currently considered a curable disease, the persistence of the physical and psychological effects of breast cancer and its treatments clearly indicate the need for more psychosocial intervention programs to reduce these effects during and after treatment [23, 25].

28.5 Functional Well-Being in Patients with Breast Cancer

Symptoms related to breast cancer and the treatment process negatively affect activities of daily living [6]. The intensity of the severity of the symptoms causes patients to lose the functionality required in their daily lives [26]. Assessment of functional status can provide a measure of an individual's ability to perform self-care and social roles in daily life. At the same time, a comprehensive assessment of the individual and the use of effective treatment and counseling approaches can improve functional status. In addition, assessment of functional status in breast cancer patients can help manage physical, emotional, and social problems and improve their QOL [6, 27]. It has been reported that patients diagnosed with breast cancer at a young age experience reduced functional well-being and QOL for reasons such as decreased social functioning, peer relationships, increased social and functional stigma, concerns about sexual problems, and inability to communicate effectively [11]. It is reported that almost all patients with breast cancer cannot return back their working life due to symptoms affecting daily life activities such as pain and fatigue, difficulty in performing daily routine and housework, and taking a long time to complete a task [26, 28]. It is emphasized that they cannot find enough energy in themselves due to sleep problems related to the side effects of treatment, they do not want to socialize, and they state that even self-care needs are a burden for them [6, 29]. In addition, it has been reported that individuals who survived breast cancer and returned to work after treatment had an improvement in their QOL [29]. It was reported that the majority of breast cancer patients who had difficulty in performing daily activities such as housework were not satisfied with the care, they gave to themselves and their families. In addition, it was found that feeling inadequate led to deterioration in family processes and negatively affected their lives [30]. It has been reported that breast cancer patients who have social support in their daily lives have a higher quality of life. It is emphasized that especially those with spousal support have significantly higher levels of adjustment to social life, participation in social activities, improved self-esteem, and have a positive impact on functional well-being [14, 31].

28.6 Social Well-Being in Patients with Breast Cancer

Breast cancer is a public health problem that causes significant changes in the life of the individual in the context of its holistic and spiritual aspects and is defined as one of the biggest traumas that a woman can experience throughout her life. Breast cancer has a negative psychosocial impact on roles and responsibilities in family and social life [9, 13]. Breast cancer patients may experience communication difficulties with their family members and others following a cancer diagnosis. However, during a long treatment process, patients often struggle to find the energy to maintain social relationships and may lack the necessary support when they need it most [14]. In addition, mastectomy, treatment, and treatment-related symptoms can cause significant problems in women's daily lives and sexual functions. Body image problems caused by multimodal treatment, such as breast loss and alopecia after mastectomy, may lead to social isolation, social behavioral changes, and negative effects on QOL. At the same time, women may experience anxiety about the possibility of disruption of family integrity or potential damage to their emotional bonds with their partners [14, 18]. In this regard, spouses should be encouraged to attend patient education sessions to increase family/spouse support and, where possible, receive professional support. Research has shown that almost half of breast cancer patients are afraid of making plans for the future because they experience uncertainty and unpredictability. Especially after mastectomy, it has been found that they experience future anxiety toward their family members and their special relationships deteriorate [2, 32]. It is stated that the impact on their work life, change in their income status, and financial toxicity due to treatment costs negatively affect family processes and the social lives of breast cancer patients. It is reported that social support provided at the stage of diagnosis improves the survival processes of patients with breast cancer and contributes positively to physical, psychological, and social adaptation to the disease [17, 18]. In addition, it was emphasized that as social support increases, QOL increases by improving social well-being and decreasing symptom severity [17].

28.7 Evaluation of Quality of Life in Breast Cancer

In women with breast cancer, life expectancy is prolonged due to early diagnosis and treatment, and accordingly, the concept of QOL has gained

Table 28.1 The features of scales used to evaluate the quality of life of patients with breast cancer

Scale name	Item/subdimension
Short form health survey questionnaire (SF-12, SF 36)	12 items 8 subdimensions
Multidimensional QOL scale, cancer version II (MQOLS_CA 2)	33 items 5 subdimensions
Functional assessment of cancer therapy-(FACT-G)	27 items 4 subdimensions
Rolls Royce QOL scale	42 items 8 subdimensions
Ferrans and powers QOL index—Cancer version	33 items 4 subdimensions
European Organization for Research and Treatment of cancer QOL (EORTC-QLQ-30)	30 items 3 subdimensions
Functional assessment of cancer therapy-breast (FACT-B)	37 items 4 subdimensions
Functional assessment of cancer therapy-breast—Endocrine symptoms (FACT-ES)	46 items 4 subdimensions
FACT-G caregiver	27 items 4 subdimensions
European Organization for Research and Treatment (EORTC-QOL-BR23)	23 items 2 subdimensions

importance. The diagnosis of breast cancer alone, regardless of the treatments implemented, may negatively affect the QOL of women [2]. Body image, functional status, sexual function, and roles in the family may be affected due to the side effects of surgical interventions, chemotherapy, and radiotherapy. The experienced symptoms affect compliance with treatment and cause changes in QOL in patients with breast cancer [3, 32]. They have to cope with many symptoms that affect their daily lives, such as pain, fatigue, nausea and vomiting, alopecia, oral mucositis, constipation/diarrhea, sleep problems, and impaired sexual function. Women who cannot cope with these side effects have a reduced QOL [2, 32]. QOL is of critical importance in all stages of cancer, including cancer diagnosis, treatment, palliative care, and survival. To this end, it is important to assess the impact of the disease and treatments on QOL at all stages of breast cancer treatment. It is not easy to measure QOL, therefore specific measurement tools are used to assess QOL. This is reported to be due to the difficulty of assessing subjective interpretations [33, 34]. Therefore, the measurement materials QOL vary according to the sample group, the application environment, the type of questionnaires used (short form, form based on patient self-report, interview, clinical application, telephone, and mail), and the general evaluation approach in the assessment of QOL. The frequently used QOL measurement tools in the literature to evaluate the QOL of patients with breast cancer are summarized in Table 28.1.

28.8 Strategies to Improve the Quality of Life of Breast Cancer Patients

Ensuring continuity of treatment and care and improving the QOL of breast cancer patients should be among the overall goals of patients' posttreatment care plans. Timely and systematic assessment of symptoms, planning, and implementation of personalized interventions for breast cancer patients who are continuing treatment will provide a better QOL for both patients and their caregivers [32, 35]. Some intervention studies conducted to improve the QOL of patients with breast cancer in the literature are summarized in Table 28.2.

It is important to educate, counsel, and support patients with breast cancer and their caregivers, regarding the effects and side effects of treatments [32, 36]. Patient education is a therapeutic intervention aimed at promoting active coping strategies to improve or maintain patients' current health status and QOL, as defined by the WHO [37]. There is evidence that the implementation of patient education programs has an impact on the QOL of breast cancer survivors. A combination of telephone and face-to-face interviews is considered to be the most effective intervention for improving QOL in both the short and long term [14, 38, 39].

Supportive care is an important part of preventing and treating the adverse effects of breast cancer. Additionally, supportive care includes

Table 28.2 Interventional research to improve quality of life of breast cancer patients

Author/Year/Country	Intervention	Evaluation of quality-of-life	Conclusion
Jassim et al. (2023)	Psychological therapy	FACT-G	It was found that women who received psychological therapy showed an improvement in QOL as well as a decrease in depression, anxiety, mood disorders, and stress
Çınar et al. (2021)	Mobile app	FACT-ES	It was determined that the QOL of women with breast cancer who underwent endocrine hormone therapy increased by 100% and their distress levels decreased by providing mobile application-based training and individual counseling services in line with their physical, social, psychosocial, and spiritual needs
Ashing and George (2020)	Telephone interview	FACT-G	The telephone psycho-educational intervention was found to be effective in improving emotional Well-being (EWB) and quality of life
Omidi et al. (2020)	Multi-group interview	QOL scale	It was determined that group-based (telegram) education had a positive effect on the QOL scores of the patients
Ashing (2020)	Mobile app	FACT-G	It found that a telephone-delivered psychoeducational intervention was effective in improving patients' QOL through symptom reduction
Juvet et al. (2017)	Physical exercise	HRQOL	Exercise was found to improve breast cancer patients' physical functioning and QOL during and after treatment, as well as during 6 months of follow-up
Galiano-Castillo et al. (2016)	Internet-based exercise intervention	EORTC-QLQ-C30	It was determined that the implementation of an internet-based, tailor-made exercise program had the effect of improving the QOL and possible symptoms of the patients

managing physical and psychological symptoms and side effects throughout the cancer journey during breast cancer diagnosis, treatment, post-treatment, and survivorship [24, 35]. Qualitative research shows that supportive and educational care interventions can have a significant and positive impact on the QOL of patients with breast cancer [25, 35]. Interventions such as yoga, pilates, and mindfulness used to improve the psychological health of breast cancer patients and survivors have been shown to have a positive impact on their QOL. QOL is an important indicator for breast cancer patients during treatment and survival. It should be addressed in all its dimensions, including physical, emotional, social, and functional aspects. Healthcare providers should provide effective, high-quality care with a holistic perspective and a multidisciplinary team approach to improve patients' QOL [13, 21, 27].

References

1. Haddou Rahou B, El Rhazi K, Ouasmani F, et al. Quality of life in Arab women with breast cancer: a review of the literature. HQLO. 2016;14:1–13.
2. Nardin S, Mora E, Varughese FM, et al. Breast cancer survivorship, quality of life, and late toxicities. Front Oncol. 2020;10:864.
3. Akezaki Y, Nakata E, Kikuuchi M, et al. Investigation of factors affecting early quality of life of patients after breast cancer surgery. Healthcare. 2021;9(2):213.
4. Fisher RS, Sharp KMH, Prussien KV, et al. Coping trajectories and the health-related quality of life of childhood cancer survivors. J Ped Psycho. 2021;46(8):960–9.
5. Tian Q, Xu M, Yu L, et al. The efficacy of virtual reality–based interventions in breast cancer–related symptom management: a systematic review and meta-analysis. Cancer Nurs. 2023;46(5):E276–87.
6. Nelwati N, Noviyani D. The effect of diaphragmatic breathing on nausea, vomiting and functional status among breast cancer patients undergoing chemotherapy. EJON. 2024;102548:102548.

7. Naeem Y, Qurat-ul-Ain A, Shafiq M, et al. Chemotherapy induced alopecia distress, body image and psychosocial wellbeing among breast cancer patients: the moderating role of locus of control. Real. 2023;6(2):357–69.
8. Kocan S, Aktug C, Gursoy A. "Who am I?" a qualitative meta-synthesis of chemotherapy-induced alopecia and body image perception in breast cancer patients. Support Care Cancer. 2023;31(4):237.
9. Bjerkeset E, Röhrl K, Schou-Bredal I. Symptom cluster of pain, fatigue, and psychological distress in breast cancer survivors: prevalence and characteristics. Breast Cancer Res Treat. 2020;180:63–71.
10. So WK, Law BM, Ng MS, et al. Symptom clusters experienced by breast cancer patients at various treatment stages: a systematic review. Cancer Med. 2021;10(8):2531–65.
11. Al-Kaylani HM, Loeffler BT, Mott SL, et al. Characterizing early changes in quality of life in young women with breast cancer. Front Psychol. 2022;13:871194.
12. Freedman RA, Partridge AH. Emerging data and current challenges for young, old, obese, or male patients with breast cancer. Clin Cancer Res. 2017;23(11):2647–54.
13. Wong WM, Chan DN, He X, et al. Effectiveness of pharmacological and nonpharmacological interventions for managing the fatigue–sleep disturbance–depression symptom cluster in breast cancer patients undergoing chemotherapy: a systematic review. Cancer Nurs. 2023;46(2):E70–80.
14. Kang NE, Kim HY, Kim JY, et al. Relationship between cancer stigma, social support, coping strategies and psychosocial adjustment among breast cancer survivors. J Clin Nurs. 2020;29(21–22):4368–78.
15. Jassim GA, Doherty S, Whitford DL, et al. Psychological interventions for women with non-metastatic breast cancer. CDSR. 2023;1:1.
16. Juvet LK, Thune I, Elvsaas IØ, et al. The effect of exercise on fatigue and physical functioning in breast cancer patients during and after treatment and at 6 months follow-up: a meta-analysis. Breast. 2017;33:166–77.
17. Dams L, Van der Gucht E, Devoogdt N, et al. Effect of pain neuroscience education after breast cancer surgery on pain, physical, and emotional functioning: a double-blinded randomized controlled trial. Pain. 2023;164(7):1489–501.
18. Lyu MM, Chiew-Jiat RS, Cheng KKF. The effects of physical symptoms, self-efficacy and social constraints on fear of cancer recurrence in breast cancer survivors: examining the mediating role of illness representations. Psycho Oncol. 2024;33(1):e6264.
19. Galiano-Castillo N, Cantarero-Villanueva I, Fernández-Lao C, et al. Telehealth system: a randomized controlled trial evaluating the impact of an internet-based exercise intervention on quality of life, pain, muscle strength, and fatigue in breast cancer survivors. Cancer. 2016;122(20):3166–74.
20. Dempsey K, Mathieu E, Brennan M, et al. Patient-reported health-related quality of life outcomes following mastectomy for breast cancer, with immediate, delayed or no breast reconstruction: four-year follow-up from a prospective cohort study. Breast. 2023;71:122–31.
21. Pilevarzadeh M, Amirshahi M, Afsargharehbagh R, et al. Global prevalence of depression among breast cancer patients: a systematic review and meta-analysis. Breast Cancer Res Treat. 2019;176:519–33.
22. Marziliano A, Tuman M, Moyer A. The relationship between post-traumatic stress and post-traumatic growth in cancer patients and survivors: a systematic review and meta-analysis. Psycho Oncol. 2020;29(4):604–16.
23. Penberthy JK, Stewart AL, Centeno CF, et al. Psychological aspects of breast cancer. Psychiatr Clin North Am. 2023;46:551.
24. Invernizzi M, De Sire A, Venetis K, et al. Quality of life interventions in breast cancer survivors: state of the art in targeted rehabilitation strategies. Med Chem. 2022;22(4):801–10.
25. Giustiniani A, Danesin L, Pezzetta R, et al. Use of telemedicine to improve cognitive functions and psychological Well-being in patients with breast cancer: a systematic review of the current literature. Cancers. 2023;15(4):1353.
26. Semra AY, Parvizi M. The functional assessment of cancer therapy general FACT-G scale reliability and validity of a Turkish version. CBU-HSIJ. 2021;8(2):198–203.
27. Rogers LQ, Courneya KS, Oster RA, et al. Physical activity intervention benefits persist months post-intervention: randomized trial in breast cancer survivors. J Cancer Surviv. 2023;17(6):1834–46.
28. Oh PJ, Cho JR. Changes in fatigue, psychological distress, and quality of life after chemotherapy in women with breast cancer: a prospective study. Cancer Nurs. 2020;43(1):E54–60.
29. Schmidt ME, Scherer S, Wiskemann J, et al. Return to work after breast cancer: the role of treatment-related side effects and potential impact on quality of life. Eur J Cancer Care. 2019;28(4):e13051.
30. Iddrisu M, Aziato L, Dedey F. Psychological and physical effects of breast cancer diagnosis and treatment on young Ghanaian women: a qualitative study. BMC Psychiatry. 2020;20(1):353.
31. Boamah Mensah AB, Adamu B, Mensah KB, et al. Exploring the social stressors and resources of husbands of women diagnosed with advanced breast cancer in their role as primary caregivers in Kumasi, Ghana. Support Care Cancer. 2021;29:2335–45.
32. Biparva AJ, Raoofi S, Rafiei S, et al. Global quality of life in breast cancer: systematic review and meta-analysis. BMJ Palliat Support Care. 2023;13(e3):e528–36.
33. Boškailo E, Franjić D, Jurić I, et al. Resilience and quality of life of patients with breast cancer. Psychiatr Danub. 2021;33(suppl 4):572–9.

34. Gavric Z, Vukovic-Kostic Z. Assessment of quality of life of women with breast cancer. Glob J Health Sci. 2016;8(9):1.
35. Williams AM, Khan CP, Heckler CE, et al. Fatigue, anxiety, and quality of life in breast cancer patients compared to non-cancer controls: a nationwide longitudinal analysis. Breast Cancer Res Treat. 2021;187:275–85.
36. Mokhatri-Hesari P, Montazeri A. Health-related quality of life in breast cancer patients: review of reviews from 2008 to 2018. HQLO. 2020;18:1–25.
37. Ashing KT, George M. Exploring the efficacy of a paraprofessional delivered telephonic psycho-educational intervention on emotional Well-being in African American breast cancer survivors. Support Care Cancer. 2020;28:1163–71.
38. Çınar D, Karadakovan A, Erdoğan AP. Effect of mobile phone app-based training on the quality of life for women with breast cancer. EJON. 2021;52:101960.
39. Ream E, Hughes AE, Cox A, et al. Telephone interventions for symptom management in adults with cancer. CDSR. 2020;6:1.

Complementary Modalities in the Management of Symptoms of Breast Cancer

29

Vildan Kocatepe

29.1 Introduction

Breast cancer stands out as a prevalent and consequential health concern on a global scale, ranking among the most common malignancies. Among women, breast cancer, lung cancer, and colorectal cancer together make up 52% of all newly diagnosed cases, with breast cancer alone representing 31% of female cancer cases [1]. The prevalence and incidence of breast cancer have been increasing, especially in developing countries, over the past 25 years [2]. In women, breast cancer ranks second among cancer-related causes of death, following lung cancer [1].

Although methods such as surgery, chemotherapy, radiotherapy, and hormone therapy are effective in treating breast cancer, these treatments bring together many complications that the patient has to manage [3]. Furthermore, despite the elevated occurrence and fatality rates associated with breast cancer, there is an upward trend in survival rates [1]. The quality of life for breast cancer survivors is crucial, and some women have reported cancer-related symptoms even months or years after completion of the treatment. Managing these symptoms is essential for improving the quality of life for patients both during treatment and in survivorship. During breast cancer treatment and survivorship, patients may experience a wide variety of symptoms such as lymphedema, reduced mobility, sexual problems, pain, fatigue, nausea, vomiting, cognitive dysfunction, depression, and anxiety [3]. The management of these symptoms may involve alternative and complementary approaches alongside pharmacological treatments [4]. Studies have shown that the use of complementary therapy is common among breast cancer patients, with a reported average of around 62% in groups under 35 years old and similarly around 60% in elderly groups [5, 6].

29.2 Complementary Health Approaches

Complementary health approaches (CHAs) are traditional practices used alongside medical treatment [7]. Complementary health approaches are used alongside conventional medical treatment, but it does not stand alone as standard treatment in its own right [8].

29.3 Complementary Modalities in the Management of Symptoms of Breast Cancer

Complementary approaches are categorized into four groups according to the method of therapy:

V. Kocatepe (✉)
Department of Nursing, Faculty of Health Sciences, Izmir Demokrasi University, Izmir, Turkey
e-mail: vildan.kocatepe@idu.edu.tr

Y. Bakar, A. Tuğral (eds.), *Managing Side Effects of Breast Cancer Treatment*,
https://doi.org/10.1007/978-3-031-75480-7_29

- Whole medical systems.
- Mind–body therapies.
- Biologically based practices.
- Manipulative and body-based practice.
- Energy healing.

29.3.1 Whole Medical Systems

Whole medical systems encompass healing methodologies that have developed over time across diverse cultures and geographic regions worldwide. Examples include ayurvedic medicine, traditional Chinese medicine (TCM), acupuncture, and naturopathic medicine [8].

29.3.1.1 Acupuncture

Acupuncture involves stimulating particular points on the skin, referred to as "acupuncture points," using slender and solid needles made of metal [7, 9, 10]. It constitutes a fundamental aspect of traditional Chinese medicine, where it is thought to alleviate energy obstructions by promoting the circulation of the essential life force known as "qi" throughout the body [9, 10].

Acupuncture is used to manage cancer-related symptoms, treat side effects of anticancer treatments, increase blood cell counts, and enhance lymphocyte and natural killer (NK) cell activity [11]. Although the precise mechanism of acupuncture is not completely comprehended, studies have shown different effects. Acupuncture has been reported to induce multiple biological responses mediated by sensory neurons in the central nervous system. It may also activate the hypothalamus and pituitary gland, leading to changes in peptides, hormones, and neurotransmitters. Thus, it has been reported to regulate blood flow and provide anti-inflammatory effects. Additionally, studies have shown that acupuncture releases opioid peptides and activates the endogenous opioid system [12–14].

Acupuncture is commonly used in managing cancer symptoms, including pain, nausea, vomiting, weight loss, fatigue, dry mouth, anxiety, sleeplessness, loss of appetite, hot flashes, chemotherapy-induced peripheral neuropathy, constipation, and diarrhea. It is often used to manage fatigue, hot flashes, nausea, and vomiting specifically in breast cancer [9–11]. In recent years, there have been numerous studies examining the effectiveness of acupuncture in alleviating symptoms associated with breast cancer. Studies involving breast cancer survivors have reported that acupuncture significantly reduces joint pain associated with aromatase inhibitors, reduces opioid medication dosage and side effects, improves menopausal symptoms associated with breast cancer, and maintains the effect of application up to 3 months after completion of treatment [14–16].

There are situations where acupuncture should be used with caution or avoided. In breast cancer patients, needle insertion into the arms from which lymph nodes were removed after surgical treatment may cause lymphedema. Additionally, acupuncture application without taking the necessary precautions in patients with suppressed immune systems may lead to infection. Moreover, acupuncture is not suitable for patients with changes in blood values related to bleeding, coagulation, or other diseases as it may cause bleeding. If the use of acupuncture necessitates the use of herbal supplements, it should not be performed in patients undergoing chemotherapy treatment, as these supplements may reduce the effectiveness of chemotherapy [9].

Serious side effects of acupuncture are rare. It is known that the reported side effects in studies are usually accidents and infections resulting from practitioner errors. Other potential side effects of acupuncture application may include pain, hematoma, fatigue, dizziness, numbness, and localized skin irritation at the needling sites. These minor side effects can be minimized with appropriate patient management, including local pressure and massage at the needling site after acupuncture application [11].

29.3.2 Mind–Body Therapies

Mind–body therapies integrate mental concentration, controlled breathing, and physical movements to induce relaxation of both the body and mind. Examples include meditation, biofeedback, hypnosis, yoga, tai chi, imagery, and creative outlets [8].

29.3.2.1 Hypnosis

Hypnosis is a method that helps individuals enter a calm and wakeful state of awareness through the use of suggestions aimed at altering perception, sensation, emotion, thought, or behavior. Hypnosis aids in preventing distraction and assists individuals in focusing on a specific idea, sensation, or memory [17, 18].

There is no consensus on any hypnosis theory, and the underlying mechanisms of hypnosis are not fully understood [17]. The process of hypnosis begins with a hypnotic induction phase, which is typically achieved using techniques such as guided imagery. Subsequently, a deepening procedure is applied using relaxation suggestions to induce mental and physical relaxation. Finally, symptom-specific suggestions are implemented, such as providing suggestions to alleviate pain. In this way, the hypnosis process aims to achieve specific goals by altering the individual's mental state [17, 19]. The application of hypnosis is influenced by factors such as the patient's psychological factors (expectations, hypnotizability), social factors (being cooperative and open to communication), and biological factors (e.g., increased theta activity following induction) [17]. Hypnosis is often used to alleviate stress, depression, pain, chemotherapy and surgery-related nausea, anticipatory nausea, and treatment-related hot flashes in breast cancer patients [10, 18].

In a randomized controlled study, it has been reported that a single brief (15-minute) hypnosis session administered before surgery in 200 breast cancer patients had therapeutic effects on pain, fatigue, nausea, and stress and also reduced the extra healthcare expenses per patient [20]. In a randomized controlled study involving sixty female breast cancer survivors experiencing hot flashes, participants in the experimental group received five sessions of hypnosis intervention per week. In this study, significant improvements were observed in anxiety, stress, hot flashes affecting daily activities, and sleeping patterns due to hypnosis intervention [21].

Hypnosis is contraindicated in patients who cannot communicate effectively, such as patients with dementia, psychotic disorders, drug addicts, those under the influence of alcohol, and those who have difficulty with understanding. Studies have not reported any adverse effects associated with hypnosis in breast cancer patients [18].

29.3.2.2 Qigong and Tai chi

The word "Qigong" in Chinese means "qi" (life energy) and "gong" (skill or achievement developed through continuous practice). Qigong is an ancient practice within traditional Chinese medicine (TCM) that combines physical movements (postures), meditation, and regulated breathing techniques [10]. Tai Chi represents the gentle movements of Qigong [22]. Tai Chi is a whole-body exercise that combines slow, fluid, subtle, curved, spiral, and sequential movements. Originating from ancient internal Chinese martial arts, Tai Chi is a practice that involves meditation and breath control alongside light to moderate-intensity physical activity. Tai Chi is an exercise that promotes harmony between the mind and body [22, 23].

Although the mechanisms of the effects of Tai Chi on biological risk factors of breast cancer are not yet fully elucidated, it is known that stress-reducing effects affect the autonomic nervous system through physical activity. These effects may involve a decrease in sympathetic activity and an increase in parasympathetic activity, along with the activation of the immune system. Proinflammatory cytokines trigger the release of glucocorticoids through activation of the hypothalamic–pituitary–adrenal axis. These glucocorticoids reduce proinflammatory cytokines and allow for the balance of T-helper 2 (Th-2) anti-inflammatory cytokines [24].

The goal of Qigong is to cultivate and harmonize the patient's spiritual, emotional, mental, and physical well-being by boosting their vital energy or life force. Among cancer patients, Qigong is frequently used to alleviate stress, fatigue, and pain, support the immune system, and improve physical and emotional balance [10].

Studies conducted in breast cancer patients have shown that Tai Chi practice reduces inflammatory responses improves quality of life, muscle strength, and shoulder function, and reduces insomnia. Additionally, it may help to alleviate fatigue, anxiety, depression, and stress [22].

29.3.2.3 Yoga

Yoga, a popular complementary noninvasive therapy, integrates physical postures (asanas), breathing exercises (pranayamas), meditation, chants, and relaxation techniques (savasana). Extensive research suggests that yoga improves diverse aspects of well-being, encompassing physical, emotional, social, and psychological dimensions, among cancer patients. Promising results have shown that yoga is a supportive intervention for alleviating fatigue, depression, stress, and sleeplessness. From a physiological standpoint, yoga plays a role in regulating the hypothalamic–pituitary–adrenal (HPA) axis, diminishing circulating stress hormones, and enhancing parasympathetic function. These mechanisms collectively contribute to stress reduction and modulation of the stress response. Furthermore, yoga influences activity within various brain structures fostering enhancements in mood and cognition. It also enhances sensory awareness, regulates autonomic input, and boosts parasympathetic activity. By engaging brain regions such as the insula, amygdala, and hippocampus, yoga improves pain tolerance while reducing distress and anxiety associated with pain [25].

29.3.3 Biologically Based Practices

Biologically based practices use natural substances and resources. For instance, vitamins, dietary supplements, botanicals, herbs, and spices such as turmeric or cinnamon, special foods, or diets [8].

29.3.3.1 Dietary Supplements

The use of dietary supplements containing vitamins, minerals, and natural products (e.g., fish oil) is more common among cancer patients and cancer survivors compared to individuals without cancer. The use of dietary supplements increases with age and is higher in women than in men. Among all cancer types, the use of dietary supplements is highest in women with breast cancer [26].

Dietary supplements should be used with caution because they contain some risks. For instance, the simultaneous use of specific vitamin/mineral supplements that include antioxidants has been reported to be associated with an increased risk of breast cancer recurrence and/or decreased disease-free or overall survival during chemotherapy. Moreover, there is still insufficient and reliable evidence to demonstrate the effectiveness of some dietary supplements. When advising patients on dietary supplements, the risks, benefits, and long-term side effects should be assessed [27]. Some interactions between anticancer agents and herbs are given in Table 29.1.

Acetyl-L-carnitine is a dietary supplement used to treat cancer-related fatigue by increasing energy levels and reducing inflammation. Its effectiveness has been proven in preventing and treating diabetic neuropathy, and therefore, it can be used for chemotherapy-induced peripheral neuropathy. However, its efficacy has not been fully established in cancer patients [10].

Soy is a plant from the pea family. Soy is used for regulating blood pressure and cholesterol levels, in the management of menopausal symptoms, preventing osteoporosis, improving memory, and treating hot flashes. However, there is insufficient evidence demonstrating the effectiveness of soy in treating hot flashes [10]. Legumes contain phytoestrogens. Soy, in particu-

Table 29.1 Lists of herb–drug interactions

Anticancer agent	Herb or dietary supplement	Interaction
Rituximab	Bilberry	Hypoglycemia
Radiation therapy	Ginseng	Increased tumor recurrence rate
Bortezomib	Green tea	Decreased anticancer effect
Sunitinib	Green tea	Decreased anticancer effect
5-FU	Green tea	Increased 5-FU serum concentration

lar, can produce estrogenic side effects through this mechanism. However, the analysis of combined data from two large studies covering more than 9500 women in total found that consuming more than 10 mg of soy per day after a diagnosis of cancer was associated with a nonsignificant decrease in breast cancer-specific mortality and a significant decrease in the risk of breast cancer recurrence [28].

29.3.3.2 Fruits

Fruits contain high amounts of polyphenols, which have antioxidant properties and may help reduce the risk of cancer. It has been observed that some fruits such as pomegranate, mangosteen, and citrus fruits inhibit breast cancer cells. Pomegranate, which contains high levels of polyphenols, has antioxidant and anti-inflammatory properties. Pomegranate extract was found to hinder the proliferation of MCF-7 breast cancer cells by prompting a halt in the cell cycle progression, specifically in the G2/M phase, while also triggering apoptosis. Mangosteen fruit could demonstrate the ability to impede the proliferation of SKBR3 human breast cancer cells and initiate apoptosis. Besides, there are studies demonstrating the inhibitory effect of apples on breast cancer cell growth [29].

29.3.3.3 Herbs and Spices

Various spices such as *Curcuma longa* (turmeric), *Nigella sativa* (black cumin), *Zingiber officinale* (ginger), *Allium sativum* (garlic), *Crocus sativus* (saffron), *Piper nigrum* (black pepper), and *Capsicum annum* (chili pepper) have the potential for cancer prevention and treatment. These spices contain essential bioactive compounds like curcumin, thymoquinone, piperine, and capsaicin. Their primary mechanisms of action encompass inducing apoptosis, inhibiting tumor proliferation, migration, and invasion, as well as sensitizing tumors to radiotherapy and chemotherapy [30].

Ginger: polyphenols found in ginger exhibit anticancer properties attributed to their ability to inhibit metastasis, tumor cell proliferation, and angiogenesis, as well as they exhibit anti-inflammatory effects. Additionally, they induce cell cycle arrest, apoptosis, and autophagy. Consequently, regular consumption of ginger contributes to natural herbal therapy for preventing and treating breast cancer, while also offering protection against the adverse effects of chemotherapy [31]. Ginger supplementation is not recommended for individuals undergoing surgery or those with bleeding disorders due to the possible aggravated risk of increased bleeding [10].

29.3.4 Manipulative and Body-Based Practice

Manipulative and body-based practices are based on working with one or more parts of the body. Examples include reflexology, massage therapy, and chiropractic therapy [8].

29.3.4.1 Reflexology

Reflexology is a practice that involves applying direct pressure to specific nerve endings in the body, stimulating the corresponding area, and aiming to reduce symptoms [32]. In reflexology, a trained practitioner applies pressure to stimulate the feet, hands, ears, and face using specific thumb, finger, and hand techniques for alleviating symptoms. It has been reported that reflexology corresponds to specific glands, organs, and other parts of the body in the feet and hands, and by stimulating these areas, symptoms can be relieved [10].

Reflexology increases circulation and alleviates symptoms through activating receptors that release oxytocin and through complex inputs and processes in the central nervous system's neuromatrix [32].

A randomized controlled study has shown that reflexology is effective in reducing nausea, vomiting, and retching, as well as fatigue, in breast cancer patients undergoing chemotherapy [33]. In another study, it has been reported that reflexology reduces treatment-related symptoms (fatigue, nausea, vomiting, pain, shortness of breath, insomnia, loss of appetite, and diarrhea) and improves the quality of life [34].

Reflexology is effective in reducing pain, insomnia, loss of appetite, nausea, vomiting, retching, and fatigue in breast cancer patients [33, 34]. Studies have reported the additional positive effects of reflexology such as decreased severity of lymphedema and peripheral neuropathy and increased productivity. Studies have also reported the side effects of reflexology such as fatigue, chills, dizziness, and fever [32].

29.3.4.2 Massage Therapy

Massage is a technique involving various pressure and touch methods applied to the soft tissues of the body using hands, fingertips, and fists. Massage includes stroking, kneading, applying friction, and stretching specific muscles [10]. Massage stimulates the neuromuscular system by systematically stimulating soft tissues, improves lymphatic drainage, relaxes muscles by speeding up blood circulation, and enhances mood by reducing heart rate [35]. Massage is used in cancer patients to promote relaxation, alleviate muscle stiffness and pain, and reduce musculoskeletal complaints [10].

Massage should not be performed on open wounds, bruises, or areas with skin disorders. Additionally, massage should be avoided in regions where tumors are present. Furthermore, application on sensitive areas due to treatments like radiotherapy should be avoided. Massage is contraindicated in the presence of embolus. Moreover, some patients with multiple bone metastases may be at risk of fractures during deep massage [10].

In a systematic review, out of five studies examined, only one reported side effects of massage such as rash, nausea, vomiting, restlessness, tremors, hypertension, and tachycardia. In another study included in the same systematic review, back pain, and increased blood pressure were reported [35].

29.3.4.3 Aromatherapy

Aromatherapy is the use of essential oils extracted from various plants (flowers, herbs, or trees) to enhance overall physical, emotional, and spiritual health. It is frequently combined with other complementary treatments such as massage and acupuncture. Massage with essential oils like rose or lavender oil is referred to as aromatherapy massage. Evidence exists to support improvement in treatment-related symptoms with regular use of aromatherapy, both with and without massage, during cancer treatment [36].

29.3.5 Energy Healing

Energy healing is based on the belief in the flow of vital energy within the body. The aim of energy healing is to balance the energy flow in the patient. Examples include reiki and therapeutic touch [8].

29.3.5.1 Reiki

Reiki, which means "universal life energy" in Japanese, is a gentle, hands-on therapy based on the belief that trained practitioners, known as Reiki masters, can transmit healing energy to another person to improve their health. It involves the placement of the practitioner's hands near or on certain parts of the patient's body while maintaining a specific therapeutic intention [37]. Reiki provides the flow of energy by activating the body's energy centers, promoting the circulation of both blood and lymph, and triggering the nervous system. Thus, it is thought to promote mental and physical relaxation [37]. Research investigating the effects of Reiki on cancer patients has indicated that it reduces pain, fatigue, stress, and depression, and improves quality of life. However, there is no study in which sufficient quality of evidence proves these effects [37].

29.4 Conclusion

The prevalence of utilizing complementary health approaches (CHA) among breast cancer patients underscores its integration into conventional care practices. However, the concurrent application of CHA with standard care may pose risks due to insufficient understanding of its associated risks, benefits, side effects, and interactions with conventional treatments. Various CHA modalities exhibit significant potential as adjunctive cancer therapies. Consequently, the healthcare system should aim for comprehensive, effective, and safe patient care that fosters interdisciplinary collaboration and incorporates evidence-based interventions from diverse sources. To ascertain the efficacy of specific CHA modalities and their suitability for integration with standard care, interventional trials may be warranted. Hence, further investigations are imperative to elucidate the impact of CHA on overall survival and recurrence rates in breast cancer patients.

References

1. Siegel RL, Miller KD, Wagle NS, Jemal A. Cancer statistics, 2023. CA Cancer J Clin. 2023;73:17–48. https://doi.org/10.3322/CAAC.21763.
2. Azamjah N, Soltan-Zadeh Y, Zayeri F. Global trend of breast cancer mortality rate: a 25-year study. Asian Pac J Cancer Prev. 2019;20:2015–20. https://doi.org/10.31557/APJCP.2019.20.7.2015.
3. Lovelace DL, McDaniel LR, Golden D. Long-term effects of breast cancer surgery, treatment, and survivor care. J Midwifery Womens Health. 2019;64:713–24. https://doi.org/10.1111/JMWH.13012.
4. Nayeri ND, Bakhshi F, Khosravi A, Najafi Z. The effect of complementary and alternative medicines on quality of life in patients with breast cancer: a systematic review. Indian J Palliat Care. 2020;26:95–104. https://doi.org/10.4103/IJPC.IJPC_183_19.
5. Hammersen F, Pursche T, Fischer D, Katalinic A, Waldmann A. Use of complementary and alternative medicine among young patients with breast cancer. Research article. Breast Care. 2009;15:163–70. https://doi.org/10.1159/000501193.
6. Neuhouser ML, Smith AW, George SM, Gibson JT, Baumgartner KB, Baumgartner R, et al. Use of complementary and alternative medicine and breast cancer survival in the health, eating activity and lifestyle study HHS public access. Breast Cancer Res Treat. 2016;160:539–46. https://doi.org/10.1007/s10549-016-4010-x.
7. The National Center for Complementary and Integrative Health (NCCIH). Acupuncture: What You Need To Know 2022. https://www.nccih.nih.gov/health/acupuncture-what-you-need-to-know. Accessed 11 Mar 2024.
8. Complementary and Alternative Medicine (CAM)—NCI 2023. https://www.cancer.gov/about-cancer/treatment/cam. Accessed 11 Mar 2024.
9. Breastcancer.org. Acupuncture 2024. https://www.breastcancer.org/treatment/complementary-therapy/types/acupuncture. Accessed 11 Mar 2024.
10. Greenlee H, DuPont-Reyes MJ, Balneaves LG, Carlson LE, Cohen MR, Deng G, et al. Clinical practice guidelines on the evidence-based use of integrative therapies during and after breast cancer treatment. CA Cancer J Clin. 2017;67:194–232. https://doi.org/10.3322/CAAC.21397.
11. National Cancer Institue. Acupuncture (PDQ®)—NCI 2024. https://www.cancer.gov/about-cancer/treatment/cam/hp/acupuncture-pdq. Accessed 11 Mar 2024.
12. Mao JJ, Liou KT, Baser RE, Bao T, Panageas KS, Romero SAD, et al. Effectiveness of Electroacupuncture or auricular acupuncture vs usual Care for Chronic Musculoskeletal Pain among Cancer Survivors: the PEACE randomized clinical trial. JAMA Oncol. 2021;7:1. https://doi.org/10.1001/JAMAONCOL.2021.0310.
13. Chen L, Lin C-C, Huang T-W, Kuan Y-C, Huang Y-H, Chen H-C, et al. Effect of acupuncture on aromatase inhibitor-induced arthralgia in patients with breast cancer: a meta-analysis of randomized controlled trials. Breast. 2017;33:132–8. https://doi.org/10.1016/j.breast.2017.03.015.
14. Hershman DL, Unger JM, Greenlee H, Capodice JL, Lew DL, Darke AK, et al. Effect of acupuncture vs sham acupuncture or waitlist control on joint pain related to aromatase inhibitors among women with early-stage breast cancer: a randomized clinical trial. JAMA. 2018;320:167–76. https://doi.org/10.1001/JAMA.2018.8907.
15. Chien TJ, Liu CY, Fang CJ, Kuo CY. The maintenance effect of acupuncture on breast cancer-related menopause symptoms: a systematic review. Climacteric. 2020;23:130–9. https://doi.org/10.1080/13697137.2019.1664460.
16. Ge L, Wang Q, He Y, Wu D, Zhou Q, Xu N, et al. Acupuncture for cancer pain: an evidence-based clinical practice guideline. Chin Med. 2022;17:17. https://doi.org/10.1186/S13020-021-00558-4.
17. Carlson LE, Toivonen K, Flynn M, Deleemans J, Piedalue KA, Tolsdorf E, et al. The role of hypnosis in cancer care. Curr Oncol Rep. 2018;20:1–9. https://doi.org/10.1007/S11912-018-0739-1/METRICS.
18. Cramer H, Lauche R, Paul A, Langhorst J, Kümmel S, Dobos GJ. Hypnosis in breast cancer care: a systematic review of randomized controlled trials. Integr Cancer Ther. 2015;14:5–15. https://doi.org/10.1177/1534735414550035/ASSET/IMAGES/LARGE/10.1177_1534735414550035-FIG1.JPEG.
19. Montgomery GH, Schnur JB, Kravits K. Hypnosis for cancer care: over 200 years young. CA Cancer J Clin. 2013;63:31–44. https://doi.org/10.3322/CAAC.21165.
20. Montgomery GH, Bovbjerg DH, Schnur JB, David D, Goldfarb A, Weltz CR, et al. A randomized clinical trial of a brief hypnosis intervention to control side effects in breast surgery patients. JNCI J Natl Cancer Inst. 2007;99:1304–12. https://doi.org/10.1093/JNCI/DJM106.
21. Elkins G, Marcus J, Stearns V, Perfect M, Rajab MH, Ruud C, et al. Randomized trial of a hypnosis intervention for treatment of hot flashes among breast

cancer survivors. J Clin Oncol. 2008;26:5022–6. https://doi.org/10.1200/JCO.2008.16.6389.
22. Luo XC, Liu J, Fu J, Yin HY, Shen L, Liu ML, et al. Effect of tai chi Chuan in breast cancer patients: a systematic review and meta-analysis. Front Oncol. 2020;10:506578. https://doi.org/10.3389/FONC.2020.00607/BIBTEX.
23. Liu L, Tan H, Yu S, Yin H, Baxter GD. The effectiveness of tai chi in breast cancer patients: a systematic review and meta-analysis. Complement Ther Clin Pract. 2020;38:101078. https://doi.org/10.1016/J.CTCP.2019.101078.
24. Huang J, Liu H, Chen J, Cai X, Huang Y. The effectiveness of tai chi in patients with breast cancer: an overview of systematic reviews and meta-analyses. J Pain Symptom Manag. 2021;61:1052–9. https://doi.org/10.1016/j.jpainsymman.2020.10.007.
25. Selvan P, Hriso C, Mitchell J, Newberg A. Systematic review of yoga for symptom management during conventional treatment of breast cancer patients. Complement Ther Clin Pract. 2022;48:101581. https://doi.org/10.1016/J.CTCP.2022.101581.
26. Hauer M, Rossi AM, Wertheim BC, Kleppel HB, Bea JW, Funk JL. Dietary supplement use in women diagnosed with breast cancer. J Nutr. 2023;153:301–11. https://doi.org/10.1016/J.TJNUT.2022.12.007.
27. Ambrosone CB, Zirpoli GR, Hutson AD, Mccann WE, Mccann SE, Barlow WE, et al. Dietary supplement use during chemotherapy and survival outcomes of patients with breast cancer enrolled in a cooperative group clinical trial (SWOG S0221). J Clin Oncol. 2019;38:804–14. https://doi.org/10.1200/JCO.19.
28. Nechuta SJ, Caan BJ, Chen WY, Lu W, Chen Z, Kwan ML, et al. Soy food intake after diagnosis of breast cancer and survival: an in-depth analysis of combined evidence from cohort studies of US and Chinese women. Am J Clin Nutr. 2012;96:123–32. https://doi.org/10.3945/AJCN.112.035972.
29. Li Y, Li S, Meng X, Gan R-Y, Zhang J-J, Li H-B. Dietary natural products for prevention and treatment of breast cancer. Nutrients. 2017;9:728. https://doi.org/10.3390/nu9070728.
30. Zheng J, Zhou Y, Li Y, Xu D-P, Li S, Li H-B. Spices for prevention and treatment of cancers. Nutrients. 2016;8:495. https://doi.org/10.3390/nu8080495.
31. Usman AN, Manju B, Ilhamuddin I, Ahmad M, Ab T, Ariyandy A, et al. Ginger potency on the prevention and treatment of breast cancer. Breast Dis. 2023;42:207–12. https://doi.org/10.3233/BD-239003.
32. Wanchai A, Armer JM. A systematic review association of reflexology in managing symptoms and side effects of breast cancer treatment. Complement Ther Clin Pract. 2020;38:101074. https://doi.org/10.1016/J.CTCP.2019.101074.
33. Özdelikara A, Tan M. The effect of reflexology on chemotherapy-induced nausea, vomiting, and fatigue in breast cancer patients. Asia Pac J Oncol Nurs. 2017;4:241–9. https://doi.org/10.4103/apjon.apjon_15_17.
34. Özdelikara A, Tan M. The effect of reflexology on the quality of life with breast cancer patients. Complement Ther Clin Pract. 2017;29:122–9. https://doi.org/10.1016/J.CTCP.2017.09.004.
35. Shan S, Lin L, Fang Q, Tian F, Guo D, Zhou Y, et al. Massage therapy significantly improves cancer-related fatigue in cancer patients: a meta-analysis of randomized controlled trials. Support Care Cancer. 2023;31:1–14. https://doi.org/10.1007/S00520-023-07926-W/TABLES/2.
36. Shin ES, Seo KH, Lee SH, Jang JE, Jung YM, Kim MJ, et al. Massage with or without aromatherapy for symptom relief in people with cancer. Cochrane Database Syst Rev. 2016;2016:CD009873. https://doi.org/10.1002/14651858.CD009873.PUB3.
37. Kuril M. Study on effect of reiki healing on breast cancer patients. Int J Sci Res. 2020;9:586–9. https://doi.org/10.21275/SR20805143216.

30 Catheter Care and Education in Breast Cancer Patients

Seda Şahan

30.1 Venous Access Devices in Cancer Patients

Patients undergo a long and complex treatment process after being diagnosed with cancer. Chemotherapy is one of the most important treatments for patients with breast cancer, which is used to treat cancer and reduce the risk of recurrence by applied intravenously [1, 2]. However, prolonged and repeated cycles of chemotherapy begin to damage the peripheral vessels over time. In addition, it is a well-known fact that chemotherapy administered through peripheral vessels can be highly dangerous due to serious side effects of this administration such as extravasation of chemotherapeutic agents, pain, and psychological trauma [3]. For this reason, a variety of catheters are preferred for use in the treatment process that offers ease of use in the medium and long-term. Central venous catheters (CVCs), peripherally inserted central catheters (PICCs), implantable venous access ports (PORTs), and venous access devices (VADs) are used to provide safe and long-term venous access [3–7].

Port catheters are implanted with open surgery and radiologic monitoring without the need for an external catheter line. It prevents the damage of peripheral vessels from irritating drugs. It also reduces the discomfort and pain associated with repeated invasive procedures in peripheral sites during the application of chemotherapy [8–11]. The subcutaneous venous port catheters are often preferred and used for this purpose because they are invisible outside of the body, well tolerated by patients, have a low risk of infection, allow patients to perform activities of daily living, and provide safe intravenous access. The device can be placed in the patient's chest, arm, or abdomen. Port catheters can remain for years and can be used primarily for chemotherapy [8, 12–14]. The PICC is placed in the superior vena cava in the antecubital region, and it is often used for long-term chemotherapy treatment [15–17].

CVCs, PICCs, and ports are used for medium- and long-term chemotherapy for breast cancer; however, these venous access routes have various advantages and disadvantages. The first obvious disadvantage of the catheters is the length of stay, PICCs have a longer length of stay than CVCs, while port catheters have a shorter length of stay [18, 19]. Port catheters are recommended for long-term use, while PICCs are recommended for short- and medium-term treatment [20, 21]. The main disadvantage of CVCs is that they must be reinserted before each chemotherapy session; therefore, the long-term use of CVCs is more prone to potential catheter-related complications [18, 22].

Ports are inserted in an operating room by an interventional radiologist. PICCs can be inserted

S. Şahan (✉)
Department of Nursing, Faculty of Health Sciences, İzmir Bakircay University, İzmir, Turkey
e-mail: seda.sahan@bakircay.edu.tr

Y. Bakar, A. Tuğral (eds.), *Managing Side Effects of Breast Cancer Treatment*,
https://doi.org/10.1007/978-3-031-75480-7_30

by specialized nurses and do not require a specific place. In addition, insertion of PICCs is faster, easier, and less expensive, whereas port insertion and removal can be complex. From this point of view, it can be said that the use of PICC is more advantageous [23, 24].

PICCs are inserted into veins with smaller diameters compared to port catheters. Therefore, slow fluid flow rate and small vessel diameter may cause thrombus formation in patients with PICCs. PICCs also have a smaller inner diameter than ports. This small inner diameter may cause the drugs to flow more slowly in the vein and consequently cause an increase in the completion of a chemotherapy cycle. In addition, the intravenous length of PICCs is longer than that of ports, which increases the likelihood of thrombus dissemination. Similarly, the smaller vessel diameter increases the exposure time of the drugs with the vascular tissue, which increases the likelihood of thrombus formation [25–28].

There is no clear information regarding the choice of venous access routes used in cancer patients. Although practice guidelines for central venous access have recently been published by the American Society of Anesthesiologists working group, the choice of the best venous access route is based on the general condition of the patient and the availability of the device, the balance of benefits and costs, and most importantly, the physician's preference [29].

30.2 Catheter-Related Complications

Venous access sites used in cancer patients can have various complications that are also similar in patients with port catheters or PICC insertion [30–33] such as catheter malfunction, accidental removal of the catheter, thrombolytic complications, and infectious complications [34–36].

In the literature, studies are comparing Port and PICC-related complications. However, it is also stated that no clear conclusion can be drawn according to the results of these studies [3, 37, 38]. A study of 8006 patients found that the incidence of complications was lower in patients with port placement than those with PICC placement [3]. In a study conducted with breast cancer patients, it was similarly reported that patients with port catheters had a lower rate of complications compared to those with PICC [39]. In another study, similar results were also found [40]. In another study, 106 PICC and port catheters were observed for complications. However, it was reported that there was no difference in the incidence of complications between the two catheters [32]. The difference in complication rates between catheters may be related to catheter care. Patients with port catheters do not require dressings after the surgical site has healed. PICC catheters, however, require weekly dressing changes. In this context, inadequate PICC catheter care may lead to higher complication rates. However, further studies are needed to confirm this conclusion.

The most important reason for fewer complications with port catheters compared to PICCs is the smaller diameter of the vessel into which the PICC is inserted. Due to the fact that the PICC catheter tip is longer than that of the port catheter, this is also shown to be an important reason for lower complications. Because the longer catheter tip may adhere to the inner wall of the vessel and prevent the passage of the drug through the catheter, the catheter may also be curved or bent the passage in a vessel, and a thrombus can stuck on the tip of the catheter [40, 41].

In a study, the complication rates seen in patients with PICC or port catheters were compared; it was reported that the complications were higher in patients with PICC insertion [31]. A meta-analysis study reported that patients with ports had a lower rate of thrombosis than those with PICCs [42].

Central line-associated bloodstream infections (CLABSI) are the most common complications associated with venous access in cancer patients. The rate of these infections is reported to be between 0.5–10 per 1000 days of venous access use. Mortality rates vary depending on factors such as the patient's pre-existing chronic conditions, the type of venous access used, and the type of microorganism causing the infection. However, an average mortality rate of 12–40% due to port-related infection has been reported in cancer patients [43–47].

On the other hand, 70% of all venous access-associated infections can be prevented with proper care [48]. Risk factors for catheter-associated infections include administration of blood products in combination with chemotherapeutic drugs or total parenteral nutrition. Another risk factor for infection is neutropenia. According to research, neutropenic patients are at a higher risk than non-neutropenic patients [49, 50].

There are several studies in the literature comparing the infection rates of PICCs and central venous catheters. The results of a meta-analysis of these studies reported that patients with PICCs had a lower rate of infection than those with other central venous catheters (RR: 0.62; 95% CI 0.40–0.94) [16, 25, 51–55].

To prevent venous access route-associated infections, the use of care packages, hand hygiene training, observation on the catheter site, and catheter care with aseptic techniques are recommended [56]. Healthcare professionals should be trained at first to prevent infections and to implement care packages. It is also expected that healthcare professionals who work with catheterized cancer patients should have specific training in the context of preventing catheter-related infections. However, it should be noted that educating patients to prevent potential catheter-related complications is a prerequisite for an improved clinical outcome in the context of patient-centred overall care [43, 56, 57].

30.3 Education in Breast Cancer: A Special Focus on Catheter Care

Patient education is essential to reduce the incidence of catheter-related complications. It should ensure that patients are aware of and in control of their catheter care, especially when catheters remain for extended periods [58].

Despite having different cancer diagnoses, most patients experience similar physical, social, and psychological challenges when catheter-related complications occur [59]. In a study, cancer patients stated that they were not ready for life after catheterization and did not have enough information about catheter care [60, 61]. Notably, some cancer patients have difficulty living with a catheter, carry psychological trauma, and therefore they feel the need to hide their catheters [62–64]. Patients reported that they felt the need to limit their social activities due to a lack of enough information on how to manage catheter care. Moreover, difficulty with self-care was another concern among patients. Because they did not know how to protect the catheter, they stated that they could not perform the usual requirements during shower while the catheter was inserted [59, 60, 65].

Most cancer patients with different types of catheters say they are afraid of experiencing catheter-related adverse events and are particularly concerned about the occurrence of infection. Patients should take more responsibility for managing the care of these seemingly complex devices themselves, often without the assistance of a healthcare professional. However, without effective information on how to manage catheters, it can cause catheter-related complications. The average rate of catheter-related complications in cancer patients is reported to be 6–25% [53, 54]. It is also shown that patients' knowledge, attitude, and practice status of daily self-care of catheters need to be further improved. Safdar et al. (2012) have shown that patients with PICC have little knowledge of catheter-related bloodstream infection, and even 50% of them lack awareness of catheter-related bloodstream infection, a life-threatening catheter-related complication [66]. In a qualitative study, patients expressed concerns about home catheter care and complications. In the study, the need to independently monitor complications at home was reported to be a source of concern for some participants. Patients expressed concern that after discharge the PICC would no longer be checked by clinicians as frequently as before.

They were anxious about whether they would be able to correctly assess the PICC to identify a complication and successfully manage a problem if it occurred. In the same study, patients expressed a need for more clinical and practical information about PICC. Most information provided to patients focused on the risks of catheter-related complications that may occur during the insertion procedure or with the device at home. While patients understood that this information was important, they also indicated that they needed information about the experience and duration of the insertion procedure and practical information to support them in adapting at home. Information to support self-management, including recognizing and responding to PICC complications, was also identified as an information need [59].

Patients with catheters experience difficulties in situations such as showering, sexual intercourse, and exercise while living with a catheter [61, 62, 65]. In a study, it was reported that care education given to patients with port catheters decreased patients' anxiety about care and accordingly increased their quality of life [33].

The main cause of patients' concerns about living with a catheter and related complications is the lack of information about catheter care. Therefore, an educational plan should be developed to meet the needs of information patients regarding catheter care to improve their quality of life, avoid social stigma, and prevent complications [58, 59, 61, 62]. In a study, it was determined that nurses' written and verbal port catheter training increased the level of knowledge of patients and improved their self-confidence in providing care [67].

For patients with catheters, providing catheter-related health education at various stages will enable patients to continue the treatment process more comfortably. Particularly during the systemic treatment process, educating patients about catheter care will reduce their anxiety. Informing patients about possible catheter-related complications and self-monitoring these symptoms will also reduce the catheter-related complications [58, 68].

30.4 Content of Catheter Care in Breast Cancer

- Hand hygiene must be ensured before catheter care. The use of gloves during maintenance does not eliminate the need for hand hygiene. Therefore, hands should be rubbed with antiseptic solutions for 20–30 s or washed with water and soap for 40–60 s.
- Dressings provide fixation of the catheter site during daily life activities; therefore, regular dressing hygiene and follow-up are important.
- The dressing should be changed weekly in case the dressing on the catheter site is clear, semipermeable, and polyurethane.
- If only a gauze pad is present at the catheter site, it should be changed 2 days after catheter insertion.
- Patients with port catheters do not require dressings after the surgical site has healed. Disinfection of the area before and after needle insertion is necessary.
- Disposable antiseptic solution bags or disposable antiseptic-impregnated swabs/wipes should be used to disinfect the port catheter site. An alcoholic chlorhexidine gluconate solution (preferably 2% chlorhexidine gluconate in 70% isopropyl alcohol) should be used to clean the catheter entry site and allowed to dry during dressing changes.
- Sterile transparent dressings are recommended for catheter care, especially for monitoring catheter-related complications. Transparent dressings securely fix the catheter, allow bathing without disturbing the dressing, and require less frequent changes than standard gauze dressings.
- Transparent dressings should be preferred, especially if there is bleeding or leakage after the surgical procedure at the port catheter site.
- The sterile gauze dressing should be monitored daily. The dressing should be changed when it becomes moist, loose, or soiled. The gauze dressing should be replaced with a transparent semipermeable dressing as early as possible.

- Each time the dressing is changed/removed, the catheter site should be disinfected with 2% chlorhexidine and 70% isopropyl alcohol, unless contraindicated. If there is a history of allergy to chlorhexidine, a 10% alcohol povidone-iodine solution should be used instead.
- Examination of the catheter insertion site is not enough to differentially diagnose bloodstream infection but can be used to detect local site infection. The catheter site should be monitored for signs of infection daily. The site should be examined for tenderness, redness, pain, swelling, and increased temperature. If these symptoms are observed, health professionals should be contacted for further examination.
- Showering is allowed after 2 days of a catheter insertion. However, waterproof, see-through drapes should be used each time to prevent water from entering the catheter area during showering. Prolonged soaking in pools or bathtubs after catheterization should be avoided. Even with waterproof dressings, water can get into the dressing and cause infection after a long time.
- Exercise can be done 1 week after catheterization, but weight-bearing exercises, especially upper-body exercises, should be done after 1 month.
- The catheter site should be protected from trauma and direct hot/cold applications.
- Pain, burning, soreness, swelling, and redness in the port area during drug administration indicate subcutaneous leakage from the port membrane. In this case, all infusions administered through the port should be stopped immediately, the port needle should be removed, and the patient's physician should be informed [29, 66, 69–77].

30.5 Conclusion

Living with a catheter is a very difficult process for cancer patients. Catheters can cause significant complications in cancer patients. In particular, the long duration of the catheter and the patient living with a catheter at home can increase these complications. Therefore, education is needed to prevent catheter-related complications and make it easier for patients to live with catheters. Patients have concerns about living with a catheter. Healthcare professionals should understand these concerns and communicate with the patient to address them. Patients should be informed about the issues they should be aware of during daily activities while living with a catheter. In particular, the issues that patients are most afraid of, such as showering and sexual intercourse, should be explained in detail. It is important to provide education on catheter care and dressings to be used to prevent catheter-related complications. Therefore, the patient's need for catheter care education should be regularly assessed, and education should be repeated as needed.

References

1. Sparano JA, Gray RJ, Makower DF, Pritchard KI, Albain KS, Hayes DF, et al. Adjuvant chemotherapy guided by a 21-gene expression assay in breast cancer. N Engl J Med. 2018;379(2):111–21.
2. Cardoso F, van't Veer LJ, Bogaerts J, Slaets L, Viale G, Delaloge S, et al. 70-gene signature as an aid to treatment decisions in early-stage breast cancer. N Engl J Med. 2016;375(8):717–29.
3. Taxbro K, Hammarskjöld F, Thelin B, Lewin F, Hagman H, Hanberger H, et al. Clinical impact of peripherally inserted central catheters vs implanted port catheters in patients with cancer: an open-label, randomised, two-Centre trial. Br J Anaesth. 2019;122(6):734–41.
4. Gorski LA. The 2016 infusion therapy standards of practice. Home Healthc Now. 2017;35(1):10–8.
5. Di Santo MK, Takemoto D, Nascimento RG, Nascimento AM, Siqueira É, Duarte CT, et al. Peripherally inserted central venous catheters: alternative or first choice vascular access? J Vasc Bras. 2017;16:104–12.
6. Veyrier M, Henry C, Decottignies A, Laouini T, Maitre S, Marthey L, et al. Design and assessment of a outpatient living with PICC-line support program: a pilot study. Ann Pharm Fr. 2018;77:62–73.
7. Nailon RE, Rupp ME, Lyden E. A day in the life of a CVAD. J Infus Nurs. 2019;42(3):125–31.
8. Güven C. Evaluation of our subcutaneous venous port catheter applications: 6 years of clinical experience. Adıyaman Univ J Health Sci. 2020;6(1):29–40.

9. Işıklı AG, Soydaş D, Önüt F, Şen H. The effect of video information before insertion of an implantable port catheter on cancer patients' fear of pain and pain levels. Cancer Nurs. 2023;10:1097.
10. Li Y, Guo J, Zhang Y, Kong J. Complications from port-a-cath system implantation in adults with malignant tumors: a 10-year single-center retrospective study. J Int Med. 2022;5(1):15–22.
11. Madabhavi I, Patel A, Sarkar M, Anand A, Panchal H, Parikh S. A study of use of "PORT" catheter in patients with cancer: a single-center experience. Clin Med Insights Oncol. 2017;11(2):1179554917691031.
12. LeVasseur N, Stober C, Daigle K, Robinson A, McDiarmid S, Mazzarello S, et al. Optimizing vascular access for patients receiving intravenous systemic therapy for early-stage breast cancer—a survey of oncology nurses and physicians. Curr Oncol. 2018;25(4):298–304.
13. Carausu L, Clapisson G, Philip I, Sebban H, Marec-Bérard P. Use of totally implantable catheters for peripheral blood stem cell apheresis. Bone Marrow Transplant. 2007;40(5):417–22.
14. LaRoy JR, White SB, Jayakrishnan T, Dybul S, Ungerer D, Turaga K, et al. Cost and morbidity analysis of chest port insertion: interventional radiology suite versus operating room. J Am Coll Radiol. 2015;12(6):563–71.
15. Gebauer B, Teichgräber U, Podrabsky P, Beck A, Wagner H. Ultrasound-and fluoroscopy-guided implantation of peripherally inserted central venous catheters (PICCs). Rofo. 2004;176(3):386–91.
16. Chopra V, Ratz D, Kuhn L, Lopus T, Chenoweth C, Krein S. PICC-associated bloodstream infections: prevalence, patterns, and predictors. Am J Med. 2014;127(4):319–28.
17. Johansson E, Hammarskjöld F, Lundberg D, Arnlind MH. Advantages and disadvantages of peripherally inserted central venous catheters (PICC) compared to other central venous lines: a systematic review of the literature. Acta Oncol. 2013;52(5):886–92.
18. Zhou Y, Hu Y, Zhang X, Zhou P, Gu Y. Evaluation on effectiveness and safety of peripherally inserted central catheters technology: an overview of systematic review. JBI Evid Implement. 2016;14(4):199–200.
19. Periard D, Monney P, Waeber G, Zurkinden C, Mazzolai L, Hayoz D, et al. Randomized controlled trial of peripherally inserted central catheters vs. peripheral catheters for middle duration in-hospital intravenous therapy. J Thromb Haemost. 2008;6(8):1281–8.
20. Akhtar N, Lee L. Utilization and complications of central venous access devices in oncology patients. Curr Oncol. 2021;28(1):367–77.
21. de Sousa DA, Spessoto AB. Peripherally inserted central catheter versus central venous catheter: it is time to use different approaches and metrics for a more useful comparison. Crit Care Med. 2021;49(1):e109–e10.
22. Robinson A, Souied O, Bota AB, Levasseur N, Stober C, Hilton J, et al. Optimal vascular access strategies for patients receiving chemotherapy for early-stage breast cancer: a systematic review. Breast Cancer Res Treat. 2018;171:607–20.
23. Martella F, Salutari V, Marchetti C, Pisano C, Di Napoli M, Pietta F, et al. A retrospective analysis of trabectedin infusion by peripherally inserted central venous catheters: a multicentric Italian experience. Anti-Cancer Drugs. 2015;26(9):990–4.
24. Wang K, Zhong J, Huang N, Zhou Y. Economic evaluation of peripherally inserted central catheter and other venous access devices: a scoping review. J Vasc Access. 2020;21(6):826–37.
25. Patel GS, Jain K, Kumar R, Strickland A, Pellegrini L, Slavotinek J, et al. Comparison of peripherally inserted central venous catheters (PICC) versus subcutaneously implanted port-chamber catheters by complication and cost for patients receiving chemotherapy for non-haematological malignancies. Support Care Cancer. 2014;22(1):121–8.
26. Royer T. Maximum flow rates achievable through peripherally inserted central catheters using standard hospital infusion pumps. J Assoc Vasc Access. 2012;17(2):78–83.
27. Lee J-A, Zierler BK, Zierler RE. The risk factors and clinical outcomes of upper extremity deep vein thrombosis. J Vasc Endovasc Surg. 2012;46(2):139–44.
28. Krein SL, Kuhn L, Ratz D, Chopra V. Use of designated nurse PICC teams and CLABSI prevention practices among US hospitals: a survey-based study. J Patient Saf. 2019;15(4):293–5.
29. Apfelbaum JL, Rupp SM, Tung A, Connis RT, Domino KB, Grant MD, et al. Practice guidelines for central venous access 2020 An updated report by the American Society of Anesthesiologists Task Force on central venous access. Anesthesiology. 2020;132:8–43.
30. Barrigah-Benissan K, Ory J, Simon C, Loubet P, Martin A, Beregi J-P, et al. Clinical factors associated with peripherally inserted central catheters (PICC) related bloodstream infections: a single Centre retrospective cohort. Antimicrob Resist Infect Control. 2023;12(1):5–9.
31. Chopra V, Flanders SA, Saint S, Woller SC, O'Grady NP, Safdar N, et al. The Michigan appropriateness guide for intravenous catheters (MAGIC): results from a multispecialty panel using the RAND/UCLA appropriateness method. Ann Intern Med. 2015;163(6_Supplement):S1–S40.
32. Herc E, Patel P, Washer LL, Conlon A, Flanders SA, Chopra V. A model to predict central-line–associated bloodstream infection among patients with peripherally inserted central catheters: the MPC score. Infect Control Hosp Epidemiol. 2017;38(10):1155–66.
33. Piredda A, Radice D, Zencovich C, Cerri M, Aventino L, Naccarato F, et al. Safe use of peripherally inserted central catheters for chemotherapy of solid malignancies in adult patients: a 1-year monocentric, prospectively-assessed, unselected cohort of 482 patients. J Vasc Access. 2021;22(6):873–81.
34. Al-Asadi O, Almusarhed M, Eldeeb H. Predictive risk factors of venous thromboembolism (VTE) associated

with peripherally inserted central catheters (PICC) in ambulant solid cancer patients: retrospective single Centre cohort study. Thromb J. 2019;17(2):1–7.
35. Madabhavi I, Patel A, Sarkar M, Kataria P, Kadakol N, Anand A. A study of the use of peripherally inserted central catheters in cancer patients: a single-center experience. J Vasc Nurs. 2018;36(3):149–56.
36. Nakaya Y, Imasaki M, Shirano M, Shimizu K, Yagi N, Tsutsumi M, et al. Peripherally inserted central venous catheters decrease central line-associated bloodstream infections and change microbiological epidemiology in adult hematology unit: a propensity score-adjusted analysis. Ann Hematol. 2022;101(9):2069–77.
37. Biffi R, Orsi F, Pozzi S, Pace U, Bonomo G, Monfardini L, et al. Best choice of central venous insertion site for the prevention of catheter-related complications in adult patients who need cancer therapy: a randomized trial. Ann Oncol. 2009;20(5):935–40.
38. Hsu CCT, Kwan GN, Evans-Barns H, Rophael JA, van Driel ML. Venous cutdown versus the Seldinger technique for placement of totally implantable venous access ports. Cochrane Database Syst Rev. 2016;8:1.
39. Lefebvre L, Noyon E, Georgescu D, Proust V, Alexandru C, Leheurteur M, et al. Port catheter versus peripherally inserted central catheter for postoperative chemotherapy in early breast cancer: a retrospective analysis of 448 patients. Support Care Cancer. 2016;24(1):1397–403.
40. Capozzi VA, Monfardini L, Sozzi G, Armano G, Butera D, Scarpelli E, et al. Peripherally inserted central venous catheters (PICC) versus totally implantable venous access device (PORT) for chemotherapy administration: a meta-analysis on gynecological cancer patients. Acta Biomed. 2021;92(5):e2021257.
41. Tamura A, Sone M, Ehara S, Kato K, Tanaka R, Nakasato T, et al. Is ultrasound-guided central venous port placement effective to avoid pinch-off syndrome? J Vasc Access. 2014;15(4):311–6.
42. Wang P, Soh KL, Ying Y, Liu Y, Huang X, Huang J. Risk of VTE associated with PORTs and PICCs in cancer patients: a systematic review and meta-analysis. Thromb Res. 2022;213:34–42.
43. Böll B, Schalk E, Buchheidt D, Hasenkamp J, Kiehl M, Kiderlen TR, et al. Central venous catheter–related infections in hematology and oncology: 2020 updated guidelines on diagnosis, management, and prevention by the infectious diseases working party (AGIHO) of the German Society of Hematology and Medical Oncology (DGHO). Ann Hematol. 2021;100:239–59.
44. Higgins M, Zhang L, Ford R, Brownlie J, Kleidon T, Rickard CM, et al. The microbial biofilm composition on peripherally inserted central catheters: a comparison of polyurethane and hydrophobic catheters collected from paediatric patients. J Vasc Access. 2021;22(3):388–93.
45. Baier C, Linke L, Eder M, Schwab F, Chaberny IF, Vonberg R-P, et al. Incidence, risk factors and healthcare costs of central line-associated nosocomial bloodstream infections in hematologic and oncologic patients. PLoS One. 2020;15(1):e0227772.
46. Milczarek S, Kulig P, Piotrowska O, Zuchmańska A, Wilk-Milczarek E, Machaliński B. Incidence of catheter-associated bloodstream infections in stem cell recipients—should we be "PICCy"? Cancers. 2024;16(6):1239.
47. Zhang Y, Wang Y, Sheng Z, Wang Q, Shi D, Xu S, et al. Incidence rate, pathogens and economic burden of catheter-related bloodstream infection: a single-center, retrospective case-control study. Infect Drug Resist. 2023;5(16):3551–60.
48. Umscheid CA, Mitchell MD, Doshi JA, Agarwal R, Williams K, Brennan PJ. Estimating the proportion of healthcare-associated infections that are reasonably preventable and the related mortality and costs. Infect Control Hosp Epidemiol. 2011;32(2):101–14.
49. Zakhour R, Chaftari A-M, Raad II. Catheter-related infections in patients with haematological malignancies: novel preventive and therapeutic strategies. Lancet Infect Dis. 2016;16(11):241–50.
50. Luft D, Schmoor C, Wilson C, Widmer AF, Bertz H, Frei R, et al. Central venous catheter-associated bloodstream infection and colonisation of insertion site and catheter tip. What are the rates and risk factors in haematology patients? Ann Hematol. 2010;89(3):1265–75.
51. Cotogni P, Barbero C, Garrino C, Degiorgis C, Mussa B, De Francesco A, et al. Peripherally inserted central catheters in non-hospitalized cancer patients: 5-year results of a prospective study. Support Care Cancer. 2015;23:403–9.
52. Bellesi S, Chiusolo P, De Pascale G, Pittiruti M, Scoppettuolo G, Metafuni E, et al. Peripherally inserted central catheters (PICCs) in the management of oncohematological patients submitted to autologous stem cell transplantation. Antimicrob Resist Infect Control. 2013;21:531–5.
53. Kang J, Chen W, Sun W, Ge R, Li H, Ma E, et al. Peripherally inserted central catheter-related complications in cancer patients: a prospective study of over 50,000 catheter days. J Vasc Access. 2017;18(2):153–7.
54. Lee JH, Kim ET, Shim DJ, Kim IJ, Byeon JH, Lee IJ, et al. Prevalence and predictors of peripherally inserted central catheter-associated bloodstream infections in adults: a multicenter cohort study. PLoS One. 2019;14(3):e0213555.
55. Campagna S, Gonella S, Berchialla P, Morano G, Rigo C, Zerla PA, et al. Can peripherally inserted central catheters be safely placed in patients with cancer receiving chemotherapy? A retrospective study of almost 400,000 catheter-days. Oncologist. 2019;24(9):e953–e9.
56. Chaftari P, Chaftari A-M, Adachi J, Hachem R, Raad S, Natividad E, et al. Improvement in the diagnosis of catheter-related bloodstream infections in a tertiary cancer center. Am J Infect Control. 2017;45(3):e34–e9.
57. Hugonnet S, Harbarth S, Sax H, Duncan RA, Pittet D. Nursing resources: a major determinant

of nosocomial infection? Curr Opin Infect Dis. 2004;17(4):329–33.
58. Xie Y, Liu L, Jiao J, Li S, Wang W, Wang J, et al. Health education and nursing needs of breast cancer patients with totally implantable venous access ports at different stages. Altern Ther Health Med. 2023;29(2):22–8.
59. Sharp R, Xu Q, Pumpa R, Elliott L, Corsini N, Marker J, et al. Supportive care needs of adults living with a peripherally inserted central catheter (PICC) at home: a qualitative content analysis. BMC Nurs. 2024;23(1):4–13.
60. Berrevoets MA, Oerlemans AJ, Tromp M, Kullberg BJ, Ten Oever J, Schouten JA, et al. Quality of outpatient parenteral antimicrobial therapy (OPAT) care from the patient's perspective: a qualitative study. BMJ Open. 2018;8(11):e024564.
61. Ryan C, Hesselgreaves H, Wu O, Moss J, Paul J, Dixon-Hughes J, et al. Patient acceptability of three different central venous access devices for the delivery of systemic anticancer therapy: a qualitative study. BMJ Open. 2019;9(7):e026077.
62. Parás-Bravo P, Paz-Zulueta M, Santibañez M, Fernández-de-Las-Peñas C, Herrero-Montes M, Caso-Álvarez V, et al. Living with a peripherally inserted central catheter: the perspective of cancer outpatients—a qualitative study. Support Care Cancer. 2018;26(2):441–9.
63. Ritchie M, Kelly LJ, Moss J, Paul J, Shaw R. Exploring attitudes towards a randomised controlled trial of venous access devices–a nested pre-trial qualitative study. J Vasc Access. 2015;16(5):407–12.
64. Twiddy M, Murray CJC, Mason SJ, Meads D, Wright JM, Mitchell ED, et al. A qualitative study of patients' feedback about outpatient parenteral antimicrobial therapy (OPAT) services in northern England: implications for service improvement. BMJ Open. 2018;8(1):e019099.
65. Kumari P, Ritchie S, Thomas M, Jull A. The patient experience of care delivered by an outpatient intravenous antibiotic service. Kaitiaki Nurs Res. 2018;9(1):18–26.
66. Safdar N, Mittelstadt K, Jacobs EA, Gaines ME. Patient awareness of the risks of central venous catheters in the outpatient setting. Am J Infect Control. 2012;40(1):87–8.
67. Piredda M. Written information improves patient knowledge about implanted ports. Clin J Oncol Nurs. 2016;20(2):28–33.
68. Lebeaux D, Fernández-Hidalgo N, Chauhan A, Lee S, Ghigo J-M, Almirante B, et al. Management of infections related to totally implantable venous-access ports: challenges and perspectives. Lancet Infect Dis. 2014;14(2):146–59.
69. Rupp SM, Apfelbaum JL, Blitt C, Caplan RA, Connis RT, Domino KB, et al. Practice guidelines for central venous access: a report by the American Society of Anesthesiologists Task Force on central venous access. Anesthesiology. 2012;116(3):539–73.
70. Murphy C, Andrus M, Barnes S, Garcia R, Juraja M, Khoury R. APIC elimination guide: guide to the elimination of catheter-related bloodstream infections. Associations for Professionals in Infection Control and Epidemiology; 2009.
71. O'grady NP, Alexander M, Dellinger EP, Gerberding JL, Heard SO, Maki DG, et al. Guidelines for the prevention of intravascular catheter–related infections. Clin Infect Dis. 2002;35(11):1281–307.
72. Mermel LA, Allon M, Bouza E, Craven DE, Flynn P, O'Grady NP, et al. Clinical practice guidelines for the diagnosis and management of intravascular catheter-related infection: 2009 update by the Infectious Diseases Society of America. Clin Infect Dis. 2009;49(1):1–45.
73. Pronovost P, Needham D, Berenholtz S, Sinopoli D, Chu H, Cosgrove S, et al. An intervention to decrease catheter-related bloodstream infections in the ICU. N Engl J Med. 2006;355(26):2725–32.
74. Rowley S, Clare S, Macqueen S, Molyneux R. ANTT v2: an updated practice framework for aseptic technique. Br J Nurs. 2010;19(5):5–11.
75. Timsit J-F, Schwebel C, Bouadma L, Geffroy A, Garrouste-Orgeas M, Pease S, et al. Chlorhexidine-impregnated sponges and less frequent dressing changes for prevention of catheter-related infections in critically ill adults: a randomized controlled trial. JAMA. 2009;301(12):1231–41.
76. Troianos CA, Hartman GS, Glas KE, Skubas NJ, Eberhardt RT, Walker JD, et al. Guidelines for performing ultrasound guided vascular cannulation: recommendations of the American Society of Echocardiography and the Society of Cardiovascular Anesthesiologists. J Am Soc Echocardiogr. 2011;24(12):1291–318.
77. Jamal MA, Rosenblatt JS, Hachem RY, Ying J, Pravinkumar E, Nates JL, et al. Prevention of biofilm colonization by gram-negative bacteria on minocycline-rifampin-impregnated catheters sequentially coated with chlorhexidine. Antimicrob Agents Chemother. 2014;58(2):1179–82.

31 Home Care Management of Breast Cancer Survivors: The Role of Caregivers

Kübra Pınar Gürkan

31.1 Home Care in Breast Cancer

Breast cancer is the most common type of cancer among women in the world. According to the data from the World Health Organization (WHO), breast cancer constitutes 23.8% of all cancers seen in women [1]. The incidence of breast cancer cases is increasing. But the 5-year relative survival rate for breast cancer is 90%. This emphasizes the need to focus on the care of patients at home as well as in the hospital [1, 2].

Home care service is defined as "the provision of health and care and follow-up services to individuals in the environment where they live with their families by the healthcare team in a way to meet their medical needs including rehabilitation, physiotherapy, and psychological treatment." It is a type of process in which many professional healthcare professionals provide care together [2, 3]. Health care services are characterized by receiving health care during the diagnosis and posttreatment care, chronic disease follow-up, and preventive health and examination services without a health problem in a home environment. Disease-related negativities or side effects can be reduced with appropriate care and treatment without changing the current conditions of the patient [4]. Home care services, which are preferred by patients in terms of providing patient-centered care, are also preferred by governments because they have many advantages in terms of health care costs. The aim of home care services is to improve the quality of life by applying the most accurate treatment with a minimal impact on the patient's daily life and minimizing the effects of the disease [5]. A study evaluating the experience of home care showed that family members of home care patients reported higher satisfaction with the overall quality of care than family members whose care was performed in an institutional setting [6]. However, the need for home care often arises unexpectedly and has quantitative and qualitative dimensions (intensity and length of care, etc.) that are difficult to assess accurately [7].

Due to the great advances achieved in cancer treatment, the treatment of cancer patients is based on outpatient care. Therefore, cancer care has shifted from the hospital environment to the home environment. This situation shortens the hospitalization period of the patients and facilitates the management of the patient at home by increasing the care responsibility of the family members, which makes them a caregiver [8]. Home care services ensure the continuation of the motivation of the caregiver and strengthen the family bonds. To provide care for individuals with cancer at the desired level, it is very important to be aware of the problems experienced by the patient and family members and to support individuals with these problems [9]. It has been reported that caring family members who take an

K. P. Gürkan (✉)
Faculty of Health Sciences Department of Public Health Nursing, İzmir Bakırçay University, Izmir, Turkey

Y. Bakar, A. Tuğral (eds.), *Managing Side Effects of Breast Cancer Treatment*,
https://doi.org/10.1007/978-3-031-75480-7_31

active role in the home care process not only want to receive services but also information about the care [10].

31.2 Being a Caregiver

People diagnosed with curable cancer may generally need temporary care before, during, and immediately after treatment, whereas people with a less favorable prognosis may need long-term palliative care [11].

Care can be provided in two different types to patients:

1. Professional (Formal) Care: Professional care is defined as care provided by public and private institutions and voluntary organizations [12].
2. Nonprofessional (Informal Care): These are the people who provide care to the individual with cancer without any fee. They have no training in this field. They usually consist of the patient's family, friends, or close environment [13]. Informal caregivers are generally defined as people who have multiple responsibilities for unpaid physical care, symptom monitoring, emotional support, undertaking housework, managing, and coordinating financial resources related to the consequences of disease and/or treatment, and all kinds of care for the patient [12].

Regardless of the quality, it is considered that the support provided by informal caregivers is equal to or more beneficial than the support obtained from other sources [14, 15]. According to reports from various organizations, more than 100 million people in Europe, Australia, and the United States provide unpaid care to a relative, friend, or neighbor in need because of old age, disability, or illness. Informal caregivers, who provide around 80% of care hours, are known to provide at least €500 billion in savings to the world economy per year [16]. Government policy therefore encourages health professionals to work in partnership with caregivers to support individuals. The importance of the roles that caregivers fulfill needs to be understood, and the impact of these roles on their lives needs to be recognized to be effective for these collaborations [17]. There are approximately five to six million family caregivers in the United Kingdom (UK) [18]. In addition, one out of every five people in the UK and Northern Ireland and one out of every 10 people in Germany undertakes the care of a sick person in their family. In the United States, more than 80% of long-term care services are provided by family members [19]. There is no clear statistical data on this situation for Turkey. Primary caregivers of cancer patients are usually unpaid, long-term, and volunteered family members, and family members who take care of their loved ones by fulfilling their responsibilities both in the hospital and at home may be vulnerable to ignoring their own needs in general [20], [18].

The American Cancer Society defines informal caregivers as an important part of the cancer team. The association lists the general tasks expected to be performed by caregivers as follows:

- Administering medication.
- Handling side effects.
- Reporting problems.
- Informing other family members and friends about the patient's condition.
- Helping to decide whether the treatment is working or not.
- Organizing patient care as part of a team.
- Monitoring of prescriptions.
- Know which tests to perform.
- Ensuring that all medical staff are informed about how the process of the patient is going [13].

It is a well-known fact that a good caregiver can be an important health resource. In most cases, it is the only person who knows the whole process and everything about the patient. Expectations from caregivers are summarized as follows:

- Do not hesitate to ask questions during doctor visits and take notes.
- Know who takes part in the cancer team.

- Learn how to communicate with the cancer team [13].

Although informal caregivers may seem simple, they may have some daily tasks that are necessary for the patient. These are

- Shopping and preparation of food.
- Feeding the patient if a patient is unable to eat.
- Helping or reminding to take medication.
- Help with bathing.
- Doing household chores.
- Payment of invoices.
- Transport to doctor's appointments, treatments, and tests [13].

31.3 Responsibilities of Caregivers According to Cancer Stages

31.3.1 Diagnosis Period

The patient's relatives as well as the patient can experience shock and anxiety at the initial diagnosis of cancer [21]. This period between the diagnosis and the treatment period is an intense period in which the relatives or family members try to adapt to their new roles and cope with their feelings of uncertainty, anxiety about the future, sadness, and grief [22]. In this period, the cancer team expects a quick decision to be made by the patient and their family members for the treatment via presenting the available treatment options to the patient. Caregivers should provide emotional support to the patient and his/her family and assume the role of a coordinator seeking information in deciding on treatment. In Western societies, the disclosure of cancer diagnosis is patient-centered, unlike in Eastern societies [23, 24]. In family-centered societies, caregivers, especially spouses and family members, can often assume a decision-making role to alleviate the patient's fear and shock at the disclosure of the cancer diagnosis [23].

For women with breast cancer, spouses constitute the majority of family support and often assume the role of a primary caregiver. Spousal support in women with breast cancer includes instrumental, emotional, and informative support. Instrumental support includes more tangible types of assistance such as helping with daily household chores, transportation, or paying bills. Emotional support includes encouragement and reassurance, listening, and understanding. Informational support includes providing advice or information about breast cancer. Spouses also have a major role during the shock and denial phase after the diagnosis of breast cancer. Emotions should be allowed to be expressed for the patient to accept the disease [22]. According to clinical experiences, family members can usually hide their concerns to prevent an additional emotional burden on the patient or each other. Though this is a commonly observed behavior, it may increase the emotional burden of the patient, caregiver, or family [25]. Another important issue is to help the patient comply with treatment recommendations. While patients generally accept the treatment recommendations, some patients may tend to need confirmation [26]. Caregivers should reach the right information at this stage.

31.3.2 Treatment Period

Immediately after diagnosis, the patient and caregiver are involved in multimodal cancer treatment, which is unfamiliar to them. At this stage, caregivers are involved in providing physical care and managing treatment-related symptoms. When complex and long-term cancer treatment begins, caregivers need to provide some professional skills (such as controlling the surgical site, administering oral medications, and regulating nutrition) to optimize patient care outcomes. Regardless of the type of treatment the patient receives, functional support is needed. The literature has also shown that a husband experiences a change after his wife's illness, including taking on more responsibility (e.g., for household activities and being a caregiver) [27, 28].

31.3.2.1 Surgical Treatment Period

It is the first stage in which patients might have various care needs and encounter the new role of a caregiver experienced by relatives and family members [9].

Household chores should be met by the caregivers until the patient adapts to his/her daily life. Some medical practices such as paying attention to infectious findings, catheter control, and preventing the development of lymphedema by taking basic precautions are of vital importance in order to ensure better postoperative wound healing. Therefore, caregivers should be trained by nurses before they are discharged from the hospital, and they should not lack information [13].

On the other hand, mastectomy may negatively affect women's breast perception and self-esteem. Therefore, the patient should be given emotional support and encouraged to express her feelings [13].

31.3.2.2 Chemotherapy Period

Patients receive their systemic chemotherapy treatment in daily oncology or outpatient oncology clinics. The duration of these treatments may vary between 1 and 6 h per day, and it is required to come to the clinic every 2–3 weeks according to the chemotherapy regimen.

Caregivers need to prepare the patient for the chemotherapy day. In this way, the patient can have a comfortable chemotherapy application, and the caregiver can use his/her time more effectively after coming from the hospital.

- The house should be cleaned, and laundry should be washed.
- Shopping should be done a day or more before.
- When going to chemotherapy, clothes should be prepared to keep the patient warm (blanket, socks).
- Books, tablets, and cards can make it easier to spend time during chemotherapy.
- Prepare healthy snacks and drinks.
- All prescribed drugs should be made ready for the patient [13].

It is also important that the symptoms that occur after chemotherapy be known and managed by the caregiver. The most common side effects seen in women with breast cancer after or during chemotherapy are nausea and vomiting, fatigue, changes in taste and smell, oral mucositis, constipation, diarrhea, infection, susceptibility to bleeding, and hair loss [29]. Informing caregivers about the side effects that may occur after or during chemotherapy should be the first step. In previous studies, the most frequently stated needs of caregivers for this period were found to be the need to know how to manage the side effects of chemotherapy (79%) in a home environment (79%) [9].

The caregiver should help to establish a daily routine for the patient during this symptomatic phase. Nonpharmacological approaches can be implemented for the patient by caregivers. These will be beneficial in terms of diverting the patient's attention. For example, listening to music, meditation, yoga, reading books, massage, or doing the patient's favorite hobbies together. The aim is here to maximize the patient's quality of life. However, in order to support the management of symptoms, nutritional balance and sleep should be regulated, and fluid intake should be supported [30].

Caregivers have important duties in symptom management. The American Cancer Society has exemplified what caregivers should do in case of infection. For example, let us assume that the patient's leukocyte count has decreased, fever has increased, and as a result, hospitalization may be required. Fever may be an important sign of infection. This is upsetting for the family and relatives and can be seen as a setback. Potential actions are expected from the caregivers such as:

- The patient may be hospitalized for a short time, and antibiotics may be prescribed for infection.
- When traveling to the hospital, pay attention to taking everything that the patient may need, including medications used by the patient for some conditions other than cancer (such as hypertension, and thyroid).
- Contacting all medical staff who are taking primary responsibility for the patient's medical condition and informing them that the patient has been hospitalized [13].

31.3.2.3 Radiotherapy Period

In the treatment of breast cancer, radiotherapy is frequently used in addition to surgery and chemotherapy. In general, it is known that 50–60% of patients with cancer require radiotherapy for curative or palliative purposes in the course of their disease [9].

In a study, it was found that the most frequently experienced symptoms during radiotherapy were fatigue, nausea-vomiting, loss of appetite, dysphagia, mouth sores, skin reactions, and regional or systemic pain. Therefore, similarly, in chemotherapy and mastectomy periods, patients will also need people to help with daily housework during radiotherapy treatment [9].

Things that radiotherapy patients and caregivers should be aware of:

- Providing sun protection in the irradiated area.
- Preferring cotton, comfortable, non-sweating clothes.
- Bathing with warm water instead of hot water.
- Cool compresses (not applying the ice directly) can be implemented to soothe the irradiated skin.
- Being aware that any lotion and/or powder should not be applied to the irradiated area except for the recommended ones by radiation oncologists [31].

31.3.3 Advanced Stage, End of Life/ Terminal Period

Due to the increasing frequency and severity of symptoms in patients in the terminal period, the duration and quality of care should also be increased relatively compared to other periods. The goal of care is maximum symptom control, minimizing the physical and emotional suffering of patients, and allowing them to pass away in dignity and peace [32, 33]. Physical, information, communication, psychological, sexual, social, financial, and spiritual needs of patients should be met. While important and comprehensive needs of both patients and their relatives arise in this period, they may often be left without help and may need to cope alone. Failure to meet the needs within the health care system leads to a decrease in the quality of care. It has been reported that caregivers are an important and integral part of the care and treatment of patients with advanced cancer and that the difficulties experienced by caregivers of patients are more than those of caregivers of patients receiving curative treatment in this period [34].

Since the symptoms of patients with advanced cancer are usually numerous, simultaneous, and severe, this situation increases the physical needs of the patients. Due to deteriorated health status and severe symptom burden, patients with advanced cancer have difficulty in performing basic activities of daily living such as dressing, feeding, moving, and bathing. In addition to physical care needs, advanced-stage cancer patients also need psychosocial care due to uncertainty and fear about the future. Since advanced-stage cancers can lead to death, they bring psychological problems such as shock, denial, anger, guilt, anxiety, depression, and stress. To cope with all these problems, advanced-stage cancer patients need emotional and psychological care. Within the scope of this care, patients should be enabled to express their feelings and face the potential consequences of the disease. Since spending most of the time in the hospital can affect the relationships of advanced cancer patients with their family members and friends, this might lead to a decrease in social life [35–37].

The spiritual and existential needs of patients with advanced-stage cancer are more serious than those of patients in the early stage of cancer. The rate of spiritual needs in advanced-stage cancer patients was found to be 72%, and it was reported that spiritual needs were supported very little in healthcare services. Around 26% of the patients stated at least one unmet spiritual need. Participation in religious ceremonies (21.1%) was the most common unmet spiritual. Among the spiritual needs of these patients, being with their family (80.2%) and praying frequently (50%) were frequently reported. It has been stated that care providers should focus more on religious and spiritual areas for patients at the end of their lives [38, 39].

Table 31.1 Responsibilities of caregivers according to cancer stages

Cancer period	Responsibilities of the caregiver
Diagnostic period	Emotional support – Supporting treatment-seeking behavior – Communication with the health team
Treatment period	
– Surgical treatment period	– Organizing household chores (cleaning, laundry, cooking, paying bills, etc.) – Monitoring the operation site – Observing signs of infection, lymphedema – Supporting the patient's self-care
– Chemotherapy	– Learning the symptoms that may occur – Organizing household chores (cleaning, laundry, cooking, paying bills, etc.) – Preparing for the day of chemotherapy – Accompanying the patient with chemotherapy – Supporting the patient's self-care
– Radiotherapy	– Household organization (cleaning, laundry, cooking, paying bills, etc.) – Supporting the patient's self-care
Terminal period	– Organizing housework (cleaning, laundry, cooking, paying bills, etc.) – Self-care of the patient – Emotional support – Supporting the patient in legal matters

It may be difficult to talk about, but legal issues can be a major source of stress for caregivers, patients, and families. Common concerns include who will manage the person's money and who will make important healthcare decisions if the patient is unable to do so. It is crucial to open these in discussion with the patient while they are still able to make choices. By doing so, the primary caregiver and the rest of the family can be clear about what the patient desires. There are proxy or complementary decision-making tools that can help the caregiver and patient. An example of this is a durable power of attorney, which allows the patient to choose a person who can make financial decisions on their behalf. (This is quite different from durable power of attorney for health care.) A durable power of attorney does not affect health care decisions [13]. The responsibilities of caregivers for women with breast cancer according to cancer stages are summarized in Table 31.1.

31.4 Conclusion

In conclusion, caregivers have different duties and responsibilities at each stage of the breast cancer process. The prerequisite for caregivers to fulfill these responsibilities depends on the provision of information that they get from the moment of diagnosis. Training of informal caregivers will improve the quality of life of women with breast cancer.

References

1. World Health Organization. Cancer Research Agency. 2022. https://gco.iarc.who.int/media/globocan/factsheets/populations/900-world-fact-sheet.pdf.
2. Regulation on the Provision of Home Care Services. 2.6.2023. https://www.resmigazete.gov.tr/eskiler/2023/06/20230602-1.htm.
3. Fadıloğlu Ç, Ertem G, Şenuzun F. Home health and care. Amasya: Göktuğ Publishing; 2013.
4. Boerma W, Genet N. Introduction and background. In: Genet N, Boerma W, Kroneman M, Hutchinson A, Saltman RB, editors. Home care across Europe. United Kingdom; 2012.
5. Oğlak S. Long-term home care services and care insurance. Turk J Geriatr. 2007;10(2):100–8.
6. Teno JM, Clarridge BR, Casey V, Welch LC, Wetle T, et al. Family perspectives on end-oflife care at the last place of care. JAMA J Am Med Assoc. 2014;291:88–93.
7. Lee K, Chaoy YJ. Psychological distress and quality of life of palliative cancer patients and their caring relatives during home care. Support Care Cancer. 2014;22:2775–82.
8. Ulgen T, Uğur Ö. Home care practices of cancer caregivers and the effect of perceived social support on care burden. Support Care Cancer. 2022;30(10):8323–32.
9. Gül E, Kalkım A, Bulut S, Sevil Ü. Quality of life and needs towards home care of patients treated with radiotherapy. Maltepe Univ J Nurs Sci Art. 2009;2(2):3–12.

10. Akdemir N, Bostanoğlu H, Yurtsever S, Kutlutürkan S, Kapucu S, Canlı Özer Z. Needs of home care services for the bedridden patient's problems living in their home. Dicle J Med. 2011;38(1):57–65.
11. Taylor C. Supporting the carers of individuals affected by colorectal cancer. Br J Nurs. 2008;17:226–30.
12. Song J, Dw S, Jy C, Kang J, Baik YJ, Mo H, et al. Quality of life and mental health in family caregivers of patients with terminal cancer. Support Care Cancer. 2011;19:1519–26.
13. American Cancer Society. Caregiver Resource Guide. Caring for a Loved One with Cancer. 2023. https://www.cancer.org/content/dam/cancer-org/cancer-control/en/booklets-flyers/american-cancer-society-caregiver-resource-guide.pdf.
14. Lindholm L, Rehnsfeldt A, Arman M, Hamrin E. Significant others' experience of suffering when living with women with breast cancer. Scand J Caring Sci. 2002;16:248–55.
15. Lauri S, Sainio C. Developing the nursing care of breast cancer patients: an action research approach. J Clin Nurs. 1998;7:424–32.
16. European Association Working for Carers. 2011. Https://Eurocarers.Org.
17. Uk C. In poor health: the impact of caring on health. London: Carers; 2004. https://www.Researchgate.
18. Wood A, Gonzalez J, Sejal M. Mindful caring: using mindfulness-based cognitive therapy with caregivers of cancer survivors barden. J Psychosoc Oncol. 2015;33:66.
19. Triantafillou J, Naiditch M, Repkova K, Stiehr K, Carretero S, Emilsson T, et al. Informal care in the long-term care system, European overview paper. Athens: Interlinks; 2010. http://interlinks.euro.centre.org/project/reports.
20. Goren A, Gilloteau I, Lees M, Costa M. Quantifying the burden of İnformal Care giving for patients with cancer. In: Europe dibona ventura. Berlin: Springer; 2014.
21. Northouse LL, Katapodi MC, Schafenacker AM, Weiss D. The ımpact of caregiving on the psychological Well-being of family caregivers and cancer patients. Semin Oncol Nurs. 2012;28(4):236–45.
22. Shaw J, Harrison J, Young J, Butow P, Sandroussi C, Martin D, et al. Coping with newly diagnosed upper gastrointestinal cancer: a longitudinal qualitative study of family caregivers' role perception and supportive care needs. Support Care Cancer. 2013;21(3):749–56.
23. Gao L, Liu JE, Zhou XP, Su YL, Wang PL. Supporting her as the situation changes: a qualitative study of spousal support strategies for patients with breast cancer in China. Eur J Cancer Care. 2020;29(1):e13176.
24. Tan MS, Narasimhalu K, Ong SY. Letting the cat out of the bag: shifting practices of cancer disclosure in Singapore. Singapore Med J. 2021;53:344–8.
25. Yıldırım NKA, Özkan M. Cancer patıents' relatıves/caregıvers: theır experıences and needs. J Ege Univ Nurs Facul. 2015;31(2):98–112.
26. Niranjan SJ, Wallace WBR, Turkman Y, Williams CP, Bhatia S, et al. Exploring the role of treatment related information and patient physician trust in shared decision making among patients with metastatic breast cancer. J Cancer Educ. 2019:1–8.
27. Chung C, Hwang E. Couples' experiences of breast cancer in Korea: a descriptive qualitative study. Cancer Nurs. 2012;35:211–20.
28. Zahlis EH, Lewis FM. Coming to grips with breast cancer: the spouse's experience with his wife's first six months. J Psychosoc Oncol. 2010;28:79–97.
29. Norouznıa S, Aydoğdu Gördes N, Somalı I. A qualıtatıve study on the problems and needs of patıents wıth breast cancer dıagnosed wıth chemotherapy. J Anatol Nurs Health Sci. 2020;23(1):127–34.
30. National Comperhensive Cancer Network, NCCN Guidline for patients. 2023. https://www.nccn.org/patients/guidelines/content/PDF.
31. Breast Cancer Network Australia. Caring for your skin after radioterapy 11.02.2023. https://www.bcna.org.au/resource-hub/articles/caring-for-your-skin-after-radiotherapy/.
32. Peppercorn JM, Smith TJ, Helft PR, Debono DJ, Berry SR, Wollins DS. American society of clinical oncology statement: toward individualized care for patients with advanced cancer. J Clin Oncol. 2011;29:755–60.
33. Elçigil A. Palliative care nursing. Gülhane Med J. 2012;54:329–34.
34. Polat Ü. Caregivers' roles and support necessities in symptom management for patients with cancer advanced. Turk J Oncol. 2011;26(4):193–8.
35. Thewes B, Butow P, Girgis A, Pendlebury S. The psychosocial needs of breast cancer survivors; a qualitative study of the shared and unique needs of younger versus older survivors. Psycho-Oncology. 2004;13(3):177–89.
36. Hashemi-Ghasemabadi M, Taleghani F, Yousefy A, Kohan S. Transition to the new role of caregiving for families of patients with breast cancer: a qualitative descriptive exploratory study. Support Care Cancer. 2016;24(3):1269–76.
37. Mandelblatt JS, Zhai W, Ahn J, Small BJ, Ahles TA, Carroll JE, et al. Symptom burden among older breast cancer survivors: the thinking and living with cancer (TLC) study. Cancer. 2020;126(6):1183–92.
38. Hampton DM, Hollis DE, Lloyd DA, Taylor J, McMillan SC. Spiritual needs of persons with advanced cancer. Am J Hosp Palliat Med. 2007;24:42.
39. Yıldırım NK, Kaçmaz N. Özkan M unmet care needs in advanced stage cancer patients. J Psychiatr Nurs. 2013;4(3):153–8.

32 Telerehabilitation in Breast Cancer: A Promising Option for Managing Side Effects

Esra Uzelpasacı

32.1 Telehealth and Telerehabilitation

Telehealth applications, which enable interaction with patients in synchronous and asynchronous conditions by using telecommunication technology in healthcare services, have grown rapidly in recent years with the development of mobile device-based healthcare technology [1]. There are telemedicine and telerehabilitation practices under the telehealth umbrella. Telemedicine is defined by the World Health Organization (WHO) as the use of information and communication technologies to protect and improve the health of individuals and communities in situations where access to health services is critical, to provide disease diagnosis and treatment, and to meet health research or health education needs [2]. Telerehabilitation is defined as the remote delivery of rehabilitation services (evaluation, application of physiotherapy modalities, control, patient education, counseling, etc.) to patients through certain procedures and protocols in order to improve their level of independence by rehabilitation specialists using a series of tools such as information and communication technologies [3]. Telerehabilitation has many advantages, such as offering an alternative and low-cost rehabilitation option to face-to-face treatment methods, carrying rehabilitation services to distant places, and being able to receive healthcare services directly at the patient's location [4, 5]. Due to these advantages, it has given a different perspective to researchers and clinicians.

E. Uzelpasacı (✉)
University of Health Sciences, Gulhane Faculty of Physiotherapy and Rehabilitation, Ankara, Turkey
e-mail: esra.uzelpasaci@sbu.edu.tr

32.2 Feasibility of Telerehabilitation in Breast Cancer

Telerehabilitation is a new concept in oncological rehabilitation. The physical and psychosocial problems experienced by cancer patients during and after the treatment period can negatively affect their quality of life, work, family, and social relationships. Telerehabilitation gives patients the opportunity to receive uninterrupted care to prevent and minimize these negative situations [6, 7]. Especially with the COVID-19 epidemic, telerehabilitation provides an innovative approach to clinicians working in this field in complying with isolation rules and minimizing hospital exposure due to the risk of cancer patients contracting COVID-19 [8, 9]. It is very important that telerehabilitation provides a comfortable, easy, and flexible healthcare service, especially for cancer patients with advanced age and comorbidities [10]. The fact is that telerehabilitation eliminates the need for travel, prevents income loss for working cancer patients, and

Y. Bakar, A. Tuğral (eds.), *Managing Side Effects of Breast Cancer Treatment*,
https://doi.org/10.1007/978-3-031-75480-7_32

meets the demands of employers [11]. Studies in the literature have reported that the advantages of the service provided to cancer patients in a virtual format, such as comfort and flexibility, increase the satisfaction level of the patients [12, 13]. Online physiotherapy services provide direct contact between patients and physiotherapists in a one-on-one or group environment [14, 15]. Multi-participant treatment environments can be created with the online video conferencing method [16]. In order to ensure patient safety in patients with some problems such as loss of balance, vision, speech, hearing, or cognitive impairment, a caregiver or patient relative may need to be present with the patient during the online session [17]. On the other hand, communication problems, especially in people with vision, speech and hearing problems, or cognitive impairment, can reduce the effectiveness of online physiotherapy consultancy [17, 18]. In addition, the inability to fully provide one-to-one and face-to-face interaction between the patient and the clinician through an online platform, the disappearance of the therapeutic effect of touch, the age barrier, technical and technological problems, and problems in patient confidentiality may also reduce the effectiveness of online physiotherapy consultancy [18]. In a study investigating the applicability of online physiotherapy services from the perspective of a physiotherapist, the areas that will benefit most from online physiotherapy consultancy from the perspective of a physiotherapist's beliefs are home exercise program monitoring and patient education [19]. However, physiotherapists' beliefs about the use of online physiotherapy services in the first examination of diagnosed patients were found to be quite low [19]. The reason for physiotherapists' low belief in this view may be that physical contact is seen as a key factor to ensure patient trust and closeness. Partially consistent with this view, telehealth has been shown to provide good validity for observational assessments (pain, swelling, range of motion, balance, and gait), but low to moderate validity for assessments requiring physical contact (e.g., some specialized tests or neurological assessments) in previous studies [20–22]. Patients think that online physiotherapy services make it easier for them to ask their questions to the physiotherapist when they have difficulty accessing a face-to-face appointment [19]. Despite all these positive thoughts, the physiotherapists in the study have weak beliefs that patients in the field of oncological rehabilitation can benefit from online physiotherapy services [19]. However, there is evidence in the literature that telerehabilitation interventions used in the rehabilitation of cancer patients provide benefits in terms of quality of life, pain management, and functional mobility [7, 23, 24]. The reason why physiotherapists express a negative opinion despite the oncological telerehabilitation gains supported by the literature may be the variable nature of the follow-up profile of oncological patients requires more surveillance. In addition, outcome measurements and telerehabilitation methods used in studies are also very important in revealing the effectiveness and feasibility of telerehabilitation.

32.3 Outcome Measurements in Telerehabilitation Applications in Breast Cancer

The selection of outcome measures used must be reliable, valid, and precise. A wide variety of outcome measures have been used in studies in the literature. The most commonly used outcome measures are quality of life scales (European Organization for Research and Treatment of Cancer (EORTC) Quality of Life Questionnaire [QLQ-C30]), disease-related functional tests (Functional Assessment Of Cancer Therapy-General (FACT-G), Functional Assessment of Chronic İllness Therapy Fatigue (FACIT-F) scale,) anxiety and depression scales (Hospital Anxiety and Depression Scale (HADS), Generalized Anxiety Disorder (GAD) scale), pain scales (Visual Analogue Scale (VAS), Cancer-Related Pain Scale), Functional Exercise Testing Scale like 6 mins Walk Test, and Timed Up and Go Test, Timed Stair Test [25].

32.4 Telerehabilitation Applications in Breast Cancer

Many different software and hardware are used in evaluation, treatment, and monitoring through telerehabilitation [25]. Virtuagym Fitness application, a mobile application called Physitrack for physical activity tracking and Fitbit wearable technology methods, online training videos, eChez-Soi telerehabilitation program, teleconference method, live video-conference methods and telephone technology, Smart After Care program, CogniMotion tele-system, and Zoom Pro applications are telerehabilitation methods frequently used in the literature and clinic [26–32]. These methods offer an alternative treatment option to face-to-face physiotherapy and rehabilitation methods for problems such as lymphedema, upper extremity movement limitation, pain, fatigue, muscle weakness, cognitive disorders, and decreased quality of life after breast cancer.

32.4.1 Telerehabilitation in Lymphedema

Before breast cancer surgery, patients receive basic physiotherapy evaluations. Afterward, patients are given a follow-up appointment at 4–6 weeks post-op. At this appointment, patients can be evaluated for signs and symptoms of lymphedema and shoulder joint range of motion. Additionally, patients can be given preventive training regarding lymphedema [33]. Attending these postoperative appointments can be difficult, especially for patients who are receiving concurrent cancer treatment and who have the burden of attending multiple medical appointments due to side effects. Additionally, access to these patient services may require long travel distances [34]. Failure of patients to attend this examination in the early period may reduce the possibility of early detection of breast cancer-related lymphedema and side effects of breast cancer treatment on the musculoskeletal system, which may lead to a worse prognosis and functional disorders in the long-term [35, 36]. These evaluations can be performed through telehealth applications, which provide similar or superior results compared to face-to-face services for a variety of clinical problems routinely managed in terms of physiotherapy [37]. In particular, it has been determined that the use of the video-conference method is successful in the evaluation and diagnosis of lymphedema in the breast cancer population [38]. In a study investigating the feasibility of providing early postoperative physiotherapy supervision, care, and education to individuals with breast cancer via telehealth, lymphedema group training was provided via telehealth and face-to-face to patients who had axillary lymph node dissection [33]. As a result of this study, telehealth provided accessible lymphedema education and assessment for individuals with breast cancer at a single time point postoperatively, with minimal technical disruption, and was associated with positive participant and clinician satisfaction and cost savings [33].

Complex decongestive physiotherapy (CDP) is a treatment method whose effectiveness has been proven in many studies in reducing the severity of edema in case of manifested BCRL after breast surgery [39]. As part of the treatment administered in clinical practice, physiotherapists who treat lymphedema often teach patients to self-massage, exercise, and self-bandaging so that they can better manage their condition in the long term [40]. In a case report regarding the application of CDP via telephysiotherapy during the COVID-19 pandemic period, 10 sessions of CDP provided by the teleconference method were applied. Each online treatment session consisted of self-manual lymph drainage, skin care, self-bandaging, and upper extremity exercises. Following completion of treatment, lymphedema severity was decreased significantly [41]. In conclusion, self-administration of CDP via telephysiotherapy may work in an educational manner for the patient and support self-management of lymphedema. In a perspective study conducted during the COVID-19 period, it is stated that a hybrid system consisting of face-to-face meetings and tele/virtual consultations may provide the opportunity to increase accessibility to lymphedema care and reduce waiting time, thus becoming a sustainable care model even after the pandemic [42]. Further randomized controlled studies are needed in this field to confirm the results.

32.4.2 Telerehabilitation for Pain and Movement Restriction

Pain and upper extremity joint dysfunction are the most common side effects of breast cancer treatment [43]. Studies recommend that musculoskeletal pain can be treated by experienced physiotherapists with active exercises, joint and tissue mobilization techniques, and assisted joint mobilization [44]. To treat neuropathic pain, it is recommended to do both aerobic and strengthening exercises twice a week for a total of 150 minutes under the supervision of an experienced physiotherapist [45]. Finally, the recommended treatment for dealing with chronic pain uses a multidisciplinary approach that includes pain education interventions, pharmacological interventions, psychological interventions, and physiotherapy interventions [46–49]. However, compliance with these programs decreases due to barriers such as the remoteness of the centers, lack of family support, and previous life habits [50]. Technological advances can help eliminate barriers such as distance, time, and cost. Considering the decrease in the quality of life of breast cancer survivors, access to programs can be increased with telerehabilitation systems that can evaluate and treat side effects [50]. In a study investigating the effect of an internet-based exercise program on pain in breast cancer patients, a telerehabilitation program was implemented using the e-CUIDATE system, an online system that facilitates the development of remote rehabilitation [48]. The e-CUIDATE system consists of a public interface and a separate private interface. The public area is the home page with up-to-date information about breast cancer. After completing the baseline assessment, participants received in-person instructions on how to access and use the private area on their own. CUIDATE research staff designed a custom exercise program best suited for each participant. This was important to increase adherence to the program. The intervention was administered by CUIDATE research staff, who used a control platform to assign and control different exercise programs. The program consisted of 3 sessions per week (on non-consecutive days) lasting approximately 90 minutes each day. The intensity and volume of physical exercise training were determined in accordance with the American College of Sports Medicine recommendations for cancer survivors. Each session was conducted online, and exercise sessions included a warm-up, resistance and aerobic exercise training, and a cool-down period. There was an area for participants to write questions or suggestions regarding their performance. CUIDATE research staff were then able to review their comments and monitor each participant's performance remotely. The system allowed participants to send instant messages and participate in video conferencing sessions. Following completion of the 8-week intervention, participants were encouraged to continue the exercise program on their own. After the intervention, significant improvement was achieved in arm symptoms, pain intensity, and pain interference results in the telerehabilitation group [48].

In a study investigating the effects of home-based rehabilitation applied with neuromodulation, computer-assisted education, and telemonitoring on pain in breast cancer patients, it was stated that the combination of neuromodulation and telemedicine interventions could reduce the pain perceived by breast cancer patients and improve their mental health more effectively than single interventions [51]. In addition, it is thought that this home-based approach will increase patients' participation in routine clinical care and reduce inequalities in access to health care. This integrated home care strategy may be beneficial for breast cancer patients who are unable to relieve chronic pain with pharmacological treatments or for those with reduced mobility or limited access to care due to geographic barriers, thereby empowering patients and reducing healthcare costs [51].

Early intervention in shoulder joint mobilization plays an important role in preserving shoulder kinematics and preventing adhesions [52].

Pendulum exercises reduce pain by distracting and oscillating. It should be performed three times a day. Guided flexion, abduction, and external rotation exercises are more effective in ROM rehabilitation than free shoulder exercises and should be prescribed from the first day after surgery. It is recommended to maintain abduction, flexion, and functional diagonal of the shoulder for at least 30 s. All these exercises can be performed through telerehabilitation [52].

32.4.3 Telerehabilitation for Fatigue and Muscle Weakness

Cancer-related fatigue is a very common and multifactorial symptom [52]. A decrease in muscle mass and strength also causes fatigue in cancer [53]. Exercise is an effective non-pharmacological method in reducing side effects such as fatigue and loss of muscle strength that may occur after cancer treatments are completed and in increasing the level of physical activity [54]. Telerehabilitation-based exercise interventions provide improvements in physical activity, fatigue, and physical performance [50]. In a systematic review, it was stated that telehealth applications were effective to increase muscle strength in upper and lower extremities as well as in the abdominal region [52]. The intervention duration of the studies included in this review ranged from 8 weeks to 8 months. Based on this, we can say that long-term tele-exercise applications should be applied to improve fatigue and muscle weakness.

32.4.4 Telerehabilitation in Cognitive Impairment

Cognitive impairment may occur as a side effect of treatments in women treated for breast cancer [55]. These patients' access to cognitive rehabilitation and psychological treatment is often limited by resources; women of childbearing age often face difficulties completing rehabilitation programs that require access to care facilities [56]. Telemedicine can offer breast cancer patients an optimal treatment option to provide cognitive rehabilitation, psychological support, and recovery [57]. Previous studies have examined the use of telemedicine to improve psychological well-being in breast cancer patients, and several have investigated the effect of telerehabilitation on cognitive deficits [8, 58]. In general, despite some inconsistencies, telerehabilitation has been reported to improve verbal fluency, processing speed, cognitive flexibility, memory, and working memory, as well as subjective cognitive functions [58].

Impairments in cognitive function after breast cancer can also negatively affect participation in daily life and quality of life. A 6-week hybrid (clinic+telerehabilitation) study in patients with breast cancer in the subacute phase shows that vocational rehabilitation provides greater improvement in the recovery of performance in primarily meaningful activities in a relatively short period of time compared to a control group receiving standard care [57]. Additionally, within-group analyses revealed improvement in regaining participation in highly demanding physical activities and cognitive abilities [57]. Providing individualized and occupation-based rehabilitation interventions as soon as possible after discontinuation of breast cancer medical treatments increases women's daily participation. Specifically, clinicians should be aware of and facilitate various self-management skills (e.g., e-health strategies) as early as possible in the rehabilitation process after BC diagnosis to develop flexible use of these skills. Integrating telerehabilitation ensures the continuation of the rehabilitation process, taking into account the consequences of women's health status, and contributes to the feasibility of the rehabilitation process.

32.5 Conclusion

In conclusion, telerehabilitation emerges as a double-edged sword, presenting both promising advantages and significant challenges in the landscape of healthcare delivery. On one hand, its integration into rehabilitation protocols offers unprecedented benefits, particularly in enhancing accessibility, convenience, and patient engagement. Through virtual platforms and remote monitoring technologies, telerehabilitation transcends geographical barriers, bringing essential rehabilitation services to individuals irrespective of their location. Moreover, telerehabilitation fosters a patient-centric approach, empowering individuals to actively participate in their recovery journey. With tailored rehabilitation programs accessible from the comfort of their homes, patients experience increased autonomy and flexibility in managing their conditions. Real-time feedback and remote monitoring enable timely adjustments to treatment plans, enhancing patient adherence, and overall outcomes. Through ongoing research, innovation, and interdisciplinary collaboration, telerehabilitation holds the promise of reshaping the future of rehabilitative medicine, transcending barriers, and empowering individuals to achieve optimal health and wellness.

References

1. Başoğlu S, Polat Ü. Kanser Hastalarına Sağlık Hizmet Sunumunda Teletıp ve Tele-Hemşireliğin Artan Önemi. Türk Hemşireler Derneği Dergisi. 2023;4(1):66–74.
2. Digital health in the Western Pacific. https://www.who.int/westernpacific/health-topics/e-health.
3. Scaturro D, Vitagliani F, Mangano MS, Tomasello S, Sconza C, Respizzi S, et al. Effect of Telerehabilitation and outpatient rehabilitation in women with breast cancer. J Funct Morphol Kinesiol. 2023;8(3):105.
4. O'Neill L, Brennan L, Sheill G, Connolly D, Guinan E, Hussey J. Moving forward with telehealth in cancer rehabilitation: patient perspectives from a mixed methods study. JMIR Cancer. 2023;9:e46077.
5. Uzelpasaci E, Ozcakar L, Ozgul S, Ozyuncu O, Beksac MS, Akbayrak T. Telerehabilitation for exercise training in pregnancy. GORM. 2023;29(1):27–9.
6. Larson JL, Rosen AB, Wilson FA. The effect of telehealth interventions on quality of life of cancer survivors: a systematic review and meta-analysis. Health Informatics J. 2020;26(2):1060–78.
7. Patel HJ, Kachhwaha R. Effect of Telerehabilitation on quality of life of cancer survivors: a systematic review. RGUHS J Med Sci. 2021;11(4):1.
8. Loubani K, Schreuer N, Kizony R. Telerehabilitation for managing daily participation among breast cancer survivors during COVID-19: a feasibility study. J Clin Med. 2022;11(4):1022.
9. Mella-Abarca W, Barraza-Sánchez V, Ramírez-Parada K. Telerehabilitation for people with breast cancer through the COVID-19 pandemic in Chile. Ecancermedicalscience. 2020;14:1085.
10. Dennett A, Harding KE, Reimert J, Morris R, Parente P, Taylor NF. Telerehabilitation's safety, feasibility, and exercise uptake in cancer survivors: process evaluation. JMIR Cancer. 2021;7(4):e33130.
11. Rocco P, Finkelstein J. Telerehabilitation for patients with cancer: a scoping review. Stud Health Technol Inform. 2022;290:543–6.
12. Seron P, Oliveros M-J, Gutierrez-Arias R, Fuentes-Aspe R, Torres-Castro RC, Merino-Osorio C, et al. Effectiveness of telerehabilitation in physical therapy: a rapid overview. Phys Ther. 2021;101(6):pzab053.
13. Chang P, Zheng J. Updates in cancer rehabilitation telehealth. Curr Phys Med Rehabil Rep. 2022;10(4):332–8.
14. Chan KO, Yuen PP, Fong BY, Law VT, Ng FS, Fung WC, et al. Effectiveness of tele-exercise programme for elderly at risk of falls. Protocol for a randomized controlled trial. BMC Geriatr. 2023;23:845.
15. Andrioti A, Papadopetraki A, Maridaki M, Philippou A. The effect of a home-based tele-exercise training program on the quality of life and physical performance in breast cancer survivors. Sports. 2023;11(5):102.
16. Baehr LA, Kaimal G, Bruneau M Jr, Finley M. Development and feasibility of a group tele-exercise program for individuals with spinal cord injury. J Neurol Phys Ther. 2023;10(1097):200.
17. Hwang R, Bruning J, Morris NR, Mandrusiak A, Russell T. Home-based telerehabilitation is not inferior to a Centre-based program in patients with chronic heart failure: a randomised trial. J Physiother. 2017;63(2):101–7.
18. Medica EM. Telemedicine from research to practice during the pandemic."Instant paper from the field" on rehabilitation answers to the COVID-19 emergency. 2020.
19. Yüceer Ş, Keklicek H. Online Fizyoterapi Danışmanlığı'nın Fizyoterapist ve Danışan Gözüyle Uygulanabilirliği. İzmir Katip Çelebi Üniversitesi Sağlık Bilimleri Fakültesi Dergisi. 2022;7(2):277–88.
20. Cottrell MA, Russell TG. Telehealth for musculoskeletal physiotherapy. Musculoskelet Sci Pract. 2020;48:102193.
21. Mani S, Sharma S, Omar B, Paungmali A, Joseph L. Validity and reliability of internet-based physiotherapy assessment for musculoskeletal disorders: a systematic review. J Telemed Telecare. 2017;23(3):379–91.
22. Richardson BR, Truter P, Blumke R, Russell TG. Physiotherapy assessment and diagnosis of musculoskeletal disorders of the knee via telerehabilitation. J Telemed Telecare. 2017;23(1):88–95.

23. Cheville AL, Moynihan T, Herrin J, Loprinzi C, Kroenke K. Effect of collaborative telerehabilitation on functional impairment and pain among patients with advanced-stage cancer: a randomized clinical trial. JAMA Oncol. 2019;5(5):644–52.
24. Mousavi AS, Kimiafar K, Sarbaz M, Mehneh MR, Abbaszadeh A, Baigi SFM. Effect of Telerehabilitation on improving physical activity in cancer patients and survivors: a systematic review. Paramed Sci Milit Health. 2024;18(2):59–74.
25. Pattanshetty RB, Athawale VK. Selection of outcome measures in oncology telerehabilitation in post-COVID times: a systematic review. Indian J Phys Ther Res. 2023;5(1):14–23.
26. Fu MR, Axelrod D, Guth AA, Rampertaap K, El-Shammaa N, Hiotis K, et al. mHealth self-care interventions: managing symptoms following breast cancer treatment. Mhealth. 2016;2:2.
27. Yilmaz RC, Kocamaz D, Fidancioğlu NA. Telerehabilitation in survival breast cancer patients: need for randomized controlled studies. Phoenix Med J. 2023;5(3):242–4.
28. Peng Y, Zhang K, Wang L, Peng Y, Liu Z, Liu L, et al. Effect of a telehealth-based exercise intervention on the physical activity of patients with breast cancer: a systematic review and meta-analysis. Asia Pac J Oncol Nurs. 2022;9:100117.
29. He Y, Han X, Zou W, Liu X, Sun N, Zhou F. Protocol: telerehabilitation programmes for patients with cancer and survivors: a protocol for a systematic review. BMJ Open. 2022;12(4):e058981.
30. Piraux E, Caty G, Reychler G, Forget P, Deswysen Y. Feasibility and preliminary effectiveness of a teleprehabilitation program in esophagogastric cancer patients. J Clin Med. 2020;9(7):2176.
31. MacDonald AM, Chafranskaia A, Lopez CJ, Maganti M, Bernstein LJ, Chang E, et al. CaRE@ home: pilot study of an online multidimensional cancer rehabilitation and exercise program for cancer survivors. J Clin Med. 2020;9(10):3092.
32. Coats V, Moffet H, Vincent C, Simard S, Tremblay L, Maltais F, et al. Feasibility of an eight-week telerehabilitation intervention for patients with unresectable thoracic neoplasia receiving chemotherapy: a pilot study. Can J Respir Crit Care Sleep Med. 2020;4(1):14–24.
33. Naumann L, Reul-Hirche H, Comans T, Burns CL, Paratz J, Cottrell M. Evaluating telehealth for the education and monitoring of lymphoedema and shoulder dysfunction after breast cancer surgery. Support Care Cancer. 2023;31(4):239.
34. Cheng AC, Levy MA. Data driven approach to burden of treatment measurement: a study of patients with breast cancer. AMIA Annu Symp Proc. 2016;2016:1756.
35. Taghian NR, Miller CL, Jammallo LS, O'Toole J, Skolny MN. Lymphedema following breast cancer treatment and impact on quality of life: a review. Crit Rev Oncol Hematol. 2014;92(3):227–34.
36. Hayes SC, Johansson K, Stout NL, Prosnitz R, Armer JM, Gabram S, et al. Upper-body morbidity after breast cancer: incidence and evidence for evaluation, prevention, and management within a prospective surveillance model of care. Cancer. 2012;118(S8):2237–49.
37. Cottrell MA, Galea OA, O'Leary SP, Hill AJ, Russell TG. Real-time telerehabilitation for the treatment of musculoskeletal conditions is effective and comparable to standard practice: a systematic review and meta-analysis. Clin Rehabil. 2017;31(5):625–38.
38. Galiano-Castillo N, Ariza-García A, Cantarero-Villanueva I, Fernández-Lao C, Sánchez-Salado C, Arroyo-Morales M. Agreement between telerehabilitation involving caregivers and face-to-face clinical assessment of lymphedema in breast cancer survivors. Support Care Cancer. 2014;22:253–8.
39. Ezzo J, Manheimer E, McNeely ML, Howell DM, Weiss R, Johansson KI, et al. Manual lymphatic drainage for lymphedema following breast cancer treatment. Cochrane Database of Syst Rev. 2015;5:1.
40. McNeely ML, Magee DJ, Lees AW, Bagnall KM, Haykowsky M, Hanson J. The addition of manual lymph drainage to compression therapy for breast cancer related lymphedema: a randomized controlled trial. Breast Cancer Res Treat. 2004;86:95–106.
41. Lytras D, Myrogiannis IS. The application of complete decongestive therapy through telephysiotherapy in the treatment of acute upper limb lymphedema after mastectomy during the COVID-19 pandemic: a case study. Phys Ther Rehabil. 2020;7(1):9.
42. Sundrasekaran A, Abdalla E, Sobani S, Shafi M, Al-Mudahka NR. Physiotherapy management response for patients with lymphedema amid the COVID-19 pandemic in the State of Qatar: a perspective study. Rehabil Oncol. 2021;39(4):E89–97.
43. Bjerkeset E, Röhrl K, Schou-Bredal I. Symptom cluster of pain, fatigue, and psychological distress in breast cancer survivors: prevalence and characteristics. Breast Cancer Res Treat. 2020;180:63–71.
44. Kannan P, Ying LH, Ngai LC, Kiu MT, Yan MT, Yan TW. Physiotherapy interventions for the management of post-mastectomy pain syndrome: a meta-analysis. J Physiother. 2022;114:e53–e4.
45. del -Rosal-Jurado A, Romero-Galisteo R, Trinidad-Fernández M, González-Sánchez M, Cuesta-Vargas A, Ruiz-Muñoz M. Therapeutic physical exercise post-treatment in breast cancer: a systematic review of clinical practice guidelines. J Clin Med. 2020;9(4):1239.
46. Lara-Palomo IC, Castro-Sánchez AM, Córdoba-Peláez MM, Albornoz-Cabello M, Ortiz-Comino L. Effect of myofascial therapy on pain and functionality of the upper extremities in breast cancer survivors: a systematic review and meta-analysis. Int J Environ Res Public Health. 2021;18(9):4420.
47. Rasmussen M. Effects of physical therapy on shoulder function and range of motion in adult women following breast cancer treatment: a meta-analysis. Fresno: California State University; 2023.

48. Galiano-Castillo N, Ariza-García A, Cantarero-Villanueva I, Fernández-Lao C, Díaz-Rodríguez L, Legerén-Alvarez M, et al. Telehealth system (e-CUIDATE) to improve quality of life in breast cancer survivors: rationale and study protocol for a randomized clinical trial. Trials. 2013;14:1–10.
49. Martínez-Miranda P, Casuso-Holgado MJ, Jesus J-RJ. Effect of patient education on quality-of-life, pain and fatigue in breast cancer survivors: a systematic review and meta-analysis. Clin Rehabil. 2021;35(12):1722–42.
50. Galiano-Castillo N, Cantarero-Villanueva I, Fernández-Lao C, Ariza-García A, Díaz-Rodríguez L, Del-Moral-Ávila R, et al. Telehealth system: a randomized controlled trial evaluating the impact of an internet-based exercise intervention on quality of life, pain, muscle strength, and fatigue in breast cancer survivors. Cancer. 2016;122(20):3166–74.
51. Conti L, Marzorati C, Grasso R, Ferrucci R, Priori A, Mameli F, et al. Home-based treatment for chronic pain combining neuromodulation, computer-assisted training, and Telemonitoring in patients with breast cancer: protocol for a rehabilitative study. JMIR Res Protoc. 2023;12(1):e49508.
52. de Rezende LF, Francisco VE, Franco RL. Telerehabilitation for patients with breast cancer through the COVID-19 pandemic. Breast Cancer Res Treat. 2021;185(1):257–9.
53. Kilgour RD, Vigano A, Trutschnigg B, Hornby L, Lucar E, Bacon SL, et al. Cancer-related fatigue: the impact of skeletal muscle mass and strength in patients with advanced cancer. J Cachexia Sarcopenia Muscle. 2010;1:177–85.
54. Wu T, Yan F, Wei Y, Yuan C, Jiao Y, Pan Y, et al. Effect of exercise therapy on cancer-related fatigue in patients with breast cancer: a systematic review and network meta-analysis. Am J Phys Med Rehabil. 2023;102(12):1055–62.
55. Oh P-J, Cho J-R. Changes in fatigue, psychological distress, and quality of life after chemotherapy in women with breast cancer: a prospective study. Cancer Nurs. 2020;43(1):E54–60.
56. Oksman E, Linna M, Hörhammer I, Lammintakanen J, Talja M. Cost-effectiveness analysis for a tele-based health coaching program for chronic disease in primary care. BMC Health Serv Res. 2017;17(1):1–7.
57. Loubani K, Kizony R, Milman U, Schreuer N. Hybrid tele and in-clinic occupation based intervention to improve women's daily participation after breast cancer: a pilot randomized controlled trial. Int J Environ Res Public Health. 2021;18(11):5966.
58. Giustiniani A, Danesin L, Pezzetta R, Masina F, Oliva G, Arcara G, et al. Use of telemedicine to improve cognitive functions and psychological Well-being in patients with breast cancer: a systematic review of the current literature. Cancers. 2023;15(4):1353.

Microbiota in Breast Cancer: A Need for Further Knowledge

33

Didem Dereli Akdeniz

33.1 Microbiota and Health

Joshua Lederberg, a Nobel Prize winner in Physiology as a molecular biologist, invented the term "microbiome" for the microbial cells that are being harbored in the human body. This invention opened a way of new insight into the human body as "it is not a solely individual organism but a complex biological system." Humans have about ten-fold of microbial cells than their own body cells, which makes them super creatures. After the discovery of the cross-talk between human cells and microbial organisms, we had to accept that our parents could inherit only a small portion of our genetic content, and most of the genes that affect our body belong to the microbiome [1, 2].

The microbiota is as unique to a person as a fingerprint and constantly undergoes individual-specific changes during one's lifespan. The gut microflora is the most studied microbiota in the human body. Many bacteria, viruses, fungi, and archaea groups live in our intestines, communicating with each other and with all our body cells, especially with our gastrointestinal epithelial cells and all other cells belonging to the immune system. The gut microbiota has important roles in many cellular and metabolic functions. These can be summarized as digestion of the foods, converting primary bile acids to secondary ones, synthesis of varied essential growth factors, and some vitamins (B and K), preventing the proliferation and infiltration of pathogenic organisms in the intestine by competing with them and acting like an immune modulator as they boost the immune system of the body through activation of immature specialized immune cells [2, 3].

Dysbiosis is the term that is used for an impaired microbiota. There are a lot of reasons that can cause the state of "dysbiosis" such as antibiotic usage, stress, an unhealthy diet, and so forth. Dysbiosis has been linked to many systemic diseases like Crohn's disease, rheumatologic disorders, obesity, type-2 diabetes, and even some malignancies. The interaction between microbiota components and host health problems has been extensively researched for nearly the last 20 years. Despite these efforts, there are still unexplained information gaps that can be the subject of many future studies. The interaction between the healthy gut microbiome and the immune system needs to be investigated in detail because the results of these studies may pave the way for new treatments for many diseases and preserve the health and vitality of the body [3, 4].

The research on this subject accelerated with the discovery of ribosomal RNA as molecular markers by Carl Woese and Norman Pace. Scientists now could examine and measure functional interactions among microbial communi-

D. D. Akdeniz (✉)
Endocrinology and Metabolism Department, Izmir Bakırçay University Faculty of Medicine, Izmir, Turkey

Y. Bakar, A. Tuğral (eds.), *Managing Side Effects of Breast Cancer Treatment*,
https://doi.org/10.1007/978-3-031-75480-7_33

ties. After this invention, two definitions were developed: alpha and beta diversity. Alpha diversity means within-sample diversity. When exploring alpha diversity, microbiologists are interested in the distribution of microorganisms within the same sample, but beta diversity is a measure of the similarity or diversities of two distinct samples. This investigates both the number of different organisms (richness) and how much they are distributed evenly in terms of abundance (evenness). Microbiologists evaluate these features by 16S ribosomal RNA analysis. When it comes to sequencing the entire genome in a given specimen for all the microorganisms, they use whole-genome sequencing. The most spectacular innovations have emerged by using new technologies like metagenomics or metatranscriptomics. The progression in microbiological culture technology in the last decade made it possible for commensal microorganisms to be culturable and opened a new window for the research of various aspects of microbiota functions or their relationship to disease that was previously impossible with computational analysis alone [2].

The National Institutes of Health started "The Human Microbiome Project" in 2008 and continued until 2017. By this project, the microbiome became a star of the scientific field, and new research started for it with industrial initiatives. The result of these investigations was the identification of 81–99% of microbial species that constitute the human microbiota. Many studies were performed to understand the association of human microbiota. Acne, atopic dermatitis, psoriasis, esophageal cancer, Crohn's disease, colitis, and immunodeficiency were the first ones that were investigated in terms of their possible interaction with gut microbiome [1–5].

At the beginning of 2014, the second phase of the Human Microbiome Project was initiated to investigate the role of microbiomes in pregnancy, Crohn's disease, ulcerative colitis, and type-2 diabetes. Today, most of the studies focus on microbiota and autism, cardiovascular diseases, and stomach cancer. Future research interests are rapidly focusing on cancer and microbiota. Gastric cancer that is induced by helicobacter infection is one of the most investigated types of cancer. Considering the treatment of cancer, William Coley, who was the frontier of these researchers, attempted to cure sarcomas in the late nineteenth century. Injection of streptococci leads to a strong antitumor response after heat inactivation. in cancer patients [2].

There are sufficient studies that the gut microbiome was proven to be a functional participant in the defense against some malignancies, and that makes it effective in treating cancer. However, we need stronger and more evidence to prove the relationship between the microbiome and tumor formation. Discovering the interactions that microbiota use to make changes in cancer induction advancement, metastasis, and response to various treatments may disclose some new protocols for diagnosis and therapy of cancer.

33.2 Breast Cancer

Breast cancer (BC) is the reason for 12.5% of all types of new cancer cases every year, and this makes it the most common cancer all around the world. Almost 13% (approximately one of every eight) of women will have the diagnosis of invasive BC throughout their lives. BC is the most common cause of death due to malignant tumors. Despite all the advancements in the diagnosis and treatment strategies, these remarkable rates persist and even go higher each year. To achieve the goal of declining mortality rates, scientists need to make more progress in understanding the unique etiology of BC and finding new prevention and treatment options [4].

In recent years, the risk of various genetic factors and biomarkers in BC progression has been revealed. The BReast CAncer (BRCA1/2) gene mutations were the first to be detected. The expression of receptors for Human Epidermal Growth Factor Type 2 (HER2) progesterone (PR), and estrogen (ER) was the second area of interest [6].

In this century, the hazardous changes in human lifestyle and environmental factors increase the risk of BC. The factors that affect the BC etiology can be an unhealthy diet, sedentary lifestyle, smoking, obesity, radiation exposure, alcohol, tobacco usage, and hormonal contraceptives.

The median diagnostic age of breast cancer is 62, which means that half of the diagnoses of BC are before the age of 62. This diagnosis is relatively rare in younger women (just 1 of 8 invasive BC); however, about two out of three invasive BC are found in postmenopausal women older than 55. The conclusion from here is that the risk of BC increases with age. Scientists could only manage to identify a few of the risks and epigenetic factors that can cause BC. Scientists continue to work intensively on innovative precautionary and therapeutic approaches for women's most important and lethal type of cancer [7, 8].

Advances in BC treatment such as breast-conserving surgery, chemo-radiotherapy, and immunotherapy have prolonged survival and increased the quality of life. However, these treatments might have serious limitations due to their low selectivity. First of all, most of these therapy methods act non-selectively and may affect both healthy and tumor cells. Even the most modern approaches used in cancer treatment carry the risk of weakness, partial or complete hair loss, cardiomyopathy, and the inability to have children. Suppression of the body's immune system and even the development of leukemia are serious side effects of BC treatment that can be life threatening. Depression is an expected result of all these factors. Eventually, side effects might overcome the effectiveness of the treatment and can cause a poor prognosis of the BC [9, 10].

For all the reasons mentioned, studies are continuing rapidly for different treatment approaches that target cancer cells only and will not negatively affect other cells of the body. Microbial elements of the intestinal microbiota have become the focus of attention because of the proven many benefits of these microorganisms on human health. If ideal culture environments can be created, producing them in large quantities with lower costs is possible. The powerful health benefits of microorganisms, ease of extensive generation, and ability to produce a broad spectrum of effective tumor-active biomolecules enable them to be used as treatment against cancer. Studies on this topic prove that the gut microbiome and the risk of malignancy are interrelated and may also change the responses to BC treatment [5].

Unrevealing this complicated interaction among bacteria of the microbiota, BC spreading, and response to therapeutic agents can help scientists develop alternatives for BC diagnosis and treatment. This brings up a new scientific investigation area and needs to explain some details, like:

- Is there any specific predisposing microbial community family that increases the risk of breast cancer and can we identify it?
- Are human microbiome dysbiosis and BC progress directly linked to each other?
- Is there any way to engine human microbiota for a better therapy response?
- Can such natural methods be integrated with traditional radio-chemotherapy to minimize the problems we are dealing with?
- Is there any specific diet plan that can help with BC treatment?
- Is pain management for BC patients possible by altering the gut microbiota, which directly interacts with and regulates the central nervous system? [11].

This chapter examines the critical evidence explaining the act of the gut microbiome in BC progression and its capacity to make changes in metabolic pathways and immunity. In addition, revolutionary information about the dynamic interaction of the human microbiome with BC is summarized in light of the latest developments.

33.3 Interaction Between the Human Microbiome and Breast Cancer

The breast microbiome refers not only to the microbiome of the breast tissue but also refers to the microbiome of the milk channels. Over the last 20 years, various studies have revealed that microbes living in breast tissue originate early in life from (1) the gut, (2) the mammary glands, and (3) breast milk. Numerous factors modulate this sophisticated mixture of microorganisms throughout a person's life. Factors can be exogenous (lifestyle and environmental actors); therefore, adaptive and endogenous (host genetics and immunity) factors are unique to each person, and some of them cannot be changed. This factor may be altered during BC. It was tried to summarize the contribution of BC risk of each element of the breast microbiome according to the studies [5].

33.3.1 Breast Cancer and Gut Microbial Dysbiosis

The gastrointestinal (GI) tract of the human body is a unique and delicate ecological system occupied by sophisticated and numerous groups of microorganisms. This structure, which contains nearly 150 times more genes than the human genome and contains nearly 1014 different microbial species, is defined as the "second Genome" of humans [3, 5].

The abundance and diversity of intestinal microflora vary according to many parameters, such as maternal microbiota, mode of delivery, breastfeeding, age, race, diet, hygiene, genetics, and the frequency of a person's exposure to antibiotics/drugs. Metagenomic and culture-based studies have revealed the presence of many different genera in the GI system such as *Bacteroides*, *Lactobacillus*, *Bifidobacterium*, *Faecalibacterium*, *Eubacterium*, *Enterococcus*, *Streptococcus*, *Peptococcus*, *Ruminococcus*, *Streptomyces*, *Peptostreptococcus*, and *Clostridium*. The microbiota is a complex ecosystem that forms a reciprocal dynamic relationship with the host rather than being a passive inhabitant inside the human body. Thanks to this, it functions as a multidimensional "microbial organ." This huge and unique organ supports nutrient absorption in the human body, metabolism of all cells, biosynthesis of essential vitamins and amino acids, detoxification of toxic and carcinogenic molecules, and the maturing and preservation of innate and acquired immunity. Human intestinal microbiota carries out these versatile functions thanks to many microbial metabolites such as short-chain fatty acids, hydrogen, carbon dioxide, methane, and ammonia. Dysbiosis means disrupting the balance in this complex structure, ultimately resulting in loss of intestinal homeostasis. This can lead to detrimental consequences for the host, including a predisposition to various malignancies. Therefore, an ideal model should be established to study the host-microbiota and disease relationship [12, 13].

Methods that can be applied to change the number of commensal bacteria in the intestines include regular consumption of pre- and probiotics and, if pathological conditions have occurred in the host, transferring beneficial bacteria from healthy individuals through fecal microbiota transplantation (FMT). The animal model studies clarified the cancer development and microbiome interactions. Furthermore, fundamental studies on humans have also proved that the effects of external factors can directly cause cancer by influencing the gut microbiota. As a result of all these, the relationship between cancer and microbiota began to be examined more deeply [14].

An early study conducted in 1976 found elevated conjugated estrogen metabolites in feces in people who use ampicillin, the first sign that active estrogen metabolism by intestinal microbes was being affected. Microbial β-glucuronidase (BGUS) in the intestinal microbiota is responsible for de-conjugating estrogen. In 1990, a study was planned considering that the consumption of whole grain foods increases the volume of stool and increases the risk of breast cancer due to the increase in BGUS activity [15].

A study in 1990 about whole-grain product consumption hypothesized that this product increased the volume of feces and changed BGUS activity, which increases the risk of BC. Microbial BGUS is the enzyme that deconjugates estrogen. This deconjugation reaction boosts free estrogen reabsorption back into the blood. And it means that much more revealing estrogens are for organs and increase the risk for metastasis [16]. Many studies have proven the involvement of estrogen levels and metabolism in BC risk, and higher levels of estrogen mean higher levels of cancer risk. After menopause, circulating estrogen levels are directly related to intestinal microbiome dysbiosis. The species that affect estrogen metabolism are Escherichia, Ruminococcaceae, and Clostridia families [17].

A case-control study comparing the gut microbiota showed that postmenopausal BC patients have less alpha diversity than healthy postmenopausal women. High levels of Fecalibacterium, Ruminococcaceae, and Clostridiaceae and low levels of Dorea and Lachnospiraceae were associated with postmenopausal BC cancer. BC clinical stage is also related to gut microbiome composition, especially Bifidobacterium density [18]. A study in 2017 proved that Bacteroidetes and Firmicutes were abundant in BC patients' microbiomes. Scientists investigating the microbiome in BC patients found that *Clostridium*, *Blautia* sp., *Bacteriodetes*, and *Faecalibacterium* species were detected more in stage 2 and 3 BC patients than those in stage 1 [18]. In animal studies, dysbiosis, even before the onset of BC, was associated with higher inflammation and can lead to metastasis. The differences in gut microbiota are seen not only in BC patients but also in many cancer types. In this context, biopsy results of patients with the diagnosis of colon cancer were shown to be related to *Fusobacterium*, a joint partner with cancer metastasis [19]. The abundance of this bacteria also seems to be related to BC metastasis. Attention has also been paid to antibiotic usage and whether it can accelerate BC growth. Some studies investigate lignan enterolactone levels in plasma. Antibiotic usage can reduce this level and thereby positively correlate with increased BC risk [20]. Colorectal, lung, and BC are important examples where the impact of the microbiome on tumorigenesis has been proven. New studies support that stomach and intestinal microbiota changes dramatically affect gastric carcinogenesis [21, 22]. However, the role of the microbiota on tumorigenesis still needs to be explored further.

33.3.2 The Breast Cancer and Breast Microbiome Interaction

The myth of sterile breast tissue has now been dispelled, and scientists have recognized that human breast tissue has a unique population of microorganisms. Additionally, breast milk is not sterile due to the baby's oral and skin microorganism profiles affecting the microbial content of the mammary duct during breastfeeding. This period does not start when the breast microbiota begins. Microbial presence is present in breast tissue from birth. 16S rRNA sequencing methods and culture studies proved that the breast tissue microbiome contains commensal microorganisms. It acts as an activator of the immune system and a degrader of potent carcinogens. Prevotella, Listeria, and Propionibacterium, members of the Enterobacteriaceae class are the components of the breast microbiome. Many scientists are investigating the role of breast microbiota in BC initiation and metastasis. The questions being studied are: i) Is there a specific fingerprint microbiome for BC? ii) Are there any specific microorganisms that are directly linked to BC? Human papilloma viruses (HPV), and Epstein-Barr virus (EBV) are microorganisms that have been proven to affect BC directly. Additionally, there is evidence showing that Retroviridea, Herpesviridea, and Coronaviridae have a direct effect on the etiology of cancer. In HER2+ BC, Nodaviridae is a specific risk factor and can be a specific biomarker for this subtype, but further validating studies are needed. A study from 2016 showed evidence of interactions among the proinflammatory cytokine interleukin-17 (IL-17), STAT3 activity (STAT3 regulates cytokine and growth factor receptors to its own target cell-like cell survival genes and oncogenes) and HPV in BC. More studies are needed to investigate the relationship between breast virome and BC [23].

Studies on the different microbial composition of breast tissue between healthy and cancerous women are still in their infancy. Regarding bacteria, one study reported that *Lactobacillus* was present in 2.2% of the microbiome of healthy breasts and 1.4% of cancerous lesions. Sphingomonas yanoikuyae is also a specific family of bacteria that is found especially in the breast tissues of healthy individuals. Currently, focused research is aimed at understanding some critical changes in the content of the breast microbiota as normal breast tissue turns into a carcinogenic structure [5]. Examinations of cancerous breast tissues have proven a decrease in the abundance and diversity of bacterial species such as *C. coccoides*, *Faecalibacterium*, *Clostridium leptum*, and the Ruminococcaceae family and an increase in *Staphylococcus* and Enterobacteriaceae [24]. Differential and weaker immune responses against cancer cells were associated with decreased numbers of *S. yanoikuaye*. This raised the idea that probiotics may be effective in breast physiology. An interesting finding about differences in breast microbiota is that patients with different stages of BC have different compositions of microbiome. Studies show dramatic differences in the breast microbiome between malignant and benign lesions. Taxonomic profiles of benign breast lesions revealed the dominance of Firmicutes and Bacteroides, while *Lactobacillus*, *Fusobacterium*, *Atopobium*, *Gluconacetobacter*, and *Hydrogenophaga* were associated with an increase in the risk of BC. Especially triple-negative BC tissue was found to be much more different than other types of BC tissues and healthy breast tissue. *Coccidiodes*, *Aspergillus*, *Geotrichum*, *Candida*, and *Rhodotorula* are the most frequent fungi families of BC tissue microbiomes [25, 26]. We need more cohort-based clinical trials to validate the subtype specificity of these findings.

However, to date, a meaningful microbial combination that will distinguish malignancy from healthy breast has not been provided. Differences in the used technologies, cohort size, and geographic location of studies might affect the results. Age, race, ethnicity, diet, and cancer stage are other factors that may affect the microbiome composition. So, more investigation to understand the composition of the breast microbiome and its diagnostic or prognostic value for BC should be conducted.

33.3.3 Impact of Breast Milk Microbiota on Breast Tumorigenesis

After birth, the baby needs to adapt to the new world. The intrauterine environment was safe, stable, and nearly sterile, but the extrauterine situation is rife with potentially harmful microorganisms. The newborn's intestinal microbiota begins to be formed immediately after birth, depending on the type of delivery (vaginal or cesarean section). The feeding method applied after that (breastfeeding or use of formula) affects the intestinal microbiota of the baby. Breastfeeding is extremely beneficial as it provides good microorganisms to the baby's intestinal system. These microorganisms enable the maturation of a baby's immune system. Breast milk microbiota is influenced by the mother's GI microbiota and the mother's skin microorganisms. Other factors affecting the milk microbiome are antibiotic consumption, nutrition, and the country where the mother lives. Geographic location, in particular, is a significant determinant of a person's microbiota. The gender of the babies, the feeding method (collection of milk and feeding with a bottle or direct breastfeeding), the breastfeeding stage, and the mother's body mass index (BMI) are among the main factors that can change the composition of the microbiota. There is a lot of evidence proving that breast milk has a unique composition. In particular, it is associated with the health problems of both mothers (breast tissue health) and babies (intestinal colonization, immune system maturation, and digestion). Studies in the literature show that breast milk microbiota (BMM) has a great diversity. The most dominant bacteria in human breast milk are *Lactobacillus*, *Bifidobacterium*, *Streptococcus*, *Staphylococcus*, *Pseudomonas*, *Corynebacterium*, and *Enterococcus*, accompanied by archaea, fungi, and viruses [27].

There are few studies on the effect of microbiomes on BC development and progression. One of these, in 2005, investigated nipple aspiration fluid from healthy controls and BC patients. This study showed significantly different microbial composition in the two groups. Further studies supported this finding, and the authors concluded that the ductal microbiome may have an essential role in BC tumorigenesis. *Corynebacterium durum*, Lachnospiraceae, *Ruminococci*, *Mycobacterium kansasii*, *F. prausnitzii*, and *Clostridium baratii* bacterial species are the bacterial species found more frequently in the breast milk of BC patients. On the contrary, *Lactobacillus salivarius* is a bacterium found to deviate from the breast microbiomes of healthy individuals [28].

The exciting thing about BMM is that the number of bacteria is sufficient to colonize the intestines of babies but does not cause any inflammatory response in the breast tissue. This is mainly attributed to Parabacteroides and lactic acid bacteria (LAB) because they can inhibit the growth of pathogenic bacteria by producing specific antimicrobial molecules such as nisin, hydrogen peroxide, or organic acids.

The abundance of microbes is not the only factor influencing the effects of microbiomes on breast health but also the interactions between them are essential and can cause or suppress tumorigenesis. The temporary presence of a bacterium may have health benefits as it can increase a certain type of IgA and immune cells.

Mononuclear cells of breast tissue contain few culturable bacteria but abundant bacterial DNA. The findings show that the same bacterial DNA can be found in mother and baby feces. Some studies show that DNA can stimulate an immune response even in the absence of live bacteria [27, 28].

33.4 Detailed Studies with New Generation Analyses on the Role of the Human Microbiome in Breast Cancer

The human microbiome project and the ability to perform advanced molecular analyses have led to in-depth information on the relationship between microbiota and BC, as in many chronic diseases. In the last two decades, many studies have been published examining the relationships of this large and newly discovered organ with cancer, such as diabetes, obesity, immunological diseases, and neurodegenerative diseases. Even now, very intensive studies are being carried out on the effects of microbiota (the GI tract and the breast itself) on cancer formation and changing drug effects in cancer treatment. It is now widely accepted that the human microbiome has an essential impact on developing and treating breast cancer [29].

33.4.1 Effects of Microbiota on Estrogen Metabolism

Apart from the known classical risk factors of BC, the effects of the amount of circulating free estrogen on breast tissue, especially in postmenopausal women, constitute an important factor for the development of BC. Phase II detoxification (especially conjugation) occurring in the liver is very important in the inactivation and removal of estrogen from the body.

The enzyme UDP-glucuronosyltransferase combines estrogens with a sulfate and/or glucuronate residue in the liver. Thus, estrogen becomes easier to eliminate from the intestines due to its evolved water-soluble nature. The bacteria in the intestine that play a role in estrogen metabolism are called "estrobolome." These bacteria produce the enzyme BGUS, which breaks down the estrogen compound that reaches the intestine as estrogen glucuronate and turns it into active-free estrogen.

The estrobolome supports optimal estrogen conjugation in hepatocytes, maintaining healthy estrogen levels in the body. Still, when imbalances occur, too much free estrogen can be reabsorbed into the circulation, resulting in much higher than normal free estrogen levels. This is an important risk factor for the development of ER-positive BC. Considerable evidence has accumulated detailing the mechanism involved in the deconjugation process by which the microbiome influences circulating estrogen levels. Studies have been conducted to investigate the role of gut microbiome structure in the regulation of urinary estrogens and their metabolites in healthy women. The ratio of estrogen metabolites to parent estrogen was found to be directly positively correlated with the density of Clostridiales and Ruminococcaceae, especially Bacterodetes density, which shows a negative correlation. The density of alpha diversity positively affects estrogen metabolism.

The estrobolome consists of groups of commensal bacteria that contain BGUS genes. In addition, BGUS is abundant in the nipple aspirate fluid of patients treated for ER (+) BC. Bacterial BGUS activity (a large number and variety of bacteria encode this enzyme in the human intestine) is an essential factor determining the function of the estrobolome. The activity of GI microbiota BGUS is positively correlated with the amount of urinary estrogen while it has a negative correlation with the amount of fecal estrogen. Studies have shown that consuming a diet rich in fat and/or protein increases BGUS activity in feces. The opposite is valid for a diet that is high in vegetables and fruit, which are rich in fiber. *Bacillus cereus* is found in high amounts in BC tissue, and this bacterium converts progesterone into 5-α-320-dione, this metabolite is known as a stimulating factor for BC [15, 16].

33.4.2 Relationship Between Genomic Stability and DNA Damage

Genetic changes, irregular mutations, chromosomal distortions, and changes in genomic structure are important factors underlying cancer metabolism. Many studies show that intestinal microbiota elements can cause DNA damage. Enterobacteriaceae and Proteobacteria cause DNA double-strand breaks (DSB) in the human genome with the microbial toxins they secrete, triggering the formation of major nuclear defects in cell division. This type of damage in cancerous breast tissue and the bacterial families has been shown (especially *E. coli*). Some bacteria can have a protective effect (e.g., Lactobacillus) to prevent DNA damage. Producing antioxidant molecules that scavenge reactive oxygen radicals (ROS), such as superoxide and peroxide, is responsible for the protective effect. Thus, it is revealed that the microbiota structure can have a positive and negative impact on the etiopathogenesis of cancer depending on the types of microorganisms it contains [30].

33.4.3 The Role of Microbiota in the Host Immune System

The mucosal immune system, a very complex and specialized structure, is seriously affected and changed by intestinal bacterial colonization. The intestinal microbiota stimulates the production of interferon (IFN)-γ by Cytotoxic (CD8+) and Helper (CD4+) T cells and thus controls the maturation and functions of the components of the gut-associated lymphoid tissue (GALT) (consisting of Peyer's patches, lymphoid follicles, and mesenteric lymph nodes). Adaptive immunity carried out by T cells is vital for recognizing and clearing cancer cells. Immune checkpoints play a critical role in the activation of these lymphocytes. Intestinal microbiota and cancer immunotherapy come together at this point, and the effectiveness of immune checkpoint drugs is directly altered by the microbial structure. The risk of BC increases significantly as a result of mild but persistent inflammation [31].

Effector lymphocyte count is associated with cancer susceptibility and is a sign of poor prognosis. The neutrophil/lymphocyte ratio (NLR) at the time of diagnosis can be used to provide information for long-term prognosis. In early-stage BC, an NLR of more than 2.5 at the time of diagnosis is considered an indicator that the risk of BC recurrence is ten times higher within 10 years. An NLR ratio above 3.3 was associated with a 44% higher risk of death within 5 years. It has been shown that the intestinal microbiota directly affects neutrophil and lymphocyte numbers. An organized communication between intestinal microorganisms, interleukin-6 (IL-6), and neutrophils has been detected in BC patients. Studies show that Toll-like Receptor-5 (TLR-5)-dependent cancer progression is accelerated by some commensal bacteria in some types of cancer that respond to IL-6. Additionally, there is a positive correlation between secretory IgA levels and BC risk. These are the findings that support the role of chronic inflammation in the etiology of BC [32].

The issue of which microorganisms in the microbiota have tumor-forming and which tumor-suppressing effects is an issue that needs to be further investigated. As a result of these studies, successful, effective, and targeted immunotherapies can be developed.

33.5 Regulation of the Host Microbiome for Breast Cancer Treatment

Understanding the relationship between BC and the human microbiome has opened new horizons for preventive and therapeutic strategies. Such new and biological treatments can significantly contribute to medicine as a preventive and side-free option to reduce the frequency of cancer. In addition, microorganism-mediated cancer therapy may provide new hope for tumors that are resistant to primary cancer treatments. This approach opens new horizons for new approaches, especially in BC [33].

This section will summarize the potential role of such microbial supplements in preventing and treating BC in various types of experiments.

33.5.1 Evidence from Cell Culture-Based Studies

Initial studies on the possible effectiveness of probiotics in the treatment of BC were carried out on various BC cell lines, and the effect of probiotics on oncogenic properties was evaluated by analysis of their cytotoxicity potency and proliferative, inflammatory, and apoptotic effects. *Lactobacillus plantarum*, a probiotic strain isolated from the vagina, was also found to exhibit time-and dose-dependent cytotoxic effects against MCF-7 cells but not normal cells (HUVEC). The same probiotic also caused apoptosis in the HeLa cell line. *Enterococcus faecalis*, another vaginal probiotic strain, suppressed the proliferation of MCF-7 cells by up to 41.27% while making no difference in the growth of HUVEC cells. Different probiotic strains with similar effects have also been identified [34, 35].

33.5.2 What Has Been Learned from Animal Experiments

The gold standard for studying a substance's effects on an organism's physiopathology is limited to animal experiments. There are many studies examining the subject of probiotics and breast cancer in gnotobiotic rodents. The tumor-shrinking effect of kefir, which is "a fermented milk drink with a sour taste, made using a culture of yeasts and bacteria" has also been shown in animal experiments for BC [36]. It has also been demonstrated in animal experiments that the use of kefir increases apoptosis against DNA damage, especially in BC, reduces the level of proinflammatory cytokines, and changes the ratio of CD4 + and CD8 + T lymphocytes. Oral use of *L. acidophilus* in mice reduces IL-4 and INF-y levels in animals with BC. Thus, the NK cell-mediated immunity against cancer was more robust, and the rate of cancer growth and the potential of new vessel formation were reduced [37]. Oral use of *L. casei* in animals also showed similar effects such as decreased IL-6 levels, and a solid anticancer effect was demonstrated with CD8+ T cells [38]. Co-administration of *Bifidobacterium* with Programmed Cell Death protein 1 ligand L1 (PD-L1) specific antibody has been proven to abolish cancer progression by enhancing dendritic cell function, leading to increased CD8+ T cell proliferation in a mouse model [12]. Similarly, studies are showing that the antitumoral activity of ipilimumab, a monoclonal antibody specific for *Cytotoxic T Lymphocyte* Antigen 4 (CTLA4) is potentiated by *Bacteroides thetaiotaomicron* and *Bacteroides fragilis* [39].

To date, cell culture and animal experiment-based studies conducted to show striking interactions between probiotic microorganisms and the human immune system, which may be in the form of stimulating the immune system to create a more substantial antitumoral effect. Normal breast tissue has a healthy microbiota that ensures a balanced immune response. However, dysbiosis in this area fundamentally alters the immune response and significantly increases the risk of BC. Increasing this risk is caused by the triggering of chronic inflammation and the decrease in the immune response. *Bifidobacterium* sp. and *Lactobacillus* sp. are beneficial microorganisms in the microbiota that can activate the immune system to destroy tumor cells and clear them from the environment. It has been demonstrated that viruses such as HPV can exhibit pro-oncogenic behavior. However, more preclinical studies are required to investigate which microorganisms are beneficial in different types of BC and which drugs can be potentiated by which bacterial structures since we face more than one type of enemy formed by more than one mechanism.

33.5.3 Clinical Study Results

It has been proven through cell culture and animal experiments that probiotics can prevent cancer growth, regulate the immune system, and activate apoptosis. However, their effectiveness in treating BC has not been fully proven in clinical trials. Clinical studies show that consuming yogurt supplemented with *L. delbrueckii* and *Streptococcus thermophilus* may be beneficial for colon and bladder cancer. A case-control study from Japan showed that soy consumption may reduce the risk of BC thanks to the isoflavones it contains. In the last decade, a group of researchers has been examining the effect of the gut microbiome in activating the immune system in BC treatment and the role of the dominance of specific organisms in this situation. These studies may provide the basis for understanding the precise role of probiotics in BC treatment. Therefore, there is still an ongoing need for further studies on probiotics to elucidate this mechanism [1, 4–6, 40].

33.6 Future Hopes

Breast cancer is a group of malignancies with different subtypes that occur due to various etiological reasons. Although personalized treatments have come to the fore in recent years, surgery is still at the forefront of treatment options for BC. This means the loss of a breast, which is part of the woman's essential self-concept, and a long course of antibiotics can affect the microbiota of the breast and also cause loss of beneficial microbiota elements that can help in the treatment of BC. The fact that many BC subtypes are resistant to classical treatment protocols reduces the chance of a complete cure. This means experiencing a deteriorated quality of life and severe side effects of prolonged treatment. The same disruptive antibiotic effect also occurs for the breast microbiota. The loss of this vital ecosystem makes women vulnerable to the risk of varied diseases. In addition, the possible positive effects of the breast microbiota on the progression of the disease and response to treatment are lost. The impact of diet on both microbiota structures is a variable that should not be neglected. There is also a close connection between breast tumor risk and dietary regimens. This highlights the importance of a healthy diet to keep the microbiome healthy. This effect is especially important in terms of ER-positive BC and changes in estrogen metabolism seen in postmenopausal women and shows a very serious correlation. Microbiota modulation for BGUS inactivation also has the potential to take its place in treatment as an essential variable in BC prognosis. In this way, the return of deconjugated estrogens to the systemic circulation via enterohepatic circulation is reduced, and the increase in circulating estrogen levels is prevented; thereafter, reducing the risk of ER-positive BC can be achieved.

The role of microbes in BC is a double-edged sword. Some bacteria have been found to promote the development of breast tumors, while others have cancer-suppressing effects. Using bacteria for therapeutic purposes can potentially create new developments in treatment protocols in the coming years. In this way, successful treatment can be achieved with low-dose radiotherapy or chemotherapy; therefore, fewer side effects can be experienced. The possibility of directly targeting cancer tissues using selective bacteria is also promising [41–43].

33.7 Conclusion

The relationship between human microbiota and BC is being investigated in detail. Today, the diagnosis of BC is synonymous with many fearful treatments for women because current treatment options cannot distinguish tumor tissue from healthy tissue, which leads to many experienceable side effects. The effects of human microbiota on BC development and treatment are becoming clearer, increasing the hopes of the development of personalized and targeted therapy. However, a large part of the microbiome structure has not been identified. Today, "omic studies" are paving the way for the rise of microbiota. In order to develop and strengthen probiotics and include them in BC treatment protocols, both industrial companies and academic institutions need to conduct intensive research and work together. This will open new horizons in our fight against cancer.

References

1. Santen RJ, Boyd NF, Chlebowski RT, Cummings S, Cuzick J, Dowsett M, Easton D, Forbes JF, Key T, Hankinson SE, Howell A, Ingle J. Breast cancer prevention collaborative group. Critical assessment of new risk factors for breast cancer: considerations for development of an improved risk prediction model. Endocr Relat Cancer. 2007;14(2):169–87. https://doi.org/10.1677/ERC-06-0045.
2. NIH HMP Working Group, Peterson J, Garges S, Giovanni M, McInnes P, Wang L, Schloss JA, Bonazzi V, McEwen JE, Wetterstrand KA, Deal C, Baker CC, Di Francesco V, Howcroft TK, Karp RW, Lunsford RD, Wellington CR, Belachew T, Wright M, Giblin C, David H, Mills M, Salomon R, Mullins C, Akolkar B, Begg L, Davis C, Grandison L, Humble M, Khalsa J, Little AR, Peavy H, Pontzer C, Portnoy M, Sayre MH, Starke-Reed P, Zakhari S, Read J, Watson B, Guyer M. The NIH human microbiome project. Genome Res. 2009;19(12):2317–23. https://doi.org/10.1101/gr.096651.109. Epub 2009 Oct 9. PMID: 19819907; PMCID: PMC2792171.
3. Zhu B, Wang X, Li L. Human gut microbiome: the second genome of human body. Protein Cell. 2010;1(8):718–25. https://doi.org/10.1007/s13238-010-0093-z. Epub 2010 Aug 28. PMID: 21203913; PMCID: PMC4875195.
4. Ma Z, Qu M, Wang X. Analysis of gut microbiota in patients with breast cancer and benign breast lesions. Pol J Microbiol. 2022;71(2):217–26. https://doi.org/10.33073/pjm-2022-019. PMID: 35675827; PMCID: PMC9252143.
5. Fernández MF, Reina-Pérez I, Astorga JM, Rodríguez-Carrillo A, Plaza-Díaz J, Fontana L. Breast cancer and its relationship with the microbiota. Int J Environ Res Public Health. 2018;15(8):1747. https://doi.org/10.3390/ijerph15081747. PMID: 30110974; PMCID: PMC6121903.
6. Kuchenbaecker KB, Hopper JL, Barnes DR, Phillips KA, Mooij TM, Roos-Blom MJ, Jervis S, van Leeuwen FE, Milne RL, Andrieu N, Goldgar DE, Terry MB, Rookus MA, Easton DF, Antoniou AC, BRCA1 and BRCA2 Cohort Consortium, McGuffog L, Evans DG, Barrowdale D, Frost D, Adlard J, Ong KR, Izatt L, Tischkowitz M, Eeles R, Davidson R, Hodgson S, Ellis S, Nogues C, Lasset C, Stoppa-Lyonnet D, Fricker JP, Faivre L, Berthet P, Hooning MJ, van der Kolk LE, Kets CM, Adank MA, John EM, Chung WK, Andrulis IL, Southey M, Daly MB, Buys SS, Osorio A, Engel C, Kast K, Schmutzler RK, Caldes T, Jakubowska A, Simard J, Friedlander ML, McLachlan SA, Machackova E, Foretova L, Tan YY, Singer CF, Olah E, Gerdes AM, Arver B, Olsson H. Risks of breast, ovarian, and contralateral breast cancer for BRCA1 and BRCA2 mutation carriers. JAMA. 2017;317(23):2402–16. https://doi.org/10.1001/jama.2017.7112.
7. Key T, Appleby P, Barnes I, Reeves G. Endogenous hormones and breast cancer collaborative group. Endogenous sex hormones and breast cancer in postmenopausal women: reanalysis of nine prospective studies. J Natl Cancer Inst. 2002;94(8):606–16. https://doi.org/10.1093/jnci/94.8.606.
8. Feinleib M. Breast cancer and artificial menopause: a cohort study. J Natl Cancer Inst. 1968;41(2):315–29.
9. Arnedos M, Vicier C, Loi S, Lefebvre C, Michiels S, Bonnefoi H, Andre F. Precision medicine for metastatic breast cancer—limitations and solutions. Nat Rev Clin Oncol. 2015;12(12):693–704. https://doi.org/10.1038/nrclinonc.2015.123. Epub 2015 Jul 21.
10. Kaaks R, Rinaldi S, Key TJ, Berrino F, Peeters PH, Biessy C, Dossus L, Lukanova A, Bingham S, Khaw KT, Allen NE, Bueno-de-Mesquita HB, van Gils CH, Grobbee D, Boeing H, Lahmann PH, Nagel G, Chang-Claude J, Clavel-Chapelon F, Fournier A, Thiébaut A, González CA, Quirós JR, Tormo MJ, Ardanaz E, Amiano P, Krogh V, Palli D, Panico S, Tumino R, Vineis P, Trichopoulou A, Kalapothaki V, Trichopoulos D, Ferrari P, Norat T, Saracci R, Riboli E. Postmenopausal serum androgens, oestrogens and breast cancer risk: the European prospective investigation into cancer and nutrition. Endocr Relat Cancer. 2005;12(4):1071–82. https://doi.org/10.1677/erc.1.01038.
11. Dieterich M, Stubert J, Reimer T, Erickson N, Berling A. Influence of lifestyle factors on breast cancer risk. Breast Care (Basel). 2014;9(6):407–14. https://doi.org/10.1159/000369571. PMID: 25759623; PMCID: PMC4317679.

12. Sivan A, Corrales L, Hubert N, Williams JB, Aquino-Michaels K, Earley ZM, Benyamin FW, Lei YM, Jabri B, Alegre ML, Chang EB, Gajewski TF. Commensal Bifidobacterium promotes antitumor immunity and facilitates anti-PD-L1 efficacy. Science. 2015;350(6264):1084–9. https://doi.org/10.1126/science.aac4255. Epub 2015 Nov 5. PMID: 26541606; PMCID: PMC4873287.
13. Armstrong H, Bording-Jorgensen M, Dijk S, Wine E. The complex interplay between chronic inflammation, the microbiome, and cancer: understanding disease progression and what we can do to prevent it. Cancers (Basel). 2018;10(3):83. https://doi.org/10.3390/cancers10030083. PMID: 29558443; PMCID: PMC5876658.
14. Rea D, Coppola G, Palma G, Barbieri A, Luciano A, Del Prete P, Rossetti S, Berretta M, Facchini G, Perdonà S, Turco MC, Arra C. Microbiota effects on cancer: from risks to therapies. Oncotarget. 2018;9(25):17915–27. https://doi.org/10.18632/oncotarget.24681. PMID: 29707157; PMCID: PMC5915165.
15. Hu S, Ding Q, Zhang W, Kang M, Ma J, Zhao L. Gut microbial beta-glucuronidase: a vital regulator in female estrogen metabolism. Gut Microbes. 2023;15(1):2236749. https://doi.org/10.1080/19490976.2023.2236749. PMID: 37559394; PMCID: PMC10416750.
16. Adlercreutz H. Western diet and Western diseases: some hormonal and biochemical mechanisms and associations. Scand J Clin Lab Invest Suppl. 1990;201:3–23.
17. Fuhrman BJ, et al. Associations of the fecal microbiome with urinary estrogens and estrogen metabolites in postmenopausal women. J Clin Endocrinol Metab. 2014;99(12):4632–40.
18. Goedert JJ, Jones G, Hua X, Xu X, Yu G, Flores R, Falk RT, Gail MH, Shi J, Ravel J, Feigelson HS. Investigation of the association between the fecal microbiota and breast cancer in postmenopausal women: a population-based case-control pilot study. J Natl Cancer Inst. 2015;107(8):djv147. https://doi.org/10.1093/jnci/djv147. PMID: 26032724; PMCID: PMC4554191.
19. Ingman WV. The gut microbiome: A new player in breast cancer metastasis. Cancer Res. 2019;79(14):3539–41. https://doi.org/10.1158/0008-5472.CAN-19-1698.
20. Knekt P, Adlercreutz H, Rissanen H, Aromaa A, Teppo L, Heliövaara M. Does antibacterial treatment for urinary tract infection contribute to the risk of breast cancer? Br J Cancer. 2000;82(5):1107–10. https://doi.org/10.1054/bjoc.1999.1047. PMID: 10737394; PMCID: PMC2374435.
21. Zitvogel L, Galluzzi L, Viaud S, Vétizou M, Daillère R, Merad M, Kroemer G. Cancer and the gut microbiota: an unexpected link. Sci Transl Med. 2015;7(271):271ps1. https://doi.org/10.1126/scitranslmed.3010473. PMID: 25609166; PMCID: PMC4690201.
22. Carbone C, Piro G, Di Noi' V, D' Argento E, Vita E, Ferrara MG, Pilotto S, Milella M, Cammarota G, Gasbarrini A, Tortora G, Bria E. Lung and gut microbiota as potential hidden driver of immunotherapy efficacy in lung cancer. Mediat Inflamm. 2019;2019:7652014. https://doi.org/10.1155/2019/7652014. PMID: 31827379; PMCID: PMC6885300.
23. Urbaniak C, Cummins J, Brackstone M, Macklaim JM, Gloor GB, Baban CK, Scot' L, O'Hanlon DM, Burton JP, Francis KP, Tangney M, Reid G. Microbiota of human breast tissue. Appl Environ Microbiol. 2014;80(10):3007–14. https://doi.org/10.1128/AEM.00242-14. Epub 2014 Mar 7. PMID: 24610844; PMCID: PMC4018903.
24. Urbaniak C, Gloor GB, Brackstone M, Scott L, Tangney M, Reid G. The microbiota of breast tissue and its association with breast cancer. Appl Environ Microbiol. 2016;82(16):5039–48. https://doi.org/10.1128/AEM.01235-16. PMID: 27342554; PMCID: PMC4968547.
25. Banerjee S, Wei Z, Tan F, Peck KN, Shih N, Feldman M, Rebbeck TR, Alwine JC, Robertson ES. Distinct microbiological signatures associated with triple negative breast cancer. Sci Rep. 2015;5:15162. https://doi.org/10.1038/srep15162. PMID: 26469225; PMCID: PMC4606812.
26. Banerjee S, Tian T, Wei Z, Shih N, Feldman MD, Peck KN, DeMichele AM, Alwine JC, Robertson ES. Distinct microbial signatures associated with different breast cancer types. Front Microbiol. 2018;9:951. https://doi.org/10.3389/fmicb.2018.00951. PMID: 29867857; PMCID: PMC5962706.
27. Kumar H, du Toit E, Kulkarni A, Aakko J, Linderborg KM, Zhang Y, Nicol MP, Isolauri E, Yang B, Collado MC, Salminen S. Distinct patterns in human Milk microbiota and fatty acid profiles across specific geographic locations. Front Microbiol. 2016;7:1619. https://doi.org/10.3389/fmicb.2016.01619. PMID: 27790209; PMCID: PMC5061857.
28. Lackey KA, Williams JE, Meehan CL, Zachek JA, Benda ED, Price WJ, Foster JA, Sellen DW, Kamau-Mbuthia EW, Kamundia EW, Mbugua S, Moore SE, Prentice AM, Kvist LJ, Otoo GE, García-Carral C, Jiménez E, Ruiz L, Rodríguez JM, Pareja RG, Bode L, McGuire MA, McGuire MK. What's normal? Microbiomes in human milk and infant feces are related to each other but vary geographically: the INSPIRE study. Front Nutr. 2019;6:45. https://doi.org/10.3389/fnut.2019.00045. Erratum in: Front Nutr 2020 Feb 19;7:12. PMID: 31058158; PMCID: PMC6479015.
29. Wang H, Altemus J, Niazi F, Green H, Calhoun BC, Sturgis C, Grobmyer SR, Eng C. Breast tissue, oral and urinary microbiomes in breast cancer. Oncotarget. 2017;8(50):88122–38. https://doi.org/10.18632/oncotarget.21490. PMID: 29152146; PMCID: PMC5675698.

30. Hanahan D, Weinberg RA. Hallmarks of cancer: the next generation. Cell. 2011;144(5):646–74. https://doi.org/10.1016/j.cell.2011.02.013.
31. Honda K, Littman DR. The microbiota in adaptive immune homeostasis and disease. Nature. 2016;535(7610):75–84. https://doi.org/10.1038/nature18848.
32. Thaiss CA, Zmora N, Levy M, Elinav E. The microbiome and innate immunity. Nature. 2016;535(7610):65–74. https://doi.org/10.1038/nature18847.
33. Motevaseli E, Dianatpour A, Ghafouri-Fard S. The role of probiotics in cancer treatment: emphasis on their in vivo and in vitro anti-metastatic effects. Int J Mol Cell Med. 2017;6(2):66–76. https://doi.org/10.22088/acadpub.BUMS.6.2.1. Epub 2017 May 31. PMID: 28890883; PMCID: PMC5581548.
34. Avand A, Akbari V, Shafizadegan S. In vitro cytotoxic activity of a Lactococcus lactis antimicrobial peptide against breast cancer cells. Iran J Biotechnol. 2018;16(3):e1867. https://doi.org/10.15171/ijb.1867. PMID: 31457026; PMCID: PMC6697826.
35. Oliveira Silva E, Cruz de Carvalho T, Parshikov IA, Alves dos Santos R, Silva Emery F, Cardoso J, Furtado NA. Cytotoxicity of lapachol metabolites produced by probiotics. Lett Appl Microbiol. 2014;59(1):108–14. https://doi.org/10.1111/lam.12251. Epub 2014 Apr 9.
36. Soltan Dallal MM, Yazdi MH, Holakuyee M, Hassan ZM, Abolhassani M, Mahdavi M. Lactobacillus casei ssp.casei induced Th1 cytokine profile and natural killer cells activity in invasive ductal carcinoma bearing mice. Iran J Allergy Asthma Immunol. 2012;11(2):183–9.
37. Yazdi MH, Soltan Dallal MM, Hassan ZM, Holakuyee M, Agha Amiri S, Abolhassani M, Mahdavi M. Oral administration of lactobacillus acidophilus induces IL-12 production in spleen cell culture of BALB/c mice bearing transplanted breast tumour. Br J Nutr. 2010;104(2):227–32. https://doi.org/10.1017/S0007114510000516. Epub 2010 Mar 2.
38. De Moreno, De LeBlanc A, Matar C, LeBlanc N, Perdigón G. Effects of milk fermented by lactobacillus helveticus R389 on a murine breast cancer model. Breast Cancer Res. 2005;7(4):R477–86. https://doi.org/10.1186/bcr1032. Epub 2005 Apr 26. PMID: 15987453; PMCID: PMC1175061.
39. Dubin K, Callahan MK, Ren B, Khanin R, Viale A, Ling L, No D, Gobourne A, Littmann E, Huttenhower C, Pamer EG, Wolchok JD. Intestinal microbiome analyses identify melanoma patients at risk for checkpoint-blockade-induced colitis. Nat Commun. 2016;7:10391. https://doi.org/10.1038/ncomms10391. PMID: 26837003; PMCID: PMC4740747.
40. Vétizou M, Pitt JM, Daillère R, Lepage P, Waldschmitt N, Flament C, Rusakiewicz S, Routy B, Roberti MP, Duong CP, Poirier-Colame V, Roux A, Becharef S, Formenti S, Golden E, Cording S, Eberl G, Schlitzer A, Ginhoux F, Mani S, Yamazaki T, Jacquelot N, Enot DP, Bérard M, Nigou J, Opolon P, Eggermont A, Woerther PL, Chachaty E, Chaput N, Robert C, Mateus C, Kroemer G, Raoult D, Boneca IG, Carbonnel F, Chamaillard M, Zitvogel L. Anticancer immunotherapy by CTLA-4 blockade relies on the gut microbiota. Science. 2015;350(6264):1079–84. https://doi.org/10.1126/science.aad1329. Epub 2015 Nov 5. PMID: 26541610; PMCID: PMC4721659.
41. De Spiegeleer B, Verbeke F, D'Hondt M, Hendrix A, Van De Wiele C, Burvenich C, Peremans K, De Wever O, Bracke M, Wynendaele E. The quorum sensing peptides PhrG, CSP and EDF promote angiogenesis and invasion of breast cancer cells in vitro. PLoS One. 2015;10(3):e0119471. https://doi.org/10.1371/journal.pone.0119471. PMID: 25780927; PMCID: PMC4363635.
42. Miller AC, Elamin EM. Use of probiotics for treatment of chemotherapy-induced diarrhea: is it a myth? JPEN J Parenter Enteral Nutr. 2009;33(5):573–4. https://doi.org/10.1177/0148607109336596. Epub 2009 Jun 25.
43. Yang J, Tan Q, Fu Q, Zhou Y, Hu Y, Tang S, Zhou Y, Zhang J, Qiu J, Lv Q. Gastrointestinal microbiome and breast cancer: correlations, mechanisms and potential clinical implications. Breast Cancer. 2017;24(2):220–8. https://doi.org/10.1007/s12282-016-0734-z. Epub 2016 Oct 5.

Understanding, Addressing, and Managing Activities of Daily Living Limitations in Breast Cancer Survivors

34

Halil Ibrahim Celik

34.1 Introduction

Breast cancer (BC) is the most common type of cancer in women, accounting for 28.2% of all female cancer cases in Europe [1]. The survival rate in BC has increased with advances in early screening, diagnosis, and treatment. However, most of the BC survivors experience short-and long-term negative consequences associated with BC and its treatments, such as physical, psychological, social, and emotional difficulties [2]. Ultimately, all these difficulties may lead to limitations in the activities and functionalities of BC survivors [3].

Defined as meaningful and purposeful functional everyday activities, the occupation is classified into nine categories, including activities of daily living (ADLs), instrumental activities of daily living (IADLs), health management, rest and sleep, education, work, play, leisure, and social participation [4]. ADLs are activities required to live independently and meet the basic needs of daily living, such as feeding, dressing, and personal hygiene. Compared to ADLs, IADLs are more advanced activities that require more complex skills and environmental interaction: shopping, financial management, driving, etc. Tables 34.1 and 34.2 provide brief descriptions of activities classified as ADLs and IADLs by the American Occupational Therapy Association, respectively [4].

34.1.1 ADLs/IADLs Limitations and Associated Factors in BC Survivors

The decrease in the capacity to execute ADLs and IADLs is extremely important for both BC survivors and healthcare professionals as it has a detrimental effect on independent living and ultimately may lead to limitations in participation, quality of life, and overall health of BC survivors [5]. In this part of the chapter, the rate and associated factors of limitations in ADLs and IADLs among BC survivors were examined in light of current literature.

Lemij et al. [6] aimed to determine changes in ADLs/IADLs performance and associated factors in BC survivors aged 70 years and older in the first 5 years after diagnosis of BC. They emphasized that approximately half of BC survivors (49%) had limitations in ADLs/IADLs. The authors noted that baseline characteristics, including age, body mass index (BMI), number of comorbidities, and ADLs/IADLs performance, had strong associations with changes in ADLs/IADLs over time. They also noted that changes in ADLs/IADLs were associated with quality of life, depression, and loneliness. Swisher et al. [7] stated that approximately 79% of BC survivors

H. I. Celik (✉)
Bilge Çocuk Special Education and Rehabilitation Center, Ankara, Turkey

Y. Bakar, A. Tuğral (eds.), *Managing Side Effects of Breast Cancer Treatment*,
https://doi.org/10.1007/978-3-031-75480-7_34

Table 34.1 The activities classified as ADLs and their brief descriptions

Activities of daily living	
Activities	Brief description
Bathing, showering	The process includes obtaining and using materials, soaping, rinsing, drying body parts, maintaining the bathing position, and transferring in the bath
Toileting and toilet hygiene	The process includes various aspects of toileting and toilet hygiene: Managing clothing, maintaining toileting position, cleaning the body, caring for menstrual and continence needs, and using equipment for bladder control
Dressing	The process involves selecting appropriate clothing and accessories based on time, weather, and desired presentation, retrieving them from storage, dressing and undressing in a specific order, adjusting clothing and shoes, and applying or removing personal devices, prosthetic devices, or splints
Eating and swallowing	The act of keeping and manipulating nutrients in the mouth and swallowing
Feeding	The process of setting up, arranging, and bringing nutrients from the container to the mouth. It includes not only self-feeding but also feeding others
Functional mobility	The process of moving from one place to another during the performance of everyday activities, such as in-bed mobility, wheelchair mobility, and transfers (e.g., wheelchair, bed, car, shower, tub, toilet, chair, and floor)
Personal hygiene and grooming	The process of various personal grooming tasks such as hair care, nail care, skin care, oral hygiene, and applying cosmetics
Sexual activity	The process of engaging in sexual activities with oneself or others, for example, hugging, kissing, foreplay, masturbation, oral sex, and sexual intercourse

Table 34.2 The activities classified as IADLs and their brief descriptions

Instrumental activities of daily living	
Activities	Brief description
Care of others	The process of providing care to others, arranging or supervising care for others
Care of pets and animals	The process of providing, arranging, or supervising the care of pets and service animals
Child rearing	The process of providing and supervising the care of a child to support his/her developmental and physiological needs
Communication management	The process of sending, receiving, and interpreting information using the equipment needed, such as phones, computers, and tablets
Driving and community mobility	The process of moving into the community using public or private transportation
Financial management	The process of planning and using finances
Home establishment and management	The process of obtaining, maintaining, and repairing personal belongings, household items, and house environments, and knowing how to seek help
Meal preparation and cleanup	Planning, preparing, and serving meals and cleaning up tools after meals
Religious and spiritual expression	The process of engaging in religious or spiritual activities, organizations, and practices for various purposes
Safety and emergency maintenance	The process of understanding and managing potential risks to health and life safety
Shopping	The process of preparing shopping lists and selecting, purchasing, and transporting items

had difficulties with ADLs, and the most prominent activities experienced with difficulty were opening a jar (76%), doing heavy housework (75%), carrying heavy objects (73%), placing objects on a shelf overhead (62%), and pushing open a heavy door (61%). Kopec et al. [8] examined the ADLs performance of BC survivors at 6 months after BC surgery and found that 32% of the BC survivors had difficulties with lifting objects >10 lb., 31% had difficulties with pushing or pulling large objects, and 19% had difficulties with reaching above shoulder level. The authors noted that sensory neuropathy, ROM limitations, and surgery on the dominant side were associated with poorer ADLs performance.

Studies examining factors associated with ADLs/IADLs performance in BC survivors pres-

Table 34.3 The factors associated with ADL/IADL performance in BC survivors

Physical factors		Nonphysical factors
Older age	Decreased shoulder ROM	Financial worries
A higher number of comorbidities	Decreased handgrip strength	Emotional distress
BMI > 25	Pain catastrophizing and central sensitization	Depression
Surgery on the dominant side	Severity of lymphedema	Loneliness
Baseline ADLs/IADLs performance	Pain	Fear of lymphedema
Sensory neuropathy	Fatigue	
Upper limb pain	ALND	

ent highly variable results. This variability may be due to key variables such as the severity of the cancer stage, type of treatment administered, age at diagnosis, and use of various tools for assessment. In a recent systematic review, upper limb pain, decreased shoulder abduction ROM, decreased handgrip strength, a higher number of comorbidities, and the presence of pain catastrophizing and central sensitization were reported to be associated with decreased ADLs performance in BC survivors [3]. O'Toole et al. [9] found that poor ADLs performance was significantly associated with increased fear of lymphedema, more pain, surgery of mastectomy, BMI > 25, axillary lymph node dissection (ALND), and emotional well-being. Fu et al. [10] studied the impact of co-occurring fatigue and lymphatic pain on ADLs and stated that BC survivors who had both fatigue and lymphatic pain experienced more difficulties with ADLs than BC survivors with only one of them. Park et al. [5] examined the association between ADLs difficulties and limb volume changes in the 1 year after BC surgery and reported that the BC survivors with limb volume changes greater than 10% experienced the most difficulties with ADLs, followed by those with limb volume changes of 5–10% and less than 5%, respectively. Furthermore, the most prominent activities experienced with difficulty were reported as taking care of children, doing yard work or gardening, carrying or lifting heavy objects, cleaning the house, vacuuming, and doing laundry. Tang et al. [11] examined the association between the surgical procedure and the ADLs performance of BC survivors 1 year after surgery and stated that the greatest decrease in ADLs performance was observed in ALND, mastectomy, and lumpectomy surgeries, respectively. Moreover, it was emphasized that the 1-year decline in ADLs performance was associated with baseline ADLs performance. Okuyama et al. [12] compared the decrease in ADLs performance of BC survivors who underwent mastectomy according to age groups (<65, 65–74, and ≥ 75 years) and found that the decrease in ADLs performance was greatest in BC survivors aged ≥75 years and was similar and lower in BC survivors aged <65 and 65–74 years. In their qualitative study, Sleight et al. [13] examined the effects of BC treatment and its side effects on ADLs/IADLs and found that BC survivors had difficulties with bathing, dressing, shopping, cooking, sexuality, and even functional mobility. Furthermore, they noted that upper-extremity mobility limitations and lymphedema, as well as financial worries and emotional distress, affected ADLs/IADLs performance.

To summarize, it is possible to say that a considerable percentage (32–79%) of BC survivors have difficulty with ADLs/IADLs, and many physical and nonphysical factors (Table 34.3) affect ADLs/IADLs performance.

34.2 Assessment Tools Used for ADLs/IADLs

Researchers often report using subscales of quality-of-life questionnaires to assess ADLs/IADLs, yet it is not appropriate to use the terms quality of life and ADL/IADL interchangeably. Quality of life questionnaires may partially include ADLs/

IADLs. For example, it should be stated that the SF-36 cannot fully assess ADLs/IADLs for BC survivors as it excludes ADLs/IADLs that are essential to BC survivors, such as cooking, bathing, and dressing. Moreover, some researchers assess ADLs and IADLs by developing a study-specific questionnaire. However, it is inevitable to use standardized tools whose psychometric properties have been examined and verified to conduct a consistent and precise assessment. The following is a summary of standardized assessment tools commonly used for ADLs/IADLs in BC survivors.

34.2.1 Canadian Occupational Performance Measure (COPM)

The COPM is a client-focused tool that is widely utilized in occupational therapy to assess a person's self-perception of their ADLs/IADLs performance. Regarding BC survivors, the COPM can be a valuable tool to assess the impact of BC and its treatment on the individual's ability to execute ADLs/IADLs. The COPM requires the individual to identify and prioritize activities that are important to them but have become challenging due to their BC diagnosis and/or treatment. The individual then rates their perceived performance and satisfaction with each activity on a rating system from 1 to 10, with 1 reflecting poor performance or satisfaction and 10 indicating excellent performance or satisfaction. By dividing the performance and satisfaction scores by the number of activities, overall performance and satisfaction scores are computed [14, 15].

34.2.2 Groningen Activity Restriction Scale (GARS)

GARS is a widely used tool for assessing disability in older adults, particularly for the ADLs and IADLs. Out of the total of 18 items in this self-report questionnaire, 11 are about ADLs, while 7 are about IADLs. The total score varies between 18 and 72, with higher values representing a greater level of disability. Four categories are identified using the total score: <19: no dependency, 19–28: some dependency, and ≥ 29: disabled [16, 17].

34.2.3 Modified Barthel Index

It is a frequently used tool to assess the functional independence and activities of daily living in various populations, including BC survivors. It consists of 10 items that evaluate an individual's ability to execute fundamental activities like feeding, bathing, grooming, dressing, bowel and bladder control, mobility, and stair climbing. The Barthel Index has a score range of 0–100, where higher values represent improved functional independence and the ability to carry out daily activities without any assistance [12, 18].

34.2.4 Katz Activities of Daily Living Scale

It consists of 6 items that assess an individual's ability to perform essential daily activities. These activities include bathing, dressing, toileting, transferring, continence, and feeding. Items on the Katz ADLs scale are scored based on the level of independence demonstrated by the individual, with 0 representing full dependence and 6 representing full independence [19, 20].

34.2.5 Lawton Instrumental Activities of Daily Living Scale

It is a valuable tool for evaluating an individual's ability to perform more complex daily activities required for independent living in society. This scale consists of 8 items that evaluate activities like shopping, using the telephone, preparing food, doing laundry, housekeeping, using transportation, handling medications, and managing finances. Each item is scored based on the level of independence demonstrated by the individual in carrying out these instrumental activities. A higher score indicates better functioning in IADLs [19, 21].

34.2.6 The Breast Cancer and Lymphedema Symptom Experience Index (BCLE-SEI) Part II

It is a validated and reliable self-report tool specifically designed to evaluate the symptoms experienced by individuals dealing with lymphedema following BC treatment. This index assesses the detrimental effects that an individual experiences of lymphedema symptoms, encompassing various aspects such as daily living, sleep disturbance, sexuality, emotional distress, social impact, and self-perception. The self-reported difficulty in performing 13 ADLs is evaluated using the ADLs subscale. Five-point Likert ratings were used for each activity. A higher score indicates greater difficulties in ADLs [5, 22].

34.2.7 The Disabilities of the Arm, Shoulder, and Hand (DASH)

It is a comprehensive tool used to assess upper extremity function and symptoms in musculoskeletal disorders. DASH is a 30-item self-report questionnaire. Each item reflects the patient's opinion on their disability due to upper limb disorders, providing insights into the impact of these conditions on daily functioning. Owing to the high number of items and long assessment time of the DASH, a new version, Quick-Disabilities of the Arm, Shoulder, and Hand (Q-DASH), containing 11 items was developed. The total scores vary between 0% and 100%, where 0 represents no disability and 100% represents severe disability [23, 24]. It can be said that DASH and QDASH are popular assessment tools for ADLs among BC survivors.

34.2.8 Shoulder Pain and Disability Index (SPADI)

It is a self-reported questionnaire designed to assess shoulder pain and disability in individuals with shoulder pathologies. The SPADI contains 13 items, which are separated into two subscales: a pain subscale comprising five items and a disability subscale comprising eight items. Each item has a score range of 0–10, where 0 represents no pain or difficulty and 10 represents the worst pain or extreme difficulty. The total score of the SPADI may vary between 0 and 100, with higher values representing more severe pain and disability related to shoulder issues [25].

As a result, some researchers' use of self-developed questionnaires or assessment tools such as DASH, SPADI, and BCLE-SEI Part II, which do not purely assess ADLs, is seen as a major problem in ADLs/IADLs assessment. We can say that it may be better to use assessment tools that focus purely on ADLs/IADLs such as COPM, GARS, the Modified Barthel Index, the Katz Activities of Daily Living Scale, and the Lawton Instrumental Activities of Daily Living Scale, in a way that is appropriate for the study population. Consequently, selecting the appropriate assessment tool allows healthcare professionals to identify patients' ADLs/IADLs difficulties, tailor rehabilitation programs to address specific needs, and evaluate the effectiveness of interventions. In addition to the standardized assessment tools mentioned above, occupational performance analysis through direct observation in the home environment or simulated occupational therapy units can also be used. However, occupational performance analysis is not addressed in this chapter, which is prepared from the perspective of a physiotherapist.

34.3 Management Options for ADL/IADL Limitations

Interventions for ADLs/IADLs limitations can be classified into two categories: compensatory and restorative approaches. Compensatory approaches are often used to adjust ADLs/IADLs limitations in situations where a full recovery is not possible, such as amputation and complete spinal cord injury. However, for BC survivors where full recovery is possible, it can also be used for an activity that the patient specifically wants to perform. To improve activity performance, restorative approaches focus on disorders in body structure and function, including pain, lymphedema, and limited range of motion, that limit activity [26]. For example, let's take a BC survivor who has difficulty performing an overhead activity due to shoulder joint ROM limitations. In an activity such as meal preparation, which is an important IADLs, the BC survivor has difficulty getting a container from a cabinet that is at an overhead level. This patient's use of a reacher to pick up a container from the overhead level is an example of a compensatory approach. Eliminating the shoulder ROM limitation of the same BC survivor with physiotherapy approaches such as soft tissue and joint mobilization/manipulation or specific exercises and making the patient able to pick up a container from the overhead level is an example of a restorative approach.

In the management of ADLs/IADLs limitations, restorative approaches should be used first, and when restorative approaches are no longer an option, compensatory approaches should be used. In some cases, using both approaches together may be preferred for a short time. However, it should be kept in mind that compensatory approaches have the potential to delay functional recovery and should be discontinued as soon as possible [27].

Restorative approaches aim to increase functionality by improving skills such as muscle strength, ROM, endurance, balance, and coordination. The most important point in restorative approaches is that the skills developed should be integrated into daily life as soon as possible [28]. Going back to our example, the patient receiving physiotherapy for shoulder ROM limitation may be asked to pick up a container from the overhead level at home or in the therapy unit. For further information on physiotherapy approaches for managing the disorders in body structure and function that are common in BC survivors and lead to activity limitation, kindly see the relevant chapters in this book.

Many BC survivors may experience physical and nonphysical (psychological, social, and emotional) difficulties associated with BC treatment, all of which may ultimately lead to ADLs/IADLs limitations. Physical difficulties such as pain, lymphedema, fatigue, ROM limitation, and sensory neuropathy are modifiable factors, and they should be monitored, prevented, and managed in physiotherapy practice. However, if nonphysical difficulties are taken into consideration, ADLs/IADLs limitations need to be addressed with the holistic approach of a multidisciplinary team that includes other health professionals as well as physiotherapists. It should not be forgotten that BC treatment requires a multimodal approach, and thus the symptoms can vary and affect each other. Hence, a management team with expertise in multiple disciplines is a prerequisite for improving ADLs/IADLs performance and is of utmost importance.

34.4 Conclusions

It is conceivable to speculate that a substantial proportion of BC survivors have difficulty with ADLs/IADLs and that various physical and nonphysical factors affect ADL/IADL performance. However, there are some concerns about the limitations of the assessment of ADLs/IADLs limitations, such as the use of researcher-developed questionnaires and questionnaires or assessment tools that do not focus on or cover entirely on ADLs/IADLs. Therefore, researchers should utilize assessment tools that are BC-specific and appropriate to the characteristics of the study population so that a consistent and precise assessment can be performed, which allows for the adaptation of rehabilitation programs to meet specific needs and the evaluation of the effectiveness of interventions. In the management of ADLs/IADLs limitations, restorative approaches should be prioritized, yet the skills developed should be integrated into daily life through activities in the clinical or home environment. It should also be kept in mind that other health professionals, as well as physiotherapists, should be involved in management as ADLs/IADLs limitations may be due to nonphysical factors.

References

1. Ferlay J, et al. Cancer incidence and mortality patterns in Europe: estimates for 40 countries and 25 major cancers in 2018. Eur J Cancer. 2018;103:356–87.
2. Keesing S, Rosenwax L, McNamara B. The implications of women's activity limitations and role disruptions during breast cancer survivorship. Womens Health (Lond). 2018;14:1745505718756381.
3. De Groef A, et al. The association between upper limb function and variables at the different domains of the international classification of functioning, disability and health in women after breast cancer surgery: a systematic review. Disabil Rehabil. 2022;44(8):1176–89.
4. Anon. Occupational therapy practice framework: domain and process-fourth edition. Am J Occup Ther. 2020;74(Supplement_2):7412410010p1–7412410010p87.
5. Park JH, et al. Limb volume changes and activities of daily living: a prospective study. Lymphat Res Biol. 2021;19(3):261–8.
6. Lemij AA, et al. Physical function and physical activity in older breast cancer survivors: 5-year follow-up from the climb every mountain study. Oncologist. 2023;28(6):e317–23.
7. Swisher AK, et al. Frequency and severity of self-reported upper extremity impairments, activity limitations, and participation restrictions following breast cancer treatment. Rehab Oncol. 2010;28(1):3–9.
8. Kopec JA, et al. Relationship between arm morbidity and patient-reported outcomes following surgery in women with node-negative breast cancer: NSABP protocol B-32. J Support Oncol. 2013;11(1):22–30.
9. O'Toole JA, et al. The impact of breast cancer-related lymphedema on the ability to perform upper extremity activities of daily living. Breast Cancer Res Treat. 2015;150(2):381–8.
10. Fu MR, et al. Co-occurring fatigue and lymphatic pain incrementally aggravate their negative effects on activities of daily living, emotional distress, and overall health of breast cancer patients. Integr Cancer Ther. 2022;21:15347354221089605.
11. Tang V, et al. Functional status and survival after breast cancer surgery in nursing home residents. JAMA Surg. 2018;153(12):1090–6.
12. Okuyama A, Takei J, Ogawa A. Perioperative treatments for and postoperative activity of daily living of patients with early-stage breast cancer according to age group: a retrospective observational study. Eur J Surg Oncol. 2024;50(2):107323.
13. Sleight AG. Occupational engagement in low-income Latina breast cancer survivors. Am J Occup Ther. 2017;71(2):7102100020p1–8.
14. Carswell A, et al. The Canadian occupational performance measure: a research and clinical literature review. Can J Occup Ther. 2004;71(4):210–22.
15. Loubani K, Schreuer N, Milman U. Participation in daily activities among working women following breast cancer. Open J Ther Rehab. 2016;04:150–62.
16. Kempen GI, Suurmeijer TP. The development of a hierarchical polychotomous ADL-IADL scale for noninstitutionalized elders. Gerontologist. 1990;30(4):497–502.
17. Suurmeijer TP, et al. The Groningen activity restriction scale for measuring disability: its utility in international comparisons. Am J Public Health. 1994;84(8):1270–3.
18. Shah S, Vanclay F, Cooper B. Improving the sensitivity of the Barthel index for stroke rehabilitation. J Clin Epidemiol. 1989;42(8):703–9.
19. van Abbema D, et al. Functional status decline in older patients with breast and colorectal cancer after cancer treatment: a prospective cohort study. J Geriatr Oncol. 2017;8(3):176–84.
20. Katz S. Assessing self-maintenance: activities of daily living, mobility, and instrumental activities of daily living. J Am Geriatr Soc. 1983;31(12):721–7.
21. Lawton MP, Brody EM. Assessment of older people: self-maintaining and instrumental activities of daily living. Gerontologist. 1969;9(3):179–86.
22. Fu M, et al. The role of symptom report in detecting and diagnosing breast cancer-related lymphedema. Eur J Clin Med Oncol; 2014. http://www.bmm-oncology.com/index.php/26-home/slider/1-home-morbi-tincidunt-sodales-neque-eu-rutrum.
23. Beaton DE, et al. Measuring the whole or the parts? Validity, reliability, and responsiveness of the disabilities of the arm, shoulder and hand outcome measure in different regions of the upper extremity. J Hand Ther. 2001;14(2):128–46.
24. Beaton DE, Wright JG, Katz JN. Development of the QuickDASH: comparison of three item-reduction approaches. J Bone Joint Surg Am. 2005;87(5):1038–46.
25. Roach KE, et al. Development of a shoulder pain and disability index. Arthritis Care Res. 1991;4(4):143–9.
26. Meriano C and Latella D. Occupational therapy interventions: function and occupations. (No Title). 2016.
27. Pendleton HM, Schultz-Krohn W. Pedretti's occupational therapy-e-book: practice skills for physical dysfunction. Amsterdam: Elsevier; 2017.
28. Gillen G, Brown C. Willard and Spackman's occupational therapy. Baltimore, MD: Lippincott Williams & Wilkins; 2023.

GPSR Compliance

The European Union's (EU) General Product Safety Regulation (GPSR) is a set of rules that requires consumer products to be safe and our obligations to ensure this.

If you have any concerns about our products, you can contact us on ProductSafety@springernature.com

In case Publisher is established outside the EU, the EU authorized representative is:

Springer Nature Customer Service Center GmbH
Europaplatz 3
69115 Heidelberg, Germany

Batch number: 10732799

Printed by Printforce, the Netherlands